THE CULTURE
OF AIDS IN AFRICA

THE CULTURE
OF AIDS IN AFRICA

Hope and Healing

in Music and the Arts

EDITED BY

GREGORY BARZ

AND

JUDAH M. COHEN

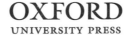
OXFORD
UNIVERSITY PRESS

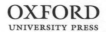

OXFORD
UNIVERSITY PRESS

Oxford University Press, Inc., publishes works that further
Oxford University's objective of excellence
in research, scholarship, and education.

Oxford   New York
Auckland   Cape Town   Dar es Salaam   Hong Kong   Karachi
Kuala Lumpur   Madrid   Melbourne   Mexico City   Nairobi
New Delhi   Shanghai   Taipei   Toronto

With offices in
Argentina   Austria   Brazil   Chile   Czech Republic   France   Greece
Guatemala   Hungary   Italy   Japan   Poland   Portugal   Singapore
South Korea   Switzerland   Thailand   Turkey   Ukraine   Vietnam

Library of Congress Cataloging-in-Publication Data
The culture of AIDS in Africa : hope and healing in music and the arts /
edited by Gregory Barz and Judah Cohen.
p.   cm.
Includes bibliographical references and index.
ISBN 978-0-19-974447-3 — ISBN 978-0-19-974448-0
1. AIDS (Disease)—Africa—Songs and music—History and criticism.
2. Music—Social aspects—Africa.   3. AIDS (Disease)—Social aspects—Africa.
4. AIDS (Disease) and the arts—Africa.   I. Barz, Gregory F., 1960-
II. Cohen, Judah M.
ML3917.A4C85   2011
362.196'97920096—dc22
2010053152

1 3 5 7 9 8 6 4 2

Printed in the United States of America
on acid-free paper

For Simon and Lucy Barz.

For Rebecca, Rena, and Gabriel Cohen.

And to all those affected by HIV/AIDS, in Africa and throughout the world, who strive to live positively each and every day.

The world at large and African leaders and our motherland in particular
Should be an example in the campaign against the AIDS epidemic
We are educating for peace, unity, and for development

Yes, everyone of Africa is on a very strong foundation
To hear the echoes almost from every home
The wind of change is blowing around,
We have all the breeze to rejoice through communication and mobilizing

Now as we enter the millennium this has to be the solution
Harmony and togetherness that's how to grow
Between traditional healers, medical doctors, religious leaders
United researching should be supported
Research institutes need to wake up to fight the epidemic

Sung by the choir of Tokamalirawo AIDS Support
Group Awareness (TASGA) Kampala, Uganda

CONTENTS

ABBREVIATIONS

ACT UP	AIDS Coalition to Unleash Power
AFSAAP	African Studies Association of Australasia and the Pacific
AIDS	Acquired Immune Deficiency Syndrome
ANC	African National Congress
ART	Antiretroviral Therapy
ARV	Antiretroviral drug or medication
AZT	Azidothymidine, drug used to delay onset of AIDS
BBC	British Broadcasting Company
BDP	Botswana Democratic Party
BHRIMS	Botswana HIV/AIDS Response Information Management System
BOTUSA	Botswana-United States Partnership
CBO	Community-Based Organization
CBPR	Community-Based Participatory Research
CBR	Community-Based Research
CDC	Centers for Disease Control and Prevention
CIE	Circus in Ethiopia
CIEYSD	Circus in Ethiopia for Youth and Social Development
CPC	Centre for Positive Care
DHAP	Division of HIV/AIDS Prevention at the CDC
DIVA	Damned Interfering Video Activists
DSGs	Data Summary Grids
FOM	Friends of Malawi
GAP	Global AIDS Program
GIPA	Greater Involvement of People with AIDS
GoB	Government of Botswana
GRID	Gay-Related Immune Deficiency
HAART	Highly Active Anti-Retroviral Therapy
HAPCO	HIV/AIDS Prevention and Control Office (Ethiopia)
HBC	Home-Based Care
HIV	Human Immunodeficiency Virus
IAC	International AIDS Conference
IDAAC	Integrated Development and AIDS Concern (Iganga, Uganda)
IEC	Information, Education, and Communication
IFPP	International Federation of Planned Parenthood
IGA	Income-Generating Activity
ILAM	International Library of African Music
IOM	International Organization for Migration
JICA	Japan International Cooperation Agency
KARP	Kagera AIDS Research Project (Tanzania)
KELC	Kenya Evangelical Lutheran Church
KIE	Kenya Institute of Education

KNUST	Kwame Nkruma University of Science and Technology in Kumasi (Ghana)
LDGs	Listening Discussion Groups
MARCH	Modeling and Reinforcement to Combat HIV/AIDS
MBC	Malawi Broadcasting Corporation
MDGs	Millennium Development Goals
MoH	Ministry of Health
MPs	Members of Parliament
MSF	Médecins Sans Frontières
MTCT	Mother-to-Child Transmission
MUDINET	Mukono District Network of People Living with HIV/AIDS (Uganda)
NAC	National AIDS Council
NACA	National AIDS Coordinating Agency (Botswana)
NACC	National AIDS Control Council (Kenya)
NACOEJ	North American Conference on Ethiopian Jewry
NACP	National AIDS Control Programme (Botswana and Tanzania)
NACWOLA	National Community of Women Living with AIDS (Uganda)
NASC	National AIDS Song Contest
NBB	National Broadcasting Board (Botswana)
NGO	Non-Governmental Organization
NOVIB	Dutch Red Cross
PADA	People with AIDS Development Association (Uganda)
PEMS	Program Evaluation and Monitoring System (at the CDC)
PLWHA	People Living with HIV/AIDS
PMTCT	Prevention of Mother-to-Child Transmission
PPAG	Planned Parenthood of Ghana
PS	Pilot Songs (category of songs discussed by Jack Allison in Malawi)
PSG	Project Support Group
PSI	Population Services International (Botswana and Malawi)
SAfAIDS	Southern Africa AIDS Information Dissemination Service
SAINT	South African Intrapartum Nevirapine Trial
SRH	Sexual and Reproductive Health
STDs	Sexually Transmitted Diseases
STIs	Sexually Transmitted Infections
TAC	Treatment Action Campaign (South Africa)
TASGA	Tokamalirawo AIDS Support Group Awareness (Uganda)
TASO	The AIDS Support Organization (Uganda)
TB	Tuberculosis
TCM	Total Community Mobilization
TFD	Theatre for Development
TRIPs	Trade-Related Aspects of Intellectual Property Rights
UNAIDS	United Nations Joint Programme on HIV/AIDS
UNASO	Uganda Network of AIDS Service Organisations
UNICEF	The United Nations Children's Fund
UNIFEM	United Nations Development Fund for Women
UU	Unitarian Universalist
UUA	Unitarian Universalist Associate of Congregations

VCT	Voluntary Counseling and Testing
VOLSET	Voluntary Service Trust Team (Uganda)
WHO	World Health Organization
WTO	World Trade Organization
ZCC	Zion Christian Church

FIGURES

ACKNOWLEDGMENTS

We are grateful for the many people who have made this volume possible.

To the many friends and colleagues who helped me see, hear, experience, and feel a variety of healing practices in ways often profound and frequently enlightening. To Vanderbilt University and its Blair School of Music and to the University of the Free State (Bloemfontein, South Africa) for continued support of my research efforts. To the countless women, men, and youth who sing, dance, dramatize, and create artistic meaning out of the scourge of AIDS in Africa. To my co-editor Judah Cohen who brought keen skills and unbounded reason and wisdom to this project—never was there a more patient partner and caring wordsmith. To one and all I acknowledge my gratitude.—*GB*

To Dr. Rebecca Cohen, research and life partner, without whom I would never have started this journey. To the 2004 members of the TASO Mbarara Drama Group, who shared the greatest of gifts by allowing me into their lives. To Gerald Paccione and Lanny Smith, who so enthusiastically opened a space for me to bring music into the discussion at the Montefiore Medical Center Primary Care/Social Medicine program. And to Greg Barz, whose invitation to serve as co-editor turned warm and meaningful conversations into a wonderful ongoing partnership. I owe deep gratitude to you all.—*JC*

To our contributors, who have waited patiently to see this collection come to print, thank you for entrusting us with your wonderful work. We hope you find the final form worthy of your considerable efforts.

Many thanks to Suzanne Ryan, whose enthusiasm, support, and interest has been instrumental in bringing this volume to Oxford's desk. Erica Woods Tucker moved this project along with a smooth and sure hand; and Caitlin Goldbaum provided invaluable assistance in the final stages of publication.

To our families: endless love for coming with us on (yet another) adventure. We are grateful for your patience when we run to our computers to edit yet another essay, or when we recruit you to listen to our next ideas. And we are grateful for your impatience when life needs to intercede. To our children in particular, at least one of whom decided, at age three and a half, to begin editing essays as well: you give us inspiration for what we do, and we love every moment that you come running into our offices seeking attention, and every time you lunge at the computer keyboard to test your newfound grabbing skills. Please continue to interrupt us.

And finally we remember in gratitude and thanks those people who live on only in memory. Your lives have taught us much; may your memories continue to show us the way.

THE CULTURE
OF AIDS IN AFRICA

1

Introduction

THE CULTURE OF AIDS: HOPE AND HEALING
THROUGH THE ARTS IN AFRICA

Gregory Barz (Vanderbilt University/University of the Free State)

Judah M. Cohen (Indiana University)[1]

> The whole village is full of diseases, that is why we suffer.
> People suffer from poverty, from ulcers, from coughing.
> But God gives us talents you cannot see.
> God gave me the talent to play the *akadongo* [plucked idiophone].
> Listen to what it says, my *akadongo* talks.
> Our children cry while suffering from polio, now AIDS came to finish us.
> It kills the beautiful, the youth and all of us who are poor.
> Where are we going to run?
>
> "Ekyalo Kyaidula Endwaire" sung by Vilimina Nakiranda (Uganda)

HOW DO YOU EXPRESS A SCOURGE?

The emergence of HIV/AIDS into the world has forced people to address this question, both personally and as part of various communities across the globe. As with other health crises, such as polio, sleeping sickness, influenza, and malaria, populations large and small have brought the expressive forms around them to bear on presenting the nature of AIDS in moral, social, local, medical, religious, and transnational terms. Yet the widespread and devastating scope of HIV/AIDS has created a particularly unique and arresting epidemiological landscape. Initially a spiral of deterioration with unknown etiology and no known cure, the disease has eventually become theoretically manageable through the use of increasingly convenient drug regimens. Yet changes have not, and do not, come easily: health interventions inevitably face broad challenges along cultural, political, and economic lines. Interactions between people and medical providers change over time, and require more than mechanical treatment. Populations have engaged in long-term struggles to find meaningful modes of action within globalized systems of relationships, knowledge, and health discourse. And throughout, people have sought ways to express the scourge.

Artistic movements around the world have given HIV/AIDS a voice, a sound, and an image: from the songs of Michael Callen, the first symphony of John Corigliano, and the AIDS activist films by John Greyson, Gregg Bordowitz and many others; to regional and national theater productions ranging from *The AIDS Show* (1984) to *RENT* (1995); to the work of numerous visual artists such as Keith Haring's 1989 "Silence=Death" (and many other works) and Maree Azzopardi's 1996 Chrysalis project; to the massive NAMES Project Foundation's AIDS Memorial Quilt; to fiction by Hervé Guibert and Andrew Holleran and a broad host of others; to the inventive, dire, and often beautiful international demonstrations of ACT UP and other AIDS activist organizations; to widely distributed international media experiences such as MTV's Staying Alive campaign; to the proliferation of local memorials and rituals, acts of memory, and acts of representation. These events, movements, and works continually emphasized the reality of "AIDS as human suffering" (Farmer and Kleinman 1989), and creative responses as contributions to a humanly organized "epidemic of signification" surrounding HIV/AIDS (Treichler 1999, 11). These works often addressed another reality as well, however. In their public dissemination, creative activity reinforced the connections between human activity, medical research and health care—forging public opinion, lobbying for research funding, recreating the meaning of being HIV-positive from within the community, and demanding access to available treatments.

The acceleration of Euro-American AIDS activism and scholarship during the 1980s seems to have benefitted from a coincident expansion of the field of medical anthropology (Crimp 1988, Mass 1994, Juhasz 1995, Román 1998, Bordowitz 2004), marked most notably with the establishment of the journal *Medical Anthropology Quarterly* in 1987 and the renaming of the *Journal of Medical Humanities* (from the *Journal of Medical Humanities and Bioethics*) in 1989. By the opening years of the twenty-first century, the increased visibility of medical anthropology, as well as medically focused subfields such as narrative medicine, medical humanities, and medical ethnomusicology (Koen et al. 2008) have begun to lay the groundwork for new ways to bring together the arts and medicine (and their constituent research agendas). Longtime advocate of medical humanities H. Martyn Evans, for example, in his recent attempt to resituate music's place within the framework of medical discourse offered an intriguing platform for future discussion. "Medicine," he noted, "belongs to music in that larger sense in which 'music' names the imaginative creation—or restoration—of order amidst our experience of chaos" (Evans 2007). Benjamin Koen, Gregory Barz, and Kenneth Brummel-Smith, meanwhile, have approached the topic from an ethnographic perspective, attempting to delineate a pluralistic field of medical ethnomusicology that brings together anthropologists, therapists, physicians, local practitioners, and others to winnow away the walls between "science" and "the arts" (Koen et al. 2008). These scholars have created significant points of departure for our discussions.

Within this confluence of literatures, however, Africa tended to receive minimal attention. Excepting the work of Louise Bourgault (2003), whenever researchers mentioned "the arts" in the same breath as HIV/AIDS, they frequently implied America; discussions of Africa and the arts in relationship to HIV/AIDS discourses more likely appeared in popular literature than in scholarship (The aWAKE Project 2002). Part of the issue, as we see it, is that AIDS emphasized a duality between Africa and Euro-America from the beginning. From one perspective, the constellation of symptoms manifested by the virus's assault on the immune system caused the Western world to view AIDS as a great leveler of civilizations. HIV, so many campaigns noted, "does not discriminate" between hosts. At the same time, paradoxically, the epidemic led people to a heightened perception of cultural and economic difference between Africa and the West (see Sontag 2001, 159–81). As described in great detail by historian John Iliffe (2006), the epidemiological narrative assigned to HIV/AIDS emphatically tied the so-called first and third worlds together: situating the disease's germination in Africa; its discovery and documentation in Europe and the United States; and the consequent international response among Western-sponsored institutions, health organizations, and pharmaceutical companies. On one level, this history justified a broad sense of partnership and action against the disease. At the same time, however, HIV/AIDS acted as an agent of differentiation: reinforcing a Euro-American self-perception of economic, intellectual, and religious superiority, particularly as Africa increasingly became the center of dire international concern. On the other side, the disparity has spurred its own responses in Africa. It has led to resistance from political leaders attempting to free themselves from a dominating Western discourse while fighting the disease; it has become a conduit for substantial international aid to African countries through such programs as PEPFAR (President's Emergency Plan for AIDS Relief); it has led to the rise of non-governmental organizations (NGOs) aiming to link together people on the ground with received knowledge from international health and aid organizations; and it has contributed to the development of "African medicine" practices on both local and national levels. Gregory Barz's discussion of the arts in Uganda as a form of HIV-related medical intervention (2006, 222–23) thus began a more significant conversation, laying the theoretical groundwork for a phenomenon as widespread in Africa as it was overlooked.

We aim to expand that conversation, showing in this volume the many pathways by which music and other expressive art forms gained prominence in Africa as agents for addressing HIV and AIDS, helping individuals and communities address the local and international conversations coursing through their lives in the process. HIV-positive Africans (or, to use one frequently evoked construction, "people living positively" in Africa) took to modes of creative expression in ways that referenced local practices and traditions, attempted to appeal to the group identity of local villages, churches, and health organizations, and connected both implicitly and explicitly with attitudes or resources seen as coming from the outside. Dedicated musicians and artists, HIV-positive and otherwise, have used their talents to represent AIDS in regional and national forums. Large-scale artistic endeavors, such as television shows and national competitions, have blanketed urban centers and rural areas alike with broad-based directives about sexual health and behavior. And various populations, both local and international, have used creative means to send their messages outside of Africa as well, especially to resource rich countries they might not be able to visit themselves (such as the United States) (National Immigration Project 2004).[2] Through these forms of expression, a "culture of AIDS" has emerged in Africa, becoming a potent medium through which Africans could create their own networks of power, express their own ideas, and tell their own stories.

Yet what does it mean to "dance" a syndrome, "sing" a medical condition, or "act out" an etiology? How can the field of medicine fruitfully engage with Ruth Stone's concept of an interrelated "constellation of the arts" in Africa (Stone 2008, 7–12)? How can artistic performance restore a sense of order to the chaos and destruction wrought by an incurable and ultimately fatal virus? And why does Africa so often represent a "different" story?

The essays in this book attempt to address these questions through rich insights into the ways communities feel, sense, and experience HIV/AIDS within the African sphere. As in other parts of the world, much of the artistic production associated with HIV/AIDS in Africa has been responsive, emerging from frameworks of health-based knowledge propagated through both internationally funded aid organizations and local practices. Those living in areas affected by the virus brought this knowledge to existing expressive conventions, resulting in new forms of signification. Broader "African" meanings of HIV/AIDS consequently emerged through patterns of communal interaction and exchange, tracking from the local to the transnational and back again.

It is important, therefore, to highlight some of the key processes through which people have established creative structures of understanding for living with, expressing, and embodying the disease, as well as some of the institutions and organizations that have contributed to and helped sustain the artistic cultures that have arisen around it.

"AFRICAN AIDS" AND "AIDS IN AFRICA"

The vast literature on HIV/AIDS in Africa that has emerged since the late 1990s lays a thorough groundwork for exploring the different ways HIV entered into creative discourses of diverse geographic areas of Africa. Iliffe notes that the first (retroactively) confirmed case of HIV/AIDS occurred in 1959 in Cameroon; and the virus eventually migrated east over the next twenty years across trucking and social routes (2006). At first, isolated to small populations and rural areas, HIV remained unknown during the 1960s and into the 1970s. Only during the late 1970s, as political conflicts, increased population motility, and forced urbanization displaced large populations within Africa, did AIDS receive significant attention and documentation on the continent. Journalist Helen Epstein has proposed that the virus found ideal conditions for a rapid spread during this time thanks to long-term, concurrent sexual partnerships frequently practiced in Eastern and Southern African populations, exacerbated by a concentration of labor (in remote mining camps, for instance) and regional armed conflicts (2007). As a result, by the mid 1980s some areas of Eastern and Southern Africa began to see infection prevalence rates among adults of up to 30 percent. Prevailing international attention on this region led to education efforts focused on "at-risk" (often seen as morally deficient) groups, such as prostitutes and young people, exacerbating the situation by adding additional levels of social stigma to the disease. The devastating landscape of AIDS that emerged in Africa thus came to display wide variation based on political, social, geographic, religious, moral, gender-related, and behavioral factors, not to mention exposure to the agendas and resources of the West; and sub-Saharan and Southern Africa in particular became the "face" of the epidemic worldwide. Cultural landscapes shifted in turn: the desperate and unchecked situations many saw around them led to a reorientation of creative expression in all levels of society.

The phrase "African AIDS," a construction propagated by the World Health Organization and others, exemplifies the dilemmas guiding AIDS assistance and research efforts in Africa. From one perspective, this approach flattens the vast array of practices addressing HIV/AIDS into a monoculture sometimes associated from the outside with primitivism and misapprehension. Seen from within, the situation is complex: Africans variously describe themselves as Africans, citizens of a specific country, part of an ethnic group, members of a locality, and representatives of a demographic, among many other groupings; each view carries its own relationships with and responses to AIDS. As one way to acknowledge the breadth of this discussion, Gregory Barz has suggested taking the perspective of "Africa and AIDS" (2006), a term that addresses the complex relationship between land, population, and virus, in doing so attempting to liberate the continent from the language of epidemiology. In this book, our perspective of HIV/AIDS in African contexts follows Barz's lead. African populations participate in (inter)national responses to HIV/AIDS while maintaining unique, local understandings, as both they and the disease constantly shift from one paradigm to another depending on their situation. Culturally defined and determined, AIDS has activated particular approaches using "Western" therapies, as well as an alternate network of "African medicine" practitioners (described via a range of terms, including herbalists and witch doctors) who provide treatments some see locally as more culturally appropriate to the surrounding population. By moving from an interpretation of AIDS "in" Africa to a model that privileges communal discourse and action, therefore, we shift our lens to the interactions taking place "on the ground." In doing so, we hope to open up a rich and vibrant window into the symbolic forms of expression practiced by Africans leading their lives in a world inhabited by HIV/AIDS.

NATIONS WITH EFFECTIVE ANTI-AIDS CAMPAIGNS (UGANDA, BOTSWANA, AND SENEGAL)

Direct Western interventions—including overpriced yet "subsidized" antiretroviral drugs (ARVs), condoms, and abstinence-only programs—have had little effect in stemming the spread of HIV in Africa. Current transmission rates throughout sub-Saharan Africa and the concomitant prevalence rates often prevent such interventions from taking root, particularly where cultural and institutional infrastructures have not been in place long enough to foster such programmatic initiatives. Yet in several African countries—particularly Uganda, Botswana, and Senegal—significant success has been achieved with effective localized anti-AIDS campaigns that drew on traditions of music, dance, and drama.

Long touted as Africa's success story in the fight against AIDS, Uganda has responded, according to Helen Epstein, to local, grassroots efforts—including those based in the arts—to stem the spread of the virus:

> During the 1980s and early 1990s, while people in most African countries were ignoring the AIDS crisis, hundreds of tiny community-based AIDS groups sprang up throughout Uganda and Kagera to comfort the sick, care for orphans, warn people about the dangers of casual sex, and address the particular vulnerability of women and girls to infection.... Their compassion and hard work brought the disease into the open, got people talking about the epidemic, reduced AIDS-related stigma and denial, and led to a profound shift in sexual norms....Warnings about AIDS [in the 1980s] were broadcast on the radio each day at lunchtime, accompanied by the beating of a drum in the traditional rhythm of warning. "When I was young, I'd lie awake all night if I heard a drum beating that way," a middle-aged Ugandan told me. "It meant a thief or a murderer was on the loose." (Epstein 2007, 160, 162)

Uganda's presidential leadership, moreover, made the epidemic an "open secret" while offering an aggressive outreach program that came to be known as ABC—Abstinence, Be faithful, and the appropriate use of Condoms. Since 2004, in part because of these efforts, Uganda's HIV prevalence rate has stayed at around 6.4% (Hladik et al. 2008).

In the late 1990s, the country of Botswana had one of the highest HIV/AIDS infection rates in the world, with one in three adults in the country believed to be HIV-positive. Since then, however, government interventions attempted to supply antiretroviral therapy (ART) to all who needed it. By 1997, localized responses to the pandemic had coupled ART with ongoing educational outreach and preventative measures. These efforts appear to have helped the country stabilize its infection rate. One of the most significant efforts in this campaign was the weekly nationally broadcast of *Makgabaneng* ("We Fall and We Rise"), a serial radio drama begun in 2001 that fused HIV prevention-related messages with high-quality theatrical production values. Supported in part by the Centers for Disease Control in the United States, *Makgabaneng* creatively manipulated the social behavior of listeners in Botswana by employing professional writers, musicians, and actors; these artists in turn created complex characters that also projected government-sanctioned and -vetted health care messages.

Souleymane Mboup, a professor of microbiology at the University of Dakar, suggested that in the West African country of Senegal early and aggressive interventions helped maintain a countrywide prevalence rate of just over 1 percent (Quist-Arcton 2001). To Mboup, the country's stability, its early response, and significant political support and involvement in outreach efforts created a broad awareness of HIV before the virus could filter widely into the population. Targeting commercial sex workers with messages heavily promoting effective condom use has also contributed significantly to the containment of HIV in Senegal. As with Uganda and Botswana, the arts have followed. International musician Baaba Maal has used his high public profile both at home and abroad to spread awareness of HIV concerns in Senegal, a country labeled as the "beacon of hope" in Africa by the United Nations. Radio dramas such as "Yen BU Diss" ("Heavy Burden"), moreover, have sought to reach specific populations while covering a variety of health issues related to HIV/AIDS.

SINGING AND DANCING HIV/AIDS WITHIN THE LOCAL COMMUNITY

In the first ethnography written about the culture of AIDS in Africa, *Singing for Life: HIV/AIDS and Music in Uganda* (2006a), Gregory Barz highlights the need to move beyond medical models in order to approach culturally bound frameworks for understanding HIV/AIDS in localized African contexts. Multiple meanings often accompany the indigenization of AIDS in a population, which in many nations is also affected by poverty, development, education, and other health care issues. By positioning interventions within the domain of general care and treatment, Barz's case studies support a broader understanding of artistic responses to HIV/AIDS. The use of music as medical intervention among women's groups, for example, and their need to "sing for life" as Barz documents, can be seen as contributing greatly to the decline in HIV infection rates in both rural and urban areas of Uganda.

Historically rooted within song and other performance texts, specific terms related to HIV and AIDS have emerged and are maintained in contemporary local performances, especially in a country such as Uganda where the disease has had such an extensive reach. Before the term "HIV/AIDS" was widely known, the virus was known in Uganda as *slim* (or *silimu*), due to its "slimming" effects on the body. The retention of such local terms continues to reference the history and the cultural position of the AIDS pandemic. The use of the term *Ukimwi* in neighboring Tanzania and in bordering Kenya indicates a similar, local nonmedical "naming." According to Barz's documentation in Uganda, audiences attending musical performances appeared much less threatened and anxious when technical, scientific, or medical "AIDS talk" was abandoned in favor of "un-translated" localized terminologies. Documentation of such terminologies within musical performances demonstrates specific ways in which local performance traditions respond to medical interventions that come from both local and foreign sources (see Barz 2006a, chapter 4). In addition, the linguistic position of HIV in arts-based contexts can effectively document historic localizations of AIDS within the general landscape of the disease.

CREATIVE EXPRESSION WITHIN NGOS AND HEALTH-BASED ORGANIZATIONS

Country-specific artistic responses have been regularly adopted by NGOs and health-based organizations. Uganda's TASO (The AIDS Support Organization), the first organized grass-roots response to the AIDS pandemic in Africa, positioned music and drama as central parts of its mission. Founded in 1987, the organization aimed to expand substantially the availability of medical and nursing care, counseling, and material assistance to the growing numbers of HIV-positive individuals in the country and their families. To emphasize their philosophy of "positive living" and self-empowerment, the TASO organization—first formed at Mulago Hospital in Kampala—initiated a drama group of its own clients to accompany medical outreach efforts to schools and communities in the cities and in the outlying areas. The skits and songs that the drama group presented, centrally vetted by medical personnel, often became the best means of communicating information about HIV/AIDS to the communities they visited. Anne Kaddumukasa, one-time director of TASO, reflected on the position of music in the NGO's out-reach efforts:

> The TASO Drama Group composes the songs, all original, together with the clients. They have not been copied from anywhere, and all these songs carry messages—about AIDS prevention and AIDS care. Songs and plays depict the treatment that society inflicts on people who are HIV infected. Surely from those dramas people always gain a lot and realize how bad it is to mistreat a person who is HIV infected and that maybe one day you may find yourself the person being mistreated.... So, music and drama has an impact.

Members of another Ugandan NGO, the National Community of Women Living with HIV/ AIDS (NACWOLA), provide counseling, emotional support, and practical assistance through a variety of initiatives. NACWOLA's Memory Project is famous globally for its efforts to educate children, often AIDS orphans, about the lives of their HIV-positive parents. The group's mem-bers also typically speak publicly and reveal their sero blood status to their families and friends in order to live positively rather than merely as one who is HIV-positive; their frequent gather-ings routinely include singing and dancing.

Among HIV-positive artists and musicians in Uganda who consistently take new direc-tions and adopt new voices, few are more compelling than Walya Sulaiman. An artist and activist who seeks to empower his community with direct medical interventions, Sulaiman continued in 2006 to use what energy he had left in his life to sing songs encouraging people to listen carefully to his messages. Sulaiman's performance group, PADA (People with AIDS Development Association, in Iganga) receives little funding yet aggressively works in the community to fight stigma. In the song, "Akawa Kangema" ("I caught the virus") Walya Sulaiman and PADA sing about the stigma associated with HIV/AIDS, specifically regarding care and treatment at local medical sites:

When I caught the virus I knew I had a real problem. Relax and I will narrate the
  point.
I used to spend the day at home mourning the disease.
I used to spend the day at home fearing.
I used to spend the day at home thinking of suicide.
But then I remembered my children.
My sister came and told me that I should go to IDAAC in Iganga.[3]
They look after many AIDS victims.
But friends, what rescued me was sensitization and counseling.

The grassroots efforts of community-based organizations such as Sulaiman's PADA weaves narrative rhetorical structures into musical contexts to educate and de-stigmatize care and treatment of the virus and disease. The testimonial approach adopted in many of the group's songs clearly affects the way in which audiences react to performances. Heads nod in agreement or hands are slapped in laughter when particular lines resonate with the audience's experiences.

MUSIC AND THE ARTS THROUGH FBOS (FAITH-BASED ORGANIZATIONS) AND TRADITIONAL HEALERS

The complementary nature of religion and medicine in contemporary African contexts has led many Africans to make use of services from a variety of healing systems, frequently drawing on multiple faith traditions. The roles of religious and faith-based initiatives in regard to HIV/AIDS care, treatment, and counseling in many parts of Africa at the start of the twenty-first century are thus quite complex, and coupled with problematic histories of interaction with the disease. Foreign faith-based organizations (FBOs) often would enter African communities with external conceptualizations of health care and medicine, as well as moral structures attached to HIV/AIDS itself; and frequently these organizations would help establish local medical clinics as a complement to their overtly religious work. Within the broad denominational sphere of organized African religions, meanwhile—each with its own concomitant interpretations, beliefs, and practices—healing practices sometimes encouraged a resistance to Western medical concepts, in part resulting from local Christian sponsorship of Western medical initiatives. Nonetheless, coalitions of Christian and Muslim community leaders in particular have jointly introduced musical interventions of faith, hope, and healing regarding HIV/AIDS in many African nations. In addition, religious, faith-based, and spiritual efforts to address AIDS in areas that government and private organizations find inaccessible have frequently drawn on localized performance practices. Such approaches reflect upon the arts as complementary medical interventions for HIV, suggesting that medical HIV/AIDS initiatives can achieve their greatest successes when supported by localized performances from religious, faith, and spiritual communities.

A few contemporary practitioners of indigenous medicine and religion (herbalists and spirit healers) continue to promote cures that the Western medical community has judged to be ineffective; but an increasing number have altered their approach to HIV to take into account broader medical practices. Since 1992, traditional healers have participated with medical doctors in retraining initiatives sponsored by THETA (Traditional and Modern Health Practitioners Together Against AIDS), a partnership initiated between TASO and the international humanitarian organization Médecins Sans Frontières (Doctors Without

Borders). Begun as a collaborative clinical outreach effort, THETA supplemented its training activities with a broad knowledge base cataloging local herbal treatments for select AIDS-related diseases and related opportunistic infections. To commemorate their first ten years as an NGO in 2002, THETA held a three-day public celebration at Kampala's National Theatre with the theme, "Music, Dance, and Drama in the Fight against AIDS." Organizations such as THETA have successfully augmented the efforts of traditional healers in regard to HIV/AIDS education, counseling, and care, while integrating them into a continuum of medical and creative expression.

CREATIVE ARTS IN EDUCATIONAL AND GOVERNMENTAL ORGANIZATIONS

Many AIDS-prevention campaigns in Africa have emphasized preventive instruction for young people. Music, dance, drama festivals, and competitions in primary and secondary schools throughout the continent consequently provide significant opportunities for the infusion of government-sanctioned messages and direct national health interventions (Rørtveit 2003). In Uganda, for example, the nationwide system of annual music competitions has included opportunities for every school in the country to perform creative dances and compose songs based on an annual theme determined in advance by the Ministry of Education (see Barz 2004, chapter 3). Similarly, PEPFAR-funded initiatives in Rwanda have organized music and sports competitions that promoted the ABC approach to AIDS prevention. Music and the arts, when used in this way, provide some of the most important HIV/AIDS-based early childhood interventions sponsored by national local governments.

AFRICA, THE ARTS, AND HIV/AIDS IN INTERNATIONAL DISCOURSES

Just as the virus in Africa has been addressed by an international web of health-related discourses, so too has an international web of the arts come to bear on the virus. One of the first prominent HIV-positive Africans to discuss the virus openly, Ugandan recording artist Philly Bongoley Lutaaya, for example, gained an international platform in part because of his exile in Sweden during the regimes of Idi Amin and Milton Obote. Though self-identified as an African artist, his residence in northern Europe connected him with a health care system and cultural fabric that engaged HIV openly. He would visit Uganda to tour, but he did much of his recording in Sweden. Lutaaya's position from Europe thus gave him latitude to speak openly on the crisis and his own health even as other African governments refused to acknowledge the subject. His final tour, moreover, became the subject of a North American documentary intended to portray AIDS in Africa (Zaritsky 1990; also see chapter 3).

Western musical representations of the AIDS crisis in Africa have also become a *cause célèbre* for creating awareness and generating financial support. High-profile artistic events across the globe have attempted to enhance the existing structures of funding, treatment, and information dissemination. One of the most visible relationships between Africa's HIV/AIDS crisis and music has been through the international popular music industry, as centered largely in the United Kingdom and the United States and manifested in South Africa. Poised as philanthropic work, the music industry's efforts have led to several mega-concerts publicly addressing AIDS in Africa; producers of these concerts consequently partnered with media companies to help collect funds from viewers and attendees for distribution to African-related AIDS organizations.

The premiere NGO venue for these benefit concerts in the first decade of the 21st century was the Nelson Mandela Foundation's 46664 campaign (named after Mandela's

Robbin Island prison number). Started in late 2002 in conjunction with the Eurythmics' Dave Stewart, 46664 brought the clout of multinational entertainment conglomerates to fundraising for Africa-centered AIDS programs. At the first concert, Stewart joined forces with Queen's Brian May to assemble a lineup of top recording artists, a series of media companies (such as Tiscali, Warner Records, and MTV), and a list of corporate donors (including Coca-Cola). The initiative also hooked into other corporate and celebrity-run AIDS initiatives, including MTV's Staying Alive campaign and Bono's philanthropic work. After a local performance in February 2003, the formal 46664 concert in Cape Town, South Africa, on November 29, 2003, officially started the initiative. Several artists who had supported the Live Aid concert raising money for the East African famine eighteen years earlier appeared in the 46664 concert, which presented an almost unsettlingly similar approach. Although actual discussions of AIDS were generally limited to spoken interludes during the concert, the concert's Cape Town location, its symbolism (a huge bust of Mandela remained onstage throughout), its strong allusions to AIDS victim and Queen singer Freddie Mercury (through May and renditions of "We Are the Champions" and "We Will Rock You"), and its appearance just before World AIDS Day gave the event a clear agenda. During the concert broadcast itself, people could theoretically dial 4-6-6-6-4 in dozens of countries to donate to the campaign. In the end, the organizers claimed, over one billion people viewed the event in part or in full.

A number of tie-in products later appeared that further promoted the experience to American and European markets. T-shirts, mugs, silicon wristbands, a three-CD recording of the event, a two-DVD version, and the Real World record *Spirit of Africa* had appeared by April 2004. The DVD set in particular included a series of one-minute AIDS-inspired videos by prominent directors, a featurette of Bono touring an African orphanage, and a romanticized *Spirit of Africa* "making-of" film that linked a Ugandan boy from the Kampala-based Meeting Point NGO with African musicians recording at Peter Gabriel's English countryside mansion. Each of these products continued to feed into other multinational AIDS awareness efforts through cross-marketing, as did a subsequent release of an original, downloadable four-track album in November 2004, just before the next World AIDS Day; smaller 46664 concerts in South Africa, Spain, and Norway in 2005; the transformation of the annual concert day into "Mandela Day" in New York in 2009; and several performances of "ambassador" artists in conjunction with 2010 FIFA World Cup festivities.

Multinational cultural flows produced by commercial conglomerates also complement events organized by nonprofit international networks such as the biannual International AIDS Conference. In 2006, the conference in Toronto incorporated numerous musical activities into its schedule, including a "Strength of Africa Concert" featuring professional African musicians such as Thomas Mapfumo, and demonstration performances of local performing groups from East Africa (including Tanzania) and Nigeria. Subsequent conferences in Mexico City (2008) and Vienna (2010) had a much smaller African representation, but nonetheless included several arts-based performances from local groups and projects in Uganda, South Africa, and elsewhere. The arts in this context became a form of presence and exchange, representing African grassroots responses to AIDS within a celebratory, international forum of activists, scientists, philanthropists and politicians.[4]

THE CULTURE OF AIDS IN AFRICA

We present this collection as an entry point into the vast worlds of expression brought forth by the presence of HIV/AIDS in Africa. The contributors whose work appears here—Africans and non-Africans, physicians and social scientists, journalists, documentarians, and educators—share a common interest in understanding the social networks, power relationships, and cultural structures inherent in creative expression during crushing and uncertain times. Still more important, they bring intimate portraits of the performers, artists, communities, and organizations that have hosted them, shared their insights, and above all tried to impart meaningful senses of their lives and actions from within a devastating epidemic.

Understanding the cultural and expressive transformations effected by HIV/AIDS in Africa requires more than a single case study, artist, art form or initiative can illustrate. People lead complex and interconnected lives, continually making choices about their messages and modes of communication as conditions change around them. Social, sexual, occupational, governmental, economic, and taste-based discourses constantly reconfigure basic questions of signification, ideology, and action. To start addressing the "Culture of AIDS," then, we begin with observation. Specific music, art, drama, radio, film, television productions, and public health campaigns offer important insight into the ways communities face crises of meaning during a pandemic. By giving them sensitive and intricate analyses, we believe, a new picture can emerge of the deep interaction that exists between the biological and creative arts.

PART I—REPORTS FROM THE FIELD

The contributors to the volume's first section compel the conversation forward by showing us how people seek livelihoods for themselves and their families through expressive commodities. The four entries presented here offer a nuanced and interconnected snapshot of the cultural landscape that AIDS has wrought in Africa—across time, space, and artistic forms (though here with an emphasis on music). Through the voices of artists, we witness a tragic duality with broader resonance throughout the book: while struggling to communicate the devastation surrounding them, artists negotiate an economy that increasingly views their HIV/AIDS work as a path toward professional viability. The people profiled here address this duality with gravity and uncertainty: at once trying to balance artistic integrity with their enhanced roles as voices of the epidemic.

John Zaritsky's film *Born In Africa* represents the first extended documentary report exploring expressive culture and HIV/AIDS in Africa. Originally aired as a quarterly update on the pandemic on WGBH's investigative reporting series *Frontline* in 1990, *Born In Africa* chronicles the final tour of popular Ugandan singer Philly Lutaaya. Lutaaya's song "Alone" became an anthem for many within the Ugandan AIDS care community, and the artist himself became recognized as the first Ugandan of any significant status to declare himself HIV-positive. The transcript presented here chronicles this significant event, but also offers early insight into the poetics of observation of HIV/AIDS: exploring how the restrictions and caution exercised on the film crew by the only sub-Saharan African government to acknowledge an AIDS crisis at the time might affect what we see. In this way, Zaritsky's work offers a window into a relatively nascent network of HIV/AIDS-based NGOs; of early attempts to "sing" the disease in Africa; and of the place international health initiatives had in addressing local HIV/AIDS agendas.

Ric Alviso's observations on Zimbabwe, meanwhile, begin to lay out some of the classic discussions of the arts' role in anti-AIDS efforts. As Alviso notes, health practitioners tend to view artists' relevant works either as a therapy aid, or as an entity that straddles the line between "education" and "entertainment." The artists who act within these expectations, however, aim to develop themselves as musicians, thus forcing mediations between originality and conformity; personal expression and group expression; and poverty and steady work.

Jonah Eller-Issacs, an audio journalist, collected numerous short interviews during several months traveling throughout sub-Saharan Africa in 2004, which he later compiled in his 2005-6 radio documentary *Singing in the Shadow of AIDS*. The voices that come through in the excerpts presented here range from those of musicians to school officials to HIV/AIDS program directors; and their stories cover a wide range of topics and positions. Eller-Isaacs finds that musical expression serves as a common thread for bringing these conversations together. His work paints an evocative picture of the landscape of AIDS in sub-Saharan Africa, presented through a lens that moves fluidly between verbal and musical communication.

Ethnomusicologist Kathleen J. Van Buren completes this section by presenting a deep-rooted travelogue of her experiences with the AIDS culture in Nairobi, Kenya and its environs. By circulating throughout several sites within a single city, she links signs, newspaper cartoons, and youth programs, with challenges facing musicians who wish to respond to HIV/AIDS. How, she asks, can musicians produce music the populace will want to hear, while at the same time living in a society that regulates messages about HIV/AIDS? Her study raises questions about the nature of cultural production in an environment where artists' work must necessarily engage numerous layers of political and cultural discourse to succeed.

While addressing a handful of areas, these four chapters open up broad routes for understanding a vast range of cultural responses to AIDS in Africa by directing our attention to the inverwoven concerns of individuals, culture industries, and international politics.

PART II—HIV/AIDS AND THE ARTS: FIRST PERSON

The role of the individual in HIV/AIDS outreach and prevention efforts in sub-Saharan Africa can often be interpreted or misconstrued as a "meddler" or "mediator," as Barz suggests elsewhere in this volume. In part II, we let these individuals turn the lens on themselves as they explain their use of music, dance, and drama to address HIV/AIDS in a variety of African contexts.

Physician Jack Allison reflects on two episodes of arts-based health intervention in Malawi. As a Peace Corps volunteer in the late 1960s, he used his musical talents to develop a series of experimental recordings and public outreach puppet shows promoting better health practices. After a twenty-five-year absence, Allison was invited back to Malawi to record popular songs on HIV/AIDS as a direct educational intervention. To Allison and his co-authors, these participatory arts-based projects delivered accurate messages more effectively in nontraditional settings, while also proving helpful in raising needed funds from abroad. Just as importantly, Allison's story offers a valuable window into the often hidden continuities between arts-based health interventions. What we see today with HIV/AIDS, in other words, may have a longer history than we think.

Annabelle Wienand presents the results of a visual and participatory HIV literacy exercise in South Africa that she herself helped to develop. The "body mapping" projects she details brought an artistic modality into the HIV educational process, encouraging community health workers, treatment literacy educators/trainers, and HIV-positive mothers to understand through their own drawings how human biology relates to the mechanics of HIV. As Wienand suggests, the complementary creative and educational aspects of the body map project led participants to incorporate knowledge about HIV in ways more effectively suited to their own needs. Yet Wienand also recounts an unanticipated benefit: through the visual medium, many participants found a comfortable place for exchanging their personal stories and experiences with HIV.

Wienand's chapter represents one of several explorations in this volume involving the collaborative and experiential educational theories of Brazilian-born scholar Paulo Freire (1921–1997). The breadth of Freire's influence here deserves note, not just because of the extent to which scholars have found his methods attractive in approaching HIV/AIDS education in Africa, but also because Freire's techniques naturally seem to incorporate the creative arts. Freire's presence in this volume attests to the significant pedagogical role the arts have taken in Africa-based HIV/AIDS initiatives, while presenting yet another layer of mediation between Africa and the rest of the world—this time through imported discourses of empowerment through education.

The last author in the this section, Mjomba Majalia, draws on his experience as a head teacher and community organizer among the Taita people of Kenya to provide an account of HIV education through drama. Mjomba notes that modern health outreach programs typically overlook relevant local sites of communication, especially as found in local schools. He consequently describes his own attempts to establish a forum for educational outreach and "candid dialogue" among primary and secondary school students. Through experiential *ingoma* (music-dance-drama) grassroots events, Mjomba pilots a forum intended to spur youth to represent their own needs in the fight against HIV/AIDS in Kenya.

PART III—HIV/AIDS AND THE ARTS: CAMPAIGNS AND RESPONSES

As illustrated through the narratives of part II, the classic international health model for addressing HIV/AIDS in Africa involves effecting change through intervention and education: to modify perceptions, personal choices, and group action (the political implications of which have also become important objects of scrutiny). Individuals work within and among communities to make this change. Yet the majority of this work is conducted by the numerous organizations on the local, state, and international levels that have mobilized to stop the virus's spread. Such efforts have often looked to well-known art forms: by using a familiar medium, goes the model, new messages can be delivered effectively and meaningfully, and compliance maximized. Whether using local forms of expression or the national mass media, researchers have thus experimented with replicable techniques for introducing safer sexual practices, reducing the stigma attached to those living with HIV/AIDS, and correcting local forms of knowledge about the virus and its spread. Along with the initiatives themselves, these organizations have generated their own social science literature, determining the metrics for measuring effectiveness, and providing blueprints for possible expansion and/or replication.

The posters that Eckhard Breitinger describes in Malawi do not necessarily represent a single campaign. Yet Breitinger's study examines the ways public visual culture reorients images, aphorisms, and cultural norms into anti-AIDS messages. Through the use of frequently seen and strategically placed public placards, Breitinger suggests, a state-sponsored campaign can transform entire landscapes of discourse to conform to desired parameters of HIV/AIDS knowledge.

Mass media resources and technology networks have also played crucial roles in allowing national and activist campaigns to communicate highly honed messages about HIV/AIDS to a receptive public. Crafted to appeal to a wide audience—with an emphasis on the young, urban, and media savvy—multimedia efforts have become central platforms for inspiring, promoting, and legitimizing a range of complementary ideas on the role of HIV in society. Abimbola

Cole and Rebecca Hodes explore the meaning of such collaborations through radio and television respectively. Cole expands existing work on AIDS-themed radio dramas by examining how contemporary music, theater, and health information came together in the 2001 Botswana production *Makgabaneng*. Hodes focuses on the long-running television show *Beat It!*—a creation of South Africa's Treatment Action Campaign, and reported to be the first television show produced by the HIV-positive community for wide dissemination. Both use their case studies to bring up important questions about how these works are created and disseminated, exploring the relationships between NGOs, producers, and consumers of self-consciously popular culture in the process.

Daniel Reed, meanwhile, compares a pair of anti-AIDS media campaigns centered in Côte d'Ivoire. Though implemented in West Africa, Reed notes, the two initiatives were begun researched and financed largely through France-based foundations. Reed's incisive chapter explores the meeting points between the local and international in the implementation of an AIDS-based campaign, while also offering insight into how these campaigns developed a specifically West African approach to HIV/AIDS prevention and treatment starting in the 1990s.

Breitinger, Cole, Hodes, and Reed take specific campaigns as their case studies. Fraser McNeill and Deborah James, in contrast, widen the circle to explore how these campaigns fit into larger discourses on the ground. In their chapter, McNeill and James describe an anti-AIDS campaign in Venda, South Africa that employs female peer educators who bring a mix of anti-apartheid, religious, and local musical styles to empower an internationally deployed health agenda. This campaign, however, has also spurred a male-centered musical counter-discourse that critiques the women's messages (along with the campaign) as manipulative and exploitative. McNeill and James's work brings the issues discussed in this section full circle, with the argument that internationally funded "interventional" health efforts themselves inevitably layer onto existing local practices of identity, class, power, and gender, and hardly exist on their own as unmitigated goods.

PART IV—CASE STUDIES: SINGLE WORKS AND ARTISTS

The next set of essays shifts the analytical lens toward specific artists and culture producers. The creative drive of individuals often produces artifacts that can become motivating forces behind change. Different artistic forms, however, bring about these changes differently: photographers, traditional musicians, playwrights, and popular musicians each employ their own techniques and networks to move, motivate, and reflect on the presence of HIV in African communities.

Michael Godby devotes his article to South African photojournalist Gideon Mendel, who has spent much of his career documenting the impact of HIV/AIDS on the people of his native country. But, Godby suggests, more than merely documenting, Mendel has served for many as a prototypical model for artist-as-activist, using his images to effect social change in arenas such as advocacy for access to antiretroviral therapies, and contributing to or fostering broader political campaigns (such as those related to the Treatment Action Campaign).

Rebekah Emanuel highlights the songs performed by Ugandan traditional singer and *akadongo* (plucked lamellophone) player Vilimina Nakiranda—cited in the epigraph to this chapter. Vilimina's song-texts reveal her to be much more than a village-based entertainer. Her songs instead show her to be a powerful advocate for women's rights and issues related to HIV/AIDS health care disparities in her rural region. Emanuel deconstructs one of Vilimina's song texts (first documented in Barz 2006a) in order to demonstrate how the elaborate codes and metaphors adopted by this artist draw on traditional values to stimulate social change through musical performance.

Zimbabwean musician Oliver Mtukudzi, meanwhile, embodies the artist's dilemmas of self-representation. Jennifer Kyker's close reading of Mtukudzi's song lyrics about HIV/AIDS reveals his compelling personal narrative and deep understanding of linguistic nuance. At the same time, Kyker cautions, these lyrics often resist the pat messages some have considered appropriate for use in HIV/AIDS campaigns. Thus, while Mtukudzi's music remains popular, it also contributes to a dialogue about the expectations of HIV/AIDS prevention campaigns, the allowance of individual expression, and the question of effectively addressing anti-AIDS messages to the public.

Aldin Mutembei documents the contributions of individual playwrights in the fight against AIDS in Tanzania. His formal analysis of two plays with central HIV/AIDS themes (one of which is his own), illustrates how the disease has caused the Aristotelian conventions so prevalent in Tanzanian drama to strain, and, ultimately, to break. In addition to changing narrative forms, Mutembei adds, individual playwrights speak to their audiences through culturally specific dramatic metaphors, providing a critical local gloss on HIV and its constituent discourses.

Mellitus Wanyama and Joseph Basil Okong'o dedicate the final article in this section to an analysis of the song lyrics of three popular Kenyan songwriters—Princess Jully, Jack Nyadundo, and Oduor Odhialo. Extensive presentations of these three performers' song texts demonstrate the artists' deep engagement with significant health care related issues in Kenya today. Particularly their use of local language terms and popular culture references evoke the threats and realities of HIV infection in East Africa.

PART V—CASE STUDIES: PERFORMANCE GROUPS

Of all the forms of expression surrounding HIV/AIDS in Africa, perhaps none has been more widespread or used in a greater variety of contexts than the amateur performing group. Recognized by many international aid organizations as a successful and replicable approach to AIDS activism, amateur performing groups (particularly drama groups) have their own history in Africa as a medium for social organization and local problem solving. Within HIV/AIDS contexts, moreover, they often serve as powerful conduits for peer instruction: dancing, singing, and delivering messages *en masse* with strength and confidence. Many also function, however, to publicize the missions of Western-sponsored NGOs. The contributors to this section thus explore a variety of amateur performing groups at the sometimes-uncomfortable meeting grounds of local and Western knowledge.

Austin C. Okigbo opens the section with his work on the KwaZulu-Natal, South Africa-based Siphithemba choir. Originally affiliated with a mission hospital in the area, Siphithemba's HIV-positive members present themselves as both agents of hope and partners in health to local and international audiences. Okigbo's detailed discussion of the group's activities and repertoire shows how its members have adopted Nelson Mandela's message of AIDS as the "next struggle" into its social, religious, and musical activities. His intimate portrait goes further, however, to desrcibe how its members use these values as the basis for mutual support and self-determination, thus helping them cope with the challenges of their own lives.

For Angela Scharfenberger, a much briefer encounter with the Young and Wise Inspirational Choir in Accra, Ghana serves as the impetus for an inquiry into the dilemmas Western researchers face in studying AIDS performance groups. While AIDS has not had nearly the impact in Ghana as it has elsewhere in sub-Saharan Africa, it has still been designated for HIV-awareness-raising resources from international health organizations. Scharfenberger argues that the singers in the Young and Wise choir take their jobs seriously, even as their experience with HIV may be limited to the campaign messages they promote. By participating in the group, however, these singers also attempt to parlay their public health-based exposure into pop stardom. This encounter between singers and researcher leads to key questions about the role of the scholar/advocate in documenting and (as a result) promoting these initiatives. Can a veneer of AIDS advocacy highlight deeply seeded ambitions among a young urban population? And how can we as scholars understand and support their actions?

Judah M. Cohen's account of the drama group at a local chapter of The AIDS Support Organization (TASO) in southwestern Uganda offers observations on the complex terrains of access that membership involves. In a setting where new health resources often come at a premium, performative forms of HIV/AIDS advocacy can offer members important opportunities for access to medical treatment, receiving international aid, high-profile exposure, attention from foreigners, travel possibilities, and increased self-worth. Any of these benefits could potentially lead to prolonged life; but they also involve negotiating a broad series of religious, moral, social, and cultural norms, each of which brings with it its own competitive resources and pressures. Joining and performing in a drama group, in other words, highlights the "expressive economy" that underlies each member's decisions, and illustrates the complexity of Africans' relationships with the promises of Western medical assistance and intervention.

Leah Niederstadt's account of Ethiopian circuses that ends this section might seem at first an outlier, particularly in relation to the first three entries. The circus phenomenon, however, which took root in Ethiopia in the 1990s through a combination of happenstance and Western support, has emerged as a key player in disseminating morality and health directives in the region—including (most prominently for our volume) HIV/AIDS prevention. Niederstadt's extensive work with these groups, and her detailed account of two major HIV/AIDS themes in circus presentations, serve as stark reminders of the breadth of expression possible around HIV/AIDS, as well as the collaborative nature that such ventures require in order to remain viable.

PART VI—POPULAR MEDIA AND POLITICS

Our last section concludes the discussion with a set of case studies that interrogate how popular media helps mediate HIV/AIDS in a variety of African contexts. By employing a range of approaches—philosophical, ethnographic, interventionist, and historical—the authors in this section underscore how underrepresented artistic forms within the landscape of HIV/AIDS expressions can also serve, even obliquely, as important vessels for understanding the disease's social and cultural reach.

Gavin Steingo contributes a triangulated focus on sexuality, HIV/AIDS, and popular music in South Africa by expounding on *kwaito*, a genre of House music that emerged in the early 1990s. Steingo's work connects the social implications of *kwaito* performance with discourses of sexual violence and rape, while offering a conception of the present that lacks a vision of the future. By providing details on the lives and careers of artists such as Zola and Khabzela,

Steingo illustrates various ways that *kwaito* implicitly parallels the sexual and social power structures associated with AIDS among South African youth.

Gregory Barz and Gerald Liu's contribution emerges from an ethnographic "experimental moment" in their research with female MCs in Uganda, during which they consciously engaged in what could be understood as a manipulation of popular musicians. Barz and Liu asked Ugandan hip hop artists known for their socially conscious rap lyrics to record music responding to their own self-described inability to achieve commercial airtime. The tracks that emerged highlight social concerns related to rape, HIV/AIDS, and specific gender issues (pregnancy, spousal abuse, and education) that speak directly to youth in Uganda in ways heretofore unachieved through other popular media. By analyzing the HIV-related rhymes of MCs Tafash and Twig through the lens of each rapper's spiritual grounding, moreover, Barz and Liu show how understandings of the disease contribute to a sense of dialogic theology and personal struggle within Ugandan hip hop society.

John C. Lwanda addresses the ways in which information about HIV/AIDS is transmitted through popular media in Malawi, in an effort to construct one of the first progressive histories of HIV responses within the popular music industry. Beyond simply delineating eras, listing musician names, and describing recordings, however, Lwanda introduces a central paradox hinted at in much of this collection: the devastation of HIV/AIDS, he suggests, led to both the growth of the Malawian music industry and, for some, successful professional music careers. On one hand, Lwanda's work highlights the artistic unpredictability of an epidemic's paths; but on the other hand, perhaps this process is more predictable than it might initially seem.

The final essay in this volume fittingly provides a literal challenge to the ways artists frame HIV/AIDS. Roland Bleiker and Amy Kay critique existing photographic representations of the pandemic, noting that attempts to present "natural" images of HIV/AIDS cultures end up cohering more to colonialist, exotic imaginings of Africa. Considering recent photographic initiatives in Uganda and Ethiopia, Bleiker and Kay actively seek new visual paradigms that avoid universalization while reducing the emotional and cultural distance between the subject, the photographer, and the observer.

Between sections, we have included other glimpses as interludes: song lyrics, a brief account from North Africa, an interview excerpt, short narratives, and a memorial. Some of these transitional moments supplement the material analyzed in the chapters, while others describe new areas deserving of greater future coverage. All, however, provide additional ways into this massive, complex, and uneven landscape.

CONCLUSION: THE ARTS AND THE CULTURE OF AIDS

The relationship between HIV/AIDS and the arts in Africa offers a multifaceted, nuanced, and deeply affective portrait, with numerous layers that we are only beginning to understand. Research presented in this volume suggests that continuing to pursue this line of discourse has much to add to the existing literature on HIV/AIDS. We cannot provide here a comprehensive portrait: this book, by its very nature, faces basic limitations in length and language, and (perhaps most significantly) depends upon the availability of existing scholars and scholarship. But we hope we present a good beginning: a launching pad for further work on the interdependence of medicine, culture, and creative expression. The more we can do to understand the coextensive nature of the healing and performing arts in Africa (and elsewhere), the richer, more relevant, and more meaningful our documentation and analysis of HIV/AIDS can become.

2

Interlude

Singing for Life: Songs of Hope, Healing, and HIV/AIDS in Uganda

Gregory Barz (Vanderbilt University/University of the Free State)

Along one of the many pathways I have taken in Uganda I met a visual artist named Francis Wasswa. Wasswa and I noted the potential for expressive culture—art in particular—to respond to HIV/AIDS at the grassroots level in Uganda. But Wasswa felt the visual arts had not yet assumed as significant a role in the struggles of community-based cooperative initiatives against HIV/AIDS as had music, dance, and drama. Several months later Wasswa presented me with several batik paintings. In his words, the largest one told a story, a narrative of devastation and disease leading to hope and healing through behavioral change in one particular rural Ugandan village. This painting stands as a testament to Wasswa's dedicated work as a visual artist. As I now follow the winding path through the painting's village scene, I see the everyday interaction between traditional healers and Christian clergy, nurses and medical workers, local business traders and ethnomusicologists—all working together. The journey begins in despair, as villagers moan and wail after consultations with herbalists and traditional healers. Hands are outstretched, and the backs of most are bent over. Further along the path, villagers visit the homes of those dying in the community while others proceed to the village's cemeteries for burials. In a clearing, drummers and musicians dance as they accompany a drama about the preparation and consumption of local brew. Off to the side, an HIV/AIDS seminar presented by medical professionals is attended only by women. I see myself—the foreign ethnomusicologist—transformed into a medical doctor in a white lab coat as men undergo voluntary counseling and testing. A white sport utility vehicle with TASO (The AIDS Support Organization) written on the side speeds along the village paths as we arrive back in the area where we started. It is

The title of this chapter is adapted from the liner notes accompanying the Smithsonian Folkways CD release: *Singing for Life: Songs of Hope and Healing in Uganda* (SFW CD 40537, 2007). Used with permission.

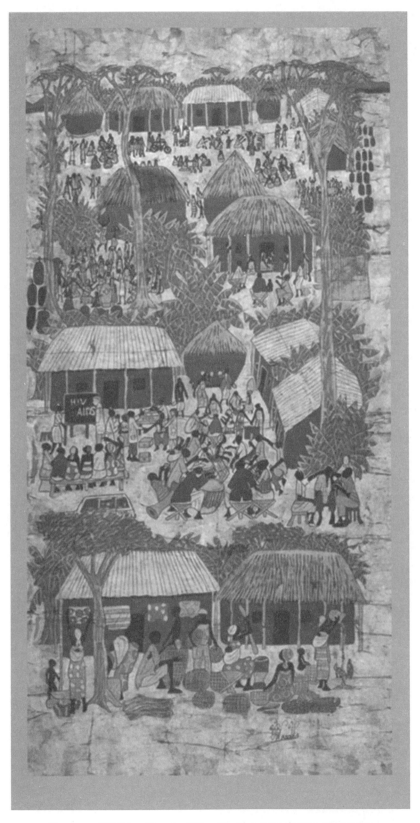

Figure 2.1 *"AIDS in a Ugandan Village,"* batik painting by Francis Wasswa

clear by the end of the metaphoric journey that everyday life in the village has responded well to the series of medical interventions along the way. Frances Wasswa's painting, *AIDS in a Ugandan Village*, is a personal story shared by many of faith, hope, and healing through the arts in a country as resourceful as it is compassionate.

AS I NOW FOLLOW THE WINDING PATHS

Vilimina Nakiranda's women's group gathers in a village clearing in the eastern Busoga region of Uganda to perform for farmers returning from a day in the fields. The women, many with babies strapped to their backs, are dressed in colorful floor-length *gomesi* with extended shoulder flaps—the everyday traditional dress of Ugandan women—and flip-flops. A group of men bring *baaki-simba, nankasa*, and *engalabi* drums over to the women. Most villagers continue to pass by until the drumming cracks an opening rhythm and the women start to dance as they sing their songs. Music, dance, and drama groups frequently sing about HIV/AIDS in Uganda today; the groups have had an enormous impact in rural and urban communities, and nowhere more important than at the grassroots. Governmental organizations in East Africa are often not able to reach out to the areas where music groups working with little or no funding have been most successful. When doctors ask women living positively with HIV why they persist in their efforts to contribute to local medical interventions, why they continue to dance when they have such little energy, the answers remain profound—Ugandan women do not want other women and youths to experience what has in many cases been forced on them. Nowadays both men and women will use whatever power they can access to initiate social and political interventions, no matter how small the reward. As a member of the Jumbo Theatre Group in Kampala suggests, music can "save":

> Music to me is food for the soul. From our African perspective, we realize that messages are portrayed better through music. When you approach something like HIV/AIDS that has such stigma and just walk up and say, "People have come to talk about AIDS," people are shy, and they will not come. But if you say, "I'm going to present a play," then you hear a song that has messages about HIV/AIDS and you're entertained, then by the end of the visit you'll think, "What did they mean?" From there someone will get the message so much faster than just coming up to a blackboard saying, "AIDS is like this!" That's why we sensitize through music, dance, and drama. People get the message very fast. I think another thing is, when we come together and sing, we get some new feelings. For example, some of us have problems. But when we are together singing, we forget our problems. So it saves us, too.

Apofia Naikoba, director of the Iganga branch of NACWOLA (National Community of Women Living with AIDS), observed, "These women have nothing left. Nothing. The words we use in our songs directly address the issue of HIV/AIDS, and people listen to us sing! People now realize the importance of condoms. Some now practice abstinence. Some seek our services for blood testing and counseling before marriage. The music we sing is not just an exercise—it excites people! They come in large numbers to join in the dancing, and if they pick some message from our songs, well, then we are successful." The Ugandan men, women, and young people devoted to creative expressions surrounding HIV/AIDS—Wasswa, Apofia, Vilimina, and others—dramatize the need for better-informed communities, dance for continued health education of youths, drum to attract the attention and participation of their communities, and sing the songs that turn people's heads. In their carefully constructed and medically informed musical performances, Ugandans today are not only singing for life, they are also saving lives!

UGANDA: A COUNTRY AS RESOURCEFUL AS IT IS COMPASSIONATE

Uganda, a land-locked country in East Africa bordered by Kenya, Tanzania, Rwanda, and Sudan, is home to numerous rural and urban communities that maintain rich histories and reflect a variety of economic conditions, geographic terrain, and linguistic and musical soundscapes. The eighteen ethnic groups of Bantu, Nilotic, and central Sudanic origins that today live in this small country represent diverse cultures that are both rooted in history and represent significant change and adaptation to modern times. The regime of infamous dictator Idi Amin (1971–79) followed by the abuses of Milton Obote in the 1980s contributed greatly to the instability of their newly independent nation. By 2011, although Uganda negotiated ongoing clashes with the Lord's Resistance Army in the north and rebel conflicts in the west, it remained a generally peaceful and politically stable country. From the soil-rich coffee and tea plantations and rice fields in the east to the Rwenzori mountain range in the west and the lush valleys in the central areas of the country, Uganda astounds with its range of geographic beauty. The cultural landscape of Kampala's urban environment, meanwhile, reflects the country's diversity. Built on seven hills, the capital city is home to a seemingly endless fleet of white "taxis," passenger buses, and speeding *boda boda* motor scooters that race across the city's paved and gravel road-ways at all hours of the day and night. Large white SUVs with the names of foreign health-care-related NGOs painted on their sides contribute to the congested downtown traffic. Street vendors hawk everything from penny candy to bootleg computer software.

Votive candles are sold on sidewalks next to newspapers from throughout East Africa. The amplified sounds of local independent churches comfortably coexist with the calls to prayer of the city's numerous mosques. The social clubs and airwaves play as much American and European popular music as local traditional and popular music. Yet many village-based cultural traditions (including music) continue to be practiced in urban contexts—taught in schools and played among families—reflecting participation in urban modernity and the persistence of rural identities.

In Uganda's villages and smaller towns, everyday life continues to present challenges. Families farm the land, growing bananas, cassava, coffee, and other cash crops to make a living. Ten-foot-tall anthills line the paths of many villages, and black bicycles imported from China add to the local soundscapes with their ringing bells. Electricity often does not make it down the network of dirt pathways that connect most rural communities, places where potable drinking water and access to necessary health care are often non-existent. In villages such as Kibaale in the eastern Busoga region, evenings are filled with local music-making and consumption of locally brewed millet beer, and many song texts tell of the hardships of everyday life.

MUSIC IN UGANDA

In a Clearing Drummers and Musicians Dance

The roots of many contemporary musical traditions can be found in Ugandan traditional culture "deep in the village," as musician Centurio Balikoowa often says. Traditional music-making continues to serve important ritual and everyday purposes in Uganda. For example, musical performances are organized for funeral rites, to communicate information through drumming patterns, to accompany labor, to console, and for educational purposes. There is also a rich diversity of musical instruments in Uganda, ranging from *ndere* flutes and pan pipes to string *endingidi* tube fiddles, *adungu* harps, and *ntongoli* lyres. Many local musical traditions draw on melodies that are pentatonic, a scale composed of five notes. Increasingly common, however, is a tendency toward the Western diatonic tuning system. In addition, drums of all shapes and sizes, grouped together or played individually, accompany plucked lamellophones ("thumb pianos") and xylophones. Village ensembles often combine instruments to form unique groups, such as the *embaire* xylophone ensemble I encountered in villages in eastern Busoga. Instruments complement singing and dancing as well as clapping and ululation—a high-pitched vocal cry manipulated by rapid movement of the tongue that punctuates musical performances throughout East Africa. Soloists Mzee Mata, Centurio Balikoowa, and Vilimina Nakiranda each offer the best of Ugandan musical performance traditions. Mzee Mata, a blind singer and *akadongo*-playing storyteller, has kept his community's history alive in the texts of his songs for most of his seventy years. Balikoowa, one of the last to be trained by the Baganda royal court musician Evaristo Muyinda, is known nationwide for his efforts to educate primary school children in elements of traditional Ugandan music. Vilimina Nakiranda, known throughout the eastern Busoga region, fuses her traditional singing and *akadongo* playing with performances that highlight contemporary social issues. Choral traditions feature local call-and-response singing styles as well as styles dependent on Western harmonies. The famous "Gampisi" song by Negro Angels Bamalayika and the song by the Kanihiro Group's song, "AIDS Has Finished Our People," offer additional examples of music used to punctuate local dramatic performances, with songs reinforcing the main themes of the plays. Instrumental, choral, vocal solo, and dramatic musical performances continue to thrive and develop in Uganda today. While popular songs and the latest dance music dominate radio airtime and the play lists of social clubs, local forms of music with socially relevant texts still meet the needs of communities throughout Uganda.

LOCAL LANGUAGES AND LOCAL MUSIC TRADITIONS

A Narrative of Devastation and Disease Leading to Hope and Healing

Ugandan songs about HIV/AIDS have appeared in a cross-section of local languages, including Runyankore, spoken among the Ankole people in the west; Lusoga, spoken by the Basoga people to the east; and English. The largest body of songs, however, are sung in Luganda, a Bantu language spoken by the Baganda people in Uganda's central Buganda kingdom that also functions as a second language for many in the country. Most songs reflect a history of sung poetic texts, and it is the lyrical nature of the songs on which most audiences focus their attention.

The breadth and volume of songs about HIV/AIDS represent a national musical response by local individuals and groups. Efforts by the government and private multinational and multilateral non-governmental organizations have failed to successfully meet the needs of the population in this global health crisis. Local languages, in contrast, often position AIDS within local cultures, specifically by referring to AIDS with labels from specific geographic regions. Centurio Balikoowa, for example, presents a litany of names associated with AIDS in his song "Abalugana." Such songs offer evidence of the contributions of musicians to the ongoing decline in Uganda's HIV infection rate at local, regional, and national levels.

The individual snapshots that follow highlight the breadth of cultural responses to HIV/AIDS in the form of music, dance, and drama in Uganda.

1. Vilimina Nakiranda, akadongo, and the Bakuseka Majja Group. Kibaale Village.
The sounds of cicadas precede the performance of this song, which I recorded outdoors in Kibaale Village in the eastern Busoga region of Uganda. "Clap and drum, and then I will narrate," sings Vilimina Nakiranda, leader of her local Bakuseka Majja women's club. The women of this group work together using music, dance, and drama to address social issues in their community. In this performance a litany of everyday health issues such as cholera, ulcers, and AIDS are situated within local contexts. The accompanying women interject responses such as "death is bad." As Vilimina Nakiranda sings and accompanies herself on an *akadongo* (thumb piano), she suggests that death is prevalent in Kibaale and does not discriminate—"death takes the educated and the ignorant, death takes the wealthy and the poor." AIDS has "finished" the local villages, and Vilimina suggests that everyone should live life to the fullest since there is no predicting when the disease will enter one's own home.

> *AIDS has finished our friends, taking the boastful villagers who contracted HIV*
> *They have searched for medicine without success*
> *Others have run to TASO, but they too have been met with defeat*
> *Others have used condoms, but they too have failed*
> *Every intervention has failed*

While a direct translation of the song text might lead us to believe that the village has lost all hope, Vilimina enumerates the ways in which local villagers have unsuccessfully addressed the AIDS epidemic in order to motivate her community to act even more aggressively. No medicine is available to her community, and as local residents turn to agencies such as TASO in the larger and more distant cities and towns, they have been met "with defeat." Condoms, Vilimina sings, have also failed. In fact, Vilimina suggests that every medical intervention in the area has failed. "The white men in Kampala have failed. The white men in America have failed."

2. NACWOLA Iganga (Led by Apofia Naikoba). Iganga Regional Hospital.
The women of the Iganga town branch of NACWOLA who meet regularly at the Iganga district hospital perform a song warning that AIDS does not discriminate. After a regular health education meeting, the group breaks to rehearse a song they will perform for various women's groups whom they will visit the following week. According to the Lusoga lyrics of "This Period of Time That We Are In" ("Guno gew mulebe gwe tulimu kat"), AIDS enters the homes of both rich and poor, adults and youth. The various symptoms are listed throughout the performance, including fever, headache, bouts of vomiting, shivering, and coughing. The song's leader, Apofia Naikoba, confesses, "This disease is difficult to describe." The song is directed primarily at young girls whom the women of the group advise not to spend time with older men and always to be mindful of the presence of AIDS in the region.

3. Meeting Point Kampala (Led by Noelina Namukisa). Namuwongo, Kampala.
Meeting Point is a medium-sized NGO in the Namuwongo slum area of Kampala run by Noelina Namukisa. I recorded their song "Is Someone There?" ("Abange ab'eno?") in the organization's front room as more and more Meeting Point clients joined the performance. Noelina Namukisa sat next to me during this song and pointed to an elderly woman who could barely walk when she entered the room, but who had found the energy to dance by the time the song had concluded. "She is dancing her disease," Noelina Namukisa stated as she slapped my hand

in laughter. Meeting Point's Learning Center, located in the so-called Soweto slums, provides shelter, educational and vocational training, and opportunities to live and grow in a nurturing community. Music, dance, and drama are central to the outreach efforts of this organization. In "Is someone there?" the singers, all clients and volunteer workers at Meeting Point, describe AIDS as a ruthless killer that has invaded the country, sparing no one in its path. Historical responses to the disease referred to as Slim [AIDS] are outlined to suggest ways in which many people have turned to ill-trained traditional healers and ended up dying in poverty.

> Chorus—*Slim has many traps through which it captures people—razor blades, needles, and others ways such as transfusions of infected blood or through contact with it in an accident. You can get Slim immediately. That is the grave. Lastly, Slim is transmitted through the "garden" that everybody likes. The owner of the garden has laid traps that you cannot miss. We all know this, but we ignore it. It is in the garden where sexual sin among the elites and the non-elites occurs. Sexual perversion is ruling the nations. It is terrible.*

4. Mzee Mata Nasani, akadongo. Kasokoso area of Iganga town.

I watch as Mata progresses down a water-filled path, clutching the arm of a younger musician as they walk toward a family compound where a makeshift recording studio has been set up in a men's drinking hut. Outside the hut, millet is spread out on a series of overlapping tarps to dry in the hot morning sun. Inside, drinking urns are stacked up along the walls next to a pile of ten-foot-long drinking straws used by the men to extract the strong traditional local brew from the urns. Mzee Mata Nasani is a seventy-year-old *akadongo* player, blind since birth, who lives in Iganga, a town located in the eastern Busoga region of Uganda. Mzee Mata—whose singing and playing style is recognizable throughout the country—is best known for having composed and recorded a song widely played on the radio that extolled the merits of the nation's newly ratified constitution in 1962. To this day, people recall Mzee Mata and the educational outreach of his political song. The songs Mata recorded in the 1990s may strike one as curious at first—songs of strange fruits enveloping entire communities, strange insects eating farm animals, and even stranger brooms that were sweeping through villages—all early references to HIV/AIDS. According to Mata, music, dance, and drama have long assumed a principal role in local medical outreach efforts pertaining to HIV/AIDS education and prevention in his area of the country:

> Music has really helped control and prevent AIDS, not only in this area but also throughout the country. People who listen to us, well, they normally change and adapt their behavior. Those who do not listen do not learn. Music has played a large role in my own community. There are songs that tell people how to protect themselves, and for those who are already sick there are songs about how to live happy and live positively. For those who have not yet got AIDS there are songs about how to be careful as they move around. Music has helped people throughout the region, preventing them from catching the virus. We even use songs to advise people how to use condoms, especially in those areas where things are not so good in terms of information about health care. We tell them that they should use condoms in order to prevent catching AIDS. Some traditional healers give out herbs; just clinics and hospitals give out tablets. But others use music to call the ancestors to come and solve the

problems. They often use music in such settings. Very many people at the grassroots have now formed groups that mirror my own group's efforts to educate, and in response to my songs people now go out and compose, also using music to change and prevent people from catching AIDS. Music controls AIDS. We have really struggled for this country, Uganda. Unfortunately, I have a feeling that AIDS has no cure, so those who do not listen to our songs and change their behavior will land in problems. Women and the youth must fight back against AIDS with their music. The youth normally listen to music and should therefore listen to us musicians who advise them to change their behavior. Those who do not listen often land in problems.

In "Emagombe newaife" ("The Graveyard is Our Home"), Mata sings in the Lusoga language about graveyards, the new home for many in the wake of AIDS. AIDS, he sings, is running us over like motorcars, like bullets piercing our flesh. In his song, the metaphor of graveyard-as-home morphs into graveyard-as-hell, a place where tolling bells beckon. Mata's narrative instills fear among his listeners: "We will not have clothes in hell. We will be provided with only one blanket. Our shirts will be torn to pieces. We will be separated from those we love, even our spouses with whom we are buried." When Mata sings, people listen.

    5. *Kanihiro Group. Kitabi Village, Bushenyi.*
The remote village of Kitabi is near Ishaka, a town in western Uganda, set in a mountainous region with farmlands cut into the inclined peaks. Primary schoolchildren commuting to school on foot share the one main road with goats and slow-moving motor scooters. Vehicles attempting the incline find the road impassable due to severe potholes. We climb the mountain to spend time with the Kanihiro Group, a local women's collective that perform for their own community and for surrounding rural communities when they have funds for transportation. Kanihiro's dramas include important messages about blood-testing sites, gender issues, and methods of HIV transmission, and they frequently conclude with a song in Runyankore that sums up the drama's central theme, such as "Silimu yaheeza abantu" ("AIDS Has Finished Our People"):

> You hear people over there yelling, others are mourning
> AIDS has finished our people, let us please protect ourselves
> It came from areas far away that we do not know
> Due to our little knowledge of the disease it spread like a bush fire when it reached
>   Uganda
> The dreaded disease has killed our children
> Those of us who were parents are now childless
> It kills both men and women, leaving behind orphans as young as those still
>   breastfeeding
> Our people are dying
> People have become infected due to promiscuity and prostitutes
> Not knowing who is infected, drinking alcohol, spending nights in discos
> These are ways people have become infected, oh, AIDS is a bad disease
> Often times the person who could have helped you has just died
> You hear a death announcement over the radio that they are taking a dead body
>   home

You spend the night in sorrow, mourning, and you bury the person the next day
If you are not at the burial, then you go somewhere to pay condolences to bereaved
  families
If you are not able to pay your condolences, then you are visiting a sick person
  elsewhere
Let us all protect ourselves against HIV/AIDS and take heed of prevention
  messages
These messages are passed along to us over the radio and screened on TV
Oh, AIDS is finishing our people, so let us protect ourselves

6. Bright Women Actresses. Bwaise, Kampala.

It is hard to escape the hustle and bustle of the urban Kampala sprawl, even as far out as the Bwaise suburb. Sewage flows down trenches lining the slums of the area, where family compounds are surrounded by large, locked steel doors. At the home of a member of Bright Women Actresses, up to twenty women typically meet to better their lives through increased involvement in health-care outreach efforts within their impoverished community. An important feature in musical performances in the fight against HIV/AIDS is the ability to trigger memory. Many CBOs (community-based organizations) that use music to communicate their messages rely on the ability of music lyrics to "stick" long after they've been sung. As one of the members of Bright Women Actresses in Bwaise suggests, the memory of a song's performance can recall the message of that particular song. And for many women who sing, this is what they hope for:

> Music has done so much, you know. People can appear indifferent, yet they will have learned something. This happens many places we've been to with this women's group. In an audience it is hard for people to go away with no lesson learned. At least one person will learn. Many listen to what we sing, and when he gets tempted to love a young girl, he remembers the songs.

In "Bannange Twajjirwa" ("We Have Been Invaded"), Bright Women Actresses opens by dispelling the myth that those who are HIV-positive brought the virus on themselves—"They are not guilty of anything, but merely the victims of the contagion, the mass murderer." According to the solo singer, who sings in Luganda, the one in a relationship who goes to work cannot trust the one who stays at home, while the one who stays home merely waits for the disease. Sadly, the song suggests, the disease begins in the womb, and it continues to "ambush" families until all are buried. According to the chorus, "Slim" causes poverty for many families, and poverty exacerbates the progress of the disease in the body. The women conclude by reminding us that their songs come with strong "medicine." The first intervention is abstinence ("Listen, youths, never give away your life to those who encourage you to have sex"). Another is to go for an HIV test ("If you are both healthy, then do not waste time"). A third is the encouragement to be faithful to each other ("Never do anything alone that you would not do if your partner were present"). A fourth is the need for protection in the form of condoms ("Use them, use condoms like shoes"). The final form the group encourages is prayer ("The last thing is to try very hard to pray, for your Creator is your doctor").

7. Negro Angels Bamalayika. Kampala.

In a dusty meeting room overcrowded with hand-soldered metal chairs at the Kampala YMCA, the members of Negro Angels Bamalayika meet to rehearse for an upcoming dramatic performance. The room's blackboards have long since fallen to pieces, and little is left of the institutional robin's egg blue paint on the walls. Roles are shuffled among members according to who will be absent or late that evening. At the end of the rehearsal one of the directors of the drama troupe asks if we would like them to perform the famous "Gampisi" song. *Gampisi*—which means hyena—became a metaphor for AIDS when it was first used as the title of a highly successful play produced by Negro Angels in the 1990s. The *gampisi* lays traps that ensnare its prey through sex, unsterilized needles, and unscreened blood. The singers, singing the text in Luganda, are fearful that they will not make it through the 1990s because they are too busy tightening their belts, constructing coffins, digging graves, and reading wills. *Gampisi* has "disorganized" everyone, especially people who used to love one another.

> 8. *Bukona Women's Group (Led by Loy Namaganda). Bupala Village,*
> *Bukona Sub-County.*

We travel in the back of a pickup truck through rural eastern Busoga along with Rev. Jackson Muteeba, the director of IDAAC (Integrated Development and AIDS Concern), an AIDS clinic in nearby Iganga town. After arriving in Bupala Village, we cut down banana branches to create an awning that will protect us all from the noon sun. As the women of the village gather to share with us the history of their performance group, children surround us. Rev. Jackson whispers in my ear, "These women will only be successful if the children continue to listen to their songs." The Bukona Women's Group suggests that all the women listening to "Silimu Okutumala" ("AIDS Finished Us") should put on the banana leaves that women in this area of Uganda typically wrap around their waists when they are in mourning. "Let's go to IDAAC," sing the women in Lusoga. *Silimu* (or "Slim") has "finished the village." The lead singer suggests that women should take their mothers with them when they go to IDAAC for HIV counseling and blood testing so that they all can raise their children for longer periods of time. The presence in the village of the visiting Rev. Jackson is acknowledged, followed in the song by a geographic mapping of the spread of the HIV virus from Kampala to Jinja, through the Mukono District, and into Iganga town. AIDS is now present in the villages of the women in the Bukona Women's Group who sing about the physical manifestation of AIDS in a graphic and direct way: "It starts with feeling cold, then there is headache, then pains in the muscles and bones of the legs, then abdominal discomfort, then diarrhea, then vomiting." Some women go for help to the local witch doctor, sings the group's leader. Those who seek out such help end up selling their land and their possessions in order to pay for treatment. The members of the ensemble, however, pledge their support if their fellow sisters go to IDAAC for treatment and help. "We used to have stigma," the song concludes. Now, however, even if women experience the physical discomfort of diarrhea, they are encouraged to "tell your friends."

> 9. *TASGA Drama Group (Tokamalirawo AIDS Support Group Awareness).*
> *Kawempe, Kampala Suburb.*

Traditional healers in Uganda utilize various forms of music, dance, and drama in their health education outreach. One group that depends heavily on its ancillary performing troupe is TASGA (Tokamalirawo AIDS Support Group Awareness), directed by Mutebi Musa. A charismatic man, Mzee Musa is passionate about marshaling as many resources as he can for the promotion of the health and well-being of his community on the outskirts of Kampala. As a recognized leader in the traditional healing community, Musa maintains, supports, and trains a music and drama group of AIDS widows and orphans that accompanies him in his outreach efforts. The members of the TASGA performing troupe frequently offer critical information for audiences concerning various medical issues confronting a given community, often elaborating on the issues already presented by the healer. According to Musa, medical and spiritual care are both integral to his healing practice:

> I began this work in 1967 when I was young. My grandy showed me the bush and herbal medicine for treating ailments among men, women, and children. That is when I started my work, and I loved it so much. I have developed over time those medicines formerly found in clay. Music and dance have played a significant role in the fight against AIDS, so much. When we go to teach, music and dance act as a trap for mobilizing people. For example, if they were to begin now, even those walking along outside would branch off. Wherever we teach, people have asked us, when we are coming back? And we also use music in treating AIDS victims. You see, when these AIDS victims are singing, even one who came very weak would be able to respond. You see, for us, our treatment is in two ways: physical care and spiritual care. When one sings, eventually she gets relieved. Sometimes she is forced to dance and forgets about the pain.

"Traditional doctors" such as Mutebi Musa contribute significantly to the overall health and spiritual well-being of many Ugandan AIDS patients. In "Fight the Epidemic," the TASGA ensemble responds to the fears expressed by Negro Angels Bamalayika by suggesting that there is reason to rejoice due to the mobilization efforts that have led to harmony and togetherness in the new millennium among "traditional healers, medical doctors, and religious leaders." The primary goal of TASGA's song, "Abange Mikwano Gyange Muvawa" ("Friends, Where Do You Come From?"), meanwhile, is to communicate the difference between HIV and tuberculosis.

> Let us start with the signs and symptoms of both as a reminder
> "Looking alike does not mean you are both related"
> TB is an English term for bacteria that infect the lungs through inhalation
> The primary difference lies is in the signs that are almost similar
> Let us give them to you and you will see
> One thing is that you can vaccinate against TB but not AIDS
> Signs, signs, open your ears
> Oh, loss of strength, skin rash, loss of weight, chronic fever, and headaches
> Abdominal discomfort, prominent superficial veins that look ugly, all are the signs
> Let us also mention the types of TB
> Abdominal TB, pulmonary TB, meningitis, and TB of the brain
> TB even causes psychoses, but the most important thing is that it can be vaccinated
>   against
> The advice that TASGA is giving you when you start any treatment is to not relax
> Destroy the friendship with TB by avoiding smoking and alcoholic drinks
> How can you avoid this pulmonary tuberculosis?
> Oh, it is possible if your children are immunized and do not spit saliva everywhere

Early treatment for those infected is important, as is completing the dose
Most important is sensitization and counseling

10. *Kibaale Village Embaire Ensemble. Kibaale Village, Busiki District.*

When we arrive in the remote village of Kibaale in the eastern Busiki region, a group of men are finishing digging the seven-foot-long, three-foot-deep trench that will support the construction of the massive, local embaire xylophone. The banana trees are being felled in the nearby banana fields to be placed along either side of the completed trough. From a neighboring family's compound, a set of large wooden keys separated by bicycle spokes are retrieved and placed on top of the banana trees. "Olumbe lwamala abanta" ("Death Killed All the People"), performed by the Kibaale men's embaire group in Lusoga, features a solo male singer who outlines the ways in which local villagers first became aware of AIDS through local councils and various media. The singer suggests that AIDS does not discriminate based on race, physical strength or stature, social status, or religious affiliation. Only at the end of the song is AIDS referenced directly with the Western term; the older, localized term, *Silimu*, is used first before it is contrasted with the more Western medical term *Ayidisi*, i.e., AIDS, a localized pronunciation (and spelling) adopted by many. This particular performance documents not only the geographic spread of the disease but also the transmission of local knowledge of HIV:

> *When I listened to the radio I first got the news*
> *Kasussa [the electoral commission] announced it*
> *As did the New Vision [English-language newspaper], they also wrote about it*
> *When you bring the Bukedde [Luganda-language newspaper], you will find that they*
> *also wrote about it, namely that in the Mukono District they got a disease*
> *Even this side of Seeta town they got the disease*
> *This death that came from Mukono*
> *Father, it has entered our area*
> *It has also entered Bbombo*
> *Listen, when it reached there, all who were there were killed*

The song later references "Sheika," a famous sheik and leader of the local Muslim community who lived in Namakoko, a nearby village. This sheik had the largest and most beautiful house in the entire Iganga District before dying of AIDS in 1998. The reference to the soil not being satisfied suggests that even the death of a powerful man will not fulfill the needs of the earth. Also mentioned is "Muzeyita," the name of a boy who first sang for me when I recorded in this village in 1999, as an indirect way for the group to inform me of the boy's death.

11. *Centurio Balikoowa and Kiirya Moses, ntongoolis. Kampala.*

Centurio Balikoowa plays the *ntongooli* bowl lyre to accompany his original composition on the theme of AIDS. One of Uganda's finest traditional musicians, Balikoowa has trained several generations of young musicians in local Ugandan music traditions. He has traveled extensively in Uganda to collect, record, and document traditional songs and dances; and his song "Abalugana" ("Those Who Have Not Settled") represents his own contribution to the effort to use music to educate others about AIDS. The song suggests that it will only be through behavioral change and ongoing education that the youth of Uganda will avoid the problems thrust on previous generations.

Abalugana bebaleta Silimu	Those not settled [with partners] brought Silimu [AIDS]
Amazima Silimu	I tell the truth about Silimu
Ogenzewa Ssebo	Where have you gone, sir?
Ogenzewa Nyabo	Where have you gone, madam?
Obolunda	My relatives
Abemikwano	And friends
Obwenzi mubuleke	Stop womanizing
Omusayi mukebbezze olabe	Go for a blood test to determine your status
Endwadde yakabi	It is a dangerous disease
Twekume	Let us be faithful
Silimu	Silimu
Mukenenya	Mukenenya [the one that makes you slim]
Kavera	Kavera [polythene bag]
Kasowole	Kasowole [the one that makes you taller]
Obbadde otya Ssebo	What is wrong, sir, that you cannot see what is going on?
Obbadd tya Nyabo	What is wrong, madam, that you cannot see what is going on?
Baganda bange	My relatives
Abanabange	My children
Ffe tunadawa	Where will we go when you are dead?
Nzembasibula	I am saying
Nti bye Mweraba	Goodbye
Endwade yakabi	It is a dangerous disease
Silimu wakabi	Silimu is very dangerous

12. MUDINET Drama Group. Mukono.

Off to the side of the main market area of Mukono town is a small, one-room office marked "MUDINET" (Mukono District Network of People Living with HIV/AIDS). Several people wait outside, forming a casual queue. As if on cue, we approach the dark office as the group inside begins to clap and sing. "I wonder what types of diseases people had a long time ago?" asks the solo singer in Luganda. MUDINET is one of the primary NGOs offering services in Uganda's Mukono District. According to their own mission statement, MUDINET depends on its songs to reach out to its large constituency as the agency "involves itself directly in the fight against HIV/AIDS by offering services such as home visiting, offering both pre- and post-test counseling, educating the community on HIV/AIDS through music dance and drama, organizing HIV/AIDS seminars, giving public testimonies" (UNASO News 2002, 8). In "Zino endwadde ezita-kyaluma kusasira" ("Such Painful, Merciless Diseases"), the drama group affiliated with MUDINET attempts to historicize AIDS in Mukono. AIDS is compared to illnesses, such as the flu, that people were able to easily overcome and even laugh off. AIDS, however, curbs ordinary activities, confusing people's bodies. There were herbs for older ailments, medicines for fevers. Now, even a fever associated with AIDS can kill.

> *Music plays in the stomach like an amadinda [xylophone]*
> *You can hear the beating drums playing loudly*

Then you end up running to the toilet due to the diarrhea that follows
It drains you until you are completely empty
And you return again like you have not yet started

13. Walya Sulaiman and PADA. CMS Trading Center, near Iganga.

At the Trading Centre along the main road approaching Iganga, Walya Sulaiman, director of PADA (People with AIDS Development Association), leads a group of local Muslims who perform songs and dramas throughout the rural area, often as the only medical outreach effort in the communities they visit. Sulaiman discovered he was HIV-positive on the death of his spouse. After losing his job because of the stigma of being labeled HIV-positive, Sulaiman dedicated all of his energy to the creation of PADA to address the endless needs of his community. For Sulaiman, drama is inherent in musical performance, so that within the act of singing the historical tradition of conveying information is reinforced. "My goal today is to tell you about my luggage, my goal today is to narrate my sad experiences." After he enumerates several of the physical manifestations of the virus's progress in this song, however, Walya Sulaiman cautions that "this luggage is too heavy." Like so many others in Uganda, Sulaiman sings his Lusoga-language songs for anyone who will listen. He believes that in order for true social change regarding sexual behavior to occur, his community needs to be nurtured in a culture of information, one in which they have the necessary tools to fight the disease.

Silimu [AIDS] is wrong, it is a wrong disease
When it wants to make you sick, it sends opportunistic infections
You feel a headache, and as that resolves the ears start to pain
When the pain in the ears resolves, backache sets in
As the backache resolves, abdominal upset sets in
As the abdominal upset resolves, profuse diarrhea occurs

14. Jumbo Theatre Group. Kampala.

The sounds of urban Kampala embellish the music of the Jumbo Theatre Group. Young people formed this group in response to the increase in HIV they found in their primary and secondary schools in the nation's capital. As one member told me, "We had to do something! People were dying all around us." The goals of the Jumbo Theatre Group are similar to those of many small-scale groups working throughout Uganda to sensitize youth in particular about HIV/AIDS. Several members of Jumbo realized after taking a HIV test how hard it was for others to go and test. They noticed that people were more inclined to go for testing after being exposed to musical interventions. Members of Jumbo began composing songs, reciting poems, and presenting plays that could help people in the same way that group members had already been helped. Group solidarity is the central theme of their song "The Struggle Against AIDS":

The struggle against AIDS should be a collective one
Should be all-embracing, a duty to me and you
Capable we are all, hands we do have
For together we can, divided we cannot

According to one member, music is a persuasive art, and as such it is one of the strongest interventions available today against the spread of HIV.

POSTSCRIPT: HIV/AIDS IN UGANDA

At the Grassroots

At the end of 2009, 38 million people were infected with the HIV virus worldwide. Of this number, over two-thirds, nearly 67 percent—or roughly 25.3 million children and adults—live in sub-Saharan Africa. The countrywide response of Uganda continues to stand out, since its initial, alarming infection rates were first documented. Uganda is the single sub-Saharan African country that has demonstrated a remarkable, constant decline in overall infection rates. Many factors have contributed to this decline, and a critical one, as I have tried to show in my book and album both titled *Singing for Life*, is music. Men, women, and children; traditional healers, witch doctors, and herbalists; as well as urban and rural residents alike all sing their response to AIDS, and they have done so for quite some time. Singing and dancing have been among the earliest interventions directed at HIV in the country. In both songs and dramas, Ugandans educate, care for, and console one another through music, as they have done for decades.

3

Born in Africa (1990):
Documentary Transcript

Written and Directed by John Zaritsky

Produced by Virginia Storring

Transcript by Judah M. Cohen

TITLE—FRONTLINE: The AIDS Quarterly[1]

TITLE on black screen—Eighteen months ago, FRONTLINE and The AIDS Quarterly set out to produce a major program about AIDS in Africa——

It is a difficult story to report.

TITLE—The facts are hard to get. Officially only 150,000 people on the continent have AIDS. But there may be as many as 4 to 5 million people infected.

And access to the story isn't any easier.

TITLE—Our producers, John Zaritsky and Virginia Storring, spent months negotiating with African governments, only to be turned down.

TITLE—Finally, one country, Uganda, gave us permission—and then, with restrictions. We were not allowed to film inside any hospital, and not allowed to film any person with AIDS—although eventually, as you will see, exceptions were made.

TITLE—But our producers were able to come back with the story of a remarkable man, who singlehandedly made his country confront the AIDS epidemic.

We call his story "BORN IN AFRICA."

Fade title out.

Fade in to an ornate concert stage. Title: KAMPALA, UGANDA. An announcer in a light suit paces the stage, announcing the entrance of Philly Lutaaya to an unseen but audibly raucous crowd.

ANNOUNCER—Ladies and gentlemen it is my *pleasure* to [unintelligible through the public address system] Philly Bongoley Lutaaya, in "Born in Africa"!

Philly Lutaaya, in a black and yellow sunburst-patterned dashiki, comes onto the stage to loud cheers and begins his show.

NARRATOR [Will Lyman][2]—In April 1988, Philly Lutaaya returned home after four years of political exile in Sweden, and instantly became the Bruce Springsteen of Uganda, with a song a new generation embraced as a national anthem.

Lutaaya, in concert, begins to sing his song "Born in Africa."

After twenty years of struggling as a third-world musician, Philly Lutaaya had finally reached the pinnacle of his career. He was now Uganda's number one pop star.

The only visual record of Lutaaya's sold-out concert tour was made by a fan on home video. But his new hit song "Born in Africa" could be heard all across the country.

Philly Lutaaya sings the second part of his song "Born in Africa."

Fade to aerial image of Ugandan plains as seen from a helicopter.

NARRATOR—Uganda was once called "The Pearl of Africa"—a fertile land where no one went hungry. But Uganda has just emerged from a twenty-year nightmare of civil war and political murder that killed a million and a half citizens. [*Images of devastated buildings.*] The savage regimes of Idi Amin and Milton Obote had also crushed economic and intellectual life. And 750,000 Ugandans, including Philly Lutaaya, had fled their homeland.

It wasn't until 1986 that peace finally began to settle on Uganda. And when Philly Lutaaya returned with his song, it symbolized for Ugandans the reawakening of hope and pride in their country.

The concert footage returns as Philly Lutaaya continues singing "Born in Africa."

NARRATOR—After his triumphant "Born in Africa" tour, Philly Lutaaya returned to Sweden to continue his recording career. It was there that mysterious ailments which had plagued the singer for months were finally diagnosed. He had AIDS.

PHILLY LUTAAYA—I was very much afraid. I knew I was in big trouble: thought about my future, my past. I felt so alone. I decided to come out if it [was] possible for me to launch a campaign, a crusade whereby some...my fellow human beings will, might be saved.

NARRATOR—Back in Uganda, Philly's older brother, A. K. Lutaaya, a conservative Kampala businessman and former captain of the national cricket team, was shocked by Philly's plans to go public.

A. K. LUTAAYA—Most people here, when they realize they'll run into this sort of problem; the AIDS disease is taken as a "hush" matter. When you catch it, you should withdraw from public eyes, and eventually you disappear, you know, you die quietly in some remote corner of some village place.

NARRATOR—Nobody knows how many Ugandans have died quietly of AIDS. But in this country of sixteen million, an estimated one million are now infected with the virus, and at least ten thousand have full-blown AIDS. In Uganda, as elsewhere in Africa, AIDS is primarily a heterosexually transmitted disease, and the infection rate is evenly divided between men and women. Despite the toll, AIDS had been a taboo subject in Uganda, a shameful secret.

And then on April 13, 1989, Philly Lutaaya became the first prominent African to publicly declare he had AIDS.

Philly's manager was Michael Daugherty, a Californian who had settled in Kampala in 1979, during the civil war. He had married a Ugandan woman, and they had two children. Over the years, the expatriate businessman had become one of Philly's closest friends.

MICHAEL DAUGHERTY—We were monitoring the press. It came, it was a bombshell. It was a big story. And the first day was handled with dignity. "Uganda's famous musician has declared he's an AIDS victim." The coverage was compassionate, it was straightforward, you know, that was it. However, day two, day three, the story changed completely.

NARRATOR—The story now was that Philly's announcement was just a publicity stunt to promote sales of his records.

ALEX MUKULU—I personally know that Philly wouldn't lie. He would have left [the] music [scene] if he wanted to make money.

NARRATOR—Alex Mukulu had been Philly's friend for twenty years.

ALEX MULUKU—And I know—we were together. We used to go without food, one day, two days, you know, but he never left [the] music [scene] for money.

NARRATOR—At the World Health Organization office in Entebbe, Adjoa Amana watched the controversy swirling around Philly, and saw an opportunity.

ADJOA AMANA—In the US, you have the.... Rock Hudson has come out; many other people who have had the disease came out to talk about it. In Uganda we have not been fortunate. In fact, on the African continent, on the African scene, we have not been that fortunate to get prominent people to talk about the disease at all, in a personal way.

NARRATOR—But when Mrs. Amana went to visit Philly, she found him badly shaken by the negative publicity.

ADJOA AMANA—And he was really feeling sorry that he had come out to say this, and basically my message to him was that "I'm sorry, it's not enough." That if you want these newspaper articles to stop, then show them why you declared. Do something.

Cut to a large open area at Kampala's Makerere University, packed with people.

ANNOUNCER AT MAKERERE UNIVERSITY—...very exceptional. For we are privileged. Privileged for the first time in this country, to have the real example of an AIDS victim...

NARRATOR—Philly Lutaaya decided to fight back. At Makerere University, the most prestigious in East Africa, he put his case.

PHILLY LUTAAYA [reading from a paper at the gathering]—I stand before you, a living example of an AIDS patient. I have AIDS and have been told that my days are numbered. I beg you, give

AIDS victims love and understanding. Don't desert us. Remember, if you do not take care, you too can [surely be in] the ranks of the AIDS victims.

NARRATOR—The speech was risky. Philly's advisors feared he would encounter skepticism and even hostility. But the audience of 5,000 students listened silently, and instead he found only respect.

PHILLY LUTAAYA [in later interview]—AIDS is here, but people wanted always to ignore it and pretend as if it was not here. So I wanted to go on shouting loud about this crisis. I did, I ignored people who were, who were calling me a liar, people who were calling me an opportunist. I knew [a] time would come when they would understand.

TITLE—"STOCKHOLM, SWEDEN"

Lutaaya, visibly thin, is being examined by a doctor.

DR. PER OLOF PEDERSEN [examining Lutaaya]—Put your tongue out. And [move your tongue] to the left. Good.

NARRATOR—Philly had returned to Sweden; but his health was now quickly deteriorating. Dr. Per Olof Pedersen:

DR. PER OLOF PEDERSEN—He had severe headache; he had severe diarrhea; was losing weight. He had fever. And he also started to get problems with his legs and feet, feeling some sort of numbness and, got sores on his soles, and that made it very difficult for him to walk.

Philly Lutaaya, holding the doctor's hand, attempts to stand up from the examination room table. He says "It's hard" and sits down. Pedersen responds as he ends the examination: "That's good. You can change [into your clothes]."

He has also been shown to have dissimilated tuberculosis with uh, tuberculosis not only in the lungs but also in the lymph glands and in the blood. And now, during the summer of 1989, it has been shown that he also has this cytomegalovirus infection. So in fact, he has had at least five, five infections or tumors that are included in the definition of AIDS.

NARRATOR—It had been six months now since Philly's AIDS diagnosis. Despite his physical condition, he was anxious to get back to his music.

In a Stockholm recording studio, he started to work on what would become the most important song of his life.

Several successive shots of Lutaaya working in a recording studio.

PHILLY LUTAAYA—I wanted to put something down, something musical, artistic, about my feelings and about the feelings of other, what I thought were feelings of other AIDS patients. The feeling of helplessness. The feeling of loneliness. I wanted to express what I felt within myself.

A Swedish woman leads a choir of other Swedish women and men. The woman snaps to the tempo, leading in the choir with the phrase "and, four." The choir, arranged in a horseshoe shape, sings together: "Today it's me. Tomorrow's someone else..."

NARRATOR—Philly ignored his doctor's advice, and worked around the clock during two months of grueling recording sessions to perfect the song he called "Alone."

PHILLY LUTAAYA—I knew, I felt I was racing against the clock, but it was a matter of time. I had work to be done, there was work to be done, and I had to do it.

Cut to a headshot of Philly Lutaaya as he sings first verse of "Alone" into a studio microphone:
Out there somewhere, alone and frightened
Oh, the darkness, the days are long.
Life in hiding—no more making new contacts.
No more loving arms goin' around my neck.

Another woman sings: Take my hand now... [*woman continues to sing under the narration*].

NARRATOR—The recording sessions took their toll. [*Fade in to Philly Lutaaya in his hospital room, an attendant unwrapping bandages from his feet.*] By August 1989, Philly was confined to bed in a Stockholm hospital. He could no longer stand because of open sores on the soles of his feet. But he was determined to return to Uganda, with the message that was in his new AIDS song.

Song fades out.

Philly had agreed to let us film his journey so his story could reach an international audience. But unexpectedly, the Ugandan government rejected Philly's request that he be accompanied by a Western film crew.

PHILLY LUTAAYA—Having been barred from being filmed in Uganda had made me more depressed, and I was really, I was down. But I really don't feel that the people of Uganda could do that to me. But this is one of the things which happened to us small people. We are frustrated always by the big ones; and they forget that they were, they were once small also.

NARRATOR—Philly appealed to Uganda's Prime Minister, Samson Kisekka. Philly wrote that getting his AIDS message to the world was his dying wish. And a few weeks later the Ugandan government approved the plan to film. But by now Philly's doctors feared he might never be able to return to Uganda.

DR. PER OLOF PEDERSEN—Couple of weeks ago, he said that "I can't even go to the toilet. I have to take the wheelchair to the toilet, because my feet they are extremely painful." I thought when I saw him a couple weeks ago that he should never be able to stand on his feet and legs again.

Cut to Philly Lutaaya in his hospital room, slowly riding a stationary bicycle with heavily bandaged feet.

PHILLY LUTAAYA [voiceover]—I'm a strong man. I don't believe in being weak or anything. Where I decide to do something I decide to do it.

NARRATOR—Philly had vowed to himself that he would not return to Uganda until he could stand on his own two feet. And in late September 1989, after six weeks in a hospital bed, Philly Lutaaya walked again.

DR. PER OLOF PEDERSEN—Three weeks ago, I thought this would be impossible. It's not due to a lot of drugs. It's due mostly due to his will to fight the disease.

PHILLY LUTAAYA [in doctor's office with Pedersen]—But I, I feel I'm getting my strength back. And I am of course I am literal[ly] excited, that [laughs] that I am going to Uganda.

DR. PER OLOF PEDERSEN [voiceover]—I wouldn't dare to talk about prognosis in terms of months or years with Philly, because he has proven that he can live much longer than we thought from the beginning.

DR. PER OLOF PEDERSEN [talking with PHILLY LUTAAYA]—So, Philly how do you feel mentally now?

PHILLY LUTAAYA—Mentally I just feel the same. I'm the same man. The same thoughts and even, creating even new songs right now.

DR. PER OLOF PEDERSEN—You do?

PHILLY LUTAAYA—Yes.

Cut to scene of Lutaaya entering his apartment and playing with his children.

NARRATOR—The next day, Philly returned to his Stockholm apartment. A single father, he had custody of his three children: Tina, fourteen; Tezzie, thirteen, and seven-year-old son John Lennon Lutaaya, named after Philly's musical hero.

PHILLY LUTAAYA [voiceover]—In my situation I always feel that in most of the things I do, the things I do and feel that, it might be my last time to do such things.

NARRATOR—The schedule for Philly's return to Uganda meant he would have only this one day at home with his children.

PHILLY LUTAAYA—I always miss my kids whenever I am away from them. But, well, this was a call for duty, and there are always sacrifices which one must take in this world.

TITLE—KAMPALA, UGANDA.

A big city in the background; in the foreground, rough structures with corrugated tin roofs. Off screen, we hear a television news broadcast.

TELEVISION NEWS ANCHOR—Good evening. Here is the news, read by Kanerie Muksha. First, are the main points. [*Cut to shot of a television set showing news footage.*] Renowned Ugandan musician Philly Bongoley Lutaaya is back home. Lutaaya's excited to launch his latest album, entitled *Alone and Frightened,* in which he calls for a collective struggle against AIDS in order to protect those not yet affected.

NARRATOR—What Ugandans didn't know was that during the flight from Stockholm, the government had suddenly withdrawn its permission for us to film Philly's activities in Uganda. There was no official explanation for the last-minute reversal. But Philly's supporters thought they knew why a Western film crew was not welcome.

ADJOA AMANA—The openness with which the Ugandan government had approached the whole AIDS problem, also brought about a lot of abuse of that hospitality, that openness, by foreign press, who came in here and tore the place apart in terms of: "Uganda is the AIDS capital of the world," or "of Africa." "Uganda is this." "All Ugandans have AIDS." Ugandans going out of the country have been subjected by all kinds of humiliation.

NARRATOR—Health minister Zac Kaheru led the opposition. In a letter, the minister explained that since Philly had lived in Sweden for five years, he should not be presented to the world as a *Ugandan* AIDS case.

HEALTH MINISTRY OFFICIAL—This is the minister of health, and under him and every AIDS control program and other experts honestly surely should have been following enough to know what schoolboys now *do* know. Ten-year-olds know that AIDS can be, you know, in your system for up to, up to ten years. And this is the myopic approach to AIDS. You know what backbiting is: instead of facing the issue, we are actually interested in finding out *where* somebody got the AIDS, you know, contact.

NARRATOR—But Philly *also* had powerful allies in the government. Dr. Ronald Batta, the minister of state of health, believed Philly's visit could have a critical impact on the future of the AIDS epidemic. Dr. Batta knew the projections. In the nineties, the number of cases would increase dramatically.

DR. RONALD BATTA—I'm quite sure as we're even talking now, some uninformed Ugandans are making love somewhere. One of them could be positive, another is negative. The disease has been transmitted. Somebody like Philly Lutaaya could come and defuse this situation for us. That's why I supported him. For two reasons: my medical profession, which says to support all patients even if you know he is going to die tomorrow; and number two is that, my interest on the big projection of the future in the 1990s. As I've told you, this case you were seeing yesterday: chicken stuff. The biggest lot will come in the 1990s, so they're trying to prevent the transmission. And I think that Lutaaya has done it for us.

NARRATOR—Two days after our arrival, as Philly dressed for the ceremony to launch his AIDS album, there was some good news. The Ugandan government had decided it *would* allow the documentary to be made. And to show its support, the prime minister would come to speak at the ceremony.

PHILLY LUTAAYA—Physically I feel tired. But I feel, spiritually I'm very much revived just by the fact that we're going to do our film. So my tiredness is likely to, to go up in, in, in the air.

Cut to Lutaaya's album launch ceremony.

PRIME MINISTER SAMSON KISEKKA [at a podium]—Ladies and Gentlemen, today's ceremony centers on Ugandan musician Philly Bongoley Lutaaya. Lutaaya declared in April of this year that he is an AIDS victim. It was a courageous move from this young man who has struggled a good number of years to develop a respectable musical career. Just at the time when the fruits of his labors were beginning to bear, fate steps in, and gives him this terrible blow. Philly, the government of Uganda appreciates your efforts. [*Applause.*]

PHILLY LUTAAYA [at same podium, responding]—Right honorable prime minister, I would like to thank you and the government of Uganda for allowing me to meet one of my final goals, and to enable me to talk to the entire world before I die. I composed this album with the hope that AIDS victims might find a few moments of solace and comfort from the music and my innermost feelings. The album *Alone* might help the healthy population of Uganda realize the importance of giving AIDS patients love and understanding. This album I have produced is a labor of love. In my condition, the recording sessions nearly killed me. But I couldn't let up because *Alone* had to be completed as my legacy to Uganda and the world. [*Applause*]

[*Audio transition to the second verse of "Alone":*]
Let's be out then.
Advise the young ones.
A new generation to protect and love.

Children singing, playing, laughing.
Let's give them everything in truth and love...

NARRATOR—That night, in Philly's old neighborhood bar in Kampala, Ugandans celebrated his homecoming and listened to his new song for the first time. In this city, where up to thirty-five percent of Philly's age group are HIV-positive, "Alone" had a powerful effect.

Lutaaya, looking frail, is in the bar leading a large number of people singing "Alone." They read from books of lyrics, smiling, swaying, and pumping their fists.

PHILLY LUTAAYA [in a separate interview]—I want to speak out, not just to sing happy songs. I, I feel like someone who represents common man status when I talk about such issues. It made me happy to bring out what other people could not bring out from within themselves.

Cut to an outdoor scene. Lutaaya and several other people are huddled around a car's front hood with several nearly empty Coca-Cola bottles. One person is playing the guitar; line by line, he accompanies another person testing out lyrics in the Luganda language.

NARRATOR—In Uganda, over half the population is illiterate. And so music is often the best way to get a message across. "Alone" was an instant hit in Kampala; but in order to ensure its success in the countryside where eighty percent of the population live, Philly and two musician friends decided to translate the song into Luganda.

The scene continues: one man plays guitar, and two others continue to translate the song. They sing the chorus together.

NARRATOR—Here on the shore of Lake Victoria, Philly found time to relax at a picnic with his friends and family. His mother, Justine Lutaaya, a retired headmistress of a primary school, had stood by her son from the time he got sick.

JUSTINE LUTAAYA [translated via subtitles]—My eldest son A. K. took a long time to tell me. He'd say Philly was sick, suffering from a fever. But I couldn't understand why such a fever continued. But he refused to tell me. So one day I got very angry and demanded some answers. Eventually my eldest son told me. Philly has AIDS. I was devastated.

NARRATOR—In the early eighties, when ignorance and fear of the disease were high, AIDS severely tested the traditional loving and supportive African family. Many Ugandans with AIDS weren't as lucky as Philly Lutaaya.

DR. ELLY KATABIRA [Senior Lecturer, Dept of Medicine, Makerere University]—A lot of families were confused. They didn't know what this new disease was. As you know a lot of our people believe in witchcraft, others don't, and so on. So, when a new disease came up, where there was no information about it, they were caught between their own safety and their love to take care of their relatives. And of course personal safety always came first. And some of them sacrificed their dignity in abandoning their relatives for their own safety.

NARRATOR—Noerine Kaleeba remembers the stigma and the isolation her family experienced during the years her husband Chris was dying of AIDS he had contracted from a blood transfusion.

NOERINE KALEEBA—The minute it is even discussed that one might have AIDS, their morality is on the table. And therefore, morality is one that Ugandans essentially hold dear. The majority of Ugandans are essentially, they are essentially God-fearing people, and immorality is not associated with God-fearing people. Therefore the first question that springs to one's mind is "I must keep this [secret]... People must not know because if they know, they will associate me with immorality."

NARRATOR—Shortly after her husband's death in 1986, Mrs. Kaleeba founded one of Africa's first self-help groups for people with AIDS and their families. Today, The AIDS Support Organization, or TASO as it is known, provides medical and counseling services for three hundred clients in Kampala and has branches in two other Ugandan towns.

NOERINE KALEEBA—Once HIV enters your house, it never leaves. Even if the individual who is physically affected dies, but the stigma lives in you for quite some time. The children of the family, the people that are closely associated will be, will have, you know, people will whisper about this particular individual.

Cut to TASO clients operating sewing machines, presumably as one of the organization's income-generating activities.

NARRATOR—TASO provides food and clothing for its clients, and jobs for those unable to work. But it still is one of the only support groups in Uganda and can help only a tiny fraction of those in need.

NOERINE KALEEBA—We accept, at least for the time being, there is no cure. But at the same time we accept and we feel quite compelled to propagate the concept that despite there not being a cure, AIDS is treatable. [*Cut to scenes of group massage therapy in a TASO center.*] The knowledge that one is infected, or that one has an illness of the magnitude of AIDS, cannot be borne by one's self. One requires a lot of support and this is what this counseling is about.

NARRATOR—A group of TASO clients and their counselors, a few of whom are uninfected volunteers, wanted to meet Philly Lutaaya. During his hospitalizations in Stockholm, Philly was isolated from other AIDS patients because of Swedish laws protecting privacy. And so on this day in Uganda he would meet, for the first time, other people with AIDS.

TASO COUNSELOR—What would you say to all of us here about its stigma?

PHILLY LUTAAYA—This stigma put to this infection is caused by ignorance. That's why I say that more, the population needs more and more education about AIDS. And people are so afraid. They're afraid. So even sometimes if they keep away from you, you don't blame them. I don't blame anyone who try to do like this [hides behind his hand], you know? It's natural. It took me a long time. And they don't want to see anyone who is HIV-positive or who has AIDS, I didn't want, I didn't know what I will see. I didn't know what I will see, and then it could make me feel worse.

TASO CLIENT #1—How did you get the courage to continue working after being told that you were positive? Were you counseled by someone, or were you, it was just self-determination?

PHILLY LUTAAYA—The first and the last time I was counseled was when I was told the result of my blood test, because I had gone to a clinic for some, something entirely different. And then they, they suspected that there was something. And then they asked me if I wanted to take a test—because it's not compulsory. I said, "Let me take the test." So when they told me the result was positive, it was, then, when there was this counseling.

TASO CLIENT #1—Were you shocked when you were told?

PHILLY LUTAAYA—Yes, I was shocked when [some affirmational laughter]. Yeah. Anyone will be. Because most people think, ah, no, no, no, they can't get AIDS. When you are told you are sick, that you are, you are HIV-positive or that you have AIDS, you must know that you still, you can still be very useful to society, to your nation, and to yourself. It's not, it's not good just to, just to give up and raise your hands and say: "Okay now, let me just wait to die." You might [wait] for five years [some laughter].

TASO CLIENT #2—As I told you before, that I fell victim in 1987, and since the day I've been with TASO, and I'm very happy with them, they are taking care of me, and the, they are taking care of, of my entire family. I don't regret [it] at all. And I'm very happy to meet you for the first time, and I pray very much to God that he keeps you alive on [your] feet. Thank you very much, Philly.

NOERINE KALEEBA [in private interview]—I don't think I could do what Philly's doing. I believe in inner powers. He must have inner power. Because, looking at him you can see he's really frail. And he's reached a level where most people that I've worked with in the last two years would just throw their hands up and say, "No." But to do what he's doing, I don't, I don't know. If I were to, put to the test, I don't know whether I could really do it, I could have the energy I need to do it. I think it is tremendous.

Fade to black, then cut to the interior of a hotel room. Dede Majoro is playing an acoustic guitar.

NARRATOR—Dede Majoro and Philly Lutaaya have been friends since they were six years old. [*Camera pans left to show Philly Lutaaya sitting next to Majoro. They sing together quietly.*] In between Philly's official appearances, they found time to reminisce about their struggles as young musicians.

DEDE MAJORO [voiceover]—Our parents saw musicians as in, guitars are taboo. As taboo, you know. Nightclubs were out of bounds, things like that. So, anything associated with nightclubs to our parents was out. They, for someone's son to be a musician those days [*Lutaaya, talking with Majoro in frame, recalls the year 1969*] is it was like losing the feller, you know? [*Majoro, in frame, responds "It's still a good song, isn't it?" Lutaaya says "Yes."*]

I think he found the only way he could express himself was through music. That's why his songs are always different. There is something unique about Philly's songs. He never was into this music where you, you sing about love all the time, girls' names, and all that, no, no. Say in about ten songs you could find one love song. Everything else was a comment, you know, his view of day-to-day problems people facing.

Lutaaya and Majoro continue singing together in frame.

NARRATOR—After a week in Kampala, Philly went back to his native village of Gomba, a tough three-hour drive from the capital. Gomba is a conservative agricultural community, and it had reacted skeptically to Philly's announcement five months earlier. Philly's family had lived here for forty-five years, and his late father was the school principal. But Gomba didn't believe Philly had AIDS. The last time Philly had been home, he was in the early stages of AIDS and appeared healthy.

PHILLY LUTAAYA—I see people coming near to look at me as if they don't believe it's me, yet now they believe, they know that I'm, I'm in big trouble. But there's nothing they can do, or, nothing they can do about it.

DEDE MAJORO [voiceover]—Most of the people who have seen Philly, believe, they quite agree, "Yes, he has AIDS." Although I've met fellows in the crowds you know, who still doubt. And they say: "Look haven't you seen Yul Brenner, actor, without hair? Well, Philly's hair is like that. It's deliberate. It's been bleached! Or, you know, whatever it is. After he goes back to Sweden, two months, the hair will grow back and Philly has earned his money."

BISHOP GEORGE SENABULYA [Gomba Diocese, Church of Uganda]—Well, in fact I have to confess, because I was among the people who were not really sure whether Philly was telling us the truth. I was thinking that where he only wanted it to announce, maybe he had been feeling some, something from somewhere to announce that. But just today I have realized what Philly announced is true.

Cut to scene of Lutaaya attending a religious service in Gomba.

NARRATOR—Over the years, the village of Gomba had experienced many anonymous AIDS deaths. But Philly had now given the disease a public face, and the community gathered to embrace its prodigal son. [*Scenes from the interior of the church, where hymns are being sung.*] In the church where Philly had been baptized, a special prayer service was held in his honor.

FEMALE PASTOR AT THE SERVICE—We are so pleased this morning for having our dear mother, Mama Lutaaya, to be here with Philly and the whole family having come here to pray, to pray with us. Here is a man who is confronted by all that he's confronted with: death, attack of enemies, anxiety, fear of anything, and yet before him there is a great a powerful, and…great God. The God he looks at, the God he looks to, the God he cries to, and He answers! This is the God I believe my brother Philly has known.

JUSTINE LUTAAYA [translated with subtitles]—When a mother has a sick child, she picks herbal remedies, washes the child and does whatever she can. But with this disease I am helpless. There is no medicine, nothing I can give to my son except for prayers. Therefore I plead to you all to continue praying for our son.

The congregation sings another hymn. Fade out.

NARRATOR—The next day in Kampala, the headlines were not about Philly's poignant return home. In a front page article, an African-language newspaper reported that on his way back from Gomba, Philly had secretly visited a traditional healer, who treated him with an expensive cure for AIDS. Concerned that thousands of Ugandans might be duped by false reports of a miracle treatment, Philly called a press conference to deny the reports and set the record straight.

JOURNALIST #1—Mr. Philly Lutaaya, today's issue of *Ngabo* carried a story that you have received a treatment from a traditional healer. Do you have any response to that story?

PHILLY LUTAAYA [reading from a statement]—It is a serious crime against humanity to so blatantly mislead the Ugandan people. False reports like this only confuse the people and hamper our battle against AIDS. Medical experts in Uganda and the world over have proven at this time that there is simply no cure for AIDS. Instead of misleading people, we need to stand together and fight AIDS with proper information on prevention, and we must look after the AIDS victims among amongst us. We must avoid cheap reporting.

JOURNALIST #2—Mr. Lutaaya, you noted that in *Ngabo* that article was, seemed to be directed to you, and you seem to be very bitter about it. What advice would you give to these people, to other Ugandans, most especially other AIDS victims who might, you know, be taken by such talk in town.

PHILLY LUTAAYA—We are free people, living in a free state, where people, where everyone is free to follow his or her own beliefs. I'm not going to tell, I mean, all that suffer don't go out to be healed by that woman or that man. But I don't believe them. I don't believe in, in these cures. Others, many people have come to me telling me: "Go, there's a *juju* man here, there's a," "This man is," "Go there," "Go there." Okay I'm really concerned about their...They're concerned, you know, they, they want me to be healed. But I don't believe in such traditional medicine. I don't know, I don't think it can help me, though I want to be healed.

JOURNALIST #3—Do you have any inkling as to when, where, and from whom you may have contracted this disease? Thank you.

PHILLY LUTAAYA—I don't.

PHILLY LUTAAYA [in private interview]—I, I am not, I don't want to back up, even if it is the most serious, even the last crisis in my life, I am not prepared to throw in the towel at all. I'll go on fighting; I'll go on, expressing the views I believe in, and I will go on trying to help the people in informing them and trying to answer their queries and everything, so that we may keep this epidemic from spreading.

Cut to gathering of Uganda's National Council of Women. Victoria Kakoko-Sebagereka is standing, speaking from a stage. Lutaaya is seated to her right.

VICTORIA KAKOKO-SEBAGEREKA—Uganda has AIDS. We call it *silimu* [pronounced "silim"]. And *silimu* is with us and among us. And it's only Lutaaya that has accepted to show us that it's here and it's up to us to know how to handle it.

NARRATOR—The chairman of the National Council of Ugandan Women,[3] Victoria [Kakoko-] Sebagereka [here pronounced "Sebareka"], had invited Philly Lutaaya to address an international conference on women's healthcare. But she ran into opposition from some delegates from other African countries who had never seen a person with AIDS before.

VICTORIA KAKOKO-SEBAGEREKA [announcing Lutaaya]—When I suggested that Lutaaya comes and talks to us, some members felt it would scare our guests. But I hope and I trust that you bear with me that for him it's a big thing to carry, but he's not carrying it for his own sake. He's carrying it for us, for you and me, and for the coming generation.

PHILLY LUTAAYA—In Uganda, fifty percent of the AIDS victims are women. Women in Uganda, in Africa, must join the battle against AIDS. When we talk about the battle against AIDS, we must forget blame. Blame is not productive. I know that I contracted the virus from a woman, but I don't blame that woman. That woman was definitely given the virus by a man.

VICTORIA KAKOKO-SEBAGEREKA [in private interview]—I feel women are more cautious and are trying to be as safe, to keep themselves as safe as possible. But with our culture, which we are trying to change gradually, women have in the past been very submissive to their husbands. You don't know who your husband has been with; he comes, you just have to accept whatever he tells you to do. But now I think if a woman, especially an enlightened woman, knows that her husband has been unfaithful, she will do everything possible not to have anything to do with him until both of them are checked.

PHILLY LUTAAYA [presenting at the meeting]—Changes must be made in our sexual behavior. For the past years we have been so free in our sexual behavior. Adultery is a serious threat to all of us, and it must stop. Adultery by either sex presents a danger to the other partner, and ultimately to the whole family. If we don't work hard, the human race is going to die.

VICTORIA KAKOKO-SEBAGEREKA [in private interview]—The young generation think it's a myth. And they think it's very far, it's very far from them. They think AIDS affect only grown-ups. And my concern is to sensitize and try and tell the youngsters that it's their age group that is more affected than the thirty-five and above [age group].

Cut to a choir of schoolgirls at Gayaza High School, singing "Do not be afraid, I am with you; I will protect you; I will save you."

NARRATOR—The Ugandan government is focusing its AIDS education effort on the five- to fifteen-year age group, which is still virus-free. [*Philly Lutaaya is shown listening to the choir.*] From primary school to university, all Ugandan students are instructed about AIDS prevention. But schools across the country were inviting Philly to visit, because they knew he would have an impact on the students they would not forget.

SISTER DR. KATHLEEN O'SULLIVAN [Headmistress, Gayaza High School]—I want to welcome all our visitors to Gayaza High School. We are the oldest girls' school in Uganda, and proud of it. But particularly today we want to welcome Mr. Philly Lutaaya. We are so grateful that he has given up this time to come and share with us and allow us to sing along with him. Mr. Lutaaya, you are very welcome to Gayaza High School. [*Applause.*]

PHILLY LUTAAYA—I wish I was just on an ordinary visit here. And I used to come and visit my sister here some years ago. But, today I have come to stand before you as a living example of an AIDS victim. This is serious. I never wanted this to happen to me. So, straightforward I would like to tell you that, I would not like this to happen to you, to any of you. The message I would like to give to you is that, let us do our best to have a virus-free young generation. It's easy to avoid getting the virus. I beseech you that, please, be careful in the way you handle yourselves. We need you.

STUDENT WITH A GUITAR [asking a question]—I wanted to know what made you decide to tell the world you had AIDS. Because most AIDS, AIDS victims don't, don't let it out.

PHILLY LUTAAYA [responding]—I wanted people, having seen me, to know that AIDS can affect anyone. Not only the poor peasants; not only the rich *mafuta mingi*;[4] not only the prostitute. But it's in all classes.

STUDENT #2—What was the reaction of your family for knowing that you've got AIDS, and what have you done to help them, um, understand?

PHILLY LUTAAYA—My eldest daughter cried. My second daughter did not cry—she's a tough girl [*he smiles; quiet laughter*]. And my young son, who is only seven years old, he didn't understand what was going on. But when I came and told my mother and my brothers, and sister here in Uganda, they were shocked. And they asked me "Are you going to take it?" I mean this, when I told them that I'm going to go public and tell the people. I said "I will take it. I can take it." So, they have been with me all the way.

STUDENT REPRESENTATIVE—On behalf of the all the girls' souls at Gayaza High School, I would like to thank Philly Bongoley Lutaaya, and we are very grateful for your presence, for your presence here at school, and would like to say "We love you." And as a token of our love we have this small gift for you. Please receive it.

Lutaaya stands up, receives the gift, and says: "Thank you very much." Applause.

Lutaaya opens his present, a Gayaza High School T-shirt with the words "Never Give Up" on the back and "Support Gayaza High School" on the front. The students sing the chorus from "Alone" in an original arrangement as Philly Lutaaya stands up and models the shirt. More applause. Philly Lutaaya joins them in singing.

NARRATOR—The highest rate of HIV infection in Uganda is found in women aged eighteen to twenty-four. And if they are poor and unemployed, they are particularly vulnerable.

ADJOA AMANA [in private interview]—Many older men are having relationships with younger women because they feel that women their own age group are already infected. And so they go after the younger ones. So you may have a situation where one man may be infecting a few of these young women. If a woman doesn't have enough to eat, and um, or doesn't have enough money to get all the nice clothing and things that she needs, and a man can offer it to her, um, a lot of these young women will go for it. This is the key message that we're passing on to women, be it rural or urban, that whatever you're doing, be proud of it. Earn a living for yourself, because one mistake can end your life.

Fade to black; then fade in to a fountain near the Kampala Sheraton Hotel.

NARRATOR—At his headquarters in the Kampala Sheraton, Philly was receiving hundreds of requests from Ugandans who wanted to meet him in person. One special request was from Philly's travel coordinator, Eddie Masoke. His brother Vincent was dying of AIDS and wanted to meet his idol. Vincent had endured a difficult two-hour journey from his village where he had been a schoolteacher. As they talked, Philly discovered that they were the same age, but that Vincent had been sick for two years longer.

PHILLY LUTAAYA [in private interview]—When I see my fellow victims, it's just like looking at myself. I know that they have gone through things I've gone through. I'm lucky no one has ever told us [laughs] what experience it is to die. But, if you know that you're going to die, better one not groan so much. Of course you regret the friends you are leaving behind in this life. I mean, the material things in the world. But you cannot just put on a sad mask and say that "I am going to die." Oh, no. That's my opinion. I would try to, to lead a happy life as much as possible.

Cut to close up of Philly Lutaaya with others surrounding him and singing "Happy Birthday." Pan out to see more people and two large heart-shaped birthday cakes with numerous candles. The frosting on the cake spells out the words "We All Love You."

NARRATOR—Philly Lutaaya turned thirty-eight on October 19, 1989. Before the party, he had privately discussed the arrangements with his brother, A. K.

A. K. LUTAAYA—He said look here. If, can ask my friends, terrible what they—let them not pity me, okay? Let us be friends. When [we] go to the party let's drink and enjoy ourselves in the short time we have.

ALEX MUKULU [friend]—With Philly it's very difficult to cry, you know. Even now, at home, he still has pain in the legs but, he still comes and gives you just one line of a joke and, you feel good, you know? You feel ashamed to kind of feel sad in his face. Because he's not.

At the birthday party, Mukulu tells the last line of a joke in Luganda. All laugh.

PHILLY LUTAAYA [in private interview]—In one way it was the best birthday I ever had in my life. I was in company with so many friends who I had known and not seen for a long time. Myself I have a little sad because—sad and happy. For I, I had not known whether I would make it to be thirty-eight. I've been sick, seriously sick, on and off, and yet, well, I made it and became thirty-eight years old, and, well I kept thinking, "Am I going to, to celebrate another birthday?"

Cut to a nightclub.

ANNOUNCER—I'd like to introduce a very special guest artist tonight ladies and gentlemen. My friend, my colleague, Philly Bongoley Lutaaya!

Music plays as Lutaaya comes up stairs to the microphone.

PHILLY LUTAAYA [voiceover]—My friends have made me what I am by appreciating my music. They have made me the biggest star in Uganda.

Lutaaya, in the nightclub, sings one of his songs.

NARRATOR—Since his arrival in Uganda two weeks earlier, Philly's fans had been clamoring for him to perform once again. Finally, in an old nightclub haunt, Philly sang a new song he had written about Kampala.

More of song, with cuts to dancers in the club.

PHILLY LUTAAYA [in private interview]—I like Kampala. It's a beautiful town. A beautiful city. And I really admire the inhabitants of Kampala—the Ugandans who come from different tribes, different corners of Uganda. And they live together, they, they've been struggling during the difficult times we've had in our nation. And I wanted to pay a tribute to the city of Kampala and its inhabitants. Also this song "Kampala" was addressed partly to people who have emigrated from Uganda, who are living abroad, and I was telling them "Tugende e Kampala"—"Let's go to Kampala." Let's go back to our town, to our country. Everything is now okay. Let's come and build our country again. So I wanted to sing to the audience "Tugende e Kampala" and I'm trying to tell them that people are coming back to Kampala.

Cut back to the performance of "Kampala." Lutaaya finishes the song; loud cheers.

PHILLY LUTAAYA—Thank you. [*He continues to speak, unintelligible due to the noise of the crowd.*]

Cut to Philly Lutaaya in underclothes in his hotel room, lying face forward, receiving a foot treatment.

PHILLY LUTAAYA [speaking to the physiotherapist]—And that, the foot has just gone down—it had, it was very swollen, the whole of it.

NARRATOR—Philly's feet and legs were still bothering him. But two Ugandan doctors had refused to treat him because they were afraid to touch an AIDS patient. Finally a compassionate physiotherapist volunteered to help. Philly's experience with the doctors was not uncommon, and the problem was on his mind when he appeared before medical students at Makerere University, Uganda's only medical school.

PHILLY LUTAAYA [addressing the medical students]—I have been told that some doctors in Uganda need to be educated and sensitized towards AIDS patients. At first I did not believe this. I'm sorry to say that it is true. I know I had to look around just to get physiotherapy when I arrived here from Sweden. In the future, each one of you will have to deal with AIDS on a professional, or at least a personal level. Treating AIDS patients is not just giving out drugs and going away. It requires a commitment from medical practitioners. I have been told that over the last twenty years about seventy-five percent of Ugandan-trained doctors have left the country to work in foreign lands. The demand for doctors in some foreign countries is high. So the temptation must be great. But I would ask you to think of Uganda first. Statistics show that there is one doctor for every thirty-seven thousand persons in our country. You are needed by your fellow Ugandans. So, do not walk out on us. Thank you very much. [*Applause.*]

NARRATOR—A shortage of doctors is only one of several crises facing the Ugandan health care system. Its hospitals are crumbling and overcrowded. Most AIDS patients will die without ever being hospitalized. Drugs and basic medical equipment are in short supply. The Ugandan government can afford to spend less than two dollars per person annually on health care. For AIDS patients, that means that life-prolonging drugs like AZT are simply not available. Ugandans also cannot afford the major weapon in the battle to prevent AIDS: the condom. Although soldiers, university students, and some people with AIDS receive free condoms from the government, they are just too expensive to become a practical solution to the AIDS epidemic.

DR. ELLY KATABIRA—A lot of people, I think probably about one percent of our population, actually, know what is a condom. So if you engage in a massive condom supply and medication it means educating literally the whole population about it.

Cut to a scene of a military band playing in the presence of Ugandan President Yoweri Museveni.

NARRATOR—When Ugandan President Yoweri Museveni came to power in 1986, he faced the task of rebuilding a country whose economy and infrastructure was in ruins. Ten percent of the population had been killed during the twenty years of civil war. AIDS was just one more challenge in a devastated land. But Museveni soon recognized the disease might become the greatest threat to his nation's survival. And so the Ugandan president became one of the first African leaders to openly acknowledge the AIDS epidemic, and understand that the only effective weapon a poor country has is public education. Since then, he's waged an all-out campaign to change Ugandans' sexual behavior. His message: Love faithfully, and stick to one partner.

The bandmaster finishes conducting the song. Cut to a market area in the middle of Kampala.

NARRATOR—In Uganda, ninety-two percent of the population regularly attend places of worship. And so the country's mosques and churches have become important allies in the president's campaign against AIDS. The Kibuli mosque in Kampala extended a special invitation to Philly Lutaaya, who was not a Muslim, to come and speak.

Exterior of the mosque. Then cut to interior: the camera pans down from above to show Philly Lutaaya speaking in front of a large crowd inside the mosque.

Lutaaya delivers his message in Luganda, as the narrator provides a translation.

NARRATOR [translating Lutaaya]—AIDS poses a special danger to Muslims and traditional African societies where polygamy is a widely accepted practice.

NARRATOR—Philly told his audience he himself had relatives with two or three wives, and he felt there was nothing wrong with that, as long as all the partners remained faithful to one another. Sex education for Muslim youngsters is not normally encouraged by religious elders. But Philly said that during the current AIDS crisis, teaching innocent children about the disease and its dangers had to become everybody's priority.

Cut to a wide shot of hundreds of primary school children at King's College Budo, sitting on benches in khaki shorts and red shirts while singing a hymn.

NARRATOR—King's College is an exclusive private school established in 1912[5] to educate Ugandan royalty, and today it still teaches the children who will become the leaders of tomorrow. When Philly Lutaaya, grandson of a Bugandan chief, returned to his former school, it was clear he regarded his campaign against AIDS as an act of patriotism.

PHILLY LUTAAYA [addressing the children]—Don't ever forget that you are Africans. You are people who were born in Africa, and you must be very proud of being an Afri, Af, Africans. Always identify yourself wherever you may go, identify yourselves as true Africans, the sons and the daughters of our grandfathers, who built the glory and the honor on which we are walking now. And when I look [*fade...*]

PHILLY LUTAAYA [in private interview]—I love Uganda most because it's my motherland. I must be very loyal, and give all I want to Uganda. I have found that I, I always miss Uganda and I am very, always very homesick when I am away from Uganda. So I decided to give my life to Uganda.

NARRATOR—As the campaign entered its fourth week, Uganda's acceptance of Philly Lutaaya had become almost universal. But at the country's most important church, Namirembe Cathedral, there was still resistance.

MICHAEL DAUGHERTY—Namirembe Cathedral is the seat of the Church of Uganda; by and large the pillars of the diocese are quite conservative. There were quite a few people in the, in the hierarchy so to speak, [who] didn't want Philly to speak, they didn't want him to sing, they didn't want his music played inside the cathedral. They thought it was a, a sacrilege or something.

NARRATOR—But Bishop Misaeri Kawuma, Uganda's most powerful religious leader, had been an early supporter of Philly's campaign, and he was determined that Namirembe Cathedral would honor him.

BISHOP MISAERI KAWUMA [to Philly Lutaaya]—I'm proud of you. May God give you the strength you need.

MICHAEL DAUGHERTY [in private interview]—But I must admit that Bishop Kawuma had the courage to face all the opposition. And you could imagine, standing up against the current, and saying: "No, this has to be done."

NARRATOR—On a Sunday in late October, Philly was invited to address the congregation, and he was also permitted to sing a spiritual song he had written called "Tumuzinze": "Let Us Worship Him."

Philly Lutaaya, in suit and tie, comes up onto the pulpit of Namirembe Cathedral to applause, and sings "Tumuzinze" in front of the congregation.

NARRATOR—Later, Bishop Kawuma would urge that Philly's spiritual song, "Tumuzinze," be adopted as an official hymn of the Church of Uganda.

Lutaaya continues to sing "Tumuzinze" with the choir.

NARRATOR—After the triumph of Namirembe Cathedral, Philly went directly to the funeral of a close friend and fellow musician, Billy Mutebi.

PHILLY LUTAAYA [in private interview]—I, I lost a, a work comrade, also, as well as a friend. He's been sick for almost two years. But we, we played together, in the "Born in Africa" show. He was my bandleader. So he was my right-hand man, as far as musical activity in Uganda was concerned.

JOHN ZARISKY [DIRECTOR, off camera]—Have you lost many friends to AIDS, Philly?

PHILLY LUTAAYA—Yes, I've lost more than five friends. Well the, the thing is that most of them, they have died of AIDS not believing it was AIDS. It was just say that "So and so has died after a long illness," or fever or diarrhea or such things, but not, they don't like to say AIDS.

Fade to black.

Fade in to aerial view of Lake Victoria from a helicopter.

NARRATOR—Philly embarked on his final mission into the Ugandan countryside aboard a government-supplied helicopter that took him into a remote rural area along the shores of Lake Victoria called Rakai. [*Views of Lutaaya looking out from the helicopter onto a devastated and empty landscape.*] The Rakai district is where AIDS first struck the country in 1982 and is the area hardest hit by the epidemic. With HIV infection rates as high as seventy percent, some villages have become virtual ghost towns. The death toll has been enormous. No Rakai family has escaped the epidemic.

RAKAI RESIDENT—My family also, I got a four children have died. Four children have died, and also I've got my two people—my brothers—their lives too also have died. [*Off-camera question: "Of AIDS?"*] Of AIDS, of course.

NARRATOR—In Rakai there are now communities populated almost entirely by the young and the old, where AIDS has virtually wiped out the middle-aged generation. Today in Rakai, two out of five children are AIDS orphans, and many cannot even afford the fee of a few shillings to go to school.

When Philly last played in one of the many nightclubs in Kyotera [narrator pronounces the city's name "Shatella"], Rakai's main trading center, it was during the early stages of the epidemic, and the town was a busy commercial stop on the Trans-African Highway.

PHILLY LUTAAYA [voiceover]—There is less, I mean nightclub life and because in those days people were so free, drivers were making that stop. And there were a lot of prostitutes around. A lot of girls, I mean—right now it's, it's a kind of a lonely place.

NARRATOR—AIDS has now virtually cut Kyotera off from the rest of Uganda, and today outside visitors are a rare sight in the devastated town.

Cut to schoolgirls dressed in blue dress-uniforms dancing and singing a welcome song to Lutaaya.

NARRATOR—Twenty-three thousand children in Rakai have already been orphaned by AIDS. Philly urged the children to learn where their ancestors had come from, so that their families' tradition and history would not disappear forever. As he had everywhere in his campaign, Philly urged the people in Rakai not to condemn the dying, but to give people with AIDS compassion and love. After his speech, a group of local musicians asked Philly to listen to a song they had written about AIDS.

Cut to Philly listening to the group, identified by held signs as "SUPER SINGERS."

[Translation of the song in subtitles:]
AIDS was inflicted upon the rebellious,
The promiscuous and the criminals.
It's terrible now because it strikes children
Who know nothing about the world.
How should we pray?
Help us father
We are perishing.

NARRATOR—Philly was stunned. The song condemned people with AIDS for their immorality. It was the very attitude he had been campaigning to change, and left him wondering whether the shame of AIDS would ever end.

PHILLY LUTAAYA [in private interview]—Just because you had sex with a, with a lady and then you, you got infected with HIV, I mean, I don't think it should be, one should need to be ashamed of it. It's just the natural course of, I mean, course of events. But people don't like to be identified with AIDS. That's that.

NARRATOR—Despite the ravages of Rakai, in most rural areas of Uganda, where eighty percent of the population lives, HIV infection rates are still relatively low. And that gives health officials a reason to hope.

ADJOA AMANA—We can save the country, because the, out of thirty-four districts, only two districts are pretty bad. The rest, it's still very much an urban problem. And so I feel that the earlier we can, the speed with which we can control from spreading heavily into the rural areas, the impact there will not be heavy at all.

NARRATOR—But in Uganda, as it is across Africa, the health of the countryside is threatened by the movement of traffic in and out of the more heavily infected cities. During the early stages of the epidemic, armies moved back and forth across Uganda, and today the Trans-African Highway, which runs through the country from Kenya to Zaire, is regarded by health experts as a transmission pipeline for AIDS. Recently, a large Kampala trucking firm reported that thirty-five percent of its drivers were HIV-infected.

In Jinja, Uganda's second largest city, Philly Lutaaya addressed a restless crowd of truck drivers. It was the most hostile audience of his campaign, but the heckling didn't stop him.

PHILLY LUTAAYA [in private interview]—I've got no secrets. I've got nothing to hide. So I speak out whenever I feel that [I] will help someone else. That's how I was brought up, and I'm not going into trouble by speaking the truth. So I kept it that way.

PHILLY LUTAAYA [addressing another rally]—It was my wish, that for the rest of the time I have left, I will try to speak to people whenever I can, whenever I have any strength.

Close-up on a small group of listeners at the rally, one of whom is holding a pamphlet entitled "AIDS: Learn the Facts."

NARRATOR—Philly Lutaaya's campaign was now in its twenty-eighth day. His health was failing, and his doctors told him he must return to Sweden for further treatment.

PHILLY LUTAAYA [continuing to address the rally]—Don't desert the victims. Try to give them good morale, try to give them support, because it's a painful experience when you know that everything is finished. When you know that all your dreams might never come true. For anyone who discovers that he's positive, please keep the virus to yourself. Don't kill other people.

DR. RONALD BATTA [in private interview]—Lutaaya's a very forceful character and dedicated to his nation. He has made a tremendous contribution in this fight. We regard him as the greatest Ugandan health educator on AIDS. From what I've just told you he's a hero. Handfuls of Ugandans have died of AIDS quietly. Lutaaya's just in a different direction. [For] that he's a hero.

The start of Lutaaya's song "Alone" begins to sound.

NARRATOR—To honor their hero, five hundred supporters from every segment of Ugandan society held a candlelight vigil on the grounds of the Kampala Sheraton. [*Lutaaya and his party are shown sitting on a balcony with their candles as the camera pans over to show hundreds of candles lit below them. A second shot shows members of the vigil, their candles lit in the darkness, marching in a long line.*] During the past four weeks, Philly had traveled the length and breadth of his homeland, and had moved the hearts and minds of a nation.

A montage of video flashbacks from the tour begins.

ADJOA AMANA [voiceover]—He brought this from out of a textbook: out of theory into reality, for the public to see him, see his family close by, to see his friends close by, and that it's alright. It's all right to have AIDS. It's not the end of the world.

MALE VOICEOVER—The ease with which you handled this, the courage which you showed, gave me personally a lot of strength.

FEMALE VOICEOVER—Lutaaya's being in Uganda has helped a lot of people. Not to always connect AIDS with immorality. Not to look for faults who brought it. Not to blame. But it has taught the Ugandans that one has to be very human to the AIDS victim.

MALE VOICEOVER #2—Anywhere you talk about Philly, they no longer look down upon him as, you know an outcast or . . . Everybody's in love with him right now. Everybody.

NOERINE KALEEBA [voiceover]—After people have seen him, there is a, a general feeling of quiet, a general feeling of uh, someone needs to, to reflect. It's as if they are, they are actually seeing AIDS with a face.

PHILLY LUTAAYA [in private interview]—This is only the beginning. The end is not in sight yet. People come out and uh, contribute to the fight until we reach total victory. A long time after my times, people are going to continue.

NARRATOR [as "Alone" fades to a stadium scene]—In the end, as in the beginning, the fans came first for Philly Lutaaya. Seventy-thousand people jammed into Kampala's Nakivubo Stadium to see their idol perform for the last time.[6] It was the largest concert audience in Uganda's history.

ANNOUNCER—Ladies and gentlemen, Bongoley was born in Africa. And he's proud of being an African. And so now he's going to sing to us "Born in Africa."

PHILLY LUTAAYA [addressing the crowd]—Allo, allo. Ladies and gentlemen, I'm giving you the last song. I would like to tell you that I'm going back to Europe on Saturday. But I'll be back in Uganda in December. And if God wishes, I shall stage a concert, at Lugogo Indoor Stadium. Thank you very much.

Lutaaya sings "Born in Africa" to the enormous crowd.

NARRATOR—On October 28, 1989, Philly Lutaaya returned to Sweden, where he was reunited with his children. Philly clung tenaciously to life, but after three weeks in Stockholm, he knew it was time to go home again. Strapped on a stretcher, he was flown to Uganda. And on December 15, 1989, he was given his last wish: to die in Africa.

At his funeral in Namirembe Cathedral, thousands of people mourned Philly. Uganda's religious and political leaders eulogized him as a shining example of the best in mankind. But Philly Lutaaya preferred a simpler epitaph.

PHILLY LUTAAYA [in private interview]—I was born to sing, to dance, and I will die a musician. That's enough for me.

Fade out as "Born in Africa" continues to play.

TITLES:
WRITTEN AND DIRECTED BY JOHN ZARITSKY
PRODUCED BY VIRGINIA STORRING
EDITOR RICHARD WELLS
DIRECTOR OF PHOTOGRAPHY MICHAEL SAVOIE
SOUNDMAN PETER SAWADE
NARRATOR WILL LYMAN
MUSIC COMPOSED AND PERFORMED BY PHILLY BONGOLEY LUTAAYA

Rolling Credits for film crews in Uganda, Sweden, and Canada.

A.K.A. Production for FRONTLINE and WGBH in association with the Canadian Broadcasting Company

AFTER CREDITS—By special arrangement, operators at the national AIDS hotline are standing by to answer questions, to refer you to resources in your area, or to provide additional information. Call toll free 1-800-342-AIDS.

4

Tears Run Dry

COPING WITH AIDS THROUGH
MUSIC IN ZIMBABWE

Ric Alviso (California State University, Northridge)

INTRODUCTION

I will never forget the first Zimbabwean band I ever saw live—the Bhundu Boys in Los Angeles at the Music Machine in 1989. Their sound and energy were incredible. With sing-along choruses and precision, interlocking guitars blasting through the club, it was almost impossible to keep from dancing. Later, when I had the chance to go to Zimbabwe, I was lucky enough to play with one of the great female musicians, Beauler Dyoko, and her band, The Black Souls, for the opening of the Zimbabwean Parliament, which commenced with a speech by President Mugabe.

I mention these artists, the Bhundu Boys and The Black Souls, because in the years since my first encounter with them, most of the members of these bands have succumbed to AIDS. This story is not unique. There are few bands—indeed few families—in Zimbabwe that have not been affected by AIDS. In this chapter, I will outline the scope of the AIDS epidemic in Zimbabwe, discuss the role of music in dealing with AIDS, and examine what, if any difference has been made by these efforts. Although music has always played an important role in dealing with struggles of various kinds, in this chapter I will show how traditional and popular music in Zimbabwe today reveal some interesting generational differences in the way music is being used to provide education, express grief, and begin healing.

AIDS AND POLITICS IN ZIMBABWE

In Zimbabwe, it is estimated that by 2009 14% of the adult population was infected with HIV (UNICEF 2010a). AIDS prevention programs are increasingly targeting young people, since one-third of those who become infected with HIV do so during adolescence. Open discussion about sex is not common in Zimbabwe. Traditional sex education was provided for boys by uncles and for girls by aunts. But with families split between the traditional rural home (where the extended family resides) and the city (where the work is) this traditional sex education does not always occur. In addition, AIDS has devastated many families: approximately 1.3 million Zimbabwean children are orphans (UNICEF 2010b). In the midst of this tragedy, music and other art forms such as theater (Communication Initiative Network 2009) are helping to fill the need for sex education and helping people cope with sickness and death. Yet the international aid that has proved so crucial to HIV/AIDS campaigns in other parts of Africa has been stymied in Zimbabwe, largely due to the activities of controversial President Robert Mugabe.

Mugabe's mass expulsion of white farmers from the country in 2002, and his 2005 human dislocation campaign dubbed Operation Murambatsvina ("Clean up the Filth"), represented two of the most visible actions of an administration that further isolated Zimbabwe from the international community. In 2003, when President George W. Bush announced $15 billion to fight HIV and AIDS in his State of the Union address, he proposed that the funds be spent in twelve African countries, in addition to Guyana and Haiti (Schoop 2003): obviously Zimbabwe was not on the list.

In late 2008, President Mugabe agreed to a power sharing deal with opposition leader Morgan Tsavangirai that allowed Tsavangirai to become the country's prime minister. As 2009 came to a close, Zimbabwe experienced a relative calm for the first time in many years; all seemed to hold their breath waiting to see if permanent improvement in Zimbabwe could take hold. While foreign aid for fighting HIV/AIDS had not improved as of the time of this writing, some cautious optimism existed that the situation might change at some point.

MUSIC AS EDUCATION-ENTERTAINMENT

I have studied music in Zimbabwe and its role in the AIDS epidemic since 1998. Musical responses to AIDS fall into three main categories: (1) as education-entertainment; (2) as therapy (i.e., the use of music to directly improve or maintain physical health); and (3) as healing (where music is used to express grief, sadness, hope, shock, or other emotions and urge action or change behavior).

Singhal and Rogers define education-entertainment as "the process of purposely designing and implementing a media message to both entertain and educate, in order to increase knowledge about an issue, create favorable attitudes and change overt behavior" (1999, 9). There is some evidence that some strategies of education-entertainment work better than others. There is good research on the effectiveness of carefully crafted television programs, plays, and dance to educate and change behavior. Certainly music can raise awareness of an issue; but Singhal and Rogers claim that music's potential remains "largely untapped and underutilized" (1999, 119). Also there are varying opinions about the power of music to change society. The BBC asked Africans the question, "Do you think musicians can help alleviate Africa's poverty? Can they help stop the spread of HIV/AIDS?" The responses were varied and revealing, but reflect attitudes that I have heard echoed by Zimbabweans. Here is a sample (Can Musicians Save 2004):

On the potential of music to deliver a message—from a Cameroonian in Italy:

Africans listen to music more than they read books or newspapers or watch TV. Musicians have the opportunity and potential to reach our people and educate them.

On confusing the message with the messenger—from a South African:

Musicians must first be proper role models and the same applies to politicians and parents. Setting examples is the ONLY language that speaks with any influence.

On the limits of music—from Lagos, Nigeria:

Music is a special ingredient in the life of every African because it creates awareness, serves as a channel for passing information and preserves our culture and tradition. Music, however, has limited usefulness in curbing poverty and reducing HIV/AIDS. Realistically, no amount of music made in Africa can bring back the billions of dollars stashed away in European banks by our thieving leaders.

On the negative influence music can have in society—from a Sudanese living in the United States:

African musicians aggravate the spread of HIV/AIDS by encouraging youths to practice more sex. Music doesn't reduce poverty either, but you can forget eating when you are in a nightclub. African music encourages HIV/AIDS.

I asked one of my closest teachers from Zimbabwe, Tute Chigamba, about music's role in addressing societal issues, and he stated that music's strongest role is to raise awareness. He noted songs by Oliver Mtukudzi, whose song "Todii?" ("What shall we do?"), talks about HIV/AIDS and urges people to prevent the scourge by changing their attitudes and eradicating the stigma associated with the disease (Tute Chigamba 2005, p.c.; see also Kyker in this volume). There is also Oliver Mtukudzi's quiet and beautiful "Mabasa" on *Tuku Music* (1999). From the liner notes:

This is a highly inspired song mourning the devastating effects of AIDS. Without directly referring to the disease, the song has enough imagery to paint the bleak picture. Tears run dry. We mourn quietly. Death has now lost meaning (because of its frequency). Funerals no longer have the necessary dignity. Everyone around us is dying. Who will sympathize with whom since each one of us has death in their homesteads daily? Who will mourn whom? Who will bury whom? Who will feed whom since the breadwinners are all dying? (Mtukudzi 1999)

The best-known Zimbabwean musician is Thomas Mapfumo, whose music galvanized the push toward independence in 1980. His 1994 *Hondo* album included lyrics for the track "Mukondombera" ("The Holocaust" or epidemic), a song that urged responsible behavior:

MUKONDOMBERA

You should stop fooling around, men,
You should stop fooling around, girls,

Beware of this plague, the illness has come,
If you are not afraid, you will perish.

Oh goodness, we are perishing,
An illness has come into this world,
Play it safe, because this world has gone bad.
This illness has come,
It is a giant whip sent down by God.

Oh God, what are we supposed to do?
God, please give us an idea.
To stop it all, stand by your spouse.

Many younger musicians tend to use humor when addressing serious topics such as AIDS in music. Simon Banda of the Zimbabwean vocal group Sunduza and Southern E Media Education & Arts (SEMEA) composed two or three highly amusing AIDS songs in the *mbube* style. In the song "Matata," a skit is performed on stage with a football team showing how AIDS is transmitted like a football from person to person. During another song there is a dance illustrating the use of condoms and the responsibilities of men. Banda's group is composed entirely of younger musicians who write in a popular (nonreligious) style of music (Phillip Weiss 2005, p.c.).

Ambuya Beauler Dyoko, whom some call the queen of *mbira* music, on the other hand is an older musician, who plays the *mbira*, a spiritual instrument. She does not play for ceremonies, however; most of her performances are in concert or nightclub settings. As the AIDS crisis worsened in 1994, she added lyrics to her song "Unozofa" ("You will die"), warning people that promiscuity would lead them to die of AIDS. Tragically, everyone in her first group to perform the song—a total of six band members—has died of AIDS, except her! She used the proceeds of the recording sales (originally on cassette) to pay for their funerals (Erica Azim 2005, p.c.).

Beauler Dyoko has also recorded a poignant arrangement of the *mbira* piece "Nhemamusasa" called "Baba Munyaradzi." Although not overtly didactic, it is at its core a plea, a cry, for responsible sexual practices (Jeff Muiderman 2005, p.c.):

NHEMAMUSASA

Baba Munyaradzi is gone
All the children they didn't want to listen
Now they must listen to what the people say
I am asking God to help us with what is happening
                    —*Dyoko (2000)*

Beauler Dyoko's niece died of AIDS, and her son died as well in 2002. Since then, she has been caring for ten children left orphaned in her family.

MUSIC AS THERAPY: THE CASE OF MHEPO

I was able to find one example of music used as therapy. The Zimbabwean Afro-jazz group Mhepo recorded the song "Zvirwere Zvichapera" in 2000. The song was designed in collaboration with naturopath Adele Smith to treat the symptoms of AIDS through musical frequencies.

The recording involved a choir of primary schoolchildren and the a cappella group Big Sister singing with the band.

Mrs. Smith's experiences with HIV-positive patients had convinced her that certain combinations of musical sounds have a positive effect on the symptoms of AIDS, and she asked Mhepo to write a song using a carefully chosen chord progression. The idea was that through listening to the song, and even better through singing it in the correct key, AIDS patients would be able to participate in their own therapy (Bridget Samuels 2005, p.c.).

UNIFEM (United Nations Development Fund for Women) funded the recording, and hoped to test the material by asking HIV-positive individuals to keep a diary documenting how the music affects their health, energy levels, and overall well-being over a period of time: i.e., what happens if they sing the song, or play the tape, say two or three times a day. This is an area where much more research is required in order to investigate the effectiveness of popular music and music in non-ritual contexts (Samuels 2005, p.c.).

ZVIRWERE ZVICHAPERA

> *We have to be the people with love for those who are sick*
> *Let us be loyal people*
> *Let us give them joy in life*
> —*Mhepo (2001)*

MUSIC AS HEALING

Mbira music is a much more common form of music-as-healing in Zimbabwe. Much of this music is performed in *bira* ceremonies where ancestral spirits are invoked, honored, and asked for guidance. Dzapasi Mbira Group, which plays for ceremonies in the rural Rwizi region of Mhondoro Communal Area, has written lyrics sung beautifully to the traditional song "Karigamombe."

Vana vangu vapera	*My children are dying*
Sekuru we dzingai mapere	*Grandfather chase away the hyenas*

The response singers repeat, "vana vangu vapera" (my children are dying) while the lead singer pleads for "Sekuru" (grandfather) to "dzingai mapere" (chase away the hyenas). But the language is indirect: they refer to the AIDS epidemic later in the song as "mukondombera," literally "the big kill" (Dzapasi 2003).

Erica Azim, who recorded this example, informed me that these lyrics are a prayer to the ancestors to help with AIDS. At *biras*—ceremonies honoring and calling upon ancestors to help a community deal with a crisis—this is exactly the kind of thing that would traditionally be prayed for, along with the prayers for rain, and other issues that seem beyond the control of the living. For most traditional Shona persons, playing the region's 22–28 key lamellophone (the *mbira*) as part of the ceremony opens a link to the spirit world. And, although AIDS is a modern problem, it is always traditional to pray and sing to the ancestors, asking for help with problems that are too difficult for the living to solve. Thus, these lyrics are a good example of ancient traditions being used to address modern issues (Azim 2005, p.c.).

ANALYSIS AND CONCLUSION

In Zimbabwe it is rare to find many songs with "direct language" about AIDS and other modern issues. The lyricists often pride themselves on their use of *tsumo* and *madimikiro* (proverbs and sayings) to get the point across. It seems to me that the older or more traditional the musicians, the more cryptic their language. Some of the younger musicians, in contrast, sing in more direct language. Thus, while a younger musician or one more oriented toward popular music might sing "Beware of this plague, the illness has come," an older or more traditionally oriented musician (*gwara*) would sing, "the places in the city that used to be parks, are now cemeteries" (Joel Laviolette 2005, p.c.). Although the language is indirect, it is a relatively obvious comment on AIDS and would be taken as such by listeners. Shona people do not commonly sing things like, "go buy condoms and use them." They are instead more likely to sing about *zvibate*, or the practice of self-control.

Of the musical examples that concern AIDS in Zimbabwe, what difference has been made? As is the case in many countries throughout Africa, music is being used to comment on, raise awareness of, and heal people from the epidemic of AIDS. But the case of Zimbabwe may show that there are many other factors that have to be in place for these efforts to make a significant difference. We have seen several countries in Africa, including Uganda, Kenya, and South Africa, where music, in conjunction with public campaigns, government support and international resources, have begun to turn the tide in HIV infection and reduction of cases of AIDS (USAID 2009). In Zimbabwe we have not seen this yet. Zimbabwe is a country dealing with many crises at this time.

A number of factors seem to be important in the success of entertainment-education. Among them are:

- Pressing social issues, which galvanize into movements with some agreement on messages that need to be brought to public attention. This often results in the formation or involvement of local organizations or interest groups.

- Artists as appropriate role models who can create a powerful message in an acceptable cultural context.

- Media buy-in along with a viable communication infrastructure for delivering the message to the majority of the public in an accessible and affordable medium.

- Strong partnerships between organizations, artists, and media; and the identification and securing of donors for large-scale problems, particularly among the international community.

- Government support or nonintervention.

In a country where the government seemed more interested in holding on to power than dealing with and helping to solve social issues, a chaotic environment reigned that affected the development of local organizations, their partnership with artists and media, and the influx of donor and international support. While there is little lack of artists and talent in Zimbabwe, there remains a climate of fear of open expression. Faced with multiple crises in Zimbabwe—AIDS, land redistribution, destruction of homes, only the most tentative political stability, effects of a multiyear drought, and continuing economic disaster that began in 1998 from the crash of the Zimbabwean dollar—they have not yet tested the boundaries of free speech with the new administration.

What does the future hold? Musicians and artists in Zimbabwe will continue to make music that has a powerful educational message about AIDS and other pressing social concerns that their people face. But in the current political and social environment in Zimbabwe, it is not surprising that AIDS continues to ravage the population with little sign of slowing. In the absence of many of the factors that seem to be important in the success of entertainment-education, the sad truth is that good music with a powerful message in and of itself is not enough to make much of a difference.

5

Singing in the Shadow of Death

AFRICAN MUSICIANS RESPOND TO
A PANDEMIC WITH SONGS OF SORROW,
RESISTANCE, ADVOCACY, AND HOPE

Jonah Eller-Isaacs

In his last days, Alec Nyirongo welcomed me warmly to his chiefdom, even as his body revealed a deep distress. His eyes were jaundiced, his handshake weak, his breath tubercular. And now, his relatives had gathered in the family compound to mourn his passing. They draped the freshly carved pine coffin with strands of bougainvillea—red, orange, yellow, magenta—death dressed in glorious spring clothes. The sobs of the widow and her fatherless children broke the chill morning air. As I walked with the family down the narrow path to the cemetery, we passed under the branches of broad acacia trees and through fields of pale yellow tobacco leaves and wilted maize.

I'd arrived in this isolated village in northern Malawi, high in the foothills of Africa's Great Rift Valley, in the spring of 2004. My aim was to investigate the ways that music was involved in the fight against HIV/AIDS. For four days, drums and voices echoed across the courtyard as the village mourned its departed chief. I asked my hosts if it would be possible for me to attend the final night of remembrance. After a long discussion, the elders decided that I could enter the mourning house.

A family member accompanied me inside and the mourners parted to make a small space for us on the concrete floor. I sat close to my escort, reeling in the rank stink of cane spirits on his breath. My eyes adjusted to the dim candlelight as I set up my microphones. Soft singing began.

The arrival of a local choir strengthened the exhausted relatives. The choir found room in the cramped space for their drums and dancing feet. The air was thick with burning paraffin and sweat. Some songs were quiet, a few voices singing hymns; some loud and energetic, accompanied by drumming and bells. Grief sat heavy in the room, but the music lightened the atmosphere, and some people smiled wanly as they sang.

Although his official cause of death was tuberculosis, it's all but certain that Alec Nyirongo was one of nearly 100,000 Malawians who died in 2004 from AIDS or AIDS-related complications, one tiny statistic in the global HIV/AIDS pandemic that has claimed more than thirty-two million lives worldwide. According to the Joint United Nations Programme on HIV/AIDS (UNAIDS), more than 11 percent of Malawi's 6.1 million adult residents (age 15–49) were living with HIV in 2007. That compares to six-tenths of 1 percent in the United States. Malawi's devastating infection rate ranks just ninth out of sub-Saharan African nations, with Swaziland topping the list at a shocking 26.1 percent.

Statistics like these are hard to put into perspective, but imagine that one of every four adults you see on the street or in the grocery store is living with an incurable disease and that access to medication is limited at best. In sub-Saharan Africa, more than 20 million people are living with HIV—slightly more than the population of the state of New York. Although sub-Saharan Africa represents just over 10 percent of the world's population, it accounts for almost two-thirds of global HIV cases.

The African HIV/AIDS pandemic has been in the news for years, but other horrors including the genocide in Darfur and the spread of H1N1 have at times upstaged it. It is easy to miss the good news that infection rates have declined in some of the worst-ravaged countries, not just because of aid from the developed world, but also because of the strong spirit of the people who live day in and day out surrounded by the deaths of family members and friends. They are finding ways to creatively rebuild their communities in the midst of disaster.

In 2002, my father, the Rev. Robert Eller-Isaacs, co-minister of Unity Church Unitarian (along with my mother) in St. Paul, Minnesota, went to Malawi with a friend. He organized the trip to reinvigorate a long relationship between the church and the Nyirongo family, which operates clinics the congregation has supported since helping Dr. Trywell Nyirongo, Alec Nyirongo's uncle, to attend medical school fifty years ago. Upon his return, my father told stories full of music. He attended an educational presentation where health professionals integrated music into their lectures. He listened to high school students sing about the painful losses of AIDS. People were searching for ways to slow the spread of HIV/AIDS, and I became interested in the possibility that this music might be a powerful agent for change.

Music is deeply rooted in many societies in Africa. It is not just a form of artistic expression; it is an arena for social commentary and oral history. Music is the language of the spirit and of the community. It made logical sense then that music-based health education could make a difference in the fight against HIV/AIDS.

I organized an independent research trip, eventually spending six months in Malawi, Tanzania, Kenya, and Uganda. For nearly the entire journey, I lived with local families such as the Nyirongos in Malawi. These families showed me endless hospitality and provided me with a gateway to understanding the realities of life surrounded by HIV. I recorded hours of music, starting with Alec Nyirongo's mourners, and heard through interviews the heartbreaking tales of loss and inspired accounts of strength in the face of overwhelming tragedy. I have tried to do justice to these stories and songs. Through a primetime radio documentary broadcast for World AIDS Day 2005 by Minnesota Public Radio, along with educational lectures I have presented at churches and schools around the country, I have presented this story as a new way for those of us an ocean away to understand the experience of living in the midst of the HIV/AIDS pandemic.

Like many Americans, I was accustomed to the mainstream media's portrayal of Africa as a desperate, monocultural continent laid waste by disasters of near-biblical proportions. Yet throughout my travels I encountered people using music to build strong and healthy communities. In the HIV/AIDS pandemic, music is a form of creative resistance, providing the hope, strength, and courage needed to stem the tide of destruction. The following stories come from a wide variety of locations and feature radically different people, but they all share a common thread. For those living in the shadow of this devastating disease, music is a way to tap into the imaginative spark that compels change. With music, we can employ the power of a single voice or join in song to heal, to educate, and to transform the world.

ROOTS AND RHYTHMS: TANZANIAN HIP HOP

In Arusha, a Tanzanian city of nearly 300,000 residents and a world away from the remote hillside villages of Malawi, there is no more common sight than a minibus, the ubiquitous means of public transport. The *matatus* covered with stickers and hand-painted messages like "No Sweet 'til There's Sweat" or "Rastaman" charge headlong into market-bound pedestrian throngs. Passengers dangle out the open doors, hanging on for dear life as the banged-up vans throttle along the dusty, potholed roads. A thumping bass line fills the air as the drivers shout and laugh with the music. A scramble of Kiswahili lingers in the air.

Before the turn of the millennium, the pounding bass might have accompanied a bouncing, melodic Congolese guitar riff. Things have changed. Today the bass provides the foundation for the most popular style of music in urban Tanzania—hip hop. The growth of Tanzanian hip hop culture, known as *Bongo Flava*, has made superstars out of the most successful lyricists. Although the influence of American and European hip hop is undeniable, I find artists in Tanzania and across Africa have claimed it as an African art form, rooting their craft in ancient African ideas of song as story, beat as myth.

Hip hop has a significant role in the lives of Tanzania's youth, and some organizations fighting HIV/AIDS in the country are harnessing this combination of rhythm and poetry to reach their target audience. One of the most prominent health organizations in Tanzania is ISHI (the command verb meaning "live" in Kiswahili). ISHI's aggressive multilevel social marketing campaign promotes the ABC model of HIV prevention ("Abstinence, Be faithful, use a Condom"). Nassoro Ally, an outreach director for ISHI in Arusha, describes the organization's strategy: "We have TV ads, we have radio ads, we use magazines, we use billboards, so it reaches a lot of youth. And for those who are not able to read and write, we reach them through our community concerts."

To further engage youth, ISHI had a group of top-selling artists record hip hop versions of their messages, and during my time in Arusha, the streets and airwaves of Tanzanian cities were saturated with ISHI's catchy theme song "Usione Soo" ("Don't Be Shy"). ISHI isn't simply promoting its messages to young people using popular music. It is also actively empowering them as artists and community leaders, inviting urban youth to help craft its messages. Even as "Usione Soo" was peaking on the charts, ISHI officials were sitting down with urban youth across Tanzania asking how young people were responding to their messages, learning what sort of slang they were using to talk about health and sexuality, and inviting them to suggest slogans that might be effective in the future.

While in Arusha, I conducted a series of interviews with ISHI officials, after which I was given a hat and T-shirt with the ISHI logo. I would walk the streets of Arusha and find the shouts of *mzungu* ("white person") typically directed at me had switched to "Ishi!" and "Usione

Soo!" Through its straightforward educational slogans and memorable pop presentation, ISHI's message has permeated the streets and made its way into the minds of freestyle hip hop artists. The poetry these artists write and improvise becomes a new language for their generation, and ISHI's campaign has helped the young artists imbue their creative production with a focus on health and HIV/AIDS.

In my search to work with these young hip hop artists, I found Aang Serian (House of Peace), an Arusha-based organization that provides cultural tours to the villages of a few of the 120-plus ethnic groups in Tanzania. It also hosts a closet-sized hip hop studio in the heart of the Arusha garment district. When I told the organization's staff about my research, they gathered their friends at the studio and started to record. I spent the next month visiting local studios, watching and listening as gifted poets gathered to put their words to paper and microphones to their lips. They integrated "Usione Soo" and ISHI's messages into their rhymes as they told stories of the tragedies and constant struggles of living a life surrounded by the HIV/AIDS epidemic.

After seeing these artists in action, it was clear to me that youth exposed to ISHI's message also understood that music, which resides in the spirit, can describe the raw experience of life, and that even adolescents can harness its power to educate each other and change society.

UGANDA: A NATION AND A POP SONG

How do you measure the impact of national trauma on a people's spirit? What is it like to bear witness to devastation? Ugandans know all too well. After the initial diagnoses of HIV in Uganda became known in the mid-1980s, it was only a short time before the virus began to tear apart the social fabric of the country. When I asked about living through the epidemic in which millions died, Ugandans responded with shaking heads and stoic eyes. James Kigozi survived and today works for the Uganda AIDS Commission:

> Oh God, it was really bad. Hospital beds were occupied by as much as seventy-five, eighty percent by AIDS patients. You could bury two, three, four people in a day, all of them known to you. In Uganda, everybody has lost somebody due to HIV. Your brother, a sister, or even a parent.

In the early 1990s, it was estimated that urban adult infection rates were as high as 30 percent—the highest in the world at the time. There are more than two million orphans now in Uganda, a country of fewer than thirty million residents. Superimposing that proportion upon the American population would mean that every single person living in New York State was an orphan, with fully two-thirds of them thought to be HIV-positive.

So it is all the more surprising that today Uganda's HIV adult-infection rate is down to 5.4 percent. Unfortunately, part of the decline in the infection rate was due to viral burnout: so many people died of AIDS so quickly that the virus couldn't propagate effectively. But Uganda also managed to bring the spread of HIV/AIDS under some control through dedicated community and government efforts to teach people the ABC method. And many people point to a single song as the beginning of this remarkable recovery.

Ugandan musical luminary Philly Lutaaya stunned the nation in 1989 when he announced that he was HIV-positive. In the climate of fear and stigmatization that often accompanies the HIV/AIDS pandemic, many Ugandans believed his revelation to be a ploy or a publicity stunt. Then Lutaaya released his album *Alone and Frightened*, and forever sealed a place beyond superstardom as a national hero. In his title track, Lutaaya not only brought his status into the limelight, but also described his emotional experience of isolation and pain:

> *Out there somewhere, alone and frightened*
> *Oh, the darkness, the days are long*
> *Life in hiding, no more making new contacts*
> *No more loving arms thrown around my neck.*

Lutaaya died in 1989, just months after releasing *Alone and Frightened*. As media specialist Joel Isabirye explains, Lutaaya's impact was immediate and tremendous: "Philly Lutaaya gave, if I am right to say, a human face to living with AIDS. He made it seem as if it was not a monstrous thing. The landmark, the most significant moment started with Philly Lutaaya, and that is when music became very significant in dealing with stigmatization in Uganda." It seemed every Ugandan I met could sing every word to "Alone." Lutaaya left a legacy of emotional honesty in music-based activism that continues today. The song and its message are a rallying cry in the fight against HIV/AIDS and "Alone" is the unofficial anthem of TASO (The AIDS Support Organization), as well as the larger community of AIDS-support organizations in the country of Uganda.

TASO is a beacon of progress in working to encourage healthy and supportive behavior. The arts are central to TASO's efforts in reaching out to individuals, teaching the ABC method, and working against discrimination. Music, says TASO official Anne Kaddumukasa, is "very instrumental in breaking the ice between the community and the people that are HIV infected."

Every TASO center supports a drama group composed of people living with HIV. The groups provide an essential outreach service and create a powerful therapeutic environment. Members attribute their full and generally healthy lives to their singing, drumming, and dancing together. Says one drama group member, Mahmoud Kayiwa: "When you come here, you rejoice, you sing, you dance, you see. So you can forget all about the AIDS. When we share each and every thing about the disease, we cannot get scared as when we are alone at home." At TASO's national headquarters in Kampala, the drama group in residence performed for President Bush during his 2003 visit.

Uganda is a living example of the power of music to transform a nation. When the HIV-positive members of a TASO drama group performed "Alone" in the central Kampala hospital, it moved me to tears. Ailing TASO clients lined the crowded halls outside the performance in their hospital beds, and it seemed that the song gave voice to their hopes—to all our hopes—to live happy, healthy lives alongside our families, to hear choirs sing songs of understanding, and for love and support in our times of need.

KENYA: FORGOTTEN VOICES

Kibera is among largest slums in all of Africa. Nearly a million residents cling to life in a long, steep valley on the west side of the Kenyan capital of Nairobi. A short walk through the neighborhood revealed brutal conditions. There is no sanitation, electricity, or running water. Plastic bags soar on the wind and sewage trickles through the streets. The corrugated iron shacks roast their residents in the stifling heat and provide little shelter from the cold nights. There is widespread malnutrition and AIDS casts its deathly shadow along the densely packed hillside.

Although Kenyan HIV prevalence rates among adults have stayed relatively low (the 2007 national estimate stands at about eight percent), the virus continues to take its toll. Those struggling with living conditions such as those in Kibera are at high risk—particularly women and young girls, who are sometimes forced into prostitution to feed their families. As in neighboring countries, AIDS is killing the most productive age groups. Parents, as well as teachers, merchants, and workers, are dying and leaving behind a generation of broken families and abandoned children. Street children wander downtown Nairobi, dazed victims in an epidemic of glue sniffing, bottles held to their drooling mouths as they beg for money in the shadow of glittering skyscrapers.

Kenyan organizations are trying to get these children off the streets and into families, schools, and healthy living environments. Few, however, are reaching out to those who are HIV-positive. Until recently, many organizations viewed outreach to orphans living with HIV as a lost cause, a waste of resources that could otherwise support those with a better chance of survival. That all changed with the founding of the Nyumbani Institute.

In 1992, the Rev. Angelo D'Agostino, an American Jesuit, began caring for a small number of HIV-positive orphans. Today, Nyumbani (the Kiswahili word for home) hosts nearly 100 children and provides off-site support to nearly 1,000 more. It is a model for respectful and effective faith-based work and a symbol of hope for the people it serves.

On my first visit, I was greeted by green gardens, colorful artwork, and screams of joy and unadulterated happiness. It was a bit of a shock. Volunteer Don Rawzi told me, "We had some reporters here. They were like, 'Oh, where are the sick kids? We want to see the sick kids!' 'Ah,' they were told, 'these are the children of Nyumbani.'"

Antiretroviral drugs (ARVs) keep the children of Nyumbani alive. They are fortunate to have access to these life-saving medications. Senior Nyumbani staff member Sister Mary Owens says:

> This is the great injustice of our world, that there is medicine available and it's not available here in sub-Saharan Africa. You see our children here. They're all healthy: sixty-two out of the ninety-four are on ARVs. And that's why they're healthy. They're living full lives. They have hope for the future. They're like normal children, planning, dreaming. That's the hope, the positive face of AIDS, and that's possible for every person who's infected.

ARVs are more effective if the person living with HIV can minimize stress, doubt, and fear. In helping the children to understand their status and raise their spirits, Rawzi—who is also a musician and producer—helped the children of Nyumbani form a choir called Watoto wa Mungu, or "Children of God." To all of Kenya's surprise, singles from the group's debut album topped the country's pop charts. The choir has brought an electric atmosphere to an already stirring humanitarian effort and has made a significant positive financial impact at Nyumbani. Watoto participants are proud of their place as a voice for their peers, as thirteen-year-old and lifetime Nyumbani resident John Mwiro explains. "I sing in the music group," he told me, "to tell the other young artists coming up they should not give up. Come forward. It's another way of explaining that you can live a positive life, a very good one."

At Nyumbani's twelfth anniversary party, Watoto wa Mungu performed an adaptation of *The Wizard of Oz*. Just two weeks before, nearly all my recording equipment had been stolen, along with my camera, credit cards, and my irreplaceable journal and fieldnotes. (My recordings, thankfully, were safe.) For two weeks I had wandered the densely packed and dangerous streets of downtown Nairobi without equipment, unable to work, wondering whether I should just go home. Strangers with ill intent followed me back to my hotel and glue-crazy beggars accosted me. It was all worth it to watch *The Wizard of Oz* at Nyumbani. Tiny Kenyan munchkins with glowing eyes performed for ambassadors. Toddlers with paper flowers on their heads struggled to sit still in their role as the scenery. Dorothy belted out, "There's no place like Nyumbani," and clicked her tattered red slippers. Angelic HIV-positive orphans sang with all their might, "if happy little bluebirds fly / beyond that rainbow / why, oh why can't I?"

THE WEB OF LIFE

News from Africa often reads like a litany of horrors: plagues of locusts, famine, rampant corruption and mountains of debt that drain resources, armies of children cajoled into atrocious crimes, even genocide committed as the international community struggles to intervene. As with many international issues, the HIV/AIDS pandemic in Africa can seem distant and advocacy unproductive. One can easily forget that there is hope and creative resistance to poverty and pandemic alike, that both local and international organizations are making progress in creating livable and sustainable conditions in Africa.

Music is a powerful idiom for education and therapy. Even more, it is a universal language that speaks to the children surrounded by the pandemic in Africa just as it speaks to us living in relative comfort. On my first Sunday in Malawi, I accompanied my host family to church. It was Pentecost, and as the preacher pointed to a verse, a neighbor helped me find the passage in English. It was Acts 2:2–4:

> And suddenly there came a sound from heaven, as of a rushing and mighty wind, and it filled the whole house where they were sitting. Then there appeared to them divided tongues, as of fire, and one sat upon each of them. And they were all filled with the Holy Spirit and began to speak in other tongues.

When the sermon ended, the congregation began to sing. I recognized the tune and sang along in a language that I barely spoke. Harmonies surrounded me that Sunday. When I came home months later, I discovered that we'd been singing Ralph Vaughan William's arrangement of the Welsh hymn "Hyfrydol." Now when we sing that hymn at my home church in St. Paul, I remember that powerful day in Malawi and I remember why the plight of people in faraway places makes a difference to us all:

> *We are builders of that city.*
> *All our joys and all our groans*
> *Help to rear its shining ramparts;*
> *All our lives are building stones*
> *Whether humble or exalted,*
> *All are called to task divine;*
> *All must aid alike to carry*
> *Forward one sublime design.*

6

Music, HIV/AIDS, and Social Change in Nairobi, Kenya

Kathleen J. Van Buren (University of Sheffield)

In 2007, UNAIDS declared that East Africa offered the "most hopeful indications" in sub-Saharan Africa that AIDS epidemics can be reversed (UNAIDS 2007b). Kenya in particular is one of three sub-Saharan countries that have experienced a decline in adult national HIV prevalence.[1] HIV rates dropped from as high as 10 percent in Kenyan adults in the mid-1990s to between 7–8.5 percent in 2007 (UNAIDS/WHO Working Group on Global HIV/AIDS and STI Surveillance 2008). Decreases in HIV prevalence are suspected by UNAIDS to come from behavioral changes, and dropping rates are interpreted as confirmation "that the epidemics can respond to specific HIV-related intervention" (UNAIDS 2007b). The dropping rates, while hopeful, prompt the questions: what interventions are being targeted at people in this region, and which of these are working? In this chapter I will consider the first question, focusing on how music is playing an integral role in HIV/AIDS interventions in Kenya. The opening section of the chapter will outline the history and status of HIV/AIDS in Kenya, and the remainder of the chapter will concentrate mainly on HIV/AIDS music performances in Kenya's capital city, Nairobi. The second question ("which interventions are working?") may not be fully answerable. Nevertheless, I will offer some suggestions on the possibilities and challenges of using music for HIV/AIDS programs. My observations on these topics stem from ongoing research (including several fieldwork trips in the 1990s, 2004, and 2007) on uses of music for community education campaigns about HIV/AIDS and other social concerns in Nairobi.[2]

HIV/AIDS IN KENYA

In his 2000 report on the national response to HIV/AIDS in Kenya, journalist Lewis Odhiambo divides the history of the Kenyan government's reaction into four stages. Between 1984 (when the first AIDS case was diagnosed in Kenya) and 1987, Odhiambo argues, HIV/AIDS was not considered a serious concern. He attributes this lack of concern primarily to the association by many Kenyans of AIDS with homosexuality (Odhiambo 2000, 92). Between 1988 and 1991, the government began to view HIV/AIDS as a potential health problem, but did not consider AIDS as more problematic than other diseases. Odhiambo notes that the public was also skeptical about the disease and that religious leaders actively opposed promotion of condoms. It was only between 1992 and 1995, writes Odhiambo, that AIDS was declared a national crisis by the Kenyan government (ibid., 93). Governmental response to HIV/AIDS is dated a little later by a 2001 Human Rights Watch report. This report states that the first national policy statement on AIDS occurred in 1997, while former president Daniel arap Moi's declaration of HIV/AIDS as a "national disaster" took place in November 1999 (Human Rights Watch 2001, 13). Increased attention to AIDS came partly because the disease was starting to be recognized as an economic and social threat as well as a medical concern. In addition, organizations in and out of Kenya had begun in the early 1990s to agitate for more governmental recognition of, and action in relation to, AIDS.[3]

Since the mid to late 1990s, there has been a significant increase in funding and mobilization related to HIV/AIDS in Kenya. Kenya has adopted a "Three Ones" approach[4] to addressing the pandemic, with the National AIDS Control Council (NACC) acting as the national coordinating authority on AIDS (UNAIDS 2007a). Other Kenyan AIDS programs come from both in and out of the country, involve a variety of governmental and non-governmental agencies, and offer a diversity of services. Services include, for example, sex education, HIV/AIDS testing and monitoring, home-based care, community mobilization, HIV/AIDS research, and policymaking. AIDS-related warnings appear on public streets (see figure 6.1) as well as in print, radio, and television media. The emphasis of many AIDS organizations has shifted from the basic message of "AIDS Kills," deemed necessary in the early days of the pandemic, to related issues that many Kenyans feel are more critical today, such as the effects of stigmatization and the plight of orphans.

Despite dropping HIV rates in Kenya, various causes for concern remain. Data suggests that rates are still as high as 13 percent in some parts of the country (UNAIDS 2007a). Urban rates (10 percent) are higher than rates in rural areas (6.7 percent), though urban rates appear to be declining while rural rates seem to be rising. Rates among women (8.7 percent) are higher than among men (4.5 percent) (UNAIDS 2007a; National AIDS Control Council and the National AIDS and STD Control Programme 2009).[5] Disparities in knowledge about HIV/AIDS throughout the country, meanwhile, are worrisome. Studies in 2003 (National AIDS Control Council 2004, 32) revealed that 50 percent of women and 65 percent of men believed that AIDS could be transmitted through mosquito bites or through sharing eating utensils.[6] Some youth in Nairobi today still argue that they are not susceptible to the disease or that they will become immune through repeated sexual activity. The high urban rates and lack of knowledge among some urban residents seem to belie the many organizations and resources that are based in cities. However, it is estimated that 60 percent of Nairobi's total population of about three million lives in low-income areas, often referred to as "slums" by scholars and residents of Nairobi.[7] While a number of organizations are targeting these areas, programs and resources do not reach all members of these communities. Furthermore, some Kenyans argue that residents of urban areas may be more susceptible to adopting harmful lifestyles and therefore to contracting HIV than their rural counterparts. For instance, men who migrate to the cities for work may seek urban mistresses, and urban youth may be more influenced than rural youth by foreign music videos and messages of promiscuity. The Kenyan government has made efforts to include sex and AIDS education in school curricula. However, these

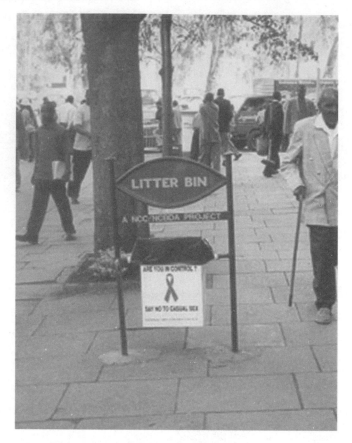

Figure 6.1 AIDS warnings in Nairobi city center. Photo Courtesy by K. Van Buren

attempts are criticized by some people as inadequate and faulty. Other issues that remain a concern within Kenya include sexual abuse of students by teachers and conflicting messages given by authorities within communities about HIV/AIDS. As Felix Wanzala of the street rehabilitation program Daraja in Nairobi comments, "The government's preaching this, churches preaching that, civic society another thing. There's no conformity on the subject." He adds, "It's one thing to educate, but who do you take as your leader?" (Wanzala Interview, Aug. 20, 2004). These and related issues are openly raised in discussions, newspaper articles, comics, and also performances (see figure 6.2).[8]

HIV/AIDS PERFORMANCES IN NAIROBI

Due to the problems noted above, efforts to promote improved HIV/AIDS awareness campaigns continue throughout Kenya. These include the efforts of musicians who—on their own and in collaboration with organizations seeking creative means of reaching audiences—draw upon music to promote social change. Because of the high number of events, I cannot give a full coverage of music performances about HIV/AIDS in Kenya. Rather, I will offer a sampling of programs to provide a sense of the extent and creativity of performances in the country, and to reflect upon some issues related to these performances. Many of the organizations and musicians mentioned in this chapter operate between urban and rural spaces (for instance, basing

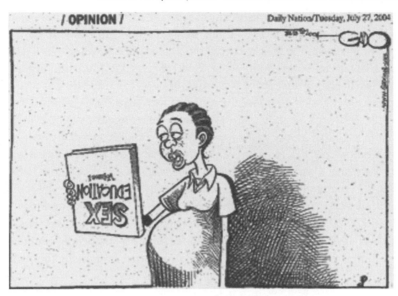

Figure 6.2 Cartoon by Godfrey Mwampembwa (a.k.a. GADO) published in the *Nation* newspaper on July 27, 2004

themselves in Nairobi, but also targeting and touring in other parts of the country). Still, urban and rural programming often involves different methods, challenges, and opportunities.[9] Thus, while issues raised in this chapter may sometimes shed light on practices across the country, this discussion focuses on events and topics especially relevant to Nairobi.

PROFESSIONAL MUSICIANS AND HIV/AIDS INITIATIVES

The extent to which Kenyan musicians should engage in music about issues such as HIV/AIDS is debated in Nairobi. At stake is both the ability of musicians to create and survive on the types of music they prefer (whether socially or politically themed or "commercial," generally defined as not primarily social or political in intent) and the extent to which musicians are viewed as capable of promoting music that is both socially and artistically valuable. Rob Burnet, former program officer for the Ford Foundation Office for Eastern Africa (based in Nairobi), suggests that there is a danger in messages dominating the creative aspects of arts. While art should push boundaries and express dissent, he argues, it has often been turned into a tool solely for conveying messages and for development agendas (Burnet Interview, May 21, 2004). While Burnet emphasizes the dominance of development agendas in the arts today, some people in the Kenyan music industry highlight the pressure that contemporary musicians face from media houses to produce "commercial" music. Prominent music producer Tedd Josiah of Blu Zebra Records suggests that social messages were more prevalent in Kenyan music in the 1980s and 1990s than today, though he—like Burnet—also argues that the social focus in the past may have impacted the artistic quality of messages (Josiah Interview, Jan. 17, 2007). Musical groups such as Sinpare, whose members describe themselves as "intellectual rappers" (Sinpare Interview, Jan. 17, 2007), speak of the conflicts they have faced with media houses that encourage them to produce commercial music rather than the message-laden music they prefer.

Despite commercial pressures, many contemporary musicians are engaging in music with social and political messages. Sometimes they do so on their own initiative, while other times they seek or are invited to collaborate with organizations promoting social change. In an article entitled "Changing Tune in Line with the Times," Clay Muganda argues that Kenyan musicians are "fast realising that there is a growing need for message-based music" (2004a, 21). As one example, Muganda describes the music of Kunguru (Eric Onguru). Kunguru's "fast-paced and danceable" *benga* beats,[10] writes Muganda, "reinforce the fact that music with social messages can still fill dance floors and need not be delivered in a preachy, slow drab manner" (ibid.). Kunguru has stated that "most of our fans are young people who face a lot of challenges and yet receive very little assistance from those of us who have the power to help them see the light." He adds, "We need to do songs that have a positive impact in the lives of our fans" (as quoted in Muganda 2004a, 21). Music producer Tedd Josiah states that organizations that seek to sponsor or collaborate with musicians are increasingly allowing musicians to "drive" the songs, rather than making the songs or issues "drive" the musicians. Popular singer Eric Wainaina argues that rather than waiting for organizations to sponsor the composition of a piece, he is seeking to write songs and then approach organizations with these songs to request sponsorship. This approach enables him to tackle the issues he wishes, in the musical styles he desires to explore (Wainaina Interview, Jan. 18, 2007).

The list of pieces by musicians addressing HIV/AIDS is extensive. One example is Kunguru's "Time for Action." The lyrics to this song are as follows (as quoted in Muganda 2004a, 21):

> *Attention, attention to all the young general in this nation*
> *You know, we've got a big population with the HIV infection*
> *Too much misinformation and misconceptions*
> *All over Africa*
> *All the way from South Africa to Nigeria*
> *Congo and Burundi*
> *Kenya, Tanzania, Uganda to Libya*
> *What do we do? What do we do?*
> *Take control tumia cd, bila haya*
> *Na usiogope, hii ni maisha usibabaike*
> (Take control, use condoms, without embarrassment
> And don't be afraid, this is life, don't talk foolishly)

Kunguru reported "good" responses to performances of the song, noting that by good he meant that "people identify with it" (ibid.).

Another example is Circute (Gerald Wagama) and Joel's (Joel Githiri) 2004 song "Juala." This song, by two cousins, blatantly speaks about protected sex. Muganda explains:

> They say they wanted to call a rifle a rifle and not a big pistol, so they decided to tell their peers about the need to have protected sex without "shooting around the target." They, therefore, came up with *Juala* which, though widely used to refer to polythene paper, also connotes a condom. *Juala's* video features a young man under pressure from his girlfriend to use a condom. He reluctantly accedes to [the] girl's demands but is too embarrassed [to] buy one in the

presence of his friends, and when he finally plucks the courage to buy one, he gets mugged on the way from the shop [but still escapes with the condoms], adding a comical twist to the otherwise educative video. (Muganda 2004a, 21)

In discussing the song, Circute argued, "We have taken it upon ourselves to encourage the use of condoms in a way not many artistes have dared (ibid.)."[11]

Circute and Joel's song has been controversial. According to one commentary by a *Nation* newspaper reader in Nairobi, passengers who had traveled with the musicians reportedly described them as "immoral imbeciles out to preach sex to the youth" (as quoted in Asiago 2004, 2). The commentator defends the musicians against the accusers, saying:

> These [passengers] are in fact the same parents who can't sit on the table with their children and openly talk to them about HIV/AIDS. If parents and elders have refused to take centre stage in the fight against this pandemic, then the only way to pass the message to young people is through blunt tracks like "Juala." Therefore those pouring scorn at the artistes should simply shut up! (ibid.)

Also defending the duo against criticism, Joel has remarked, "We are not encouraging immorality, we are just being realistic" (as quoted in Muganda 2004a, 21).

James Ayugi and Frank Faraji (a.k.a. Famous jei and Funny p) of the hip hop group Border Klan have also been active in promoting HIV/AIDS awareness. For some time, they worked in collaboration with Grace Center International, a faith-based non-governmental organization (NGO) that focuses on AIDS issues. The musicians performed at events organized by Grace and assisted with office tasks and events, and in return Grace helped James and Frank with recording fees. However, James and Frank have also registered Border Klan as a self-help group, joined up with another performer (Xzane, or Kennedy Okech), written various proposals involving AIDS education for which they have sought funding, and toured the nation giving performances. The lyrics of their song "Balaa" ("Troubles"), in Kiswahili and Sheng (slang mixing English, Kiswahili, and other languages; see Samper 2002, 94) and set to a background track of synthesized ostinato patterns, address a variety of issues related to AIDS, including the promiscuity of youth, parental concerns, lack of knowledge among many Kenyans concerning their status, the high number of infected Kenyans, the fact that the disease has "defeated" scientists, problems of alcohol and rape and witchcraft, and the need to get tested, practice fidelity, and plan for the future (Border Klan Interview, Sep. 15, 2004). The musicians target Kenyans at large, but also reference select groups such as teenagers and men. The chorus of the song offers a set of questions, each followed by the repeated answer "Balaa" ("Troubles"):[12]

Uki hanya hanya beste kuna nini?	If you are a prostitute, there's what?
Balaa	Troubles
Uki kosa kuaminika kuna nini?	If you can't be trusted, there's what?
Balaa	Troubles
Uki freak bila sox kuna nini?	If you freak without sox there's what?
Balaa	Troubles
Kuna nini? Balaa. Ukimwi ndiyo?	There's what? Troubles. AIDS, yes?
Balaa	Troubles[13]

Other musicians are also active in composing and performing about HIV/AIDS. Designated by the United Nations as a Millennium Development Goals ambassador, vocalist Lydia Achieng Abura has worked with musicians such as Miriam Makeba, Youssou N'Dour, Koffi Olomide, Manu Dibango, and Bono in recording and performing songs in various parts of Africa about poverty and AIDS ("A Strategy to Promote the Millennium Development Goals in Africa" n.d.; Ngaira 2004, 21). Eric Wainaina, who moved from gospel music to music addressing social and political issues in an effort to reflect national concerns as well as those of faith, has collaborated with the NGO Primary School Action for Better Health (PSABH) on an HIV/AIDS peer education program targeting Nyanza province (Wainaina Interview, Jan. 18, 2007). A song composed for this program was incorporated into the syllabus of the national Kenya Music Festival, which I will discuss shortly.

Musicians from outside Kenya also participate in performances in the country to promote AIDS awareness. One example is Edward Kabuye, a Ugandan drummer and dancer who was based in Nairobi for over ten years. Kabuye was director of the Talking Drums of Africa, a group comprising Kenyan and Ugandan neotraditional and "fusion" musicians. In 1998, the Talking Drums of Africa was awarded first prize in the dance-drama category of the USAID-funded National Youth World AIDS Day Drama Festival held in Nairobi. Set in rural Buganda (in Uganda) and featuring diverse Ugandan, Kenyan, and other African musical and cultural elements, the group's entry included four pieces that combined music, dance, and drama: (1) "Ssekabembe," in which a sick man laments his poor health; (2) a section referred to by Kabuye as "the medical part," during which community members fall ill and seek aid from traditional and "modern" doctors; (3) "Towone," a song of mourning with lyrics that translate as "You won't survive, you really won't. You're going to die...Because there are no cures"; and (4) "Ayowei," an invigorating display of drama, dance, and drumming that involves a medical doctor offering a condom demonstration and the community celebrating with a sense of renewed hope for the future (Kabuye Interviews, 2001, 2004; The Talking Drums 1998).

A final example of work by non-Kenyans comes from Kijani Kenya Trust, a Kenya and UK-based nonprofit organization which organizes arts events in Kenya featuring internationally renowned musicians to promote awareness about and raise funds for HIV/AIDS and conservation projects. In 2007, the Kijani Kenya Trust program featured performances by the Cape Town Opera, the Guildhall Strings from London with the Nairobi Chamber Choir, and jazz performances by Kenyan musicians; and in 2009 the program included performances by Kenyan musicians Eric Wainaina and Suzanna Owiyo and by the London Adventist Chorale. The organization has reached over ten thousand people and raised more than thirteen million Kenyan shillings for charitable projects ("Kijani Kenya" 2009, Mwaniki 2007, 29).

CHILDREN'S AND YOUTH PROGRAMS

In addition to performances by professional musicians, HIV/AIDS works are also performed by amateur musicians. Across Nairobi, numerous schools and children's centers use music to speak about AIDS and other concerns within their communities. Describing these children's groups, Festo Wang'ele, formerly with Childlife Trust (an umbrella organization that works with children's centers across Nairobi), has commented:

> They use the music to...create awareness among the society. Because one
> good thing is most of the songs they do in the institutions, they are thematic,
> you know. You'll find them talking about drugs. You'll find them talking

about... HIV and AIDS. You'll find them talking about female genital mutilation, even child labor. That's one good thing that we do. Because you know they create awareness amongst themselves.... That's what I've actually seen. (Wang'ele Interview, Jul. 28, 2004)

Visitors to schools might remark that performances by different groups appear similar. School group after school group will address the same themes. Even the same phrases seem to appear in multiple pieces. In some cases, though not all, this repetition reflects the fact that students at numerous schools are following the Kenya Music Festival program.

KENYA MUSIC FESTIVAL

The Kenya Music Festival is an annual event featuring zonal, divisional, district, and provincial competitions leading to a national competition.[14] One report estimated attendance at the August 2004 national competition at four thousand people per day (*Sunday Nation* 2004, 40), while another suggested that over ten thousand students and teachers attended (Njagi 2004, 6). Groups at many educational levels participate (from nursery, primary, and secondary schools to colleges, technical training institutions, and universities), performing in a diversity of artistic styles. The 2004 festival, for instance, featured performances in 484 categories of vocal and instrumental music, dance, and elocution, performed in African, Western, and Asian performance styles and in a variety of languages (Kenya Music Festival Foundation 2004, 1–4; *Sunday Nation* 2004, 40).

While the objectives of the event as outlined in the festival syllabus largely focus on the artistic development of students and of Kenya's cultural heritage, the competition also features "special compositions" (songs and recited verses) on set themes. Themes have included: in 2004 and 2005, reproductive health and "fight against HIV/AIDS" (Kenya Music Festival Foundation 2004, 17–26; Kenya Music Festival Foundation 2005, 20–22); and in 2006, "worth the wait," to help reduce rates of HIV/AIDS and other STDs as well as unwanted pregnancies (Kenya Music Festival Foundation 2006, 27–28).[15] The 2004 festival syllabus notes that youths competing on the theme of AIDS "will be playing a role in sensitizing the public on important issues affecting the society" (Kenya Music Festival Foundation 2004, 26). A majority of the audience members at the festival are students, though judges, students' families and friends, and other guests are also present. In addition, winning compositions are sometimes adopted by sponsoring bodies (Kidula 1996, 74), and winning groups may perform for government officials or charity events following the festival. Leading up to the festival, meanwhile, student groups rehearse and perform pieces in their schools and communities. By doing so, they introduce audience members to and remind themselves about some of the issues affecting their communities.

The type of imagery associated with AIDS in school performances can be striking. Since teachers often compose and choreograph pieces, the resulting imagery can represent the perspectives of adults as much as that of youths. On August 9, 2004, for instance, thirteen groups competed in choral verses on the theme of HIV/AIDS. These were spoken, rather than sung, verses. However, verses were spoken in distinctly melodic patterns, with performing groups producing similar patterns of rising and falling speech tones and phrases. In their performance, Huruma Girls High School from Nairobi spoke in English of a "dark and mysterious pit," an "unconquerable monster breathing death," and a "monster like Goliath." St. Agnes Shibuye High presented a piece entitled "The Invisible Monster," in which students spoke of the "monster that Lucifer has put together," and implored people to "say no to sweet honey," "flee away from cheap, unprotected honey," and "stop spreading the monster like bush fire." Menengai High School students asserted that it is "time to raise...armor in readiness for battle": "men, cover your heads with helmets," and "women, close your doors." Reflecting global politics of the time, students from Chemelil Academy from Nyanza urged audiences to "arm the nuclear weapons" to destroy the "monster of mass destruction." Arguing that Kenyans knew that the disease is a danger, the adjudicators for the session emphasized that the challenge today is to create performances that can retain audience attention and provide additional information on coping with the epidemic. They praised the innovative imagery of many groups, and stated that they were less impressed with groups that presented detailed information about AIDS, much of which would already be familiar to audiences.

KASPI CHILDREN'S CENTRE

Due to a lack of funds or for other reasons, not all schools participate in the Kenya Music Festival. Still, even schools that do not compete often follow the festival syllabus and perform for guests and community members. Two pieces from a 2004 performance at Kaspi Children's Centre, a non-formal school in Nairobi,[16] offer an example of the form, content, and presentation of thematic performances prepared by many school groups. Entitled "AIDS is a Destroyer" and performed in English, the first piece was a choral verse. The different fonts (bold and normal) of the transcription below reflect the contrasting inflections of the students' voices: **bold font** demonstrates rising pitch and volume, while normal font indicates falling pitch and volume. The accompanying hand and body motions of the students are indicated in parenthesis.

First student:

> **AIDS is there**
> From the East and West
> **North and South** (pointing different directions)
> **Killing farmers, teachers, pupils, doctors and nurses** (the student makes a slashing
> motion across her neck along with each word)
> **Killing doctors**
> And leaving orphans behind

Second student:

> **Death everywhere**
> We hear sad songs (in thinking pose, with finger on chin)
> **The strong and the healthy** (flexing arms)
> Are dying, dying, **and dying** (crouching lower and lower with each word "dying")
> **Covered with the earth** (covering head)
> Never to work again

Third student:

> **Others in various stages** of feeling ill (arms crossed on chest)
> **Attacked by infection after infection**

*(The second student intervenes with a fit of coughing and a sneeze, which makes
the young pupils in the audience giggle)*
*And no longer to do even a touch of **what** they once do (shaking her hand to signal
no)*

Fourth student:

> **AIDS is a killer**
> *AIDS is a murderer (shaking his finger at the audience, and then making a
> sweeping motion with his hands)*
> **My teachers, parents, and our guests**
> **Stand tall and shout**

The four students in unison:

> **Halt** *to AIDS (they raise their fists in the air)*
> **Fight it by all means** *(they punch the air with their fists)*
> **Because** *it can kill anyone (they slash their arms crosswise across their bodies)*

The second piece on AIDS, which was introduced as a drama-song entitled "AIDS," was performed by two female students, one of whom pretended to be a boy. As the a cappella song
unfolds, the "boy" bumps into the girl with a backpack on center stage. Rubbing her arm where
the "boy" had knocked into her, the girl says in a frustrated tone, "Hello, do I know you?" At
this, the song begins. The "boy" sings:

> *Will you come for a walk with me? Please come.*
> *I've got plans for you and for me. Please come.*
> *I will give you gifts, sweet things, and promises,*
> *Hugs and kisses and all that's in the world.*
> *Will you come for a walk with me? Please come.*

During this solo, the girl with the backpack tries to ignore the "boy," turning her back to him
and crossing her arms as if not interested in what he is saying. However, the "boy" is persistent.
He grabs her hand and tries to turn her around. The girl sings:

> *I've been warned about people like you, my friend,*
> *Who promise the world of sweet things that have become as the end.*
> *I've got plans of becoming a doctor—*

At this point the "boy" interjects, "What?" He looks shocked. The girl continues, undaunted by
his remarks:

> *A pilot, a colonel, and teacher.*
> *I don't believe that your plans*
> *Are going to help with me do that.*

Now the two students face the audience and, switching into Kiswahili, sing together:

Ukimwi tuvute chi	Let us pull AIDS down
Lazima tuvute chi	It is necessary to pull it down
Ukimwi tuvute chi	Let us pull AIDS down
Mimi na wewe rudi	Me and you, let us go back

(The students point to themselves and then at each other during this last phrase, and then they embrace.)

While the Kenya Music Festival provides much stimulus for schools to train students in the arts and to explore particular themes such as HIV/AIDS through performance, and school staff offer further support for the arts (for example, by including music in lessons and seeking opportunities for arts workshops for their students), how much students learn from thematic performances such as those described in the above sections is debated. Genres and themes featured at festivals are often chosen by festival organizers and organizations that sponsor the festival, and individual pieces performed by students may be composed and led by teachers rather than students. This leaves some audience members wondering how much children are being challenged creatively. Concerns are also raised about student comprehension of themes in pieces that they recite or perform, but which they may never fully own (in that they have not instigated or developed the performances). Such worries became particularly apparent when, in 2004, some students were arrested at the national festival for possession of alcohol while their peers performed on themes such as drug abuse as part of the competition. This scandal elicited numerous articles in the national press about the problems involving youth in contemporary society as well as the social and artistic impact of the festival on youth (see, for instance, Otieno 2004, Macharia 2004, Muganda 2004b).

OTHER YOUTH PROGRAMS

As Festo Wang'ele points out, school groups can also perform thematic pieces that have not necessarily been influenced by the Kenya Music Festival.

> We can't just say most of them do it because they are preparing for the festivals. Because...not all the teachers or even the managers know much about the national music festival. They know very little. But surprisingly enough, you know when an issue—like now an issue of HIV and AIDS is very, very, it's very hot, that anybody who does not talk about it, you are like you're nowhere. So that's why they look at it....They go with the current affairs. (Wang'ele Interview, Jul. 28, 2004)

Furthermore, many programs that offer support to children in areas other than, or in addition to, schooling also engage in performance to promote AIDS awareness. One children's group that has performed locally and internationally about HIV/AIDS is affiliated with Shangilia Mtoto wa Afrika (literally, Rejoice Child of Africa), a street children's home and program based in the low-income community of Kangemi. In July 2004, twelve children from Shangilia traveled to Thailand to perform at the Fifteenth International AIDS Conference. This trip proved educational not only for the performing group and its audience in Thailand, but also for members of Shangilia who remained in Nairobi. As Shangalia's director Japeth Njenga explains: "Some of our children here [in Nairobi] are HIV-positive, and the other kids used to be very scared of them, but the kids who went to Bangkok have returned to end the discrimination (against) and stigmatisation of the AIDS orphans" (as quoted in Taylor 2005). This change came in part from meeting people in Bangkok who were also HIV-positive.

Individual youths are also seeking to compose and perform pieces about HIV/AIDS on their own.[17] I met Martin, a.k.a. Young Messenger, in 2004 through the Kawangware Street Children and Youth Project in the low-income community of Kawangware. Like many of his peers, Martin was captivated by hip hop and eager to succeed as a musician. His goal was greater than fame: his mission was to use music to teach audiences about life in his community and to demand change (Young Messenger Interview, Aug. 27, 2004). Borrowing resources from a local church, and accompanied by other youth in the community, he performed one of his compositions for me. He was backed by the sound track for "Still D.R.E." (featured on hip hop musician/producer Dr. Dre's 1999 album 2001), a piece whose original lyrics chronicle Dr. Dre's successes in the U.S. hip hop scene. Martin's piece tells a different story: of homeless people, HIV/AIDS sufferers, and the apathy of community members who are complacent about the people dying around them. He shifts gracefully between personas and topics: "They're living on the street, no shoes to wear / Just a piece of rubber plastic wrapped around their feet…" and later, "I'm not yet dead, and I still wanna care / But everyone stops, just to tell / A lonely baby I will always be / All because of this thing / Called HIV." His friends join in the chorus, which forces listeners to consider their responses to the problems around them (Young Messenger Interview, Aug. 27, 2004):

> *I close my eyes and I start to cry*
> *Before you ask me why, just tell me why*
> *You are sitting on the chair*
> *Tell me that you care*
> *Why homeless souls are dying everywhere*

Having now moved on to country music, which he perceives as equally popular and less frequently performed than hip hop in Nairobi, Martin continues to try to impact his community through music. He is one of many youths in Kenya who seek to do so.

OTHER HIV/AIDS PROGRAMS

Among the variety of other HIV/AIDS performances in Nairobi are music and puppet shows,[18] such as those run by Family Programme Promotion Services (in collaboration with Doctors Without Borders) in low-income communities such as Kibera, and the Kawangware Street Children and Youth Project in Kawangware. These two programs use puppet skits to convey messages about issues such as HIV/AIDS, but incorporate recorded or live music to attract and engage audiences. Churches also promote HIV/AIDS performances, including the Kenya Evangelical Lutheran Church (KELC), which has developed a multifaceted HIV/AIDS strategic plan with activities targeting prevention and control of transmission, provision of care and support, and AIDS awareness and stigma reduction. While the arts do not figure formally into the KELC policy, many parishes employ drama or music in addressing HIV/AIDS. According to Wilfred Otene (Interview, Jul, 28, 2004), HIV/AIDS program coordinator for KELC, drama is used especially within rural communities, where seminars are not effective due to language barriers with English and Kiswahili and where performance can improve communication. On occasion, performances also include singing. Music is given particular emphasis by choirs in local KELC parishes. The extent to which choirs address HIV/AIDS, however, depends on the interests and strengths of the individual parishes.

Other community events in Kenya also incorporate performances about HIV/AIDS. At World AIDS Vaccine Day held on May 18, 2004, drama, poetry, and drumming performances by young adult groups were featured alongside speeches by scholars and dignitaries involved in experiments to develop an AIDS vaccine. Performances about HIV/AIDS were also included in activities related to the World Social Forum held in Nairobi in January 2007 ("Nairobi 2007: World Social Forum" 2007).

ASSESSING MUSIC AND HIV/AIDS INITIATIVES

Residents of Nairobi have years of experience with viewing, organizing, implementing, being targeted by, and critiquing a diversity of HIV/AIDS projects. Through performances at commercial venues, schools, churches, and community events, as well as through recordings and proposals for sustainable education programs, musicians in and out of Nairobi are demonstrating their commitment to raising awareness about AIDS and to creating positive change within their communities. They, and the community organizations with which they sometimes collaborate, are thinking creatively about how to reach audiences with vital information on prevention and care. They hope not only to address AIDS, but also to affect a range of equally critical concerns within their communities—from poverty, to family relations, to gender issues—often inextricably linked with AIDS.

Scholars involved in music, communications, and education research suggest various reasons why music programs may be effective in promoting HIV/AIDS awareness and stimulating behavior change. Many ethnomusicologists argue that music (or musical individuals) and societies can mutually impact each other (see, for instance, Seeger 1979; Abu-Lughod 1986; and Sugarman 1997). Music scholars working in Africa highlight the long history of uses of music for educational purposes in Africa.[19] Communications scholars, active in researching and promoting "entertainment-education" projects in Africa and elsewhere, suggest that such projects may be more effective in enhancing knowledge about an issue than in changing behavior, yet also note that increased knowledge can stimulate audiences to join programs that can enable change (Singhal and Rogers 1999, 13).[20] Further clues as to why music programs may be effective come from Brazilian philosopher and educator Paulo Freire, who has famously argued for a "problem-posing" approach to education (fostering collaboration, critical thinking, and empowerment) rather than a "banking" system (featuring teachers who impart knowledge and students who memorize and regurgitate it; Freire 1997[1970], 52–67; hooks 1994, 5). Some performances may be no better than banking systems of education—even if the narrative is wrapped in a creative disguise. Yet many projects also seek to break the divide between educators and students, stimulating critical thinking within communities by involving audience members in performances or in discussion following performances.

Many of the people with whom I have spoken in Nairobi argue that efforts to address HIV/AIDS through performance arts, including music, can be effective. Anne Bittock, of Grace Centre International in Nairobi, argues that performances allow for greater personal, physical, emotional, and intellectual engagement by community members than lecture-based programs. Some people view the arts generally as "the easiest way" to communicate to audiences (Bittock Interview, May 31, 2004) and as more effective in reaching audiences than communicating messages "dry" (Ochango Interview, Aug. 10, 2004). Individuals suggest that performance may be particularly effective in addressing sensitive topics such as AIDS. Gathecha Kamau, country coordinator for the Youth Employment Summit Campaign Kenya, argues that bringing in a doctor to speak about AIDS would only frighten audiences, and particularly groups such as young girls. Artists, however, may be given more attention by audiences and can imaginatively communicate about AIDS-related issues (Kamau Interview, May 4, 2004). Finally, while many performers involve multiple arts in performances, and may shy away from calling themselves only musicians or dancers or actors, music is described by some musicians as being performed and received by people more "naturally" (Border Klan Interview, Sep. 15, 2004) than other arts.

Despite its potential effectiveness, however, using music for HIV/AIDS interventions presents a number of problems. Erasmus U. Morah, UNAIDS country coordinator for Kenya, agrees that "there is, has been and will always be a role for the arts, including music," in HIV interventions. The challenge, Morah argues, is in "isolating, interpreting and attributing [that] role" (Morah E-mail, Feb, 19, 2007). Multiple performers have suggested to me that addressing HIV/AIDS through music is more complex and difficult than addressing other social issues. Edward Kabuye argues that the difficulties of addressing this disease relate to the nature of humans (who succumb to sexual desires, even if they know better, and who may deny their illness), the nature of the disease (involving lengthy periods in which people appear healthy), and the problem of social pressures (gender differences, poverty, etc.). Aside from the topic of HIV/AIDS, there are other challenges: resources are scarce, funding is often limited,[21] and questions are raised about the styles of performance musicians choose. Debates about the artistic and social value of hip hop, and its ability to reach older as well as younger audiences, are especially heated. Furthermore, HIV/AIDS initiatives in general are met with skepticism by audiences. Numerous people with whom I conversed in Nairobi reacted similarly to questions about the extent of HIV/AIDS knowledge among Kenyan audiences and the need for further HIV/AIDS work, whether through music performance or through other means. On the one hand, there is a feeling that more "deep" information about HIV/AIDS is needed within communities. On the other hand, there seems to be a backlash against AIDS-related work. Because numerous initiatives have been targeted at different communities, many people in Nairobi have become weary of the continual focus on AIDS and the ongoing intrusion into their lives by AIDS-related organizations and campaigns. This weariness extends into music-making, with some school administrators opting not to have their students perform songs about AIDS because so many other schools are doing so (J. Simiyu Interview, May 13, 2004). Further issues raised by audience members and performers concerning HIV/AIDS programming in general and music performance in particular include songs frequently taking a "snapshot" of AIDS, pinpointing it but not treating it in depth; performances often occurring only once, rather than as part of an ongoing, holistic AIDS program; performers not always appearing well informed about the epidemic, and passing on incorrect information or providing poor examples through their own behaviors; sponsors not always knowing who they are targeting and thus not necessarily helping the situation on the ground; and sponsors sometimes not taking music and musicians seriously, perceiving them as distributors or messengers rather than fundamental players in the development agenda. Public skepticism about the effectiveness of AIDS campaigns has worsened in Kenya, moreover, due to a number of corruption scandals that have erupted in and out of the government.[22] Thus, despite the potential for music to promote social change, musicians and organizers of HIV/AIDS initiatives may need to work harder and be even more creative in the future than they have been in the past.

STEALING ELEPHANTS, CREATING FUTURES

> My father told me if you steal, steal big. One day I stole an elephant. And when I was asked why I stole an elephant, I told them that my father told me if you steal, steal big. (Moses Ouma, 13, resident of Mathare, quoted in Wong 1999)

Spoken by a child in the low-income community of Mathare, these words speak of a spirit that lives throughout Nairobi. To me, these words relate not to the stealing of material goods, but rather to a daring to dream, to be creative, to defy the odds. They speak of stealing what may sometimes seem most improbable: a future. The examples in this chapter offer a glimpse of the efforts of some musicians to "steal" just that. These are people, I would suggest, who dream big and who use music to help turn those dreams into reality. Through their performances, these individuals highlight the problematic realities of contemporary life and suggest a world of possibility (the ability to be tested, be faithful, practice safe sex, etc.). As these musicians attempt to shape their communities through performance, their performances too are shaped by the social, cultural, and political contexts in which they work. The challenge for musicians today, as stated by the Kenya Music Festival adjudicators discussed earlier in this chapter, is to continue to make performances attractive, well informed, and relevant. Many musicians accept this challenge. They press on in their efforts to use music to build new lives for themselves and for members of their communities.

7

Interlude
Nyimbo Za EDZI
(Songs About AIDS)

E. Jackson Allison, Jr.

Returned Peace Corps volunteer E. Jackson (Jack) Allison is a medical doctor who specializes in emergency medicine and public health. He created the following six lyrics (in English and Chichewa), at the request of Project HOPE, in cooperation and collaboration with Peace Corps/ Malawi and the Malawian government, which he performed in concert in Malawi and released as an album in 1995. The full recordings have been posted on Jack Allison's page at http:// afriendofmalawi.com/.

For the full story behind these compositions, please see Allison's entry in this volume.

COMPASSION, CARE AND LOVE

What we need is compassion, care and love for people with AIDS
What we need is compassion, care and love let's find a way
To teach our families about AIDS
Let's teach them today
By showing compassion, care and love for people with AIDS

Wodwala EDZI ndi munthu ngati ife tomwe	A person with AIDS is just like us
Timusamale ndithu wodwala EDZI	We must take care of a person with AIDS
Wodwala EDZI amafuna chikondi ndi chisamaliro	A person with AIDS wants love and compassion
Wodwala EDZI ndi munthu ngati ife tomwe	A person with AIDS is just like us

KANSALU KOFIIRA

Kansalu kofiira mwavalaka kakutanthauza kuti mukudziwa munthu amene ali ndi EDZI kapena anafa ndi matenda a EDZI.

(*Wearing a red ribbon means that you know someone who has AIDS or someone who has died from AIDS.*)

YOU CAN'T GET AIDS FROM A HANDSHAKE

You can't get AIDS from a handshake
You can't get AIDS from holding your sister's hand
You can't get AIDS from a handshake
No you can't!
No you can't!
You can't get AIDS from a handshake
You can't get AIDS from shaking your brother's hand
You can't get AIDS form a handshake
No you can't!
No you can't!

EDZI sichilango chochokera kwa Mulungu	AIDS is not a punishment from God
Matenda sichilango chochokera kwa Mulungu	No disease is punishment from God
EDZI ndi matenda wogwira aliyense	Since AIDS is an illness which can affect anyone,
Ndipo kupewa ndi udindo wa aliyense	It's everyone's duty to be involved in AIDS prevention
EDZI simatenda olodzedwa mfiti...	AIDS is a disease which has nothing whatsoever to do with witchcraft...

USE A CONDOM!

Use a condom, to protect yourselves
Use a condom, to protect your health
Use a condom, show respect for your lover
Use a condom, show respect for yourself
Use a condom, show respect for one another
Use a condom, to protect yourselves
Use a condom, to protect your health

Aphiri, kodi mukudziwa ntchito ya kondomu?	Mr. Phiri, do you know what condoms are used for?
Kondomu imateteza kumatenda osiyanasiyana	Condoms prevent many diseases
Kondomu imateteza kumatenda opatsirana	Condoms protect us from venereal disease

Kondomu imateteza kubereka kosakonzekera	Condoms prevent unwanted pregnancies
Komanso mondomu imateteza kumatenda aja oopsya a EDZI	Condoms are especially important in protecting us from the terrible disease of AIDS

ATSIKANA MUZINGOTI TOTO!

Chenjerani ndi EDZI	Be careful of AIDS
Ganizirani za EDZI	Think carefully about AIDS
Atsikana nonse	All girls and young women
Chenjerani ndi EDZI	Be careful because of AIDS
Muzingoti Muzingoti TOTO!	Just say No! to sugar daddies
Atsikana chenjerani	Girls be careful
Atsikana ganizirani	Girls think
Atsikana chenjerani ndi EDZI	Girls be careful because of AIDS

KUTCHINJIRIZA

Kutchinjiriza anthu onse	We must protect all of our people
Kutchinjizra anu athu	We must protect our children
Nthenda ya EDZI ndi yoyipa	Because AIDS is a very bad disease
Nthenda ya EDZI ndi yoopsya	AIDS is a terrible disease
Kupewa EZDI ndi udindo wa alimi	AIDS prevention is the duty of the farmer
Kupewa EZDI ndi udindo wa asodzi	AIDS prevention is the duty of the fisherman
Kupewa EZDI ndi udindo wa adalaivala	AIDS prevention is the duty of the driver
Kupewa EZDI ndi udindo wa aphunzitsi	AIDS prevention is the duty of the teacher
Kupewa EZDI ndi udindo wa abusa	AIDS prevention is the duty of the preacher
Kupewa EZDI ndi udindo wa azipani	AIDS prevention is the duty of political parties
Kupewa EZDI ndi udindo wa amai	AIDS prevention is the duty of the mother
Kupewa EZDI ndi udindo wa abambo	AIDS prevention is the duty of the father
Kupewa EZDI ndi udindo wa atsikana	AIDS prevention is the duty of the daughter
Kupewa EZDI ndi udindo wa anyamata	AIDS prevention is the duty of the son
Kupewa EZDI ndi udindo wa anthu onse	AIDS prevention is the duty of everyone in Malawi

8

Using Music to Combat Aids and Other Public Health Issues in Malawi

E. Jackson Allison, Jr. (SUNY Upstate Medical University)

Lawrence H. Brown, III (Anton Breinl Centre/James Cook University)

Susan E. Wilson (East Carolina University)

BACKGROUND

My personal foray into health education began as a trainee with the United States Peace Corps in 1966. During a two-week field exercise with the Centro de Salud (Health Department) in Mexicali, Baja California, Mexico, a fellow trainee and I produced and performed a puppet show in Spanish for five- and six-year-old children who were about to receive mandatory immunizations as a prerequisite for attending school. The show's message contained simple information about what the "shots" were for, that the procedure would be brief, and that their pain would be comparable to that of a mosquito bite or less. The children were enthralled with the puppets. They really paid attention and laughed heartily at our silly, honest humor. The public health nurses were delighted. They had never before experienced children who cried significantly less during the immunization process, which was also much more efficient in terms of time and orderliness. We trainees were pumped![1]

Our group of Peace Corps volunteers arrived in Malawi, southeastern Africa, in January 1967. Once posted to our assigned villages, our initial task was to perform a survey to determine what foods were available locally for children to eat. Our major charge was to run an under-fives' child welfare clinic where we weighed the children on a scale and plotted their weight and head- and chest-circumference over time. We also provided immunizations against diphtheria, pertussis (whooping cough), and tetanus on a regular basis, and against measles and smallpox less frequently.

Clinics were held twice a week for three months, until the caseload warranted dropping back to a weekly schedule. Other parallel activities included performing cooking demonstrations with two goals: first, getting more protein and vitamin C into the children's diet by encouraging the addition of pounded peanut flour and a crushed tomato to the traditional maize porridge; and second, getting mothers to feed their children three times a day instead of just once. We also got involved in convincing mothers to boil drinking water, convincing the population to protect local water supplies, and helping to dig latrines and getting folks to use them. It was truly demanding, yet gratifying work.

After I had been in Malawi for three months, I discovered that I could write music! I recorded the first of sixteen songs and jingles in April—"Pirikitsani Nchenche," a song that implored parents to brush the flies from their babies' eyes in order to prevent eye disease. It was recorded with the Jazz Giants, one of the most popular bands in Malawi, and became an instant hit. The next month we recorded "Ufa wa Mtedza," which asked mothers to put peanut flour in their children's maize porridge and feed it to them three times a day if they wanted them to weigh a lot on the scale. "Ufa" quickly became the number-one song on the Hit Parade in Malawi and remained so for the next three years.

A unique project developed over the success of my music in Malawi that has been documented elsewhere (Allison 1977). I received an educational grant from Colgate-Palmolive to tour the entire country under the aegis of the Ministry of Health to perform a traveling health education rock 'n' roll road show. Every morning I would give half-hour presentations at four local elementary schools on the virtues of vector control—flies, mosquitoes, roaches—utilizing a flannel graph, a papier-mâché handheld puppet, and one or two of my songs. I also informed the teachers and pupils where I would be performing that evening.

Approximately two hours before sundown, I would begin playing a combination of traditional and Western rock 'n' roll to help draw a crowd. At nightfall we would crank up a generator that provided power for the lights and microphones. All of my performances, including my songs, were sung in Chichewa, a Bantu language akin to Kiswahili. After being introduced by the local chief and the health assistant, I would begin talking about my songs. I always started each show with "Ufa wa Mtedza," since it was the most popular song in the country. Other songs in the program included "Brush the Flies Out of Your Babies' Eyes," "Boil Your Drinking Water," "TB," "Rabies is Fatal," "The Best Food for Your Children is A Mixture," "Make War on Ignorance, Poverty, and Disease," "Self-Help Schemes Help to Build the Country of Malawi," and "Wash Your Hands After Going to the Latrine."

The real star of the show was the puppet *Bambo Umoyo*, which literally means *Mister Health*, but which translates as *Father Well-Being*. Before I sang each song, the health assistant and I would explain in detail its intended message: describing why it is important, for instance, to brush flies from our babies' eyes. After I sang the song, *Mister Fab*, the representative from Colgate-Palmolive, would begin asking five or six questions about the message of that song and invite one person at a time to come on stage to speak answers into the microphone. Then *Bambo Umoyo* would pop up in the puppet theater to pass judgment on each answer in a semi-serious way. To put it mildly, the puppet's interaction was powerfully engaging and *always* stole the show. These performances were built around repetition and reinforcement. Prizes such as toothpaste and toothbrushes, hand soap, and detergent, were given away for correct answers, congruent with the theme of promoting better health; and we repeated the Q&A session after the last song was sung. Each show lasted until around midnight, performed completely in Chichewa. During this five-month tour, which focused on rural villages and towns throughout Malawi, we taught forty thousand students and teachers and reached twenty thousand attendees during the nightly shows.

Upon my return to Malawi twenty-five years later, I was interviewed separately by two Malawian reporters who reminded me that I had chatted with and sung to them when they were students. Then they each spontaneously sang a song I had performed that day ("Brush the Flies..." and "Self-Help Schemes..."). Needless to say, I was completely undone, on the verge of tears. Since writing my first song in Malawi in 1967, I have now written over one hundred songs and recorded over seventy of them. My songs have garnered over $150,000, and my wife, Sue Wilson, and I have donated every cent to various charitable causes. The CD *Nyimbo za EDZI* (*Songs about AIDS*) raised over $30,000, which has been used to help feed Malawian children who have been orphaned because their parents have died of AIDS.

HIV/AIDS, 1994

My return to Malawi after twenty-five years was precipitated by the first telephone call I ever received from the country in July 1994. I actually received three back-to-back calls, admonishing me to return to Malawi to head up a mission to combat HIV/AIDS. Since I was on sabbatical from the Department of Emergency Medicine, Brody School of Medicine, East Carolina University, I was available. The project I became involved with was funded primarily by the international social health organization Project HOPE, with assistance from Peace Corps/Malawi. I signed a contract to write, produce, and record three songs about AIDS awareness, education, and prevention, yet ended up with six songs, three in Chichewa, and three in Chichewa and English. I spent my first week in Malawi auditioning bands for the project, and selected two groups out of two dozen. We spent the next two weeks in rehearsal. Additionally, we hosted a 2-1/2-day workshop where I lectured on and demonstrated how to write educational songs and jingles. During that time, I supervised the writing, development, and eventual recording of a myriad of artistic offerings—songs (traditional music from the village, and Western rock 'n' roll), dances (traditional and modern/interpretive), poems, storytelling, and dramas.

We recorded my six *Songs about AIDS* at the Malawi Broadcasting Corporation (MBC), incidentally on the very same equipment I had used to record my other songs back in 1967, '68 and '69. The official launch of the mission was held at the Mt. Soche Hotel in Blantyre, the commercial capital of Malawi. MBC recorded this event as well, which was attended by three hundred guests and dignitaries. The evening featured my six *Songs about AIDS*, interspersed with performances from other creative art forms. Fittingly the guest of honor from the Malawian government was the minister of sport and culture, a gentleman who had taught our group Chichewa during a one-month crash course held in Puerto Rico before we reported to Blantyre in January 1967. The launch was such a rousing success that it was decided that regional contests—Northern, Central, Southern—would be held for the best contributions in each category. These regional contests have also been quite successful, for the winners' entries continue to be featured on MBC.

EVALUATION

Evaluation is a perennial problem for projects in the developing world, which tend to be rather modest in scope and grossly underfunded, if indeed funded at all. We performed a modest evaluation following the mission of 1994. Using a structured questionnaire, we surveyed a convenience sample[2] of 691 urban and rural residents of the Lilongwe (Capital) District at twenty sites over a one-week period. Our primary goal was to measure the penetration of AIDS awareness/education/prevention songs aired on MBC following the program's official launch in November 1994 through August 1995, and to delineate the perceived messages from both my six pilot songs (PS) about AIDS and entries from the National AIDS Song Contest (NASC).

The results were encouraging: 77 percent of the respondents said that the radio was where they had learned the most about AIDS; 93 percent had heard a song about AIDS; and 87 percent indicated that they had heard at least one of my six pilot songs. Of the latter, 62 percent said "avoid promiscuity" was the message they had remembered from the songs, and 27 percent said that "use condoms" was the message. Furthermore, 78 percent of respondents had heard of the NASC; 70 percent said that the song contest's primary message was "avoid promiscuity," whereas 22 percent identified "use condoms" as the main message. We concluded that "[t]he PS and NASC reached a significant percentage of Malawians in Lilongwe District. These songs played a role in reinforcing the message on the primary methods of preventing AIDS (Carpenter 1996).

HIV/AIDS, 2005

In 2004 I received an invitation from the U.S. State Department to return to Malawi. I was asked to tour the entire country for a month to sing and speak about AIDS awareness, education, and prevention. The tour would be sponsored by the United States Embassy and the United States Peace Corps in Malawi. At first I resisted, explaining that although I was healthy and energetic, realistically I was almost 61, and doubted whether the proposed tour would be well received. As in 1994, I was told that Malawians *still* had a fondness for "Ufa wa Mtedza," as well as the *Songs about AIDS* collection, and that I should not fear.

Logistically, I could not make the trip to Malawi until June 2005 because I wanted to wait until our son, Josh, had been graduated from the University of North Carolina at Chapel Hill. After my arrival, however, I rehearsed with a group of musicians that called themselves the National Health Education Band, gave three major concerts, and held two shorter sessions in the capital of Lilongwe. Although each performance featured *Songs about AIDS*, we opened and closed with "Ufa wa Mtedza." The total attendance for all these events exceeded ten thousand people.

What was so unique about this tour is that we auditioned over seventy-five groups who wanted to be a part of these performances concerning AIDS awareness/education/prevention, including a one-man band. Although I was the major "draw" to attract local people to attend, each event lasted 2-1/2 hours and featured many of the arts—various dance troupes, dramatic presentations, poetry, storytelling, posters, and music of all sorts, including choirs—leading to enthusiastic audience participation.

DISCUSSION

The important link between the arts and health is well established. Not only can the arts be used to make health environments more attractive—for example, hanging pictures and playing music in stairwells increases the use of stairs (Boutelle 2001)—but they have also long been recognized as an effective tool in health education and health promotion. Art is more than paintings or music, however. Music (Carpenter 1996); video (Chavez 2004); graffiti, dance and music videos (Peres 2002); theater (Seguin 1996, Evian 1992); puppetry (Allison 1977, Wilson 1986, Friedman 1992); storytelling and drama (Cueva et al. 2005) are just some of the art forms that have been used in health promotion.

Participation is a consistent theme in the success of arts as a medium for health promotion (Thomas 2004, Wiehagen et al. 2007, White 2006, Chavez 2004, Peres 2002, R. Davis 2003). A collaborative approach helps to create personal connections to the message (Thomas 2004), and ensures culturally sensitive and appropriate content (Evian 1992, Chavez 2004). As a result, art-based health promotion efforts can more readily bridge racial, cultural, linguistic, and educational barriers (Friedman 1992), increasing comfort with the presented material and, thus, changing behavior more effectively (Cueva et al. 2005). Successful participatory art-based health promotion efforts have been reported for many diseases in diverse cultures from around the globe, including HIV/AIDS in Africa (Evian 1992, Carpenter 1996, Seguin 1996, Friedman 1992); HIV and STDs among imprisoned Brazilian youths (Peres 2002); HIV and STDs (Seguin 1996); and cancer (Thomas 2004, Wiehagen et al. 2007) in North America (including indigenous Alaskans) (Cueva et al. 2005); women's health issues among Aboriginal Australian women (S. Davis 2003); and tobacco use among children (R. Davis 2003).

An important aspect of participatory art-based health promotion is the ability to deliver health messages in nontraditional settings. A Johannesburg, South Africa theater-based AIDS education program, for example, reached more than twenty-thousand people through presentations "...at factories, canteens, clinics, parks, and community events" (Evian 1992). Measuring the impact of art-based health promotion efforts can be difficult, as it does not lend itself to more traditional research methods. The Centers for Disease Control and Prevention (CDC) Division of HIV/AIDS Prevention (DHAP) in the United States has designed and implemented the Program Evaluation and Monitoring System (PEMS), which is intended to provide "accurate and timely data to monitor and evaluate federally funded HIV prevention programs...in a consistent, efficient, and effective manner across the United States" (Thomas 2006, 74). Unfortunately, data collection and data management remain significant problems throughout Africa. The CDC has also developed an instrument "...to assess HIV/AIDS knowledge and four attitudinal dimensions (Peer Pressure, Abstinence, Drug Use, and Threat of HIV Infection)...validated for use with Spanish-speaking students in El Salvador" (Zometa 2007, 231). However, whether this instrument will have applicability in Africa remains to be investigated. Furthermore, the role of health education and how best to present it, including incorporation of the arts, currently comprises three rather disparate concepts. Researchers must take a more holistic view of health and health effects, recognizing the importance of social, educational, and economic benefits, even in the absence of frank changes in behavior or improvements in health status (White 2006). Additionally, process evaluation should be considered as important as impact and outcome evaluation (White 2006). A ten-stage model of conducting community-based research (CBR) from Alberta, Canada, has been developed (Harris 2006) that has yet to be validated in Africa. Indeed, by bringing in the principles of community-based participatory research (CBPR)—engaging stakeholders, soliciting funding, creating shared ownership, building cross-cultural collaborations, etc.,—researchers can actually contribute to the *creation* of art-based health promotion efforts as well as their evaluation (Chavez 2004, Wiehagen et al. 2007).

Yet to be sorted out is the interrelationship between Western medicine and African traditional medicine in the prevention of HIV/AIDS, much less the care and treatment of people with first the early symptoms, followed by the disease. Although it has been noted that "the use of traditional practitioners as a choice of health care is attributed to both the strengths and weaknesses of this system of health care" (Summerton 2006, 15), it has also been recommended that "...joint workshops should be conducted with traditional and western practitioners to demystify traditional healing practices" (Summerton 2006, 15).

Perhaps the awarding of the first ever Nobel Prize in Global Health awaits the prescient researcher who succeeds in bringing both camps together to foster meaningful, focused, validated health education, i.e., the best *educational vaccine*, for the prevention of HIV/AIDS, through utilizing music, dance, drama, poetry, painting, videos, and/or storytelling, in combination with a titrated tincture of medicinal magic. Until that august time, hope does indeed continue to spring eternal.

THE FUTURE

So much more needs to be done, and can be done, regarding health education about HIV/AIDS internationally. Utilization of the arts will continue to enhance more formal educational offerings, especially for less fortunate villagers. Personally, I would welcome the opportunity to work in other Bantu-speaking countries in East, Southeastern, and Central Africa, specifically having my *Songs about AIDS* translated into those Bantu tongues and having them recorded by local recording artists. Based on the anticipated success of such a project, I would then welcome having *Songs about AIDS* translated into Spanish, Arabic, French, and other languages in a concerted effort to reach even more people internationally. The basic age-old problem is funding. Those who have tried to wrest money from major funding sources, especially the Gates Foundation, know that it can be an insurmountable challenge.

Another triad yet to be investigated is that involving medical-religious-artistic partnerships. The question arises as to how the arts might fit into educating patients about the four premises of the health belief model as discussed in detail by Bennett (2009): an individual must be convinced that (1) he or she is susceptible to the disease in question, (2) the disease has severe consequences, (3) these consequences can either be prevented or treated effectively, and (4) "the benefits of illness prevention or treatment regimens outweigh the costs or burden of these regimens" (Bennett 2009, 36–37).

Yet, again, villagers themselves need to be invited to help solve the pervasive international problem of HIV/AIDS. We are convinced that their collective wisdom needs to be heard, and expressed—through dialogue *and* the arts—in order to bring to the fore the sage adage: "an ounce of prevention..." as advocated by Shortell (2008).

9

Visual Approaches to HIV Literacy
in South Africa

Annabelle Wienand (University of Cape Town)

INTRODUCTION

South Africa's HIV epidemic remains one of the worst in the world with an estimated 16.9 percent of adults aged 15–49 living with HIV (Shisana et al. 2009). At the time of this study, a number of HIV literacy campaigns aimed to increase public knowledge in an attempt to reduce the spread of the virus. This chapter identifies the essential role played by community health workers and treatment activists who provide HIV education in their communities and assist the state health care system. The aim of this study was to complement existing initiatives with the development and evaluation of a visually oriented and participatory HIV-literacy workshop. The central focus of the workshop was the creation of life-size drawings based on tracing around a human body which provided a template for a series of participatory exercises. These "body map drawings" enabled the participants to develop their knowledge of human biology in relation to HIV prevention, care and treatment.

The workshop was conducted with a sample of forty participants from three separate groups (community health workers, treatment literacy educators/trainers, and HIV-positive mothers). The health workers, educators, and trainers were approached to take part in the study after initial meetings with the organizations they worked for identified the need for further training in the biomedical aspects of HIV. The group of HIV-positive mothers were involved in the project because they matched the socioeconomic and educational background of the clients the health workers and educators work with on a daily basis. In this way, the study could achieve some insight into how the end target audience would respond to the techniques and content of the workshop.

The workshop was evaluated using a mixed-method approach, including multiple-choice questionnaires, participant observation, analysis of the body map drawings and semi-structured in-depth interviews. While most of the participants had been previously exposed to at least some of the biomedical content of the workshop, the use of visual and participatory tools and techniques was something new. A visual and collaborative learning style was found to be effective because it presented the material in a practical and straightforward way that people could readily apply to their lives and work environments. The significance of this finding is that visual and participatory approaches to HIV literacy are shown to have the potential to help facilitate a better understanding of HIV prevention and treatment. Given the small sample size, further research is needed in order to verify and extend the findings to South Africa's general population.

BACKGROUND

At the time of the study, five years after the South African government's commitment to provide universal access to antiretroviral therapy (ART), it was estimated that less than half the South Africans requiring ART were receiving it (Nattrass 2007). A number of non-governmental organizations involved with providing ART in South Africa have stepped in to assist the public sector by actively recruiting and training lay people to prepare and support ART patients. These community health workers, also known as treatment literacy practitioners and community adherence workers, help nurses and doctors in clinics and hospitals. I was interested in their role as HIV educators, not only within the clinic context, but also in facilitating support groups and other forms of peer education. The workshop project described in this chapter was developed to train such people and to enable them to potentially use visual techniques in HIV education contexts within their organizations and communities.

The development and implementation of the drawing-based workshop was built on the premise that ordinary people can, and more importantly want to, learn the science of HIV. One of the lasting legacies of colonial and apartheid rule is that a large number of South Africans lack basic education, including knowledge of human biology. Without knowledge of cells, how can a person understand the existence of a virus? And without knowledge of viruses and other pathogens, how can a person make informed decisions with regards to their general health, and in particular the treatment and prevention of HIV?

The workshop intended to build on the existing knowledge of the workshop participants[1] and enable them to find ways to explain human biology, the science of HIV, and other social issues to their clients and people in their communities. Given its biomedical emphasis it is important to clarify that the workshop did not aim to undermine indigenous understandings of health and illness; rather, it aimed to provide information that many South Africans have been denied, either in the past or currently, due to continued disparities in schooling, especially with regard to the sciences. As previously mentioned, the participants were familiar to a greater or lesser extent with the biomedical content of the workshop. Exercises that addressed social issues, such as accessing social support and the challenges of disclosure of HIV-positive status, were new to them. The use of visual and participatory tools and techniques employed in the workshop were also novel to most participants. The participatory style of the workshop thus fulfilled the dual purpose of exposing the participants to biosocial information, while also training them to replicate the workshop in other contexts, such as HIV-positive support groups, youth groups, and voluntary counseling and testing (VCT) clinics. In this way, the workshop intended to provide training in participatory and visual learning styles in order to assist the participants with their work as HIV literacy educators and trainers.

PARTICIPATORY AND VISUAL APPROACHES TO ADULT LEARNING

Given the interactive nature of the workshop, it is important to consider the influential work of education scholar Paulo Freire. The last twenty years have seen the adoption of Freire's notion of critical consciousness (1997) by a number of projects working within the domains of social justice, adult education, health, grassroots mobilization, and participatory action research (Minkler and Cox 1980, Campbell and MacPhail 2002, Campbell 2003, Cornwall and Jewkes 1995). The dissemination of Freire's ideas has coincided with a shift from "top-down" approaches for addressing social issues to more community-based and participatory interventions. The influence of this change in approaches can be seen not only in development literature, but also in a number of international declarations promoted by the World Health Organization, including the Ottawa Charter and the Jakarta Declaration (Campbell 2000).

Freire promoted participatory approaches to adult education as the key to empowering people and giving them the necessary skills to challenge current limitations in their lives. Freire resisted the traditional power hierarchy evident in the teacher/student relationship where the student was perceived as passive, while the teacher actively "teaches." He proposed instead that adult learners bring a wealth of lived experience and knowledge to the learning process and should ultimately drive their development of new knowledge and ways of understanding. In Freire's model, the teacher acts as a facilitator and guide, while the learners are actively engaged in the learning process. This philosophy was built on the premise that "liberating education consists of acts of cognition, not transferrals of information" (1997, 60).

Freire proposed that adult learners need to develop critical consciousness, which included skills of inquiry, problem solving and creative ways of challenging circumstances that currently limit their life situations. The learning process was not an academic exercise, but rather a way of equipping adults with skills to engage in social action and improve their lives. In a similar way, Mezirow's ideas of critical reflection and transformational learning (Mezirow 1991, Mezirow et al. 2000) enable adult learners to question their assumptions about their life situations and to make positive changes to improve their circumstances. Both Freire and Mezirow identified group conversation as a tool for developing awareness and an increased sense of agency with adult learners. Their goal, they claimed, was achieved by addressing real-life situations within the learning environment: an approach that shares similar principles to peer education and support group settings.

When considering Freire's theory of critical consciousness it is useful to see the development of critical consciousness not as an end in itself, but rather as a necessary skill for initiating social change. In the case of HIV literacy it can be seen as increasing people's awareness of the conditions and norms inhibiting them from making decisions that prevent HIV infection. Critical consciousness can also help HIV-positive people understand how to live productive lives. Campbell (2003) echoes this sentiment in the following statement:

> Critical consciousness is a precondition for the collective renegotiation of sexual and social identities in ways that are less damaging to sexual health, as well as for the development of confidence and empowerment to be able to engage in safer sexual behaviour. (Campbell 2003, 133)

Both Freire's theory of critical consciousness and Mezirow's transformational learning offer participatory approaches to adult learning that support it as an active process. They both view adult learning as an agent for social change that enables individuals and their communities to develop solutions to existing challenges and limitations.

This project approached critical consciousness through a visual lens. Various visual forms of mapping and drawing have long been employed in different disciplines including psychology, geography, sociology and anthropology to record information such as natural and urban environments, local resources and social structures. In particular, Participatory Research practitioners have made extensive use of mapping and drawing as a tool for accessing local knowledge and stimulating social action. In this way mapping and drawing techniques support a "bottom-up" approach based on locally defined priorities, while acknowledging indigenous knowledge and skills (Cornwall and Jewkes 1995).

Two visual tools were used collaboratively in the course of the workshop: body map drawings and the Visual Body Map chart. The creation of life-size body map drawings was the key focus of the workshop and was the basis for most of the exercises. The Visual Body Map, an educational tool depicting all the organ systems in the human body in overlaid acetate sheets, was used as a reference.[2] To create the body map drawings, a workshop participant's body was traced onto a large piece of brown cardstock. Then, over the course of the workshop, the participants would work in small groups (of about five individuals per group) to fill in their body maps. These group drawings were used to capture the participants' existing knowledge, as well as to record new information presented in the workshop via the Visual Body Map or through other interactive exercises.

The most obvious advantage of using visual techniques is the unambiguous, straightforward, and direct presentation of concepts and information. Visual communication offers certain advantages and limitations compared with verbal or written forms, which rely on literacy or sharing a common language in order to be understood. Cornwall (1996) suggests that the key principle of visualization techniques, such as drawing, is that they offer ways of collectively producing and representing information in a form that encourages debate and analysis. The participatory nature of the process also creates new understanding by drawing on the diverse knowledge and experiences of those taking part. In this way, visual techniques engage in social action by actively encouraging people to explore and represent what they know, which "can validate them as knowledgeable, active subjects capable of interpreting and changing their situations themselves" (1996, 95). The creation of body map drawings offers an advantage in recording perceptions of HIV/AIDS and biomedical facts, because it develops appreciation of differing understandings of health and illness, as well as understandings of social issues separate from the physical experience of the disease.

In two separate studies that encouraged adult patients to draw their illness conditions, Guillemin (2004) assessed the potential role of drawing as a tool to develop conceptions of how individuals experience ill health. Guillemin interviewed her participants, asked them to draw "how they visualized their condition" (2004, 276), and then discussed with them what they had drawn. In this way the participants were able to explore their emotional responses to their condition, develop a better understanding of their illness, and, in some cases, gain a more positive outlook toward living with it. Guillemin argues, as a result, that "the act of drawing necessitates knowledge production, with a visual product as an outcome" (2004, 272).

Harrison (2002) approaches the use of drawing as a visual methodology from within the field of sociology of health and illness. She not only notes the long history shared by art and medicine, but also comments on the increased emphasis on recording the ways patients themselves interpret and attribute meaning to their experiences of being healthy or sick. She goes on to suggest that visual approaches are participatory by nature and that "for participants the sense of being more active, of having some control over the research process, also gave them greater control over their illness" (Harrison 2002, 862). The collaborative and participatory nature of visual methods thus challenges traditional models of knowledge production (Harrison 2002).

Brice Heath (2000) approaches the educational potential of visual methodologies from the perspective of neurobiology. She argues that when both viewing and creating visual images, there is interplay between visual and expressive meaning within the brain. This process assists in learning because images serve to recall information stored in the brain through prior experience and enable the learner to verbalize the new information to which he or she has been exposed. Consequently, Brice Heath suggests that the use of visuals assists the learning process and also stimulates conversation. "[T]he visual and the verbal reinforce one another in the sustained and adaptive learning necessary to increase learning from the theories of others and to build strength in one's own theories" (Brice Heath 2000, 124).

Throughout the world cartoons and illustrations have been used to promote understanding around HIV and AIDS, as well as other health-related issues. In the South African context, where almost two-thirds of the population cannot read basic health education materials, visual media are often seen as a solution. Arbuckle (2004) refers to the positive response to the *Mkhize* picture story, which is part of the *Learn with Echo* adult literacy educational newspaper supplement, as further evidence of the efficacy of visual methodologies. However, the same research shows that visual literacy cannot be taken for granted: non-literate people often experience difficulties in understanding certain visual conventions that use perspective to depict scale, size and movement, as well as concepts such as thought and speech bubbles. The lack of illustrated educational material in developing countries such as South Africa thus means that child and adult learners alike have limited opportunity for developing complex visual literacy skills, which are sometimes dependent on being able to read in the first instance or being exposed to visual materials such as comics. Despite their appeal, then, illustrated educational materials are not automatically easily understood by illiterate audiences.

In her work with women in Zimbabwe on developing understanding about sexual and reproductive health, Cornwall made extensive use of drawing techniques to gather popular and indigenous knowledge (Cornwall 2002). Each woman in the study drew in the sand with a stick to illustrate her understanding of how the female reproductive system worked. Cornwall later copied the drawings in her note book. She realized the importance of engaging with the women's existing knowledge as a starting point, before introducing the biomedical model, in order to address problems experienced by both the village women and local clinic staff. In this way Cornwall's use of drawing is similar to the development of the body map drawings in the workshop assessed in this chapter. The emphasis of the body map workshop lay not in anatomical accuracy, but rather in generating as much information as possible about the human body, including lay understandings of the body.

While artistic creation is often seen as an individualistic exercise, collaborative visual production has been used for both therapeutic and educative purposes. With their involvement in community art projects, Karkou and Glasman (2004) promoted the suspension of any aesthetic or artistic value judgments of what constitutes "good" art in order to enable both learning and healing to take place. They argued that by making the level of skill irrelevant, greater social inclusion and participation was achieved. In my workshops, I thus looked to frame the process of creating the body map drawings not as an artistic exercise, but rather as a way of reinforcing and recording the learning process. Participants were free to depict the body and parts of the body in any way they chose without having to consider anatomical correctness or aesthetic beauty.

This section has addressed the relative advantages and challenges of using visual and collaborative methodologies. It has also described how drawing in particular can be used as a way of encouraging people to learn more about health and illness, as I will now show in my own project's context of HIV literacy.

WORKSHOP DEVELOPMENT

The intention of the body map drawing workshop was two-fold. Firstly, it aimed to increase the knowledge of the participants. Secondly, it was designed to serve as a "train-the-trainer" style workshop so that on completion of the workshop, the participants would be able to run similar workshops in contexts such as youth groups, church groups and support groups. A manual was developed in order to keep the content of the workshop consistent, and to serve as an HIV education resource. This manual contained factual information about HIV, as well as step-by-step instructions to assist educators and community health workers in running future workshops.

In the course of the manual development, the workshop was piloted with three HIV-positive adults who had attended support groups themselves and subsequently been trained to facilitate psychosocial support workshops for HIV-positive people to increase knowledge about HIV and how to better manage their health. Two of the three participants were ART patients who exhibited excellent knowledge of treatment options, as well as valuable first-hand experience of the personal challenges of living with HIV and taking ART. Their knowledge was particularly useful and informed exercises in the workshop that addressed social support, disclosure of HIV-positive status and access and adherence to ART. The piloting of the workshop also enabled me to test different exercises, some of which were discarded in the process.[3] After necessary changes had been made to the workshop manual, I approached four more HIV literacy facilitators and adult educators for further comment and feedback.

The workshop was designed so that it could be run as either nine separate one-hour sessions or as a two-day training. I met with people and organizations involved with running HIV-positive support groups and learned that support groups typically meet for one- or two-hour sessions either once or twice a week. The two-hour sessions usually allocate one hour to general conversation and counseling, and another hour for discussing educational topics. Those groups that met twice a week had a similar approach, dividing the time between "sharing" and educational sessions. This arrangement encouraged the development of one-hour sessions that could be easily incorporated into existing support group structures.

In order to assess the potential effectiveness of the workshop, I approached different organizations working in HIV literacy training and offered to provide workshop training free of charge with the understanding that participants would be invited to take part in voluntary interviews afterward. I facilitated two-day workshops with three different groups (TAC, HOPE Cape Town, and a group of HIV-positive mothers). While facilitating these workshops the manual was viewed as a working document; I updated it following the running of each respective workshop. Once all three workshops had been completed, final changes were made to the manual based on the recommendations of workshop participants, as well as my observations of what had failed and what had worked best.

All workshop participants were given a copy of the workshop manual on completion of the training. "Fact File" sections within the manual provided detailed information about the human body and HIV/AIDS and were designed so that facilitators could refer back to facts covered during the workshop. Workshop participants were encouraged to use both the training and the manual as sources of information and ideas that could be adapted to their daily work needs. For example, individual exercises could be taken from the workshop and used as stand-alone activities without the need to create a body map drawing. This arrangement was intended to encourage the use of individual exercises in other contexts, such as VCT sessions, clinic waiting rooms, and schools.

BODY MAP DRAWING WORKSHOP CONTENT AND TECHNIQUES

The body map drawing workshop was spread over two days and relied on visual and participatory approaches to present the HIV literacy material. The first day concentrated on the participants' understanding of human biology and how the body is affected by HIV/AIDS. The second day focused more specifically on living with HIV. It addressed social aspects of the disease and practical knowledge of care and treatment options. Home-based care, nutrition, and hygiene were discussed together with when, how, and where to access primary health care and medical treatment, including ART. The combination of seemingly separate issues, such as nutrition, social support, and ART, was based on an inclusive approach to HIV literacy where the biomedical aspects of HIV were viewed together with the social and practical challenges of living with the virus.

At the start of the workshop I had the outline of my body traced on a piece of brown cardstock as a way of demonstrating how to create a body map drawing. Each participant was then given a pen and asked to add all the information they knew about the human body. This exercise immediately demanded the engagement of the workshop participants and made the collaborative and relaxed nature of the workshop clear from the start. It also provoked a humorous response from the group, which helped them put aside their fear of making "mistakes" when drawing and encouraged them to view the process as a fun way to learn. On another level the exercise proved a useful means of assessing the level of knowledge in the group.

As previously mentioned, the workshop was run with three different groups, consisting of Treatment Action Campaign (TAC) treatment literacy educators and trainers, HOPE Cape Town community health workers, and HIV-positive mothers. The TAC, in addition to campaigning for issues related to public health and care for people living with HIV, provides treatment literacy in communities throughout the country, and produces the newsletter "Equal Treatment" in an attempt to increase knowledge of HIV- and AIDS-related issues. HOPE Cape Town, a nonprofit organization that employs twenty-two full-time community health workers in the Western Cape, teams with lay people to provide service and care in conjunction with government clinics. The group of HIV-positive mothers was drawn from a clinic affiliated with HOPE Cape Town; they had limited educational background, and their knowledge of HIV/AIDS was largely a product of clinic appointments.

At the beginning of the workshop participants were encouraged to form groups of four or five in order to create the body map drawings. Each group produced a single body map. One person in each group served as a model for tracing around and creating the template for the body map; participants would later fill in this map with collaborative drawing, writing, and collage exercises. An example of one such exercise was asking each group to put together a homemade puzzle (a photograph cut into pieces). The participants were asked to think of anything in the human body that could be compared to a puzzle, with smaller pieces making up a whole. This "puzzle exercise" developed the participants' understanding of how different organs make up systems (e.g., the heart, veins, and arteries in the circulation system) and also illustrated the cellular composition of the human body.[4] In another exercise, each participant was given a photocopy of a road map of the greater Cape Town area and asked to trace the route they had taken that morning from their home to the workshop venue. The participants were then asked if the exercise made them think of anything inside the human body that could be compared to a road network. This started a discussion about the circulation system followed by the nervous system.

The first day of the workshop focused on the systems of the human body. A series of exercises enabled the participants to ask and answer questions about the functions of each system and how they work together. For example, when discussing the digestive system, the absorption of both nutrients and medication was explained in relation to diet and antiretroviral therapy. The Visual Body Map was used to demonstrate the way nutrients and medication leave the stomach and enter the blood and circulatory system. In this way the biology of the body was explained both generally and also with a specific focus on how HIV and AIDS affect it. Participants were encouraged to choose the level of detail they wanted to engage in with the material.

The second day focused on HIV transmission and how the virus compromises the immune system. The group marked and labeled areas on their body maps where HIV can enter the human body and wrote short descriptions of how the virus could be transmitted in each instance. The group also compiled a list of all the ways HIV cannot be transmitted, such as sharing a meal or embracing an HIV-positive person. Opportunistic infections were discussed and all areas in the body that could be affected by such infections were clearly labeled, along with available treatment options and home or traditional remedies. By looking at their body map drawings it was easy to locate which parts of the body were affected by which illnesses and what treatment options were available.

From the beginning participants were asked to contribute and share their knowledge and expertise in their groups. The Visual Body Map was initially absent from most exercises when the groups discussed their understandings of how the human body works. It was then later displayed to clarify questions and further explain relationships between the different parts of the body and how HIV and AIDS affect the healthy functioning of the human body. In this way the Visual Body Map was used as a reference source, as opposed to the starting point of the body map drawings. The participants were not expected to replicate the Visual Body Map in the drawings, but rather to choose what they thought was important to remember. Given the portable nature of the Visual Body Map, it was easy to hang up or remove according to need.

The immediate relationship between the Visual Body Map and the participants' own experiences of their bodies and health and illness further encouraged questions and learning. The Visual Body Map has no labels. The exclusion of written language not only simplified the presentation of human biology, but also encouraged participants to take ownership of the material and ask and answer questions verbally in their everyday language, as opposed to academic or medical language (which would have imposed itself if written labels had been placed on the Visual Body Map).

Exercises using both the Visual Body Map and the body map drawings encouraged the participants to add new material about human biology directly to the relevant areas on their group drawings. The space surrounding the traced outline of the body was filled with other exercises that involved pasting objects onto the cardstock. Some of the exercises, like the two described above, illustrated biomedical facts, while others addressed social and practical issues. The end result was a densely packed drawing of the human body with sketches of parts of human anatomy, information on the functions of different organs and systems, explanations of how HIV and AIDS affect different parts of the body, advice on healthy living, resources for social support, and treatment options.

One of the ways nutrition was discussed was in an exercise that involved cutting out pictures of food items from local supermarket advertisements and pasting them onto the body map drawings. The pictures of the different foods could be grouped into possible meals, encouraging debate on how to maintain an inexpensive yet practical balanced diet. Apart from foods available in supermarkets, the participants also wrote up the components of traditional meals in a group exercise. In order to emphasize that good nutrition need not be expensive, another exercise encouraged participants to describe their typical meals over a course of a week.

In addition to discussing a balanced diet, the participants were also encouraged to think more generally about food preparation. Apart from ensuring that the nutritional value of the food is retained and that food is not overcooked, the storage of foodstuffs was also discussed. Participants were informed about the importance of basic household hygiene, such as washing hands and food before cooking and keeping food covered and if need be, refrigerated. This discussion evolved into a debate on how to ensure a relatively germ-free home environment to help prevent opportunistic infections. Participants also discussed cheap and effective ways of preventing HIV transmission in the context of providing home-based care, such as using diluted bleach as a disinfectant. Socioeconomic obstacles to health, such as living in an informal settlement and unemployment, were also discussed, because many people are constrained by their living conditions.

Many of the participants had been trained as counselors or provided counseling as part of VCT services at the clinics where they worked. Workshop exercises that focused on social support and the challenges of HIV-positive status disclosure were thus particularly useful tools to assist them in addressing real life challenges, such as concerns about disclosing an HIV-positive status to a family member in order to access antiretroviral treatment.[5] One particularly popular exercise involved tracing around both the left and right hand. In the one hand, participants would list all the people who provided them with support; in the other, they would write the names of all the people who they supported. This resulted in a discussion of different kinds of support, including financial, emotional, spiritual, and material, among others. Participants said this exercise would prove useful when providing VCT, as well as in support group contexts.

Preparation for ART, the different options available and potential side effects to medication were also covered in the workshop. Factors that contribute to the spread of HIV/AIDS, such as socioeconomic conditions and gender inequality, were discussed in varying depth depending on the group. In this way the workshop aimed to increase biomedical knowledge about HIV/AIDS, while also addressing some of the social aspects of the disease.

Once the workshop was complete I photographed the body map drawings for more careful analysis. The body map drawings provided an unmediated and direct documentation of the learning process. While most exercises were recorded on all body map drawings, the way in which they were done and the degree of detail depended on each group. The level of engagement with the workshop process was immediately evident by looking at and comparing the body map drawings of the small groups within the same organization and between the three larger groups. I used this visual analysis of the completed body map drawings, together with interview responses and participant observation, to develop an understanding of how the workshop training was received.

RESEARCH METHODOLOGY

The research methods included observation of the workshop participants, administering questionnaires, evaluating the completed body map drawings, and conducting semi-structured group interviews on completion of the workshop. As demonstrated by the choice of observation and interview techniques, the methodological approach to this research project was predominantly qualitative with the exception of some descriptive, quantitative data collected in a questionnaire.

Qualitative processes, such as conducting interviews and participant observation, enabled me to get an in-depth understanding of how the participants responded to the workshop material and techniques. This approach increased the validity of the study, which was important given the relatively small sample, but left further study to be done to determine the reliability of the results within the greater South African context.

In the course of the project, I researched, developed, facilitated, and evaluated the workshop. It is often recommended that external groups or individuals conduct project monitoring and evaluation (Rossi et al. 2004), based on the premise that an external assessor will be impartial and provide a more balanced and objective report. For these reasons I made use of external workshop facilitators, educators, and academics in the earlier phases of the workshop development. However, I decided to facilitate the workshop because it would allow me to observe participants myself. Participant observation enabled me to record responses to the workshop content, tools, and techniques while the workshop was in progress. These observations contributed to further modifications to the workshop structure and content, with an eye toward improving its effectiveness.

At the end of the second day of the workshop, participants were asked to take part in a voluntary questionnaire. Nearly all agreed to fill in the questionnaire, but some people were unable to attend the second day of the workshop or had to leave before the end in order to catch transportion home. The questionnaire was designed to collect information about the workshop participants' educational background, previous training, and work experience and their current work environments and needs. This data served to gather background information that would shape the content of the follow up interviews and help contextualize participants' responses to both the workshop content and the visual and participatory techniques used to present the material. The data I collected enabled me to calculate averages and percentages in order to compare the three different groups with regards to level of formal education and general knowledge of HIV/AIDS and ART.

The questionnaire was written in English and translated into isiXhosa to limit errors due to language-based misunderstandings and also give the participants a choice of language. The majority of workshop participants were isiXhosa first-language speakers who communicated confidently in English, albeit with grammatical errors. It is interesting to note that most participants elected to fill in an English questionnaire, despite it being their second or third language. The questionnaire consisted almost exclusively of multiple choice questions, as well as the opportunity to write alternative answers to some questions when the choices did not correspond with their experience.

After the workshops, a majority of participants also agreed to meet with me for a group interview. Having established a relationship with the workshop participants, I believed it was important that I conduct the interviews to gather their opinions of the workshop and receive further recommendations. While it can be argued that the participants may have responded more positively than they would have done if someone else was interviewing them (because they might not have wanted to offend me), it is also likely that employing an alternative interviewer could have introduced more room for misinterpretation of the questions. Workshop participants, moreover, may not have been as willing to give as much of their time to someone they did not know.

I decided to interview participants either in pairs or groups of three or four, rather than individually, in order to encourage informal discussion. The rationale behind this decision was based on observing the camaraderie and humor evident during the running of the workshops. The participants appeared relaxed and confident expressing their views in front of their peers and colleagues. It was important that the participants felt comfortable and that the interview process proceeded more like a conversation, rather than a test of their knowledge or level of workshop participation. I took every effort to ensure a relaxed environment while guiding the interview conversation by asking questions and then allowing participants to talk among themselves.

The completed body map drawings were also present during the interview process. In this way, both the participants and I could refer to specific exercises recorded on the drawings. The participants were not interviewed in the same groups that created the body map drawings, so a number of drawings from different groups were typically viewed at the same time. I used the interviews to gain further clarity on how the participants had responded to the different exercises in the workshop. I was also able to check the validity of the questionnaire data by asking similar questions and cross-checking the answers I received.

EFFICACY OF VISUAL LEARNING

The creation of body map drawings is both visual and participatory by nature. In order to assess if visual approaches to HIV literacy are effective, participants from TAC and HOPE Cape Town were asked in their follow-up interviews to relate the workshop experience to their work as HIV literacy educators and trainers and community health workers. They were asked to describe how they could potentially use the visual exercises demonstrated in the workshop. In particular, they commented on the Visual Body Map and the creation of the body map drawings. The group of HIV-positive mothers was asked additionally if the use of visual material and drawing had increased their knowledge of health and illness in relation to HIV and AIDS.

One of the dominant themes to emerge in the course of the interviews was the way visual learning was particularly powerful within the context of illiteracy or low literacy environments. The community health workers in particular noted the lasting legacy of apartheid educational policy that has left many South African adults with very poor formal education. In the course of interviewing the community health workers, both Darryl and Maryanne (HOPE Cape Town) made references to the educational gaps found both among many of their patients and closer to home within their own families.[6] In Maryanne's words "Yes, adults are not aware of their body parts, because some of them don't even know where their lungs is...because [in] those days there wasn't much school" (Interview with Maryanne, February 2007). When discussing the lack of formal education within his own family, Darryl noted the potential for the use of visuals to assist with the learning process:

> [I]f you look at the area where most of us come from...[our] parents...left school since they were grade four [or] something. They will tell us that and...that's where the charts get in...because you can show it to them...My parents, my mommy actually, if you show it to her she will pick it up quicker. (Interview with Darryl, February 2007)

In the interviews it emerged that some of the community health workers and HIV literacy trainers and educators already used drawing as an educational tool.[7] The way that drawing can develop a person's understanding of HIV and the human body was described by Maryanne (HOPE Cape Town). She suggested that verbal explanations have a limited impact on people, especially if they have a low level of education:

And now sometimes I draw to show them...the body and then show them this is where it [HIV] can enter...because you get people that...can't write and read...so it's better that you use the drawings so now they understand what you are talking about. Because if you just telling them this is HIV...when you finish talking you will realize that that person actually knows nothing because now you are asking him a question, but he can't answer...so that's why I am using the drawing. (Interview with Maryanne, February 2007)

Another advantage of using visuals is the absence of medical terminology. This eliminates the power dynamics inherent in using jargon or academic language. The following comment comes from another HOPE Cape Town participant who had never used drawing as an educational tool, but had previously employed other participatory techniques such as role-play activities. Amanda explained why she thought drawing would be useful for HIV literacy education:

[I]t was simple because not all of them are literate and the examples we use when we do the drawing...makes it simple for the person to understand...their own bodies better, how the body functions...Because most of the time they are listening to you...but you don't know how much do they know...But if they are part and parcel of doing it themselves...if there is one who doesn't want to talk, it makes her also to be part of it...when we do the drawing...people will understand. (Interview with Amanda, January 2007)

Amanda also commented on drawing's ability to encourage participation and enable learners to demonstrate their new knowledge in the process. This is an important aspect of the learning process since it reinforces new understandings and also enables the facilitator to see whether or not participants have understood what has been discussed. Amanda also noted the potential for drawing to include reserved participants who lack confidence in expressing their opinions verbally, but are able to do so visually. She went on to identify the way that medical language can exclude people from understanding how their bodies work, making it difficult for them to engage with medical practitioners.

Charmaine (HOPE Cape Town) also identified the way that medical language immediately creates a power dynamic between those who can understand and speak it and those who cannot:

It's a nice way of getting to know about HIV in a...way that suits them...Because in training sometimes the words is up there [difficult] and we can't really talk together...And if you are illiterate you don't want to hear those words...because it scares you...The struggle is going to be there because some [people] feel maybe inferior. (Interview with Charmaine, February 2007)

In these examples, the community health workers supported the use of drawing as an HIV education-tool based on their previous experience and knowledge of how the people who attend their clinics and support groups typically react to medical language and information. Their projections proved to be true when compared with the responses of the group of HIV-positive mothers. While the mothers were able to read and write at a basic level, on the whole they did not have extensive formal educations. The group of mothers was drawn from an HIV clinic where two HOPE Cape Town community health workers were employed. In this way they provided an insight into the educational needs of the clients that the community health workers would see on a daily basis.

The mothers emphasized the ease with which they could learn visually. When asked if they thought that the creation of body map drawings had confused their understanding of how the human body works, Noluthanda replied:

> No, I think by drawing it is clear more than [if] you are taught... When you see it in drawing it is clear. You understand it more... because maybe if you learn about something that you don't see it's not easy to understand, but then you see it and it's easy to understand. (Interview with Noluthanda, April 2007)

The simplicity of learning about the human body with the creation of body map drawings and the use of the Visual Body Map was affirmed by two other mothers, Selena and Joy. In Selena's words: "We enjoy it because you can see such and such a part" (Interview with Selena, April 2007). They both drew attention to the ease of discussing illness and opportunistic infections by simply pointing out the different parts of the body that are affected. They suggested that by seeing where a particular organ is found in the human body, they could more readily understand the relationship between different organs and the way that the systems in the body are interconnected. The need to show people the part of their body that is causing their illness or show which organ is being affected by HIV was also echoed by Chantal from TAC:

> [S]ometimes [you] educate people about their body or their immune system and sometimes people don't actually understand what... you are saying about their bodies inside... and... that map will be very useful if you can use it in the clinics or in any training... You can exactly show the person that is the thing that is wrong. (Interview with Chantal, November 2007)

Similarly, Sipho (HOPE Cape Town) emphasized the need for patients to understand the interconnected nature of the human body, because it clarified the relationship between the immune system and the way that HIV affects the entire body. Like Chantal, Sipho also referred to the Visual Body Map and the simplicity of the visual representation of the human anatomy:

> I think all the exercises were very good, but the map... was good in the sense that... you also saw the interconnectedness between the veins, your immune system and... the cells with the body map. (Interview with Sipho, January 2007)

TAC trainer Nolwazi also noted the potential for the Visual Body Map to clarify the relationship between the immune system and the other systems in the body. The importance of understanding the link between the immune system and the rest of the body was considered vital by many of the workshop participants because in many ways it appeared to be the key to explaining how HIV and AIDS affects a person's health. Nolwazi believed that it was important for people to understand how the body works when it is healthy, before they learn about illness and infection. She believed that the use of visual education techniques such as the Visual Body Map and the body map drawings simplified this explanation enormously:

But first explain what is happening…without opportunistic infections, without HIV…It's important to show again how HIV attacks our bodies, especially…the different systems when we are doing the visual mapping…Then the person will see "OK if my immune system is not working that means other systems will be affected." (Interview with Nolwazi, November 2006)

Apart from the simplicity of using visual representations of the human body to educate patients and people from their communities, a further advantage of using the Visual Body Map and body map drawings is that they enable participants to relate the information that they are exposed to in the course of the workshop with their own bodily experience. By tracing around a human body as a starting point for the creation of the body map drawings, the connection between the drawing and the participants' own bodies was emphasized. This association highlighted the relevance of what the participants were learning while also reinforcing the personal nature of the participatory exercises. Sipho commented on this relationship:

[Y]ou can relate it to yourself because it was…[about] our own bodies, because we did our own drawings. So it was a reflection of our selves, as well as our anatomies and what is happening within our body systems…I find it very relevant…with what we are doing there at the clinics in the communities. (Interview with Sipho, January 2007)

Another community health worker, Celeste, also affirmed the ease with which people who had no biological or anatomical knowledge of the body would be able to relate to the material presented in the workshop. In reference to the potential use of the Visual Body Map, Celeste noted: "But then they will say 'That is my body, so if there are veins then I must also have veins.' So then it will let them wonder what is happening to [their] body" (Interview with Celeste, February 2007). In a similar way, her colleague Amanda noted the empowering potential of being able to show and explain to clients what is happening inside their bodies. Amanda commented on the importance of patients being able to "see it themselves," as opposed to being told they have a particular illness and leaving the clinic without having a basic understanding of the implications of their diagnosis. She explained:

It makes it easy to understand, because now they know what is going on in their body and how the HIV travels. How do I get pain and swollen? Why do I get a pain here? What are they talking about with a liver? Where is this liver? Sometimes people don't even know the first thing…And I think it is much easier so that you can even explain and show and they see it themselves, what it is all about. (Interview with Amanda, January 2007)

Apart from the advantages of people being able to relate the workshop material directly to their health and that of their clients, the usefulness of the body map drawings to illustrate complex concepts was further explained by TAC trainer and educator Nolwazi. She used the specific example of explaining the difference between HIV and AIDS using the body map drawings:

[S]o if you draw a human body that means you are able to show the people everything…where are the opportunistic infections that build up to AIDS. So

> it is very simple for a person to understand. Because the thing is out there;
> they do not know the difference between HIV and AIDS. And then when we
> have a human drawing we will say "OK this person is HIV-positive..." And
> then you place the opportunistic infections and then you say "This is AIDS."
> And so it is very simple and nice. (Interview with Nolwazi, November 2006)

This comment affirms the direct nature of visual learning and the use of body map drawings. Nolwazi went on to discuss ways the body map drawings could be used to demonstrate potential side effects that ART patients could experience. She suggested that if people were shown the areas on their bodies that could potentially be affected by side effects, there would be less fear. By being able to isolate the exact area, such as the example of the feet being affected by peripheral neuropathy, Nolwazi believed that patients would be able to grasp the idea that side effects are localized and can be controlled. She said that often patients think side effects can kill them and that this perception could potentially be changed by explaining the exact nature of the side effect, where in the body it is found, and how it can be avoided or treated.

Maryanne (HOPE Cape Town) commented on the potential for the Visual Body Map to be used to help explain medical procedures to patients and reduce their anxiety. For example, she suggested the use of the Visual Body Map in VCT sessions would make it easier for her to explain the need for a blood sample and to test for HIV antibodies:

> You can even use it in the [VCT] counseling...because a lot of people are
> scared because of the test and they don't know what's going to happen now.
> So...you can show them the [visual] body map and you can show them "OK,
> this is what's going to happen. There's your veins. Sister [nurse] just wants a
> little blood." And it makes it easier. (Interview with Maryanne, February
> 2007)

The creation of the body map drawings included a range of other visual exercises that did not use drawing to illustrate a particular concept. The response to the exercise involving the choice of healthy foods and meals, for example, was positive, because many of the participants noted the practical value of it. One of the community health workers, Pumla, suggested it would encourage debate not only on what foods to include, but also how the food was prepared:

> I also like your information...about the food. You give us papers so each and
> every person must go and take the picture and put the balanced diet. So it was
> easy for us because now we see there is [a picture of] chicken and you just cut
> it and put [paste] it down and then finish all the different types of food. So
> it...also makes us interested. (Interview with Pumla, January 2007)

Her closing remark about how the cutting and pasting held their interest is worth noting because it highlights the advantages of using material from real life, such as advertisements. As with the other exercises in the workshop, this exercise also involved group discussion. Pumla's response illustrates how in the course of the workshop the use of visual methods led to collaborative learning and group debate. The creation of body map drawings in small groups intended to ensure the involvement of all workshop participants and enabled them to drive the learning experience. In this way it was hoped that the information generated in the workshop would be relevant to their needs and could be used in their community work.

CONCLUSION

In this chapter, I recounted the planning and implementation process of a workshop that tested the potential for visual tools and techniques to be employed in South African HIV literacy programs. Three different groups attended the workshop: community health workers, HIV literacy educators and trainers, and a group of HIV-positive mothers. A mixed-method approach to data collection was adopted. This chapter focused specifically on the content of in-depth group interviews as a way of evaluating the potential successes and failures of a visual approach to increasing biomedical knowledge about HIV and AIDS, as well as social issues related to the disease. On the whole, the participants spoke positively about the ways the Visual Body Map and the creation of body map drawings facilitated learning within the workshop context. They also described how visual exercises and the Visual Body Map could be used in their work. In particular, they identified VCT, support groups, youth groups, work with schools, and counseling sessions as places where they could potentially make use of some of the workshop exercises, if not create the entire body map drawing.

The most obvious barriers to the implementation of the workshop were the cost of the materials and the lack of time. Every effort was made to keep the materials affordable, with the use of brown cardstock, chalk, colored pens, and wood glue. Nonetheless, the materials still require some funds, as well as time to collect and transport them to the workshop venue. Both HOPE Cape Town and TAC own their own Visual Body Maps and the educator's guides that accompany them, facilitating the ability to implement the body map drawing workshop as well as other educational activities. Despite the fact that the organizations owned their own Visual Body Maps and material expenses were kept to a minimum, however, the issue of having the time to run the workshops remained a serious obstacle. This was confirmed when many participants spoke frankly about the demands of their work and the fact that they are already overextended. The additional time needed to organize and facilitate a workshop appeared to be such a serious restraint that it looked doubtful as to whether future workshops could be run by the participants independently.

However, five months after facilitating the body map drawing workshop with the TAC treatment literacy educators and trainers, I was invited to attend the joint Western and Eastern Cape annual TAC training, where I conducted a morning session that used body map drawings in order to increase knowledge about human biology and how HIV affects different parts of the body. This suggests that the small group who initially received the training saw its value and wanted other members of their organization to be exposed to the body map drawing workshop. Furthermore, a follow-up visit ten months after the workshop was facilitated with the HOPE Cape Town community health workers revealed that some had in fact made use of the workshop exercises. One had created body maps with a youth group he led. The rest of the health workers said they referred to the workshop manual in education sessions. While the participants may not have gone on to conduct complete workshops, therefore, it appears that they did use the skills and information they received during the workshop, as well as some of the exercises. These observations suggest that if visual tools and techniques are introduced on an organizational level, there is increased opportunity to use them, and consequently they will more likely be implemented in the field. Such results depend on follow-up support by the organizations in the form of further training, as well as the availability of materials and the allocation of sufficient time for leading visual and participatory HIV literacy sessions.

In conclusion, the use of visual and collaborative approaches to learning was shown to be effective in presenting HIV literacy material in a straightforward way that people could readily apply to their lives and working environments. The significance of this finding is that visual and participatory techniques and tools helped participants develop understanding of the biomedical aspects of HIV in a way that was relevant to participant needs. Given the density and complexity of the biomedicine of HIV, it was exciting to see how the creation of body map drawings developed real understanding of human biology in relation to HIV prevention, care and treatment. However, given the small sample size, further research is clearly needed on the value of visual and participatory methods in HIV literacy contexts in order to explore the extent to which these findings apply elsewhere.

One of the unexpected outcomes of the research was the extent to which knowledge genuinely flowed in both directions. Participants learned about human biology, but they taught me about their lived experiences and their understandings about what needed to be done to combat the AIDS epidemic. Their views shifted my understanding of how HIV/AIDS impacts the daily lives of South Africans, especially those in socio-economically marginalized communities, and shaped the work and research I went on to do. Participatory learning methods thus have the potential to educate both the participants and the educators.

10

Ngoma Dialogue Circles (Ngoma-DiCe)

COMBATING HIV/AIDS USING LOCAL CULTURAL PERFORMANCE IN KENYA

Mjomba Majalia (St. Augustine
University of Tanzania)

INTRODUCTION

Throughout my fifteen years experience as a high school teacher, head teacher, and community leader in Kenya, I have observed many rural development projects fail mainly due to ineffective communication between social change agents and the people. In most cases, the *watu wa maendeleo* (Swahili for "social change agents") used local chiefs' meetings as a means to disseminate development messages. During such meetings, the urban-dwelling change agents would ceremoniously arrive in a convoy of big airplane-like cars, extraordinarily dressed, and exuding with sophistication. From a "high" table, distanced from the community, they would address the people as if they were empty vessels to be filled (Freire 1970). After lecturing and sloganeering, the change agents would leave ceremoniously pending a repeat of similar rituals.

In these *barazas* (assemblies), opportunities were rarely provided for the people to air their views so their needs and concerns could clearly be identified and addressed. Communication was clearly linear, top-down, expert-driven, and non-negotiable (Ascroft and Masilela 1989). My informal evaluation, through everyday interactions with the people, fairly consistently revealed that the community's discourse had little to do with the social change message being delivered from outside. Not surprisingly, the village gossip emanating from such *barazas* paid more attention to the convoy of big airplane-like cars, the urban aura, the dress of the change agents, and the pomp that took place that day. This was to me an indication that *watu wa maendeleo* more often than not fostered the wrong or unintended buzz among the target population.

For example, the introduction of a hybrid rooster that was meant to "better" the local chickens in Wongonyi village (I was a head teacher and local leader in this community from

1993–1997) never really took off. Instead, the effort failed because the communication strategies adopted by the concerned government officials ignored the people's local knowledge, ideas, feelings, cultural values, and messages in existing folk media. Consequently, government officials never managed to have a clear understanding of the strong cultural undercurrents and local myths that militated against introducing anything labeled "hybrid"; rather, Wongonyi's residents alleged the initiative to be a way for the government to implement family-planning measures.

In addition, the community held deep-seated beliefs about the hybrid rooster as less flavorful than the indigenous breed, more prone to diseases, more expensive to maintain, and not part of the local culture. My informal conversations with some of the government officers on why they thought the project failed revealed a fairly consistent prevailing attitude that it was because of the people's ignorance, laziness, and anti-development mindset. In my opinion, the hybrid rooster project in Wongonyi failed because the government officials did not adequately immerse themselves in the village. Had they done so, they would have been able to create dialogue and share information directed toward mutual understanding, mutual agreement, and collective action.

One of my major tasks, as a head teacher and local leader in Wongonyi location (an administrative region in Kenya), was to sensitize and mobilize the community to participate meaningfully in school development projects. Cognizant that a top-down communication approach alone may not be effective, and being a native as well as a teacher of creative traditional dramatized dance, I decided to experiment with some of the indigenous communication channels. Music and dance have been used since time immemorial among the Taita, the ethnic group found in Wongonyi, to entertain and educate the young in preparation for adult roles. Therefore, by having students inventively insert appropriate change messages in commonly used local Taita and Swahili cultural performances, I found out that they could effectively "talk" from within the experiences of the community and hence establish good rapport. Through a process called *kumaza*, which consists of a combination of drama, dance-song, talk-singing, poetry, and call-and-response, the students made their problems known to the community through respectful, nonthreatening, entertaining, and stimulating dialogue.

For the illiterate members of Wongonyi community, who constituted the majority, I observed that the repetitive and circular communication inherent in Taita cultural dance performances assisted in articulating and visualizing the central ideas of development messages. Since the creative dance-songs were based upon the locally spoken Taita and Swahili languages, moreover, the people could easily comprehend and understand the social change message being delivered. Finally, the vibrant drumbeats and repetitive call-and-response nature of the dance-songs were stimulating and hard to ignore, and thus naturally invited participation. This kind of involvement was especially true for the majority of the village women, who initially would start by "responding" to the "calls" from their seats; as the performances progressed, however, they shot up to participate actively in the dances, hence vicariously internalizing the message.

These observations and experiences invariably challenged me and raised a number of questions. Why are the indigenous, time-honored, and culturally relevant communications channels within rural communities in Kenya usually downplayed or totally ignored in communication for social change? Why are literate and Eurocentric communication approaches such as lecturing, brochures, posters, and so forth, valorized over the oral Afrocentric approaches such as dramatized dance-songs, poems, *mashairi, sarakasi,* etc., especially in rural communities where Eurocentric approaches seem to be ineffective? Is it that oral African-centered communication approaches lack the capacity to carry modern social change messages, such as family planning and HIV/AIDS prevention? Finally, given the fact that these indigenous, participatory communication modes are still alive and vibrant in many rural communities in Kenya, how can they be creatively utilized to effect social change?

PURPOSE OF THE STUDY

I initiated my participatory communication research to overcome three major challenges in designing HIV/AIDS intervention programs aimed at the youth in Kenyan schools:

1. Move away from the top-down lecture/teaching/preaching approach and make the intervention program more participatory at all stages of development.

2. Minimize the cultural distance between health promoter (teacher, health professional, AIDS activist, etc.) and the health receiver (youth).

3. Find appropriate language(s) for articulating HIV/AIDS in a realistic and intelligible manner for youth, i.e., a verbal and non-verbal communication channel that could assist in achieving shared meaning between health promoter and health receiver.

SIGNIFICANCE OF THE STUDY

This study put in place a school-based HIV/AIDS intervention program that tested ways *ngoma* (local cultural performances in Kenya that include song, dance, poetry, talk-singing and proverbs) could be used to mobilize youth in Kenyan schools so they could take ownership of the fight against HIV/AIDS. The results of this work provide substantive ideas for further study and theorizing on problem posing, entertaining, creative *ngoma* as a participatory communication strategy. By valorizing the thoughtful practical application of African-centered cultural media/resources, I argue, we can enhance young people's abilities to solve their own problems. This study also adds insights on the rhetorical agency of local cultural performances and their immense potential to organize and mobilize for social change within grassroots communities in Africa.

STATEMENT OF THE PROBLEM

The HIV/AIDS epidemic in Kenya presents a number of challenges for young people. Candid discussions about safe sex, condom use, and HIV/AIDS are still a cultural taboo. Unemployment, poverty, parental death from AIDS, and other harsh social realities often place the youth in a vulnerable position. After a slow start, the Kenyan government finally began to take some measures to combat the epidemic. In late 1999, President Daniel arap Moi declared the epidemic a national disaster and set up the National AIDS Control Council (NACC). This council helped mobilize and coordinate resources for preventing HIV transmission and providing care and support to the infected and affected people in Kenya (NACC 2001). After many years of resistance to school-based HIV/AIDS intervention programs, especially on the part of religious organizations, the Ministry of Education finally distributed curriculum material for both primary and secondary schools in 2001. These materials offer basic facts about HIV/AIDS, and include a teacher's guide listing objectives and main points to be covered in the various lessons.

Teaching about HIV/AIDS may have been helpful in increasing awareness, but more participation and involvement of the youth was needed for effective social change. Research findings based on twelve school-based sex education programs from developing countries around the world indicated that "chalk and talk" was not enough (Scalway 2001). For example, in Zimbabwe researchers compared a lecture on AIDS prevention with a session in which students put a condom on a model and practiced negotiating condom use. When interviewed four months later, those who took the practical skill course knew more about condoms and reported having fewer sexual partners than those who attended the lecture only (Scalway 2001).

Sexual health and HIV/AIDS are emotional and sensitive topics, which more often than not increase the already existing cultural distance between resource providers (teachers, health professionals, parents) and young people. Effective communication between the two thus becomes almost impossible, a situation exacerbated by two major issues. One issue is the generation gap that emanates from age differences. It is customary for the youth in African societies to show great respect toward their elders. Consequently, there are various sensitive topics such as menarche, wet dreams, sex, and HIV/AIDS that young people find extremely difficult, if not impossible, to discuss with adults. The other issue is education itself, which can be linked to differences in socioeconomic status, expert knowledge, and position in society. In general, those who are educated and work for the government or other reputable organizations in Kenya—such as medical practitioners, engineers, and teachers—tend to be alienated from the general public.

From my experiences as a high school teacher and head teacher in Kenya, I am aware that young people tend to detest authority figures, especially those that show no concern for their welfare. In addition, while using the current official school system of reward and punishment to diffuse HIV/AIDS prevention information may increase awareness, it may not be effective in securing widespread adoption and practices among the youth. Kothari and Kothari (1997) argue that when health receivers distrust or are afraid of the health promoter then bonding problems arise, leading to a lack of both the understanding and cooperation required to deliver high quality health services. Therefore one major challenge in designing HIV/AIDS intervention programs for the youth in Kenya has been finding ways to bridge the cultural gap between the resource providers and the young people.

Another challenge in designing HIV/AIDS interventions for youth has been finding an appropriate language to articulate the disease in a manner that reflects young people's reality. This challenge requires finding verbal and nonverbal communication channels that could assist in creating shared meanings between health promoters and young people. A statement by male representatives from an AIDS Committee of Mathare Youth Sports Association in Kenya is indicative of this need. These representatives clearly state that resource providers need to "start teaching about AIDS in our school curriculum—in a language understood by the youth" (Scalway 2001, 7).

Available literature (Human Rights Watch 2001, Nduati and Kiai 1997, Onyango 2001, UNAIDS 2001, Singhal and Rogers 2003) and my personal experiences as a native of Kenya indicate that HIV/AIDS is not only viewed differently from a Western perspective, but is also viewed differently from one cultural group to the other. These differences, some subtle, others conspicuous, stem from preexisting cultural groupings such as adults vs. youth, medical vs. non-medical/public, male vs. female, literate vs. illiterate, rural vs. urban, coastal vs.

upcountry, and Luo vs. Taita. Studies continually suggest that effective communication is difficult when two parties have different cultural values associated with health and disease, and point to the need to use trained interpreters or intermediaries in order to provide health services efficiently (Fadiman 1997, Katalanos 1994, Kothari and Kothari 1997, Kaufert and Putsch 1997).

To make a dent in the fight against HIV/AIDS infections among the youth, then, intervention programs need to acknowledge and be sensitive to these underlying challenges. Airhihenbuwa (1995) laments the valorization of Eurocentrism in the production and acquisition of health knowledge and behavior, coupled with the continued suppression of cultural expressions of non-Western peoples. He strongly advocates for the inscription of local culture at the root of all health promotion and disease prevention programs, at least in some manner that legitimates local culture's importance in public health praxis. Airhihenbuwa points out:

> This process of engaging teachers/interventionists and students/audiences in the production of meaning, value, pleasure, and knowledge should be central to the mission of health promotion and education. It is only through such dialogue that varied cultural expressions and meanings are affirmed and centralized, and the production of cultural identity can be legitimating and empowering relative to promoting individual, family, community, and societal health. (1995, xiv)

Onyango (2001), in advocating for a cultural approach in HIV/AIDS prevention and care, asserts that when creating a health intervention, the target group's own cultural resources should be considered as a building framework for strategies and sustainable social action. Singhal and Rogers (2003), meanwhile, posit that HIV/AIDS interventions should go beyond the conventional mass media to include other culturally situated expressions. They use as their example *khangas*, the traditional fabric wraps commonly worn by women in East Africa, which are now used to carry HIV prevention messages.

UNAIDS' local responses, moreover, emphasize convincing a target audience to see HIV/AIDS as their *own* problem, rather than as a government agenda (Singhal and Rogers 2003). The purpose of such facilitation is to empower local actors to take responsibility for finding solutions to their AIDS problem in a fashion that is appropriate to them. I consequently believe that the young people in Kenyan schools, provided with resources, are capable of controlling the spread of HIV/AIDS among their peers. Like any other cultural group, Kenyan youths have the innate potential to bring about their own change in response to HIV/AIDS, as long as they are provided with what I describe as "activation energy" to get them mobilized. Consonant with the cultural approach advocated by the UNAIDS communication framework, my own participatory communication research aimed to investigate how the ubiquitous local *ngoma* performances in Kenyan schools could be used to conscientize and empower the youth to own the fight against on HIV/AIDS. The following research questions guided this study:

Research Questions

- How can *ngoma* be used to carry and convey current social change messages on HIV/AIDS prevention to the youth in Kenyan schools?

- How can *ngoma* be used to trigger and sustain candid dialogues on HIV/AIDS among the youth in Kenyan schools?

- How can *ngoma* be used to introduce the youth in Kenyan schools to a critical form of thinking about HIV/AIDS so as to transform their attitudes?

- How can *ngoma* be used to mobilize the youth in Kenyan schools to shift from the position of **spectator** (passive beings) to the position of **spect-actor** (active beings) so as to take ownership of the fight against HIV/AIDS?

- How can *ngoma* be used to reduce the cultural distance between HIV/AIDS resource providers and youth in Kenyan schools?

YOUNG PEOPLE AND HIV/AIDS

HIV/AIDS has triggered national emergencies around the world. In any society, most infectious diseases tend to kill those who are weak such as the old or infants. AIDS, however, "like war, kills those in the prime of life. Indeed, in one way it is worse than war. When armies fight, it is predominantly young men who are killed. AIDS kills young women, too" (*Economist* 2000, 177). At the time of doing this study, Human Rights Watch (2001) reported that twenty-two million people had died from the scourge and over thirty-six million were infected, which meant that the worst was yet to come. With 80 percent of the twenty-two million deaths occurring in sub-Saharan Africa, AIDS had become a problem of unprecedented magnitude in the continent.

Young people are vulnerable to HIV/AIDS infection because of risky sexual behavior, high incidences of drug abuse, and lack of access to coherent HIV information and prevention services (UNAIDS 2001). Young women in particular are more likely to become infected, since they are susceptible to sexual violence, coerced sex, and unequal power relationships. When conducting its 2001 study, UNAIDS (2001) reported that in nearly twenty African countries, 5 percent or more of women aged fifteen to twenty-four were infected. Exposure to conflicting messages through television, family, school, and religious institutions about sex, HIV, and behavior that is immoral, fashionable, or irresponsible often leaves young people confused about HIV. Hence lack of proper knowledge about AIDS may lead to decisions on sexual health and partnerships that are based on superstition, harmful gender stereotypes, the latest youth culture, or some other form of non-scientific information (Scalway 2001).

Since there is no known cure for AIDS, prevention is one major intervention strategy being used to curb the scourge. The fact that HIV is mainly transmitted through sexual contact implies that communication for social change, at both the individual and community levels, is an important element in the fight against AIDS among young people (Singhal and Rogers 2003). But what is communication for social change?

COMMUNICATION FOR SOCIAL CHANGE

A working paper produced by the Rockefeller Foundation (Figueroa et al. 2002), "Communication for Social Change: An Integrated Model for Measuring the Process and Its Outcome," defined participatory communication as the social process where people come together to define who they are, what they want, and how they can obtain what they want. Groups with common interests jointly construct messages for improving their existential situations and changing unjust social structures. Participatory communication for social change therefore focuses on using direct, grass roots, many-to-many communication, using models that spring from the affected communities (Gray-Felder 1999). It is communication that gives voice to the previously unheard and communication that has a bias towards local content and ownership.

Scholarship points to two major approaches to participatory communication. One is Freire's (1970) pedagogy of dialogical communication; the other evolves from the ideas of access, participation and self-management articulated in the UNESCO debates in the 1970s (Servaes 1996). My research project was based on the first approach, developing substantive ideas from Freire's (1970) and Boal's (2000) comprehensive theoretical and practical body of knowledge, and combining those ideas with entertainment-education theory (Singhal and Rogers 1999).

Freire's Pedagogy of Dialogical Communication

Freire's *Pedagogy of the Oppressed* (1970), which introduces individuals to a critical form of thinking about their world, has been widely applied in various participatory communication approaches. His theory is based on the conviction that every human being, no matter how "ignorant" or "submerged" in a "culture of silence" is capable of looking critically at the world in a dialogical encounter with others. Provided with the proper tools for such dialogical encounter, the individual can gradually perceive his or her personal and social reality, and deal critically with it. In this process, the old paternalistic depositor-depository relationship, where the teacher is the depositor and the learner a depository, can be overcome.

In Freire's proposed pedagogy of the oppressed, the teacher/social change agent is no longer an authority, but a facilitator: someone who both learns and teaches in dialogue with other fellow learner-teachers. In the conscientization process, Freire used a photograph, a picture, or a drawing representing the existing reality to initiate a discussion. The participants would be encouraged to question why things were as they were, what could be done to rectify the situation, and so forth. Communication channels thus helped generate dialogue, allowing people to talk to and understand each other. This method therefore moved away from the conventional top-down development communication approach, which Freire described as perpetuating the culture of silence of the dispossessed. It has since had wider application in entertainment-education communication strategies (Singhal and Rogers 1999) and Boal's *Theatre of the Oppressed* (2000).

Entertainment-Education Strategy

Entertainment-education is a strategy that has applied Freire's methods in an attempt to make mass-mediated messages more participatory. By purposely designing and implementing a media message to both entertain and educate in order to increase knowledge about an educational issue, people who engage in this strategy aim to increase favorable attitudes and thereby bring about social change (Singhal and Rogers 1999). These messages can stimulate dialogue among audience members, moreover, creating opportunities for social change at both individual and community levels. For example, analyses of *Tinka Tinka Sukh*, an entertainment-education soap opera in India (Papa et al. 2000), suggested that a more participatory strategy could lead to behavior change based on the degree to which audience members publicly react to media characters and discuss them with other audience members. Reflecting on the educational themes present in a media program can also help viewers recognize behavioral alternatives in their lives. This interaction creates a socially constructed learning environment in which people evaluate previously held ideas, consider alternatives, and identify steps to initiate social change.

Boal's Theatre of the Oppressed

Boal began developing his Theatre of the Oppressed in 1956, at the Arena theatre in São Paulo, Brazil. Influenced by Freire, Boal developed a series of imaginative theatre exercises to transform the theatrical experience from "monologues" of traditional performance into a "dialogue" between audience and stage. Boal's interactive, dialogic, problem-posing, reflective, and conscientizing techniques have since been used by labor, community organizers, and educators all over the world as participatory tools for democratizing organizations, analyzing social problems, and transforming reality into direct action. Boal employed Freire's methods on a major scale for the first time in his experiments with the People's Theatre in Lima and Chiclayo, Peru. He worked with ALFIN, a literacy campaign that began in 1973 with the objective of eradicating illiteracy in Peru (Boal 2000).

Aware that teaching an adult to read and write posed a difficult and delicate problem, the ALFIN project formulated two principal aims. First, to teach literacy in both a participant's first language and in Spanish without forcing the abandonment of the former in favor of the latter. Second, to teach literacy in all possible expressive languages, especially the artistic ones such as theatre, photography, puppetry, film, and journalism (Boal 2000). To Boal, theatre constituted a language capable of being utilized by any person, with or without artistic talent, to mobilize passive beings or spectators into "spect-actors," activated spectators/audience members who take part in the action. His work has precipitated the wide use of local theatres and cultural performances as participatory communication approaches to social change.

As a teacher and dancer-choreographer with many years experience in creative cultural dramatized dance performances in Kenya, I envisioned great potential in the role that this approach, through the medium of *ngoma*, could play in organizing and mobilizing for social change in my own community.

Problem-Posing, Entertaining, Creative *Ngoma* for Social Change

Ngoma, a local cultural performance practice in Kenya, refers to a diverse musical setting involving a combination of drum, song, poetry, drama, dancing, and storytelling. To some, *ngoma* is an avenue where differences are aired and then defended, resolved, or stabilized in less threatening ways (Gunderson and Barz 2000). Like other cultural performances in Africa, it is not a separate art but part of the whole complex of everyday life. Based on the indigenous oral languages, *ngoma* contains a mosaic of information and skills meant to be "entertainment in the sense of involved enjoyment; it is moral instructions; it is also a matter of life and death and communal survival" (Thiong'o 1986, 23).

Turner's *Anthropology of Performance* (1987) posits that cultural performance functions as a special form of public address and rhetorical agency. According to Turner, it is through cultural performance that many people both construct and participate in public life. This assertion is particularly true for the poor and marginalized people denied access to middle-class public forums. For example, in my ethnic group, the Taita from the coastal region of Kenya, cultural performances such as the dance *ngoma ra mwazindika* act as venues for public discussion of vital issues important to the community, as well as arenas for gaining visibility and staging identity. Therefore *ngoma* provides basic rhetorical structures that allow the people to engage in dialogue and self-reflection.

A further elaboration on a specific type of *ngoma ra mwazindika* that dwells on the theme of hunger or *njala* among the Taita should provide a better picture. This practice is a local cultural performance that articulates a hunger situation and provides tips on how to cope in the future. Through entertainment-education (i.e., drama, dance, song, poems, and talk-singing), the performers try to show the audience all that is experienced during the hunger period convincingly, and provide "solutions" in case hunger should strike members of the audience. Such articulation not only helps capture a difficult situation but it also suggests helpful motives for the people to embrace in confronting their trials. Similarly, since the dance performance invites participation in its rhythms, it enables the people to process the situation actively. By having *wachemshangoma* (performers) engage the audience through an entertaining and participatory call-and-response fashion, organizers can vicariously assist the people in understanding the dangers of hunger.

Ngoma was officially revived in the Kenyan school curriculum during the 1980s to promote cultural creativity, entertainment, and education, while shaping young people's cultural identities. The fact that *ngoma* is inherently dialogic and theatrical in nature, and is already entrenched in Kenyan schools, made it an ideal medium for this participatory communication research project.

METHODOLOGY

My project involved participatory communication research, a form of inquiry in which participants and researcher generated knowledge together through collaborative communicative processes. The roles of the researcher and the researched constantly changed, with the interaction aiming to foster a meaningful pedagogical environment for all participants. Participatory researches do not follow rigid designs; thus they challenge investigators to be inventive about the range of methods that could be used by the people themselves (Tandon 1981).

I conducted my research in the Murray Girls and Kenyatta Boys High Schools in the Taita/Taveta district in Kenya. These schools are full boarding schools, where students study for three months at a time before going home for a one-month holiday. Over 85 percent of the student population comes from the coastal province, and most are fluent in Swahili, English, and a native language. (Native languages spoken by the different ethnic groups in the coastal region of Kenya are quite similar and can be understood by a majority of people across the groups.) The ages of the students ranged from fourteen to twenty-one years, and they came from a variety of socioeconomic backgrounds. The two projects, one in each school, ran concurrently for a period of six months (April–September 2003) and a total of about seventy-five participants (seventy students, two teachers, two research assistants, and one researcher) were involved in the exercise. Ethnographic methods of collecting data that included writing thick descriptive fieldnotes, participant observation, informal conversations, in-depth unstructured interviews, and video and audiotapes served a crucial part in this study.

In this investigation, I intended to use my insider status in multiple contexts (native, former teacher and administrator in several schools in the area, youth leader, *ngoma* teacher/ performer, father, and community leader) to establish trust and rapport, which were crucial prerequisites for conducting such a study. Since "a village raises a child" in the Taita district, I also felt compelled to go and give back to my community that has contributed a lot to make me what I am today.

RESULTS OF THE STUDY

Letters of introduction, copies of my research permit from the Kenyan government, personal vita and other relevant documents were sent to the principals of the two schools in April 2003. This initial contact led to telephone calls about two weeks later, and an appointment to visit the schools when they opened in early May. Due to the location of where I stayed and its proximity to Kenyatta high school, I was able to meet informally with Kenyatta's principal, a former colleague and friend, several times before the date of appointment. This early interaction was instrumental in setting the ball rolling much earlier in Kenyatta than in Murray.

In the first week of May I had my first formal meeting with the principal of the Kenyatta school. His reception was warm and cordial. I made it clear to the principal the purposes of my research project and what I required from the school. He was enthused by my research idea and suggested I work with the Peer Guidance and Counseling club. Then he introduced me to the patron teacher in charge of the club, and we set an appointment to meet the student committee responsible for running the club's affairs.

On my next visit, I met the student committee. This was a brief meeting lasting about forty minutes where we got to know each other and set a date for officially meeting the entire club membership. During this meeting day, the patron introduced me to the club members and excused himself. What transpired is better stated by these notes from my field notebook:

> There were about 40 students in the room. They introduced themselves giving their name and class. It was a mixed lot consisting of students from form one to four [roughly equivalent to American grades nine through twelve]. A majority was in upper level classes and they were prefects, dormitory captain, games captain, entertainment captain etc.; they held some responsible position in the school...The main purpose of the club is to counsel others. This is done either in a group or one-on-one. How? Teachers recommend discipline cases to them. They also give speeches and do short drama skits during general school assemblies on some Fridays to counsel the others on various issues affecting them...The members got some basic training on guidance and counseling through the teacher-in-charge and a local community-based organization that came in once to provide some basic training. The club has been on for six years.

During this first meeting with the club members, I introduced myself in detail and made it clear that I was on their side. I stated the purposes of the research and made apparent that despite my status as a teacher and head teacher in several schools in the area for many years, I was now a student like them who is out to share and learn during this particular participatory study. I also clearly spelled out to them that the project cannot be carried out without a sense of mutual understanding and trust among all participants. I then helped facilitate discussion and provided a lot of room and time for questions so as to clarify any issues that were not clear to them. Many asked questions about my life in Kenya, but showed particular interest in my time in the United States. There was apparent heightened eagerness on the part of the club members to study one day in the United States.

I proceeded to show the club members videos of my creative *ngoma* work in the United States and other works by other artists. At the end of the forty-five-minute show, I asked for ideas on how we could get started formulating creative *ngoma* pieces for our project. My field-notes capture the kinds of ideas that were forthcoming on that day:

> Many ideas came out. One student talked about having a picture of his girl-friend on one hand and a textbook opened, as if reading it, on the other. From this depiction he would create a discussion by asking his fellow students which one is good for us? Another suggested having some drumming on the background while rapping messages on HIV/AIDS prevention. His rationale was that rap is really the "in-thing" among the youth in the school and hence bound to compel their attention. There was also a suggestion about using popular musical beats by famous Kenyan artists in the background to sing message[s about] HIV/AIDS. The popular beats would surely be a good atten-tion-getter for the youth. Some other suggestions were about having mixed discussions between boys and girls as the youth involved both sexes. I thought about having Murray girls coming over some weekends to Kenyatta to have joint sessions...It was decided that they students write ideas on creative *ngoma* pieces on paper that come to mind and pass them to the chairman any-time along the coming weeks. We agreed to meet twice a week.

It wasn't until the end of the second week of May that I had an opportunity to meet the principal of Murray Girls School. I described the purposes and requirements of my research project, and she recommended I work with the True Love Waits club members. This club consisted of about forty girls who met every Wednesday to discuss various issues concerning their well-being. They also worked on promoting abstinence among themselves and their peers. I was intro-duced to the patron and set a day to meet the members of the club.

The following Wednesday, at my meeting with the True Love Waits club members, I talked about my study and what I required from them just as I did with the boys in Kenyatta. I also delved into the virtues of working hard, the determination to succeed in life against all odds, and the hope that I would challenge and inspire them to follow in my footsteps. This is part of what I told them:

> [Y]ou can see I do not have three eyes, or three legs, I am just like you born and raised in the villages of Taita. If I did it you can also go to study in the U.S. All you need is to dream big...The girls seemed really captivated and got some good rapport with the message sinking well as indicated by the questions aris-ing. How did you get your way round in America? How can I apply for Universities there? Can you help me?

Students are usually respectful of teachers and adults to the point of fearing and being suspi-cious of them. My gut feeling is that this kind of interaction was crucial in clearly revealing my intention to them, indicating that I was totally on their side in this participatory research in order to gain their trust.

The next meeting with the True Love Waits club members was a challenge but it did finally work out, as this excerpt from my fieldnotes indicates:

> I meet Faith, a trained peer counselor working as my research assistant. As we drive to Murray, the car overheats because of the steep climb. We stop and let

it cool. At Murray, first I was told that I could not meet the girls; I insisted that the headmistress had assured me to come this day. T[he] teacher on duty was not very cooperative. [I] sent word with a student and some members of the club were found. Once gathered in a classroom, I introduced the business of the day. I showed videos of my work in the U.S. to boost their morale and provided fertile grounds for ideas to flourish...[Their] response was very positive judging from levels of applause and hands clapping after the show. One girl said she wants to do a dance in Giriama, her native tongue. Another girl emphasized being proud of their culture and not aping the west. Faith, my research assistant, introduced herself to the students. She also seemed enthused by the videos and talked about working with the girls in getting ideas for their creative *ngoma* pieces.

In both schools, it was during these initial meetings that I planted the seeds for developing creative and entertaining *ngoma* pieces that problematized the HIV/AIDS situation. The idea was for the students to try and come up with a *shairi* (poem), *ngoma ya kitamaduni* (traditional dance-song), *wimbo* (song), or *sarakasi* (skit) that was three to five minutes long and had the capability to trigger a heated dialogue among their peers.

Decoding of the Project Site

Once the participants had agreed to the participatory communication research project, I worked on establishing a rapport with them. My main activity during this phase involved several visits to the project sites with the aim of understanding the dynamics of the school community. I observed the everyday lives of the group members and their routines. I also learned, through informal conversations with the students, how they interacted in their class sessions, their dormitories, the dining hall, and the places where they spent their leisure time. In addition, I held informal conversations with some teachers, especially those involved with the Peer Guidance and Counseling club in Kenyatta High School and True Love Waits club in Murray Girls.

During this phase, the students and I also settled on some key details for the project. In line with Boal's work, we decided to use all spoken languages for creating the *ngoma* works: Swahili, English, and *Sheng* (a slang-like mix of English, Swahili, and native tongues). In cases where native tongues were used in creative *ngoma* pieces, the user would translate the central idea of the message into either one of the other two languages. After a couple of meetings, we also settled on meeting times to fit their busy curricular and extracurricular schedules: Mondays and Sundays for Murray meeting sessions, and Tuesdays and Saturdays at Kenyatta. Weekday sessions were short, about one and a half hours, because students were tired after a long day in class and they had to have time to prepare for supper and evening study. On the weekends we met during the afternoons. These sessions were longer, about two and a half to three hours, during which they were more relaxed and seemed eager to do something other than schoolwork. While initially our meeting location varied, we eventually found ourselves able to use the same room with relative consistency.

We also discussed how large should the group be, who else should be part of the dialogue circles apart from the club members, and how the evaluation of the creative *ngoma* pieces should be done. Ultimately, we decided that having more than forty members could be counterproductive for an effective dialogue circle; such a size would not give adequate time to everyone to actively participate within a two-hour session. We also agreed that health professionals, HIV/AIDS activists, and resource persons could be invited to share their experiences and provide facts and knowledge on the disease. However, due to lack of funds, professionals were not involved in these projects apart from the research assistants and patrons of the concerned clubs. Finally, we also looked at three options for evaluation procedures: (1) having brief evaluation meetings after each session, (2) holding longer meetings after a couple of sessions, and (3) holding an evaluation workshop at the end of the whole exercise. The members settled on the first option. Thus, after each *ngoma* circle, we held brief meetings to evaluate the sessions citing what worked, what did not work and what needed improvement during the next meeting. The meetings also served to clarify my role as a co-enactor, organizer, and coordinator of the whole project, as I worked toward creating an enabling atmosphere of trust, rapport, and bonding between all the participants.

My most important task during this phase was to come up with themes for the creative *ngoma* pieces they were at work on. To begin, I interviewed the members to find out what educational campaigns on HIV/AIDS they had encountered in their respective communities, including posters, notices, announcements, and lectures. At Kenyatta I then asked them to take some of the themes that they dealt with during Friday morning assemblies, where the counselors would come out to make short speeches or skits, and creatively attempt to insert them in the *ngoma* pieces. Other questions that I tried to investigate concerned the school community "gossip," and the manner in which the group members talked about their reproductive health and HIV/AIDS. I also asked whether group members knew of any deaths/sicknesses of other members through direct or indirect relation to AIDS. What were their imagined lifestyles in a world of HIV/AIDS?

I found out that the club members in both schools were fairly well-informed on matters of HIV/AIDS: fully conversant with its modes of transmission and aware that there was no cure. Both schools had shown videos on the dangers of contracting HIV/AIDS, including *The Silent Epidemic* (sponsored by UNICEF Kenya and produced by Ace Communication Studios), a twenty-minute video depicting horrifying pictures of HIV/AIDS-related ailments. Both clubs were also aware of the magazine *Straight Talk*, a monthly pull-out from the *East African Standard* newspaper devoted to teen reproductive health, HIV/AIDS, and other issues pertaining to young people. Some of the True Love Waits club members in Murray had published short articles in this magazine. I also came across a resource book used by the True Love Waits club patron titled *Bloom or Doom*, which provided some tips on preventive measures for HIV/AIDS for the youth in schools. It was produced by the Kenya Institute of Education (KIE), a government body in charge of curriculum development in many Kenyan institutions of learning.

After a number of visits (approximately six at each project site) and many discussions emanating from the agreed-upon protocol, participants began to base their problem-posing, entertainment pieces on a number of themes: peer pressure, parental and other authority figures' pressure to conform, societal norms and values that put pressure on the youth, teenage pregnancy, boy-girl relationships, abortions, adoptions of orphans, support person/groups for the youth, drug abuse and its effect on youth, sexually transmitted diseases such as AIDS, and adolescence/secondary development. It is important to note that during this phase, the development and testing of creative *ngoma* pieces took place at every meeting, even as the participants themselves felt frustrated from the lack of resources and the pressures of other school and social commitments. Here I outline two of the scenarios as recorded in my field notebook:

> Fatuma presents a Giriama song; call and response is evident and so is the drumming. After the dance, she explains the central idea in English—that it is warning the girls on HIV/AIDS. It is very dangerous, it is killing many par-

ents and orphans are out there not getting their basic needs. She warns the girls to be very careful about how they carry themselves out there.

Christine Zighe and Susan Wawuda do a short skit in Swahili mixed with *Sheng*. The story line is about a strict mother who doesn't allow her daughter to go out for discos. Girls were laughing, which seemed like the story resonated well with them....This may be because it touched on a subject common to most teenage girls, mother-daughter conflict.

Ngoma Dialogue Circles

The objective of these *ngoma* dialogue circles was to present, through problem-posing, entertaining, creative *ngoma*, issues on HIV/AIDS that challenged the club members to think critically. During these sessions, participants sat in a large circle. Each session usually started with a dance-song; call-and-response mode was used to create a non-threatening and enabling atmosphere for stimulating dialogues (Gunderson 2000). *Wachemshangoma* (peer educators) were employed to problematize and spark group discussion around the controversies stemming from HIV/AIDS issues. The creative *ngoma* pieces that followed each took about two to three minutes. Each episode triggered a heated debate that lasted between fifteen to twenty minutes. The group members were asked to respond in any agreed-upon language as long as it was intelligible to the others. *Wachemshangoma* also helped the group transition to the next creative *ngoma* piece after the discussion seemed to slow. I coordinated and facilitated direction of the dialogue when needed, making efforts to represent HIV/AIDS-related themes familiar to the youth so that the club members could easily recognize the situations and hence their own relation to them. These themes included mother-daughter conflict, Matatu-mania,[1] and boy-girl relationships. There were various kinds of creative *ngoma* pieces presented in English and Swahili, including short skits, songs, poems, parables, and dramas.

Here I capture a scene of the Matatu-mania creative *ngoma* piece during the video-filming session at the Murray Girls School (all creative *ngoma* pieces were filmed during one session of about five hours in each school):

Preamble: Dance song begins with calls from dancer and responses from the audience members. This is used to set the mood for discussion. The song comes from the Giriama community. The central idea is that someone had been infected by AIDS, therefore the girls needed to be careful about the disease.

Matatu-mania: Scene one (A three-episode creative *ngoma* piece in Swahili). The scene starts with the *matatu tout* [conductor] shouting the vehicle's destination in characteristic fashion of the trade. A beautiful schoolgirl in uniform appears and the *tout* stops to admire her. The *tout* approaches her. Greetings are exchanged and he goes ahead and tries to seduce her. There is a typical boy-girl interaction and the short episode ends with the *tout* asking the schoolgirl to meet him the next day (scene runs for about two minutes).

The actors paused to trigger discussion by asking the participants what they thought would happen next. Would the schoolgirl show up the next day for the date? If so, they were to give a reason for their answer. It was made clear that there was no correct answer and all that was required was a personal opinion. As schoolgirls who might be faced by such situations, they were asked to decide what they would have done in this particular case. A heated discussion ensued, and the striking thing about most of the statements made was that they started with *kama ange-likuwa mimi*, meaning "If it were me." I feel this phrase put students in the position of the actor, forcing them to think critically of appropriate actions that they would have to take in such a scenario. Consider some of the statements that were made and the ensuing dialogue:

> *Mimi naona hangeenda, ana mwambia ili mambo yaishe.* (I do not see her going, just bluffing the guy to leave her alone.)

> *Mimi naona vile msichana alikuwa anajibu alikuwa anamwambia atakuja ili mambo yaishe.* (I think the way the girl was answering she will not show up. She just wants to get it over with and that is why she is said yes.)

> I think she will go because she wants money. *Touts* have a lot of money.

> She will go because she wants to get free lifts from the *tout*.

> She will go so that she can boast to other friends.

> She will go because school girls are always easily influenced by *manamba* (*touts*) especially Tudor *manambas* who put on designer clothes.

FACILITATOR: *Kwa nini manamba aende na mtoto wa shule? Kwani wana nini kinacho wavutia wasichana wa shule?* (Why do *touts* tend to lure schoolgirls easily into having sexual relations with them? What attracts schoolgirls to them?)

RESPONSE: Great cars, new cars, good music, fashion, designer clothes, schoolgirls want to be associated with *touts*. *Touts* have money, for the quick cash.

The dialogue went on for about fifteen minutes before the second episode, lasting about two minutes, came in. During this episode, the *tout* is seen waiting for the schoolgirl. He is cursing and wondering why the girl was taking so long to show up; but then the girl finally shows up. There is the typical boy-girl interaction. They agree to go somewhere as long as it does not take long because the schoolgirl says she does not want to be late. They leave the stage and trigger the question: What do you think they had gone to do and why do you think so? Another fifteen-minute discussion ensued before episode three. Episode three is a doctor-patient scene. The schoolgirl is seen coughing and looking terribly sick. The doctor takes some tests and calls in the mother. The mother wails and the episode ends. The trigger question here was: Why do you think the mother of the girl wailed after getting the results from the doctor?

Recording of *Ngoma* Dialogue Circles and Viewing of Tapes

I recorded *ngoma* dialogue circles for research analysis during a one-day session. Another day was designated for viewing the recorded tapes, for celebrating the end of the research project, and for distributing small tokens to all club members. I noted during the viewing that the participants expressed great interest in watching their own presentations:

> Excited to see themselves on tape, themes and messages resonated with them
> as the creative *ngoma* depicted the social world/AIDS in a manner intelligible

to them. [I thus] felt that this could be an efficacious strategy to reach other youth because they could see their peers on tape, [and] relate to the message. [I]t is more sensitive to their feelings, entertaining, non-threatening and thus can make them open up/candidly discuss [and] enrich the discourse on HIV/ AIDS.

Some of the comments by the participants quoted verbatim tell it all:

I believe that this presentation will really help other youth[,] especially [in developing] the skill [of] dealing with family matters. I hope parents will start understanding us youth and also give us the freedom we need. The advice we get will help us and other youths. Thanks you so much Mr. Mjomba for giving us the chance to air out our view. Have a nice time!

I had a great time. I learnt a lot and was taught a lot. It was actually my first time to act and be taped. I think that what the youth are doing is great. We have to get things out in the open and create awareness. We youth have to get our priorities straight. I am glad you gave us that opportunity to air our views.

According to me the whole thing was fun and I learnt a lot. It was a lifetime opportunity to have the youth to share ideas in a cooperative way. My main prayer is that this play may educate many youths because [these] kinds of things happen all over the world and destroy many youth[s]. I hope you will also enjoy the whole tape.

It has been wonderful for the exposure you brought to us. Some like me was able to get courage that I can do something despite all circumstances i.e., whether a big crowd of people is present or not. I have been able to believe in myself that I have confidence and also I have realized if I can perfect the talent then I can be better placed in such activities. Thanks for your exposure.

There are several deliverables that could be taken from these tapes. They could be used for further training in other schools, or used as catalysts for new *ngoma* dialogue circle projects. While they do not describe the HIV/AIDS situation comprehensively, nor do they provide a how-to manual to be memorized by the youth in other schools, the videos do show youth problematizing the HIV/AIDS situation for critical self-reflection. Intended to embody challenges for rousing critical consciousness, they should therefore be regarded as part of a dialogue between learner and facilitator. Other group members, in studying the *ngoma* circle videos, engaged in the discourse that emerged during the project around youth and HIV/ AIDS prevention. In this way, they delved into each video's meaning and established a relation between the video under discussion and various aspects of the young people in the world of HIV/AIDS. Further reflections, themselves carried out through *ngoma* dialogue circles, could also be taped to give rise to new videos proportionately more critical, pluralistic, and rich in their themes. This continued exchange can go a long way in helping young people develop their own forms of self-expression around HIV/AIDS, as well as other issues that impact their lives.

Finally, since creative *ngoma* is not a new concept among the rural communities in Kenya, there is immense potential for it to be used to impact the communities around the schools through outreach programs. The *wachemshangoma* could be asked to get out into the villages to perform for their parents and other villagers in order to trigger and sustain meaningful dialogue on a number of issues. I believe this approach could kick-start processes of bridging the ever-increasing gap between schools and the communities they serve.

FINDINGS

From the data so far analyzed from this participatory research project, I feel there is great potential for *ngoma* to be used for grassroots organizing and mobilizing for social change. In particular, as I have shown, this form can be used as a communication tool for conscientization and empowerment of youth in Kenyan schools to own the fight against HIV/AIDS. This goal could be accomplished through:

1. High level inventiveness that makes *ngoma* able to adopt new social change messages on HIV/AIDS without distorting, exaggerating, or trivializing the facts.

2. Making it entertaining to the youth. There is a lot of potential buried in the youth, thus there is a need to let them come up with ways of making issues palatable for their peers.

3. Full involvement of the youth at all stages of development of the creative *ngoma* (which is imperative), as well as the use of peer educators (*wachemshangoma*).

4. Packaging creative *ngoma* as a parable (akin to a two-minute well-thought-out advertisement) that stirs the imagination of the youth so as to kick-start processes that lead to their discovering facts and/or truths on their own. Youth can easily relate to parables, since these have been used in African societies by the old to engage the young in figuring out social issues. When used to pose provocative problems, *ngoma* can carry with it with the stimulus for young people to mobilize.

CONCLUSION: LESSONS LEARNED

There are a number of lessons that could be derived from this exercise. For purposes of this chapter, I will mention just a few:

- Valorizing African-Centered Communication: There is immense potential for *ngoma* as a participatory communication strategy that valorizes thoughtful, practical application of Afrocentric traditional media/cultural resources, thereby boosting a grassroots community's capacity to solve its own problems. Creative *ngoma* involves a communication process that is not alienating or threatening, but rather biased towards local content and ownership.

- Democratizing: The emphasis of this approach is on dialogue, debate, and negotiation rather than persuasion and the transmission of information from external technical experts. It makes intervention programs more participatory at all levels of development: educating, entertaining, stirring thinking toward mobilizing for action (problem-posing), and utilizing peer educators, thus basically handing over the means of production to the people in accordance with Freire and Boal's work.

- Empowerment: This approach inherently relies on the innate potential of young people (in Kenya) to control and bring about their own change in response to HIV/AIDS by attempting to provide resources and activation energy for them to actualize their gifts. The use of *ngoma* thus places greater emphasis on getting the target audience involved in perceiving HIV/AIDS as its own problem, rather than as a government agenda. It originates the communication processes within the experiences of the target group, gives full respect to that population's values, and aims to empower individuals as well as the collective to initiate their own change.

- Providing Skills for Social Change Agents: Social change agents need to have the ability to understand target audiences in terms of the context and culture in which the people live. This requirement means that facilitators must have the capability to effectively decode local cultural manifestations through active listening and keen observation of what is happening within and without the target audience, as well as readiness to be a co-enactor. Knowing who is doing what to whom and how it is affecting the group must complement an ability to communicate clearly and effectively. Social change agents must therefore seek a thorough knowledge of the local conditions, community issues, and cross-cultural issues in order to have a hope of success.

II

Interlude
To Sing of Aids in Uganda

Judah M. Cohen (Indiana University)

FROM *DOCTORS FOR GLOBAL HEALTH REPORTER* V. 9, #1 (SPRING/ SUMMER 2005)

On July 10, 2004, I was in an audience of several hundred in a small village in southwest Uganda as sixteen HIV-positive patients sang, danced and acted out a message of hope in the face of the AIDS epidemic. In a rectangular brick assembly hall with a corrugated steel roof, the Drama Group of the Mbarara branch of TASO (The AIDS Support Organization) gave their presentation in both English and Runyankore (the local language).

The performers, who are TASO clients, sang choral songs, rousing the audience to fight AIDS, to get tested for HIV, and to remember that everyone—including priests, doctors, and school headmasters—is susceptible to the disease. They enacted a thirty-five-minute drama showing both how HIV is transmitted and how people with HIV should be treated. They presented a "folksong" dramatizing the story of a woman ostracized by her family because she had HIV. One member of the group gave a personal testimony on how he acquired HIV and what he was doing to live with it. In between segments, the group's director answered questions about HIV from the audience. Then the group closed by dancing the region's folkdance, leaving the crowd on its feet cheering.

A remarkably large portion of the afternoon used music as a means of communication. This is important to consider because the medical world, while receptive to music, has created a literature that treats it overwhelmingly as a form of therapy, or as a way to alleviate pain. Yet such a limited definition of organized sound hardly does the topic justice. As I saw in my work with the TASO Mbarara Drama Group during the summer of 2004, music is itself a form of communication deeply embedded within a community's cultural values. In this case, it plays a valuable role in helping communities negotiate the often contradictory messages they are hearing about AIDS.

A TASO Drama Group presentation is typically about three-hours long and takes up the afternoon at the village or secondary school where the group performs. After a brief introduction, the group begins with a series of four to five minute-long choral songs. Most of these songs have direct, simple titles and lyrics (such as "Fight, Fight AIDS" and "Let's Get Together, AIDS Cannot Win"), follow a verse-chorus format, have an upbeat tempo, and are almost as often in English as they are in Runyankore. Members of the Drama Group typically perform these songs in two rows while wearing khaki uniforms and TASO logo or red ribbon lapel pins. The only instruments they use for the choral songs, if they use instruments at all, are percussive: usually drums and sometimes a small box-shaped shaker.

One of the most powerful examples of this genre that I witnessed was a choral version of Ugandan pop star Philly Lutaaya's 1989 song "Alone." Lutaaya, who died of AIDS in the same year, was one of the first public figures to raise awareness about the disease. "Alone" has since become an anthem for AIDS workers across Uganda. Watching the Drama Group members perform with their hands on their hearts to a hushed audience, it became clear to me that this song (and others in its genre) provided a medium for listeners and performers to connect with a national, mass-mediated style—one that is helping contextualize the epidemic as something that is itself widespread and international.

Later in the afternoon, the drama group presents what it calls the "folksong." Performers, typically wearing traditional costumes, line up in a single semicircle behind a set of drummers, and provide sung commentary on a story that individuals act out in front of them. The story the TASO Mbarara Drama Group developed for 2004 provides a good example of a typical plot: a wife and husband are feeling weak and sick, but do not know why. The husband conjectures his malaise must be spiritual payback for stealing and eating a cow. Enter three friends, accomplices in the crime, all scratching furiously to indicate they too have been stricken with disease. The group calls in a "witch doctor," who gives them potions, scores their skin and uses incantations in an attempt to cure them. But, warns the chorus, while some people rely on this kind of treatment, it does not work. Instead, you should go to your local TASO center or AIDS clinic where you can now be treated with antiretroviral drugs (ARVs). The folksong ends with all the characters dancing to indicate ARVs coursing through their system, and thanking outside sources (such as American-funded NGOs) for making them available. Throughout, the folksong presents a sense of localness and an intimate knowledge of the region's musical and folk practices.

The final segment of an afternoon presentation is the folkdance, described to me as a way for the group to celebrate and communicate its vitality to the audience. Words and melody, while present, are regarded as less important here than the form of the piece and the drumbeat that controls it. Throughout my time with the group no one tried to translate the lyrics sung behind the folk dance to me; the words eventually become inaudible anyway. Audiences consistently react vociferously to the dancers' movements and pack in close to the stage in order to indicate their interest. That such activity takes place in a show devoted to HIV/AIDS awareness highlights the breadth of cultural expression used to frame and deliver the message.

I provide here only a glimpse into the deep and complex relationship music has with AIDS in Ugandan society. Not only is music a crucial factor in disseminating information about HIV/AIDS, but it also helps Ugandans provide information about AIDS research and treatments available in a culturally robust context. It also represents another reality in understanding the way those infected by the virus tell of the AIDS epidemic in their country. Music in this context is not a "therapy," nor is it a way to alleviate pain. Rather, it serves an important role in negotiating community values that will likely lead people to make crucial choices about their own health. Understanding how music factors into the lives and activities of those whom it surrounds would go far in bringing doctors more intimately into the cultures and lives of the people they so much want to help.

12

HIV/AIDS Poster Campaigns
in Malawi[1]

Eckhard Breitinger (University of Bayreuth)

My first contacts with HIV/AIDS and the use of theater and the arts in AIDS education and prevention date back to 1986. In the wake of the civil war in Uganda, a mysterious disease spread rapidly that was named *slim* according to its most striking symptoms. Patients slimmed down to skin and bones with skin rashes, coughs, and diarrhea. They sought help and medical attention, but the health stations in the rural areas were in ruins. The medical services had collapsed; whatever was left in hospitals, clinics, and health stations—drugs, syringes, and bandages—had been stolen by soldiers. It soon became known that *slim* was a sexually transmitted disease and it was recognized by official health policies under its proper medical term: Acquired Immune Deficiency Syndrome, or AIDS. The direct connection between the spreading of the disease and the political situation of civil war in Uganda was all too obvious, given the robbing, raping, and marauding soldiers and a famished, impoverished, devastated civilian population that fled the battle zones and took refuge in ill-equipped camps. When the new Ugandan government was established under Yoweri Museveni, it addressed the issue of AIDS squarely, opening a general debate through all the formal modern media as well as traditional oral media. Uganda's open information policy concerning AIDS led to two significant consequences:

1. Since the HIV/AIDS issue was discussed widely and openly, Uganda was perceived as the country in Africa most badly affected by the disease. Worst case scenarios were drawn up for the southwestern region, the Rakai District in particular. After the devastations by the civil war, the district was now threatened to be even further devastated by AIDS: entire villages and regions had been depopulated, and other areas were threatened by a demographic disaster that would leave only young children and the elderly alive.

2. With its open HIV/AIDS information policy, Uganda became the only African nation that succeeded in lowering the rate of new HIV/AIDS infections.

The majority of African governments pursued a different information policy, either denying the existence of the HIV/AIDS threat—or at least its prevalence—and blaming the occurrence of AIDS on foreigners, as something that had been caused and spread by tourists and refugees. The most striking case of this dishonest information policy took place in South Africa, surprisingly so due to the "enlightened" strategies the South African government had taken in other political fields, such as its post-apartheid reconciliation policy. Thabo Mbeki publicly denied the connection between HIV and AIDS, between being infected with the virus and actually becoming a victim of the disease. In 2009, South Africa remained one of the countries with the highest rate of new infections.

I am not suggesting that there is a direct causal relationship between the Ugandan information policy and the reduction of the infection rate, or South Africa's denial policies and the drastic increase of the infection rate. This assumption would be too simplistic. One must certainly consider that the effect of information policies and the spread of the disease depend on a variety of different factors: cultural, political, and economic. Governments obviously assume that the existence and the spread of HIV/AIDS conflicts with or contradicts attempts to generate a positive national identity; yet they also weigh their actions in light of the realities of the epidemic on the ground.

Uganda became a model for other African nations in its utilization of the arts and mobilization of a variety of cultural activists to enlighten ordinary people about the dangers of HIV/AIDS. The country's campaigns concentrated on rural areas and disadvantaged sections of the urban and peri-urban population in Kampala. In the late 1980s, the government launched the first AIDS drama competition for primary and secondary schools, followed by general theater competitions on the regional and national level; hundreds of theater groups participated. Philly Lutaaya, Uganda's internationally known pop-singer, returned to Uganda for a farewell concert tour in 1989. His song "Alone and Frightened" became the anthem of HIV/AIDS campaigns in the early 1990s. Philly Lutaaya performed not just in a big concert at the National Stadium, but also in schools and at his birthplace, always presenting himself very forcefully in his double function as AIDS victim and AIDS campaign cultural activist. His farewell tour also acquired a kind of model character in its combination of compassion for the victims and the determination of the educator—he attracted the emotional attention of his audience as a private individual while presenting his audience with the rational analysis of a public health advocate.

Uganda also designed an advertising campaign for condom use that was integrated into a broad and diverse publicity campaign organized by the Kabarole Basic Health Services Project in the Kabarole district (near the border with Congo). The Kabarole Basic Health Services Project distributed its own condoms under the name of *Engabo* ("The shield"). The campaign's idea to link the fight against AIDS with the old Toro warrior tradition meant to emphasize how protection against AIDS could well function within the principles and values of their target population's own culture. Thus people could easily identify with the campaign through a product, i.e., a condom, that they could consider specific to their area and, it was hoped, reduce the reluctance of the male population toward condom use.

All these different strategies and cultural activities in the AIDS campaigns had been first designed and tested in Uganda. Ten to fifteen years later, many of these strategies have been adopted in other countries. With non-governmental organizations taking a major role in the campaigns against AIDS, campaign techniques have become professionalized, involving professional designers, artists. and advertising agencies.

Since the late 1990s the focus of HIV/AIDS campaigns has shifted toward southeastern and southern Africa. One of the ill-advised and negative examples of government policies was Mbongemi Ngema's *Sarafina II*. Mbongemi Ngema, commissioned by his friend in the Ministry of Education, designed a stupendous show that toured the country in a luxury bus and performed to urban audiences. Yet the show never engaged in a dialogue with the spectators—a typical top-down or cargo-cult methodology. Other campaigns that have promoted a bottom-up approach, or that have attempted to spur dialogue within a target population, have proven more successful models.

South Africa's neighbors, and Malawi in particular, have always been tied to developments in South Africa due to the large number of migrant workers. They worked on contract in the gold mines, or as domestic or agricultural workers. When they returned home to their families they brought not only the money they had earned, but also the diseases they contracted. After the 1994 elections in South Africa, the number of returnees in Malawi increased drastically. In response, by the late 1990s, various Malawian NGOs had started AIDS education campaigns with hand-painted posters, and promoted song and dance performances by traditional dance troupes in the villages (Wolf 2006). Apparently dissatisfied with the impact of those HIV prevention activities, in 2003 the government of Malawi launched a massive publicity campaign on AIDS education with a series of posters. One set of giant posters—6 x 2.5 meters—covered the general messages of the campaign (promoting AIDS testing in particular). Smaller size posters that addressed specific situations of risky behavior, and concentrated on condom use, provided supplemental messages. These posters displayed the logo of *Chishango*, also meaning Shield (see figure 12.1), the "national condom" of Malawi.

Photographs on the posters emphasized a sense of realism, and, judging from the visual style and setting, all originated from the same graphic design studio. The positioning of the posters on solid metal stands and in metal frames further revealed the campaign to be the work of a professional advertising company. The placement of the extra large posters in highly trafficked strategic places of the town, such as the central bus station, the clock tower, or the T-junction of Zomba's main road and the central market road, indicated that this campaign was designed to address an urban audience. This arrangement was further enhanced by the smaller posters, located at important intersections such as the main road and College Road, the main entrance to the bus station and taxi park, or the intersection where the road to the government

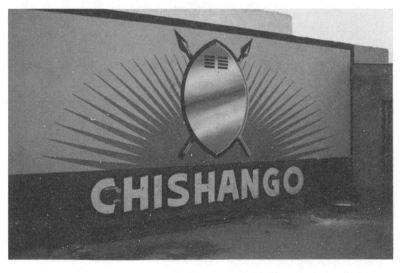

Figure 12.1 Chishango mural painting

buildings branched off: strategic intersections where two or more streams of public traffic or main pedestrian routes merged. All the locations of the posters ensured high and frequent visibility by the general public. The motifs on the posters further underlined the urban milieu as the main target of the campaign. Pictures of well-dressed women and partying men in bright button-down shirts roasting meat on a *braai* (barbeque), all aimed to appeal to the aspiring middle class in Zomba, Blantyre, or Lilongwe.

Our observations are based on the poster campaign in Zomba itself, the former capital of Malawi and a university town. The giant poster at the crossroads of Main Street and Market Street shows the former Head of State Bakili Muluzi with a general admonishment to Malawians to change their sexual behavior: *"AIDS is Killing Africa. Malawians Change YOUR Behaviour Now! Let Us Save Our Country."* This personal statement by Muluzi, who was President of Malawi from 1994 to 2004, suggests both a personal concern and an official political position as Head of State, signalling that the government of Malawi professes an official Malawian AIDS policy. The National AIDS Commission (NAC), which was in charge of the poster campaign, acted on behalf of government in the formulation of its official AIDS policies.

The giant posters address basic issues in the state's 2004 AIDS campaign (see figure 12.3). The images in the posters match the verbal messages. The poster showing a group of younger people propagates the need to go for AIDS testing to achieve certainty about one's personal HIV status: *We have already gone for voluntary counselling and testing of HIV. NOW IT'S*

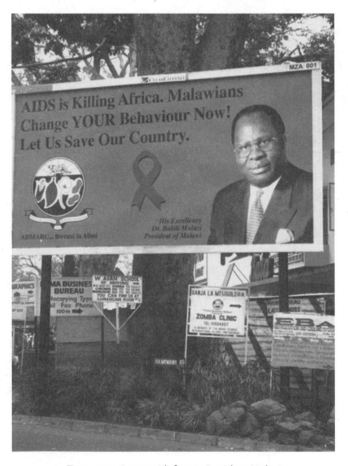

Figure 12.2 Poster with former President Muluzi

PRESS RELEASE

THE GOVERNMENT OF THE REPUBLIC OF MALAWI

2004 WORLD AIDS DAY COMMEMORATION
1st DECEMBER 2004,
MCHINJI COMMUNITY CENTRE GROUND

The **Government of Malawi** through the **National AIDS Commission (NAC)** and **Malawi Network of AIDS Service Organisation (MANASO)** wishes to remind the general public that 1st December is World AIDS Day and **will be commemorated at Mchinji Community Centre Ground in Mchinji District.** This Day aims to call upon individuals, families, communities, organisations, faith communities and governments through out the world to renew their commitment in the fight against HIV and AIDS.

The theme for this year's campaign is *Women, Girls, HIV and AIDS.* It explores how gender inequality fuels the AIDS epidemic, and is conceived to help accelerate the global response to HIV and AIDS by encouraging people to address female vulnerability to HIV. This year's World AIDS Campaign, with the slogan 'Have you heard me today?' seeks to raise awareness about, and help address, the many issues affecting women and girls around HIV and AIDS. Malawi's local slogan for the campaign is *Support Women and Girls: Fight HIV and AIDS.*

In Malawi more women than men are infected with HIV. According to 2003 National AIDS Commission HIV/AIDS Report, out of 760, 000 infected adults aged between 15 to 49 years, 58% were women. In 2003, there were about 36, 000 new female AIDS cases compared to about 25, 000 male cases. Among young people aged 15 — 24, there are six HIV positive girls for every one young male infected with HIV. At the same time, more women and girls than men and boys are burdened by the challenge of providing home care, and more girls and women are more prone to sexual and physical abuse than the male counterparts.

Why focus on women and girls?
The following are some of the reasons why this year's campaign is focusing on women and girls:
1. More women and girls are particularly vulnerable to HIV infection and to the impact of AIDS than men and boys.
2. Some women and girls face sexual violence such as rape, which exposes them and their perpetrators to HIV infection.
3. Most women and girls do not enjoy the same rights and access to employment, property inheritance and education as men and boys.
4. In most communities women and girls are always expected to care for the sick and orphans thus increasing the burden of care on them. Some girls are even pulled out of school to care for orphans or sick relatives.
5. Poverty affects women a great more seriously than men and yet the majority of them have no economic skills to improve their situation;
6. Many cultural practices such as wife inheritance, death cleansing and those related to marriage affect women and girls negatively more that they do affect men or boys.
7. Information design, content and distribution mechanisms do not always consider the needs and situations of girls and women.

Expected Achievements
This year's campaign seeks to achieve the following:
1. Increased awareness on the factors and practices that perpetuate vulnerability of women and girls to HIV infection and impact of AIDS.
2. Increased HIV and AIDS sectoral interventions that will address issues that affect women, girls, men and boys.
3. Increased number of political, religious and traditional leaders that speak out against practices and behaviours that contribute to HIV infection among women and girls.
4. Increased resource mobilisation and allocation towards HIV and AIDS interventions addressing women and girls by various stakeholders.
5. Increased number of men and boys actively involved in home-based care and the care for orphans.
6. Reduced incidences of gender-based violence.

The Government, through the National AIDS Commission and MANASO is, therefore, appealing to individuals, families, traditional and religious leaders, politicians, organisations, development partners, donors and government departments to:
1. Participate in the national function marking the Day on 1st December 2004 in Mchinji and in Regional and District World AIDS Campaigns.
2. Mobilise resources for the World AIDS Day and the regional and district campaigns.
3. Advocate for establishment and implementation of HIV and AIDS interventions that protect women and girls from new HIV infection; promote their equal access to treatment and reduce the impact of HIV and AIDS on women and girls.
4. Support people living with HIV and AIDS and those affected by the disease.

For more information on the commemoration for the Day and the whole campaign, please contact:
The Executive Director, National AIDS Commission, P. O. Box 30622, LILONGWE; Tel.: 01 770 022; Fax: 01 767 249, E-mails:chibwanab@aidsmalawi.org.mw; chizimban@aidsmalawi.org.mw; telekac@aidsmalawi.org.mw OR National Co-ordinator, MANASO, P. O. Box 2916, BLANTYRE; Tel.: 01 635 046; Fax: 01 621 984, E-mail: manaso@malawi.net or visit www.unaids.org/wac2004

SUPPORT WOMEN AND GIRLS, FIGHT HIV AND AIDS!!!

Figure 12.3 2004 World AIDS Day press release

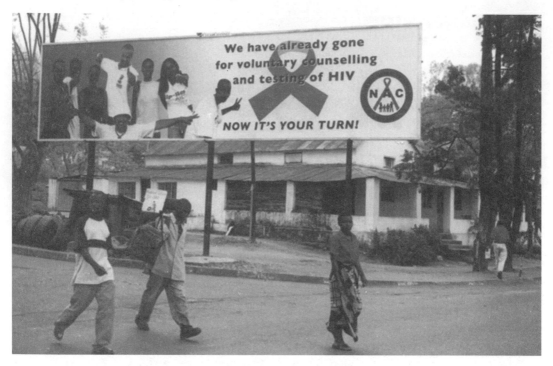

Figure 12.4 Calling for AIDS tests; poster located on Main Street, Zomba

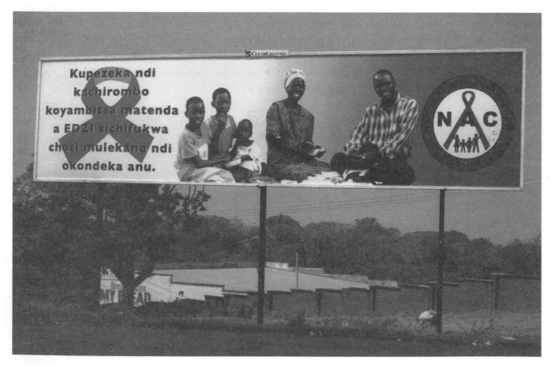

Figure 12.5 Poster at the Central Bus Station, Zomba

YOUR TURN! The message implies of course that one should adjust one's sexual behavior to one's personal HIV status (see figure 12.4) This poster was placed at an intersection of Main Road (opposite the Muluzi poster). The second giant poster was posted at the far end of the local bus station. It shows members of a (nuclear) family combined with the appeal of how to deal with HIV/AIDS victims within the family. The Chichewa message reads: *Kupezeka ndi kachirombo koyambitsa matenda a EDZI sichifukwa choti mulekane ndi okondeka anu* (Finding that the virus leads to AIDS is no reason for you to hate/shun your friend/beloved). The appeal to solidarity with HIV victims within the family is also an appeal to maintain traditional social links and responsibilities (see figure 12.5).

One set of posters seems conceived as two complementary pairs that address specific, gendered audiences. The first poster shows two smartly dressed young men, one in a European-style shirt, the other in a kind of African shirt, exchanging their worldly wisdom about the hazards of sex in the age of AIDS: *Amwene, sungangomukhulupirira mkazi wamba pankhani yogonana* (Brother, you cannot just trust a woman on appearance alone). The respondent in the poster draws the pragmatic conclusion from this awareness of sexual risk behavior: *Ndikudziwa, ndichifukwa chake ndimagwiritsa ntchito makondomu nthawi zonse* (I know, that's why we use condoms every time) (figure 12.6). The female version of this poster, with the identical verbal

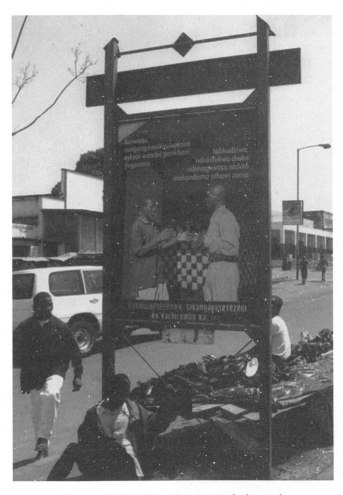

Figure 12.6 "Men's" poster opposite the bus park

message, figures even more prominently. It is one of the giant size posters, showing two well-dressed women—European style, and immaculately coiffed—exchanging the identical insights on the risk of sexual encounters: *Sungangomukhulupirira mwanuna wamba pankhani yogonana* (You cannot just trust a man on appearance alone). And the logical consequence: *Ndikudziwa, ndichifukwa chake timagwiritsa ntchito makondomu nthawi zonse* (I know, that's why we use condoms every time). With the extra large size of the women's poster, the advertisers obviously convey their intention to specifically and even more forcefully address women with their messages (figure 12.7). Another significant feature of this poster is its particular location. It stands at the upper intersection of Market Street, towering above the first market stalls, directly adjacent to the great mosque in Zomba. Based on my observations, worshippers regularly headed for the mosque for their Friday prayers without being irritated by the poster. It is difficult to imagine that the same poster could be raised next to a Christian church or chapel without highly vocal protest from both the church authorities and the congregation.

The "women's" poster at the bus terminal (figure 12.8) inadvertently appears in an evocative real life context. The road along the bus station houses small shops and businesses, including two coffin shops and undertakers who logically put up their advertisements along the street. This accidental juxtaposition of the poster for AIDS prevention and the twenty-four hour service of the coffin shop is highly ironic, but also very realistic, and reminiscent of one of the major AIDS preventions slogans: *AIDS has no cure* and *AIDS kills*.

The implied and underlying message of potentially misleading appearances is taken up once more in the concluding statement of all these posters: *Kukhulupirirana wamba sikunga-kutetezeni ku kachilombo ka HIV* (Just trusting each other cannot protect you against the HIV virus). The term *kachilombo* provides a remarkable example of how African languages manage to transliterate medical, technical, or scientific terms into elegant and precisely coined phrases

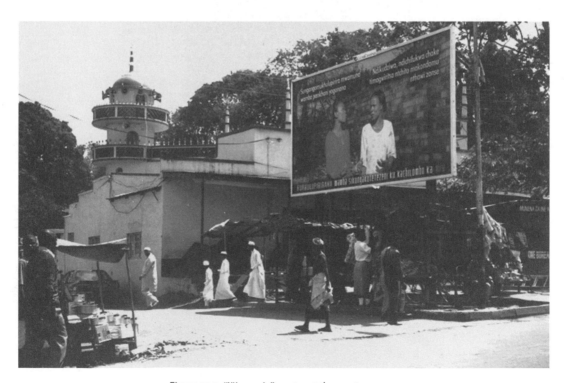

Figure 12.7 "Women's" poster at the great mosque

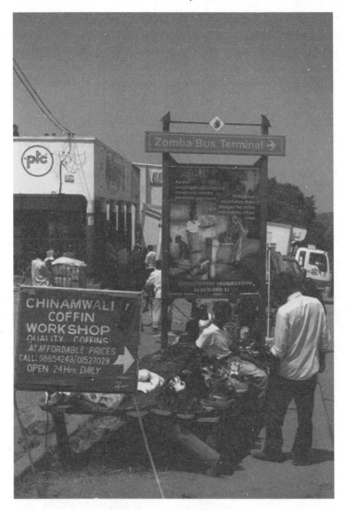

Figure 12.8 "Women's" poster at the bus terminal

through allegorical or proverbial figurative speech. *Kachilombo*, standing for virus, literally means "tiny monster," i.e., something that you cannot see at first glance but something of whose presence you should better be aware and beware. Translating a medical/scientific term into a figurative or even proverbial phrase reduces the rationality, i.e., the "coldness" of the scientific fact and infuses an emotional and affective quality of compassion to the HIV threat.

The same linguistic and pictorial pattern repeats itself in a second pair of posters. The first poster shows two women in modest dress who are obviously meant to look like village beauties, brandishing a kind of village upper-class fashion dress. They have gathered at a standpipe, drawing water—a typically female activity in the rural and peri-urban locations (figure 12.8). We are still dealing with the same picture (figure 12.8) with the coffin shop ad on the left and the two women at the standpipe on the right. They engage in the identical dialogue as their urban counterparts: *Sungangomukhulupirira mwamuna wamba pankhani yogonana* (You can't trust a man on appearance alone). *Ndikudziwa, ndichifukwa chake timagwiritsa ntchito makondomu nthawi zonse* (I know, that's why we use condoms every time). If we adhere to the argumentative strategy of the publicity campaign designers and managers, we must conclude that the issue of AIDS presents itself identically for all walks of life, independent of gender and class, for men and women, for city dwellers and country folks, and therefore needs to be addressed by the same verbal messages.

The specific targeting of particular groups—male/female, rural/urban—occurs in the pictorial messages represented in the *Chishango* posters. Some of the *Chishango* posters refer to the differences in communication styles between town and country through their pictorial representation, their use of language (English vs. Chichewa) and their use of figurative speech. The poster targeting urban youth, for example, shows a group of partying young men in casual but stylish dress with baseball caps and branded T-shirts, gathered around a *braai*. The message *Talk Lifestyle—Talk Chishango* is striking in its blunt directness. It aggressively states the good life aspirations of the city yuppies and deduces as a logical consequence the use of condoms. We don't see any females nor hear about partners; only about partying and, implied, about sex (see figure 12.9).

The rural counterpart (see figure 12.10) operates on a completely different strategy: We see a middle-age couple in front of some traditional village function with dancers wearing feathery headpieces. Their dress is modest, the pose of the woman signals shyness, and the image of a man pushing his bicycle expresses humbleness. The verbal message does not come as dialogue between the actors in the poster, but as a distanced third person observation: *Okaona Nyanja Anakoana Ndi Mvuu Zomwe* (If you see the lake be prepared to see hippos) (figure 12.10). This phrase follows the neo-proverbial speech technique. It maintains the structure and the illustrative

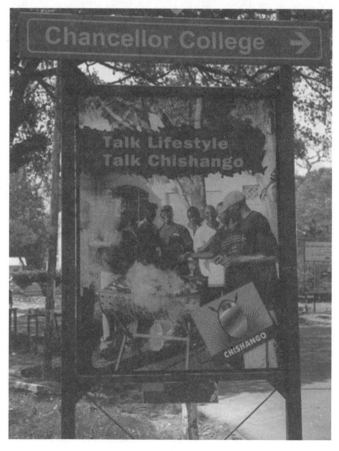

Figure 12.9 Urban yuppies enjoying life

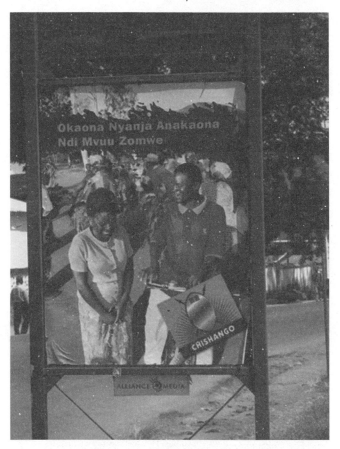

Figure 12.10 AIDS and rural festival atmosphere

logic of the proverb, but it creates a new proverbial sequence of images that stand for a new social and personal challenge. The pleasure of going to the beach on Lake Malawi is combined with a warning of the dangers of enjoying these pleasures. Hippos look gentle and phlegmatic, but they are one of the most dangerous animals; more fatal accidents result from encounters with hippos than with any other animal. The neo-proverb about the lake, hippos, and the danger of AIDS provides another example of the adaptability and flexibility of the indigenous languages; of how Chichewa manages to retain its earthbound, traditional flavor and yet communicate a forceful warning against the new challenge of HIV/AIDS.

The slick professionalism of the AIDS Commission and the PSI/Chisango poster campaign appears to meet squarely the lifestyle aspirations of the better-off urban population. In the rural areas, however, simple hand-painted posters can be found more frequently. These posters use the same materials and decorative styles as the signs for barbershops, beauty parlors, or dressmaker studios. Plywood or presswood boards and cardboard plates from packaging boxes serve as bases for simple iconographic paintings. Since they intend to convey simple messages in an unmistakable fashion, these posters use a visual idiom that is at the same time realistically direct and abstract like a pictogram.

Some of the NGOs, such as ActionAid, seem to find this kind of popular style of rural graphic design more attractive and more appropriate for their particular target groups. They apply it in a more refined mode in design and printing technique even in the urban and peri-urban context. The poster shown in figure 12.11 forms part of the program used in schools and universities to teach "life skills," comprising AIDS awareness and knowledge about risky behaviors.

The viewing angle of this poster conveys the most essential part of its message. As spectators we follow the eyes of a female student looking back over her shoulder watching a couple of other students obviously heading for the bushes to have sex. The boy brandishes the latest fashion in hair cut and happily puffs his cigarette. He is doing his utmost to appear cool. Together with his girlfriend he is playing up to the stereotype of the "popular couple": the popular boy and the popular girl within the peer group. The girl in the foreground, from whose perspective we are witnessing the scene, figures as the "unpopular girl," the one left behind as being unattractive or dull. The message of the poster, *Achinyamata musatsanzire makhalidwe oipa a anzanu* (Don't spread bad behavior to your friends) gives another twist to the standard setting of textbook illustrations: Being popular and playing with this popularity has become risky in the times of AIDS. Being not so popular and less insistent on finding acceptance in the peer group might prove much wiser. It reveals a good command of the appropriate life skills.

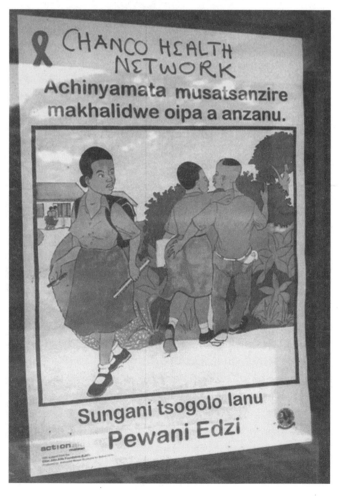

Figure 12.11 AIDS poster

Looking at the poster campaigns cannot tell us much about the posters' effectiveness. Pinning down quantitative evaluations of behavior change, particularly of changes in sexual behavior, is probably one of the most difficult exercises in any empirical study in public health. But the posters tell us much about concepts and ideas that might be effective and persuasive in the AIDS campaigns. By displaying moral, ethical, and aesthetic values that are current in sections of Malawian society, they offer one strategy for government intervention in a multi-front battle against a devastating and vexing pandemic.

13

Contemporary Uses of the Musical Arts in Botswana's HIV/AIDS Health Education Initiatives

THE CASE OF THE RADIO SERIAL DRAMA

MAKGABANENG

Abimbola Cole (University of California, Los Angeles)

INTRODUCTION

Radio serial dramas occupy an integral role in public education campaigns. They are vital in curtailing negative behaviors, encouraging positive change, and promoting social development. Due to their tremendous potential and overwhelming transformative possibilities, serial dramas are recognized as an innovative approach to information dissemination.[1] The undeniable appeal of such serials seals their position as tools in evoking societal change by addressing fluctuating economic, political, and social dynamics.

The Archers, which is widely cited as the first existing issue-based serial, entertained British audiences from its genesis in 1951, when it became a mouthpiece for information regarding topics such as environmental conservation and health (Singhal et al. 2002, 6). Its pioneering efforts served as a benchmark for ensuing serial dramas broadcast in India (*Tinka Tinka Sukh*), Kenya (*Ndinga Nacio*), Nepal (*Cut Your Coat According to Your Cloth*), and Nigeria (*Story, Story*) that tackled a vast array of subjects such as crime, cultural mores, family values, gender, and religion (see Adam and Harford 1999, Sharan and Valente 2002, Singhal 1990, Sood 1999 and 2002, and Sood et al. 2004).

Developments in radio serial dramas ignited a transcontinental movement to introduce them as a method of engendering discussions about increasingly significant social matters like HIV/AIDS. In the wake of the burgeoning world pandemic, which became a global concern of monumental proportions, radio serials addressing the topic flourished in Afghanistan (*New Home, New Life*), Peru (*Bienvenida Salud!*), and St. Lucia (*Apwé Plezi*), sparking a new-found awareness about the global impact of HIV/AIDS (see Noar et al. 2009, Rogers et al. 1999, Sypher et al. 2002, Valente et al. 1994, and Vaughan et al. 2000). There was a profound need to create radio serials in sub-Saharan Africa, the area that contained 10 percent of the world's population and two-thirds of all HIV infections at the time I began my research (NACA 2005, 8). This stark reality led to the establishment of HIV/AIDS radio serials in Gambia (*Fakube Jarra*), Ethiopia (*Journey of Life*), and Tanzania (*Twende na Wakati*). And in Southern Africa, where HIV/AIDS prevalence rose at an alarming pace, formidable serials took shape in South Africa (*Soul City*, which entailed a television and radio serial as well as other forms of marketing such as brochures, pamphlets, and public service announcements); Zambia (*Gama Cuulu*); and Zimbabwe (*Mopani Junction*), prompting radio serial drama enthusiasts to label them a "new effective tool for social change" (Lee 2004, 1).[2]

For Botswana, a small country that once possessed one of the world's highest HIV/AIDS prevalence rates, radio serial dramas represented a new tactic for transmitting HIV/AIDS health education messages that presented background information and strategies for curbing HIV/AIDS transmission. The radio serial drama *Makgabaneng*, sponsored by the Botswana-United States Partnership (BOTUSA), Botswana Ministry of Health (MoH), and the United States Centers for Disease Control and Prevention (CDC) Global AIDS Program (GAP), rapidly became a method of conveying messaging about the pandemic to the public.[3] Broadcast in all of Botswana's health districts, the serial drama was touted as a successful way for Batswana, the people of Botswana, to gain essential details about HIV/AIDS. The serial drama was a drastic change from the early days of the pandemic in Botswana when AIDS was labeled the "radio disease" in the late 1980s because it was "widely publicized on radio, but had not been experienced by most people" (Ingstad 1990, 29). By the turn of the century it was known that Batswana were encountering situations where, as the adage goes, they were either affected or infected by HIV/AIDS. *Makgabaneng* emerged as part of a creative countrywide HIV/AIDS response. Due to its cost-effectiveness and the expansive reach of radio, it metamorphosed into a preferred format and medium for packaging HIV/AIDS messages (Mead 1998, 1; Ministry of Finance and Development Planning 2003, 361–62).[4]

Makgabaneng premiered on Botswana's airwaves in August 2001 and contributed to the national media response to HIV/AIDS. Complementing countless information, education and communication (IEC) efforts constructed to combat HIV/AIDS in Botswana, *Makgabaneng* provided a new "arts sector" approach to HIV/AIDS education espousing HIV/AIDS awareness and behavioral change (Fidzani Interview, Jul. 13, 2004). Since its inception, studies about *Makgabaneng* have elaborated on the transformative aspects of the serial, especially how it acted as a tool for behavioral change and social development (see Galavotti et al. 2001, Mooki et al. 2004, Pappas-DeLuca et al. 2004, Pappas-DeLuca et al. 2008).[5] While these studies investigated the practical aspects of the radio serial drama such as its listenership demographics, reach, and scope, one essential component of *Makgabaneng* has yet to be explored—the manner in which the drama functions as a contemporary musical arts based program in the age of AIDS.[6]

Using the case of *Makgabaneng*, I will examine the serial drama's role as a contemporary form of musical arts education capable of conveying health care objectives and details related to psycho-medical care (Nzewi 2004, 67) as described in Botswana's national HIV/AIDS goals and policies. I will provide an overview of the radio serial drama, its cultural context, and its significance in Botswana's national life and community. Then, I will reveal the ways in which *Makgabaneng* establishes communities of listeners whose lives are intertwined with the imagined worlds of the serial drama's characters (Abu-Lughod 1993 and 1997, Gunner 2000a and 2000b).

I draw upon field research in the musical arts conducted in Gaborone, Botswana's capital city, in 2004, which included a visit to the *Makgabaneng* studios, face-to-face interviews with several staff members, and personal communication with actors. My goal here is to provide a glimpse of how *Makgabaneng* functions as a contemporary musical arts endeavor reflecting everyday situations in Botswana that raise national consciousness about HIV/AIDS.[7]

RADIO, THE MUSICAL ARTS, AND HEALTH EDUCATION

Makgabaneng is rarely considered a musical arts-based program; rather, it falls within the broad classification of "communications." Nevertheless, its use of music and dramatic narrative provides a different concept of the serial, illustrating that it is part of a holistic matrix of creative arts applied to teaching Batswana about HIV/AIDS (Stone 2000, 7; Kwami et al. 2003, 261). Music scholars have examined the significance of the musical arts in mental, physical, and spiritual education, and suggested that, among other things, they make contributions to health management and sex education (Bebey 1969, 2; Nketia 1974, 36; and Nzewi 2003, 15–19).[8] Armed with what has been deemed "musical arts knowledge," communities can consider pressing issues and enter into transformative dialogues about social issues and social reform (Nzewi 2004). Ultimately this sustains the overall "health of the community" (Thiong'o 1999, xiv).

The maintenance of community health demands that the musical arts remain relevant in the face of developmental challenges such as HIV/AIDS. Contemporary music and drama performances critique and supply plausible solutions to HIV/AIDS-related matters among women and youth (Barz 2002, 2004, and 2006a; Namukisa 2002). It is believed that these contemporary arts emerge from scenarios that form the "basis of social life" (Nketia 1995, 1). Yet in the face of developing technologies, these musical arts projects also require "accelerating the transfer of knowledge skills and repertoire from traditional environments into contemporary settings through educational programs and the media" (Nketia 2001). Thus, radio becomes a useful conduit for contemporary musical arts in HIV/AIDS health education initiatives.

There is a long legacy of educational radio programming in Botswana. Radio functioned as a tool to distribute pertinent information to the community since its advent in Botswana in 1934.[9] Public information broadcasting began in Botswana in 1937, when the country's first station, ZBN-Mafikeng, was founded (Botswana National Broadcasting Policy 2003, 7). Initially, the radio station aired nine hours of music and news Sunday through Friday. Throughout World War II (1939–1945), radio enabled Botswana to learn of how local soldiers were faring overseas. The Botswana Department of Education assumed control of ZBN-Mafikeng following the war. In subsequent years, the country's radio scene underwent substantial changes, the most notable being the creation of independent stations in the early 1960s, shortly before Botswana, then known as the Bechuanaland Protectorate, gained its independence in 1966.

The turning point for radio in Botswana was its coverage of independence week, or the week surrounding the first national elections in 1965, during which the national station aired an unprecedented sixty hours of election coverage. Botswana's meager radio station had never before accomplished such a feat. After the elections, Sir Seretse Khama, the nation's first president, declared at his swearing-in ceremony: "Broadcasting can bridge distances in space, time and knowledge itself. Radio can stimulate discussion among the people and assist in the process of democracy. People from one end of Botswana to the other can hear the opinions of their fellow countrymen, drawing [them] together as a nation" (Khama quoted in the Botswana National Broadcasting Policy 2003, 13).[10] Sir Khama's remarks signaled the necessity of radio in nation building and ushered in a variety of radio programming, including educational school and agricultural broadcasts, at the newly renamed radio station, Radio Botswana. Radio Botswana ultimately relocated to Gaborone to continue its legacy of educational broadcasting.

In 1992, a second commercial radio station, Radio Botswana 2 (RB2), was established and educational broadcasting expanded even further.[11] This new station began with coverage limited merely to Gaborone and its immediate surroundings, but emerged as a national broadcaster in 2001. Two years later, RB2 matured into a station with twenty-four hour broadcasting services. In the midst of these developments in government-controlled radio, two private stations, Gabz FM and Yarona FM, made their debuts. From their modest beginnings in 1999, these stations have flourished and secured national licensing from Botswana's National Broadcasting Board (NBB). RB1, RB2, Gabz FM and Yarona FM comprise the four main stations. Additionally, a fifth radio station, Duma FM, began broadcasting in 2007.

Over the past three decades, radio in Botswana has reflected the view that broadcasting is capable of "creating a national culture, a [national] identity, and an independent and unified nation" (Chopyak 1987, 451).[12] Pre- and post-independence radio broadcasting has operated as a vehicle for bolstering public awareness about the country and current events. RB1 and RB2 remain two of the most listened-to stations in the country (Thapisa 2003, Thapisa and Megwa 2002).[13] Their firm positioning in the national broadcasting landscape made these stations the ideal future home of *Makgabaneng*.

THE ESTABLISHMENT OF THE RADIO SERIAL DRAMA *MAKGABANENG*

In 2001, Radio Botswana 1 and 2 featured a new educational radio initiative, *Makgabaneng*. This radio serial drama's title means "rocky road" in Setswana, one of the local languages of Botswana. Its motto, "*re wa re tsoga*," which also appears in Setswana, translates into the phrase "we fall and we rise." Broadcasts are typically fifteen minutes long and the goal of *Makgabaneng* is to "promote prevention through the 'abstain, be faithful, condomise' (ABC) message; encourage voluntary HIV counseling and testing; prevent mother-to-child HIV transmission; and persuade Batswana to offer care and support to people living with HIV and AIDS" (Pappas-Deluca et al. 2004).

Through its unyielding commitment to HIV/AIDS awareness and education, *Makgabaneng* is considered a form of entertainment-education programming, which Arvind Singhal has described as "a performance which captures the interest or attention of an individual, giving them pleasure, amusement, or gratification, while *simultaneously* helping the individual to develop a skill to achieve a particular end by boosting his/her mental, moral or physical powers" (Singhal 1990, 2). *Makgabaneng* staff concur that the radio serial drama appears in a format that is "emotionally engaging and entertaining" (Galavotti et al. 2003).[14] Relying on overlapping storylines to promote education and transform behavior, *Makgabaneng* is "trying to cater for Botswana by casting stories in four different situational contexts: a big village or home, the farm or cattle post, the city, and youth" (Mooki Interview, Jul. 29, 2004).[15] Within these coexisting contexts there are themes such as orphanages, alcohol consumption, physical abuse, and communication issues that indicate the impact of HIV/AIDS on various segments of society in Botswana (Tembo Interview, Jul. 15, 2004).[16]

HIV/AIDS IN BOTSWANA

Botswana is a small landlocked country bordered by Namibia, South Africa, Zambia, and Zimbabwe. Nearly 2 million people inhabit this sparsely populated country, dwelling mainly in the cities in the eastern region.[17] Botswana has maintained a growing economy and is governed by the Botswana Democratic Party (BDP). The country has a rich supply of natural resources including copper, diamonds, and nickel. Furthermore, Botswana has managed to dedicate a quarter of its annual budget to educating its citizens. Despite these various national accomplishments, the HIV/AIDS scourge threatened to reverse Botswana's progress.

HIV first emerged in Botswana in 1985. During the early years of HIV/AIDS in the country, there were only a few isolated cases. Anthropologist Benedicte Ingstad notes that there were 107 cases of HIV by 1987 (Ingstad 1990, 29). The first AIDS-related death was recorded in 1986 and World Health Organization (WHO) statistics indicate that by 1989, there were 49 Batswana living with full-blown AIDS (ibid.). Between 1985 and 1991, moreover, only 178 cases had been reported in the country (Barnett et al. 2002, 5). In time, the numbers continued to grow. Figures from the 1995 *Sentinel Surveillance Survey* confirmed that 23 percent of 15- to 49-year-olds were HIV-positive (Ministry of Health 1997, 8). Statistics from Botswana's *National Development Plan (NDP) 9 2003/04—2008/09* revealed that in 2001 HIV prevalence rates gathered from pre-natal clinics among pregnant women was at 38.8 percent (Ministry of Finance and Development Planning 2003, 22). The data on HIV/AIDS acquired from these clinics did not represent the total number of infections. Still, given the size of Botswana's population and the rate at which HIV and AIDS was developing, a new approach was needed to tackle the mounting pandemic.

One of the turning points in Botswana's HIV/AIDS response was the realization that further measures had to be taken to mitigate its spread. Institutions targeting HIV/AIDS were established as early as 1985, when the National AIDS Control Program (NACP) was founded. Screening for HIV began at local hospitals the following year. The *Short Term Plan* (STP), the first detailed plan for controlling HIV/AIDS in Botswana was implemented in 1987, ushering in the *Medium Term Plan I* (MTP I) in 1989 to 1993 and the *Medium Term Plan II* (MTP II) for 1997 to 2002. In the interim, the government of Botswana prepared sentinel surveillance reports to assess national HIV prevalence, the first of which was published in 2000. There was also a Presidential Directive around 1993 to design a *National AIDS Policy* (Government of Botswana 1993, Ministry of Health 1997, ix).[18] Beginning in 1992, policymakers on HIV/AIDS-related matters were steered by the National AIDS Council (NAC), the highest ranking body on HIV/AIDS in Botswana, which was governed by the former President of Botswana, His Excellency Festus Mogae, and a body of multisectoral in-country representatives.[19] Their motivation was to focus on the "three ones": one AIDS framework, one AIDS coordinating organization, and one monitoring and evaluation mechanism (NACA 2005, 14–15).[20] Further HIV/AIDS guidance was offered by the National AIDS Coordinating Agency (NACA), the "secretariat to NAC" at the forefront of the war on HIV/AIDS, which was established in 1999, and the AIDS Coordinating Unit (ACU), a branch of the Ministry of Local Government, that followed in 2000 (NACA 2005, 15; ACHAP 2006, 7).

NACA was instrumental in the preparation of Botswana's HIV/AIDS strategy, the *Botswana National Strategic Framework (NSF) for HIV/AIDS 2003–2009*. In this document, the nation's ten national HIV/AIDS objectives were presented. Among these objectives were increasing HIV-prevention behaviors; decreasing the transmission of HIV from HIV-positive mothers to their babies; increasing the productivity of persons living with HIV/AIDS

(PLWHAs); and seeking total implementation of HIV/AIDS activities across the country (NACA 2003, 10). NACA also outlined five national goals involving preventing HIV infection: offering ample care and support; fortifying the national HIV/AIDS response; handling the psycho-social and economic impacts of the pandemic; and pursuing a supportive legal and ethical environment (NACA 2003, 9).

HIV/AIDS goals and objectives from the *NSF* operated in tandem with other national strategies such as Vision 2016 and the Botswana Millennium Development Goals (MDGs). The Vision 2016 initiative was a detailed plan that was penned in 1997 to make Botswana "an educated, informed nation; a prosperous, productive and innovative nation; a compassionate, just and caring nation; a safe and secure nation; an open, democratic and accountable nation; a more an tolerant nation; and a united and proud nation" (Presidential Task Group 1996, Johnson 2000). Pillars from Vision 2016 were supported by the overarching principles of democracy, development, self-reliance, unity, and *botho* (humanity). Tenets from Vision 2016 carry over into various aspects of national life, especially long-term endeavors to combat HIV/AIDS, arriving at an "AIDS-Free Generation" and zero HIV/AIDS transmissions by the year 2016 (Presidential Task Group 1996, Government of Botswana/UNDP 2001).

Vision 2016 was not drastically different from another closely related policy, the MDGs. After a meeting where 189 countries convened with United Nations officials, the MDGs were concretized. They were established to "eradicate extreme poverty and hunger; achieve universal primary education; promote gender equality and empower women; reduce child mortality; improve maternal health; combat HIV/AIDS, malaria and other diseases; ensure environmental sustainability; and develop global partnership for development" (Government of Botswana/United Nations 2004, 9). Elements of the MDGs were widely recognized and integrated into national programs to emphasize their significance in advancing the national understanding of these matters.

Adherence to the *NSF*, Vision 2016, and the MDGs helped *Makgabaneng* evolve into a growing HIV/AIDS health education phenomenon. Prisca Tembo, the person responsible for coordinating and budgeting for *Makgabaneng*, shared that the storylines for *Makgabaneng* were written "in line with what NACA has in place," which demanded consulting the national HIV/AIDS targets, executing extensive national research, and inserting data into scripts to convey information to listeners that corresponded to national aims (Tembo Interview, Jul. 15, 2004).[21]

Prior to the debut of *Makgabaneng*, national research was conducted to ensure that the topics of the shows would be relevant to audiences. Classified as "formative research" by staff at the serial drama, the countrywide investigation sought to uncover what the main issues are and what people felt and thought about HIV/AIDS (Mooki Interview, Jul. 29, 2004). This sort of research demanded building a framework for the show that was built upon a standard entertainment-education "values grid" and focused on twenty-four themes including the ones mentioned above (orphanages, alcohol consumption, physical abuse, and communication) (Singhal and Rogers 1999, 58). These themes functioned as a springboard for further ideas for *Makgabaneng*'s Modeling and Reinforcement to Combat HIV/AIDS (MARCH) framework.

MODELING AND REINFORCEMENT TO COMBAT HIV/AIDS

MARCH was intended to "promote behavior change through showing people how to change and reinforcing their efforts to change" (Mooki et al. 2004). Additionally, it gave "accurate information," increased audience members' "perceived relevance," shaped "outcome expectations," boosted "self-efficacy," aided "listeners in developing skills," and helped listeners "plan and strategize and create supportive environments" (Rametsi et al. 2003).[22] The main way that MARCH operated was through character modeling that "provide[d] examples of people, behaviors and situations and shows how these can be changed" (Galavotti et al. 2003). Modeling worked in conjunction with reinforcement, which helped individuals "personalize" the models provided (ibid.). As in the case of many other radio serial dramas, the characters were created to fit positive, negative or transitional roles. Positive characters were people who always do the right thing, negative characters consistently engaged in the wrong behaviors, and transitional characters fit somewhere in between the two extremes (Mooki et al. 2004). Out of these three types of characters, the transitional one best mirrored the behavior of the everyday person (ibid.). The major lessons of *Makgabaneng*, however, came from the positive characters that were given functions as role models.

The six scriptwriters working on *Makgabaneng* took these character types and traits into account when writing the storylines for each episode. They had two to three days to produce six weeks of character storylines; then the scripts were subjected to eight stages of development (Mothowamadimo Interview, Jul. 27, 2004). First, the writers engaged in research on contemporary issues that a character would encounter and gathered enough information to build a script. Next, they inserted some kind of conflict or character barriers into the story so that the character has certain things that they will have to overcome. The barriers were conceived in terms of what is facilitating them. Following this step, there was a period of writing, refining, and discussing the storyline with a committee. Finally, the script was rewritten with more precision, sent to the managing editor and completed.[23]

Makgabaneng staff members believed that "the art of scriptwriting" involved listeners finding "characters emotionally compelling and entertaining" (Mooki et al. 2004). Scriptwriters carefully developed characters to make sure that they were believable and that the scenarios were convincing. Whatever decisions the writers arrived at determined the responses of listeners. Listeners were expected to identify the repercussions of the negative characters' behavior as well as the benefits of the positive characters' behavior. Likewise, the transitional characters wavered "between the positive and negative values"; positive characters typically "embod[ied] positive values and are rewarded"; and negative characters "embod[ied] negative values and are punished" (Vaughan et al. 2000, 149). *Makgabaneng* used character modeling and the creation of fictitious scenarios to give listeners the vital skills they needed to deal with real-life situations.

Planning tools were crucial features in expediting the scriptwriting process. Such tools were used to assist writers in "creat[ing] characters that listeners can identify with" and "ensur[ing] that the characters face similar situations and struggles as audiences" (Mooki et al. 2004). Paired with data summary grids (DSGs) capturing information obtained during the initial formative research process, one tool called "pathways to change" identifies the possible "barriers" and "facilitators" for each *Makgabaneng* character (Mooki et al. 2004). It was devised to be played as a board game evaluating social facilitators (Fs), social barriers (Bs), personal facilitators (Fp) and environmental barriers (Be) that shape the actions of characters on the show.

Another indispensable planning tool was the "character trajectory planner" that revolved around characters' behavior and how transitions in behavior impacted the storylines. The planner was centered on the fact that "characters move through stages of change—from recognizing the need to change, forming an intention to change, trying the behavior, overcoming obstacles, and eventually maintain[ing] the new behavior" (Mooki et al. 2004). Staff discovered the significance of constantly consulting the planner to monitor each character's developments. However, there have been isolated cases where the planner was neglected; in one case a character was cast as pregnant for thirteen months, an error that led to scripting inconsistencies. Nonetheless, when the planning tools were applied correctly, they could produce realistic characters that listeners came to admire and viewed as role models.

AN EPISODE OF *MAKGABANENG*

Character modeling and planning in *Makgabaneng* can best be understood through the narrative from an episode of the serial. This segment of my chapter explores the "Masego and Cecilia Disclosure" installment, focusing on how music, special effects (indicated as "FX" below), and narrative combine to tell the tale of a young pregnant woman, Masego, who has just discovered that she contracted HIV from her lover, Thabo, and needs the consolation of a close friend, Cecilia. While episodes of *Makgabaneng* generally air in Setswana, there are occasions where stories such as the "Masego and Cecilia Disclosure" are recorded specially in English. A transcription of an excerpt from the episode is provided below:

[MUSIC: *Makgabaneng* theme song]

[FX: Rain and thunder]

[MASEGO: Crying]

CECILIA: Masego, Masego, what's wrong? Why are you crying? Masego, what's wrong? Please don't scare me like this. Tell me. What is the matter?

MASEGO: Cecilia, it's the end for me.

CECILIA: What do you mean?

[FX: THUNDER]

CECILIA: What end?

[FX: CAT'S MEOW]

MASEGO: My life, Cecilia. I went to the clinic this morning and I got my HIV test results.

CECILIA: Oh my God! What are you trying to tell me, Masego?

MASEGO: Cecilia, I'm HIV-positive [sobbing]

CECILIA: Oh my God! Shhh...

[MUSIC: ELECTRONICALLY SIMULATED SOUNDS OF A CHOIR]

CECILIA: This sure is serious. However, know that all is not lost Masego. At a time like this all you need to do is to have faith and trust in God.

MASEGO: What?! Cecilia, I'm telling you I'm HIV-positive. How can God help me with that, heh?

CECILIA: Please, please, Masego. Please.

[FX: DOOR CLOSES]

CECILIA: Don't talk like someone with no faith.

MASEGO: Woman, are you deaf? In fact, you know what, you're right. I don't have faith, heh. I have the HIV virus.

CECILIA: Please, Masego. Please, friend. Know that I will always, always be here for you.

MASEGO: What have I done to deserve this from God, heh? What have I done?

CECILIA: Baby, you haven't done anything wrong.

[FX: THUNDER]

CECILIA: And please don't talk to me like that. You've done nothing wrong.

MASEGO: Cecilia, are you aware of the fact that Thabo just gave me the death sentence, huh? So simple and easy...

CECILIA: Sego, that's not true. You know, being HIV-positive does not mean death. Please. Please, Masego leave everything in the capable hands of the almighty God.

MASEGO: But Cecilia, they say God only helps those who help themselves.

CECILIA: I know that's what they say, but remember I'm also here for you. Always.

MASEGO: As for me and my bad luck...

CECILIA: Masego, please. This is not the end of the world. All this is doing is giving you a chance to think through your life affairs—taking your status into consideration.

MASEGO: What life Cecilia, huh? What life? Do I even have a life? Please get real! You know if it was just the case of the baby alone it would be easy, for I would tell the baby its father was run over by a train, but as for the HIV virus...

CECILIA: Masego, please...

MASEGO: Eh-eh...

CECILIA: Please try to understand how fortunate you've been for having had the wisdom to test before it was too late, huh. This gives you time to learn to take care of yourself.

MASEGO: But how will that help me? I'm dying anyway.

CECILIA: This is our way, all of us. We all face the same fate.

MASEGO: Don't give me that, Cecilia. Stop talking like the counselor that I saw this morning at the clinic.

CECILIA: As for that dog, Thabo...Anyway, don't you think it's a good idea to tell him so that he also can go for a test. You know...

MASEGO: Testing for what?! Where do you think I got the virus from?

CECILIA: No, no, Sego. No, baby. I didn't mean it like that. I just meant telling him to test so that he too can know his status, you know. We don't want him going around spreading the virus now. Or do we?

MASEGO: Well, that's his problem! I want nothing to do with that hooligan...ever!

CECILIA: I understand what you mean, Masego. But...

MASEGO: As far as I'm concerned, he will only get to see the child when I'm dead and buried.

[FX: THUNDER]

MASEGO: As long as I live I will never let him near my child.

There were definite indicators in the scripted speech acts for how this storyline transpired. Masego visited a clinic to find out her HIV status, a decision that showed her investment in her health. By making a trip to the clinic in the early stages of her pregnancy, it is obvious that Masego planned to continue receiving medical care over the duration of her pregnancy. One can assume she anticipated taking the available drugs to prevent mother-to-child transmission of HIV. All of these factors made Masego a positive character.

In contrast, Thabo was clearly depicted as a negative character because he infected Masego with HIV. Masego announced that Thabo gave her "the death sentence" and called him a "hooligan." Cecilia supported this view, calling Thabo a "dog," yet she also suggested that Masego notify him that she is HIV-positive. Towards the close of the episode segment, Masego hinted that Thabo would probably resist the idea of getting tested for HIV, even if he learned that she was infected with the virus. This implied that he was irresponsible and had no interest in his health.

Unlike Masego and Thabo, Cecilia was the transitional character in the story whose behavior had the potential to shift to either positive or negative. Once Cecilia discovered that Masego was HIV-positive, she could have shunned her, thereby transforming herself into a negative character. However, Cecilia remained supportive, telling Masego that she "will always be there for her," and emphasizing the fact that Masego could find strength through her relationship with God.

Stories such as that of Masego reinforced the two main behavioral change objectives of *Makgabaneng*: positive prevention and care (Mooki Interview, Jul. 29, 2004). Positive prevention offered encouragement to young people to adjust their behavior and get tested for HIV so that they know their status. Care required undergoing any sort of therapy that might be necessary to live a full life as a person living with HIV/AIDS. This went hand in hand with the national sentiments for people to get tested and learn their status. Hence, *Makgabaneng* promoted both individual and community-level health education. The personal decisions that a listener made after listening to the serial drama were deeply rooted in external cultural and societal factors, which determined the proper course of action.

PRODUCING IMAGINARY COMMUNITIES THROUGH SOUND

The juxtaposition of music, sound effects, and narrative accentuated the character modeling elements in the "Cecilia and Masego Disclosure" episode. Although this episode of *Makgabaneng* was not "music-heavy," as Suruchi Sood characterized the Indian radio serial drama *Tinka Tinka Sukh* ("Happiness Lies in Small Things"), music and sound effects constituted a major part of the show (Sood 1999, 31). Brando Keabilwe, a local musician and radio DJ at Gabz FM, was responsible for producing all of the music and sound effects for the show. He devoted four days to producing each episode of *Makgabaneng*. Recording the episodes took anywhere from eight to forty minutes (Keabilwe Interview, Jul. 27, 2004). Once this had been accomplished, Keabilwe commenced the most complicated aspect of the show, editing the recording using the popular computer program ProTools. Keabilwe shared that his main concern at this phase of the show was to "make things as convincing as possible" (ibid.). At times, this called for recording additional sounds from the city and inserting them into the recording. This happened in circumstances where Keabilwe needed the sounds of a donkey cart or a chorus of people singing at a funeral.

I witnessed Keabilwe's sound production first hand when he recorded an episode featuring Spokes, D.T., and Thabo, three male characters on *Makgabaneng*. The episode told of an employee who suspected he was sick with HIV. At a certain point in the script, there was a bar scene. Right before my eyes, I saw a bar created through the sounds of clinking glasses on a tray and Keabilwe's insertion of electronically generated crowd sounds catalogued in his sound files. When he played back the original in-studio recording, with the additional crowd sounds and clinking of glasses layered over it, it was clear that he was able to concoct a very realistic sounding scene.

The role of music in *Makgabaneng* extends far beyond the realm of sound effects. Theme music indicates the beginning of each chapter. It is also used to heighten the mood of a scene. For example, when the ethereal electronically produced music started in the "Masego and Cecilia Disclosure" following Masego's announcement that she was HIV-positive, it demonstrated the sudden emotional shift. At this key moment in the episode, the choir music added to the tension of the situation, emphasizing the volatility and sensitivity of Masego's confession to Cecilia.

There is a longstanding belief that radio has the ability to "motivate people by building on aural/oral traditions and stimulate the imagination better than video or television" (Adam and Harford 1999, 3). It has long been deemed a "theatre of the imagination" (Berger quoted in Tshamano 1993, 13).[24] Even the managing editor of *Makgabaneng*, Maungo Mooki, was convinced that radio is not merely "about accessibility," but encompassed getting "people to internalize" the serial drama's messages and making "the listener visualize" what is taking place (Mooki Interview, Jul. 29, 2004). Thus, a community of radio listeners would take collective interest in particular elements of a program as they are forced to envision a "theatre that exists in the mind" (Crook 1999, ix).[25]

Scholars Lila Abu-Lughod and Liz Gunner elaborate on this notion of imagined radio communities as it relates to radio serials and television serials (Abu-Lughod 2005, 8; Gunner 2000a, 217), pointing out that listeners become engrossed in the stories of fictional characters, often entering into a world where they identify with them and can learn from their experiences. Abu-Lughod underscores the idea that serials are imbued with political and social messages, functioning as part of overarching governmental projects, as was the case in the Egyptian serials that she investigated—*The White Flag, The Journey of Mr. Abu al-'Ela al-Bishry* and *Hilmiyya Nights* (Abu-Lughod 1993, 1997, and 2005).[26] Consequently, in the instance of serials, imagined communities are constructed by listeners who carefully follow the programming and immerse themselves in the fictional lives of characters.

LISTENERS AND REINFORCEMENT ACTIVITIES

According to figures appearing in surveys assessing listening patterns, 50 percent of respondents admitted to listening to *Makgabaneng* at least once a month and 45 percent tuned in at least once a week (Pappas-DeLuca et al. 2003). These criteria corresponded to the categories of regular and committed listeners, respectively. One of the ways that *Makgabaneng* aimed to attract these listeners and retain them is through assorted community reinforcement activities designed to foster discussions amongst listeners (Mooki et al. 2004). There were four main modes of reinforcement for the radio serial drama: listening discussion groups, contests, public listening spots, and road shows. Such activities contribute to *Makgabaneng's* popularity because aspects of the serial are widely debated by the public, thereby becoming integrated into the mainstream (de Fossard 1996, xii).

One of the activities that elicited such discussions was the establishment of listening spots, locations where people congregated across Botswana to listen to and interrogate aspects of *Makgabaneng* (Mooki Interview, Jul. 29, 2004). The primary goal of listening spots was to explore different dimensions of the radio serial drama such as supplying "accurate information about HIV/AIDS," practicing "new skills that may be required in avoiding HIV/AIDS infection" and "supporting those infected and help[ing] participants apply messages of the drama to their own lives" (Rametsi et al. 2003).

Another reinforcement activity was listening discussion groups (LDGs), gatherings of five to fifteen individuals participating in moderated dialogues about *Makgabaneng* with field officers. The organization Total Community Mobilization (TCM) teamed with *Makgabaneng* staff to carry out bi-monthly discussion groups. They played excerpts from the radio drama and stimulated conversations by asking questions about *Makgabaneng* such as: What was said in the scene? Are there people like this in your community? And, What would you do in this situation?[27] Group members used these discussion cues to give their own evaluations and interpretations of the serial drama.

LETTER-WRITING CONTESTS

Another mode of *Makgabaneng* listener analysis is letter-writing contests. One of the first contests occurred in 2002 to commemorate the one hundredth show. After placing Setswana advertisements in newspapers and on radio, inquiring "Who is your favorite character?" and "Give two reasons that encouraged Masego to go to test for HIV," listeners wrote in to *Makgabaneng* staff. Within a period of two weeks, 3,633 letters came flooding in (Tembo et al. 2003). Prize *Makgabaneng* T-shirts were given to the first fifty letter writers who provided the correct answers to the second question.

Staff members noticed a series of interesting trends in the letters. According to data compiled, 78 percent of letters came from women and twenty of the leading letter-writing communities were rural (Tembo et al. 2003).[28] Additionally, listeners gave frank answers about the characters, the circumstances they encountered, and how these scenarios impacted their lives. Out of a batch of three hundred randomly selected letters, a range of insightful comments was accumulated.

As in the case of similar radio serials, fans' letters provided "insights" about how *Makgabaneng* "affects the audience" (Law and Singhal 1999; Singhal and Rogers 2002). Letters about the "Masego and Cecilia Disclosure" demonstrated keen audience awareness about HIV/AIDS such as the fact that Masego tested for HIV in order to "protect her unborn child" and "because she got encouragement from others" (Tembo et al. 2003). Consequently, the audience feedback was a sign of what has been labeled a Freireian "empowerment-education" approach to data presented in radio serial dramas (Sood 2002, 167). Thus, listeners inadvertently adopted Paulo Freire's concept of problem-posing education and "dramatization acts" where all information undergoes a process of critical contemplation before it is internalized (Freire 1970 and 1994). The essence of empowerment-education called for listening to HIV/AIDS messages woven into the narratives of the radio serial drama, critically considering their significance, and then applying them into actual situations. For instance, after hearing *Makgabaneng* broadcasts about Masego going to test for HIV/AIDS and enrolling in a PMTCT program while supported by clinic counselors and a friend, listeners might see the value of her actions.[29] As one listener wrote, "I like Masego when she says she wants to go for an HIV test...because even me, it taught me to test for the disease because it kills" (Tembo et al. 2003). Other listeners favored Cecilia in this scenario, stating, "Cecilia at all times gave Masego advice on the importance of her education, rather than just sitting back and seeing her delayed by the nice and short-time things of the moment" (ibid.).

IPOLETSE INFORMATION HOTLINE

Masego's plight triggered further audience response through the *Ipoletse* information hotline, the call center responsible for responding to inquiries about HIV/AIDS and Sexually Transmitted Infections (STIs). There was a period in 2003, when the storyline involved Masego seeking PMTCT to prevent transmitting HIV to her unborn child. On April 23, *Makgabaneng* staff aired an epilogue titled "Masego's Epilogue," encouraging listeners to follow her example, and supplying the *Ipoletse* hotline number for listeners who wished to talk about the matter with someone. An overwhelming number of calls poured into the hotline. Within five days after the epilogue aired, over 1,600 calls were received, signaling the intense desire of audience members to mull over the topic at hand (Galavotti et al. 2003).

Research on the *Ipoletse* hotline indicated that before the month when "Masego's Epilogue" was broadcast, there were generally not more than two hundred calls per day (ibid.). However, when the epilogue first aired, and was later rebroadcast, the call volume skyrocketed. Evening and weekend *Ipoletse* hotline closings prevented some callers from responding. Nevertheless, the call volume showed that callers felt strongly enough about the topic to create a dialogue and probe for further answers.

CONCLUSION

In his dissertation on HIV/AIDS preventive behavior in Botswana, Boga Fidzani encouraged the construction of "a wide array of preventive and curative strategies to bring [HIV infection] to a halt" (Fidzani 2003, 3). *Makgabaneng* is one of the many preventive approaches that have been formed in the country. It fuses HIV/AIDS health education models and behavioral change programs to transform national perceptions of HIV and AIDS. As Elizabeth Gunner elaborated in a 2005 lecture, the musical arts are a way for communities to make sense of the challenges of their present circumstances and to see their way to the future (Gunner 2005). Contemporary musical arts education initiatives are doing just that in today's contexts.

The musical arts remain "principal tools of many local initiatives and the media that disseminate information, mobilize resources, and raise societal consciousness regarding issues related to HIV/AIDS" (Barz 2006a, 3). *Makgabaneng* actor Ben Ngwato echoed these sentiments, noting that the musical arts, and drama in particular, equip communities with the skills needed for survival, thereby providing Botswana with the "roots" for "empowering" themselves (Ngwato Interview, Jul. 27, 2004). As a mode of dramatic interpretation, *Makgabaneng* is etched firmly into Botswana's multisectoral HIV/AIDS response, fulfilling its duties in health education efforts.

Maungo Mooki believed the serial drama operates as a "gateway to behavioral change" that can make considerable contributions to Botswana's HIV/AIDS epidemic (Mooki Interview, Jul. 29, 2004). With the urgent move to eradicate HIV/AIDS in Botswana by 2016, the fiftieth anniversary of Botswana's independence, *Makgabaneng* has certainly opened the gate to new possibilities for reversing the devastation of HIV/AIDS in the country. The last set of national HIV/AIDS statistics indicated that national HIV prevalence decreased to 17.1 percent, triggering speculation that heightened HIV/AIDS health education campaigns like *Makgabaneng* are helpful in the national HIV/AIDS prevention strategy (NACA 2004, 14). Based on *Makgabaneng*'s various accomplishments and successes, members of the staff team are convinced that the "trajectory" of the serial drama is "endless," and they plan to continue producing it for years to come until the war on HIV/AIDS in Botswana is won (Tembo Interview, Jul. 15, 2004).

14

"We Are the Loudmouthed HIV-Positive People"

"*SIYAYINQOBA/BEAT IT!*" ON SOUTH AFRICAN TELEVISION

Rebecca Hodes (University of Cape Town)

INTRODUCTION

In 1999, a program was piloted on South African national television that focused on issues facing HIV-positive people. *Siyayinqoba/Beat It!* began as a small-scale production, but grew rapidly over its eight seasons. From 2003 to 2006, it occupied a prime slot on a national channel where it was watched by over a million viewers a week. The program, closely aligned to the Treatment Action Campaign (TAC) and Médecins Sans Frontières (MSF), has innovated ways of addressing HIV-related stigma through its normalization of the disease and its portrayals of a diverse array of HIV-positive participants. It has also cultivated HIV status disclosure through its frequent broadcast of rousing "treatment testimonies," including accounts by participants in South Africa's mother-to-child-transmission prevention and public antiretroviral (ARV) treatment programs (Robins 2006, 316).[1]

Beat It! has reflected developments in the socio-political and medical spheres surrounding HIV and has echoed the workings of the treatment access movement in South Africa. Through a description of the discursive strategies used by the show, with a particular focus on the show's role in the 2000–2002 activist campaign for prevention of mother-to-child transmission (PMTCT) treatment programs, I will suggest that Beat It! harnessed television's ability to demystify complex issues relating to HIV. Under the rubric of "positive living," Beat It! presented the many ways in which HIV-positive people could maintain a healthy lifestyle, most importantly through being informed about prevention, transmission, and treatment. Capturing and conveying the most significant developments relating to HIV in South Africa between

1999 and 2006—during which *Beat It!*'s first six series were broadcast—the program's mirroring of the political campaigns of HIV activist organizations provides an important record of the contemporary history of HIV politics during this time.

BEAT IT! PREHISTORY

During the 1980s, AIDS frequently featured in newspaper headlines and electronic media across the globe (Altman 1986, 19). These media constructed what Simon Watney (1987, 145) has termed a "punitive palisade" around HIV, with the disease represented as "just desserts" for immoral behavior—particularly sexual perversity and promiscuity. Paula Treichler (1999, 315) has examined how television coverage of the epidemic in the United States relied on hackneyed, pathos-heavy storylines, which presented audiences with predictable narrative trajectories and stymied broader public identification. As a result of activists' resistance to denigrating media representations of people with HIV/AIDS at the end of the 1980s, however, new media discourses were constructed. Part of the work of the American AIDS Coalition to Unleash Power (ACT UP), for example, was to intertwine art and politics. The use of protest paraphernalia, including stickers, posters, and videos, formed a distinctive visual aesthetic and propelled ACT UP to the position of one of the United States' most visible social movement at the end of the 1980s (Epstein 2005, 176). DIVA (Damned Interfering Video Activists), a media offshoot of ACT UP, used the medium of video to publicize the movement's grievances. Its establishment led to the invention of new cinematic approaches to AIDS, and to the growth of activist media distribution networks (Horrigan 1993, 168).

By the close of the nineties, HIV activism had become increasingly organized and assertive, in South Africa as elsewhere. A core group of activists and health care workers had founded TAC in 1998, primarily to fight for access to Highly Active Antiretroviral Therapy (HAART) in the public sector. The introduction of this treatment had drastically decreased AIDS mortality in wealthy nations since 1996. But while Europe and the United States saw an 84 percent decline in death rates from AIDS between 1997 and 2001 as a direct result of access to HAART, AIDS mortality in the global south continued to escalate (Iliffe 2006, 149). HIV testing and the mobilization of broad-based support for public access to ARVs now took on new imperatives. Activists were confronted with the daunting task of reforming public opinion about HIV as a disease of shame and death when, for the majority of HIV-positive South Africans, this remained the stark reality.

In his analysis of the role of television in democratic participation, Groombridge argued that current affairs-based participatory programming forms "the basis of socially relevant adult education" on television, helping people to formulate opinions and stimulating social action (1972, 220, 240). In this sense, the medium of television is well suited to a large-scale public education about HIV, including the possibilities for long-term survival with the disease. The participatory format of *Beat It!*'s episodes drew on television's interactive dimension to challenge taboos and to encourage public engagement with HIV-related issues. *Beat It!*'s use of the support group as its primary focus engaged viewers, both through its communicative format and its content. The show also included frequent calls for audience involvement through letters and telephone calls to the *Beat It!* offices or the National AIDS Helpline. Challenging stigma became one of *Beat It!*'s central themes, encapsulated by content producer Michael Rautenbach's assertion that the show's primary messages hinged on "openness, stigma, 'positive living.' That you don't have to die" (Rautenbach Interview, Apr. 24, 2007).

By exposing and confronting many forms of HIV-related stigma, from social discrimination to self-stigma, the show could then promote strategies for resisting prejudice through disclosure and "positive living."

THE NORMALIZATION OF HIV IN *BEAT IT!*

Beat It!'s normalizing tactics assumed a variety of forms, from the subtle to the overt. A demystifying image could be as casual as a bowl of condoms or ARV pillbox left nonchalantly on a table, or as forthright as a support group member's disclosure of her HIV-positive status on a busy commuter train. Television provides an ideal medium for this kind of normalizing: it has been regarded theoretically as one of the most quotidian forms of mass media, both in terms of content and reception. This is due to its ability to broadcast the lives of ordinary people into the private spaces of viewers' homes (Biressi and Nunn 2005, 9–10). And while the lives of ordinary people have long been a preoccupation of documentary filmmakers, the rise of reality TV has seen the massive popularization of programs about the interior lives of others. *Beat It!*'s focus on the support group—members of the South African public discussing intimate aspects of their HIV-positive lives—cohered with the genre of reality TV. In order to normalize HIV, the program used the "demythologizing function of film," with its peculiar ability to capture reality and thereby to foster understanding of complex subjects (Rosenthal 1980, 5). Through constant portrayals of a diverse range of HIV-positive people who talked honestly about matters ranging from the banal to the most private, the show sought to desensationalize the disease. In explaining how *Beat It!* differed from earlier representations of HIV in South African media, content producer Cilla Blankenberg stated:

> [Y]ou see people in their homes with their kids, in their communities. It's far less stigmatized...We have every kind of person on the show. But, it's very South African, it's very true to real life here. It doesn't pretend to be anything you haven't seen with your own eyes in the street, or in a rural area or in an urban area...It is very real. (Interview, Apr. 17, 2007)

The program's producers thus believed in the importance of its verisimilitude as a point of differentiation from older media representations of HIV/AIDS. Episodes presented HIV-positive people as living healthy, active, and ordinary lives, and portrayed a slew of seemingly ordinary activities in order to underscore the vitality and normality of the program's HIV-positive participants: from lifting weights in a gym, to overseeing their children's homework. One of *Beat It!*'s presenters described the show's attempts to demystify the disease in the following terms:

> We were normalizing it and part of the things we did was to convey that: "We're ordinary people by the way, we can laugh, we can joke. Just because you are HIV-positive doesn't mean you have to stay put, eat salads, take your medication and live as if you were in a straightjacket." (Nhlapo Interview, Mar. 20, 2007)

Beat It! also confronted arguably the most heavily stigmatized practice relating to HIV—the subject of "sex and the positive person" (2004, ep. 20). This episode examined the intimate lives of serodiscordant couples, and exposed taboos relating to sex and HIV-positive people. The everyday images of couples at home, together with their assurances that their sex lives were

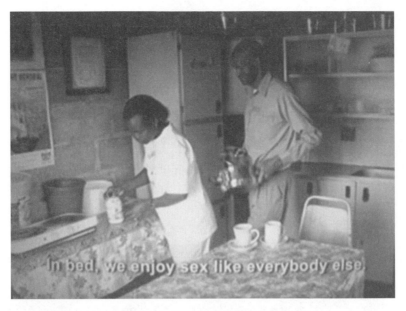

Figure 14.1 Image of couple at home

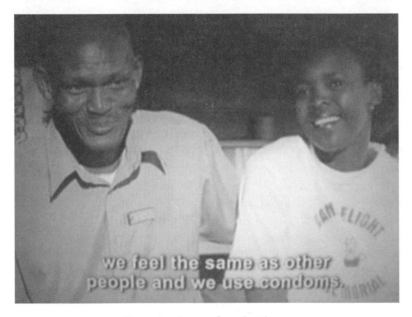

Figure 14.2 Image of couple at home

pleasurable and "like everybody else's" conveyed a normalizing message about the possibilities of safe, sensual sex within committed partnerships (see figures 14.1 and 14.2).

LANGUAGE AND DISCLOSURE

Rosenberg (1992, xiii) described disease as an "elusive entity," relying on "a generation-specific repertoire of verbal constructs reflecting medicine's intellectual and institutional history." In the historical construction of the HIV/AIDS pandemic, language initially obscured the fact of heterosexual transmission in its medical inscription of the disease as "Gay-Related Immune Deficiency" (GRID). Thus, in a very real sense, the language used to talk about HIV/AIDS has defined both the meaning of the disease and the nature of public responses to it.

Descriptions of HIV/AIDS in the South Africa media of the 1980s were strongly influenced by frameworks from abroad. A *Beat It!* presenter recounted how, in the South African media, HIV "was presented as death, dirty...a scourge, something that people get punished with for their wrongdoings" (Nhlapo Interview, Mar. 20, 2007). Media accounts of modes of HIV transmission were confusing, with nebulous references to the "exchange of bodily fluids" instead of straightforward explanations. The vagueness of these descriptions did not calm fears of casual contagion, nor did it educate the public about precisely which sexual acts put one at risk of transmission. In contrast with older media, *Beat It!* has aimed explicitly to oppose stigmatizing language and to encourage HIV-positive people to disclose their status. A content producer explained:

> [T]he thing about *Beat It!* is that nobody hides. It's HIV-positive people on TV. We talk about sex...it becomes normalized and it becomes something you can watch on TV after lunch at half past one on Sunday. It's not taboo...All the other information is almost secondary to the fact that "We are the loud-mouthed HIV-positive people!" (Blankenberg Interview, Apr. 17, 2007)

The very first episode of *Beat It!* was a watershed in the history of HIV in South Africa, as it featured fifty HIV-positive people disclosing their status openly on national television. The aim of this mass disclosure was to break the silence and stigma surrounding the disease, which had led to the murder of HIV activist Gugu Dlamini in 1998 after she disclosed her HIV-positive status on a radio broadcast. In a later episode, presenter Mercy Makhalemele described openness around HIV as a primary reason for *Beat It!*'s existence:

> We started the program because we knew that there are thousands of people living in silence with HIV, no one to talk to, no one to share with, to confront many challenges of living and surviving with HIV. (2000, ep. 12)

Every episode of *Beat It!* began with disclosure, as the presenters introduced themselves and stated that they, as well as all the other members of the support group, were "living positively with HIV." Disclosure was often depicted as an important means of challenging stigma and of coming to terms with an HIV-positive status. In an episode from the 2005 series, Edwin Cameron, a South African judge living openly with HIV/AIDS, described the role of disclosure in combating HIV stigma and denialism:

> I think we've had a silent epidemic. There are so few voices in the epidemic...The more people who speak out, whether they are business people, soccer players, entertainers or politicians...it will help a lot with stigma. As soon as we see that our leaders begin to speak about the normalization of this disease, we don't have to treat it as something scary and horrible. (2005, ep. 22)

Beat It! also drew on the authority of key state figures to encourage HIV disclosure. The public admissions of high-ranking political families (including the Mandelas) regarding their relatives' deaths from AIDS were lauded by the support group for fostering a culture of HIV-openness. But the program placed greater emphasis on the disclosures of a range of ordinary people who proclaimed the benefits of being open about their status. In episode four from the 2004 series, a documentary insert entitled "Learners beat HIV" featured the following dialogue between HIV-positive school-goers who had been invited onto the show as guest participants:

> Babalwa Tembani: I decided to disclose my status and show that HIV is here, especially for us youth. Because every Saturday in Khayelitsha you see us bury the youth who've died of AIDS. So no one forced me to disclose, I did it on my own.

> Nwabisa Njaba: First I disclosed to my class, and then to the whole school. After that, students came to me with their problems. Then we formed the AIDS Task Team at my school.

This exchange emphasized the importance of disclosure in educating others about the disease and in addressing HIV-denialism and misinformation among young people. In Njaba's assertion that she has become a source of authoritative advice for other students, she conveyed one possible benefit of disclosure. *Beat It!* broadcast frequent confessions by support group members that relayed other transformative aspects of disclosure. In a program from the 1999 series, support group member Faghmeda Miller recounted:

> Before, I was a very shy person. I never used to go out. But today I go out in the community and I speak about HIV and AIDS, and I can say that it has changed my life for the better. And I just want to talk about it. I just want to tell everyone: "It's okay, when you are HIV-positive you're not going to die now. Life goes on." (2000, ep. 5)

Beat It! participants testified to the transformative effects of living openly with HIV in numerous other episodes, subverting perceptions of HIV as a mark of death and disgrace. However, a prerequisite for accessing the possible benefits of living openly with HIV is disclosure of one's status. In certain episodes of *Beat It!*, the impetus to disclose approached mania. In an early episode from *Beat It!*'s first series, a man named Benjamin Borrageiro was profiled. Borrageiro, who died of AIDS shortly after this episode was filmed, issued the following advice:

> I suggest to everybody, talk about it if you've got it. Speak about it immediately, because the longer you hold it inside, the quicker you are going to die. Because you will be living a lie. (2000, ep. 9)

This emphasis on the public confession of one's HIV status has been criticized as one of the more alienating practices of treatment activists (Steinberg 2008, 317). But although certain episodes of *Beat It!* conveyed a kind of "disclosure fever," presenting openness about the disease as a necessity for survival, an acid test of friendship and an essential matter of self-respect, the program also contained many messages that countered the notion of disclosure as a panacea for HIV-related problems. Episodes included more ambiguous accounts of disclosure experiences, or portrayed experiences that were overtly negative. A statement by support group member Prudence Mabele conveyed some of this ambiguity:

> I like the fact that I'm open. I'm talking to people, and I educate people. But I'm talking to you out there, you say I am dead... I am *isidumbu* (a corpse). You call us by names like that... If you show your face it is like some kind of germ. (2003, ep. 5)

In many episodes, members of the support group cautioned viewers to ensure that their HIV disclosure would not endanger them in any way. Some shows also featured the testimonies of women who were persecuted as a result of their HIV-positive disclosure: these informants were beaten by their partners, expelled from their houses, ostracized by their communities and, in one instant, forced to have a "traditional" abortion through immersion in a bath of toxic herbs. Thus, while disclosure was portrayed as an important and empowering aspect of the "positive lifestyle," the harsh realities of persistent stigma were confronted by the show as well. *Beat It!* participants also asserted the right of people with HIV *not* to disclose, to keep their status a secret (2005, ep. 9). Support group member Anthony Fernandes encapsulated this in his assertion that: "Disclosure is up to you, there's no bloody law that says you have to disclose! I say it makes it easier, but it's still your personal choice" (2004, ep. 6).

Episodes issued practical advice to viewers regarding aspects of disclosure, ranging from how to tell children that they were HIV-positive, to legal rights regarding disclosure in the workplace, problems facing openly positive teachers and students, and the importance of disclosure in effective adherence to ARVs, including PMTCT. The program advised a "go-slow" approach in certain circumstances, thereby modulating "disclosure fever" with reminders of the shocking impact that disclosure may have on loved ones.

Beat It!'s overall approach to HIV disclosure was summarized by the "Take Home Messages" of the 2005 episode devoted solely to the subject (2005, ep. 1):

- There is no "right way" or magic formula to disclose.

- Disclose when you are ready and it feels right for you.

- Disclose gradually over time to the people you feel comfortable with.

- Prepare for disclosing by talking to someone you can trust, like a counselor.

- Contact support groups and organizations for help.

THE PROMOTION OF THE "POSITIVE COMMUNITY"

Television allows its audience a privileged view into the lives of its subjects and, in terms of the recent popular explosion of reality programming, has spawned a new culture of exposure, confession and witnessing (Biressi and Nunn 2005, 107). This is applicable especially to what has been termed "therapeutic television," in which ordinary people share graphic details about their lives with a talk show audience. *Beat It!* mirrored many of the conventions of a TV talk show, particularly in terms of its intimacy and its reflection of the ordinary lives of HIV-positive South Africans. It also tapped into a history of South African media-based community affiliation, including community radio that promoted awareness of and engagement with the social and economic problems faced by black communities (Hadland et al. 2006, 36–37). In its diversity and its connectedness, the *Beat It!* support group presented viewers with a microcosmic community of HIV-positive people: support group members, guests, and people profiled for the documentary inserts were drawn from the public. Moreover, in the show's frequent reminders that HIV-positive people are just ordinary South Africans, in the intensity of the experiences that the program portrayed, and in the intimacy of its informants' on-screen confessions, *Beat It!* strove to encourage audience identification with the "positive community." The director of *Beat It!*, Jack Lewis, explained: "It was clear that in South Africa in 1999, the HIV epidemic was giving way to an AIDS epidemic, and *Beat It!* aimed to do something that was pretty well unparalleled…use the national media to echo a movement on the ground that was seeking to secure and promote the rights of people living with HIV and AIDS" (Lewis Interview, May 23, 2007). Affection between the support group members was another of the program's overt strategies for representing a tightly knit "positive community." Every episode ended with footage of members hugging each other and their studio guests. Especially in episodes in which the show's participants had argued, the closing footage of the hug confirmed that mutual respect and affection, rather than antagonism, had prevailed. An example of the empathy the show portrayed between the members of the "positive community" was encapsulated in an interview with HIV activist Queenie Qiza. Qiza (figure 14.3) made the following statement of solidarity:

> I'd like to say to the community: be strong, be supportive, be active, like me! [She is shown joking and laughing energetically with a friend.] I love all those who are HIV-positive like me. Live on, and don't be discouraged! Continue with your lives, do not be afraid. Enjoy your life! (2000, ep. 4)

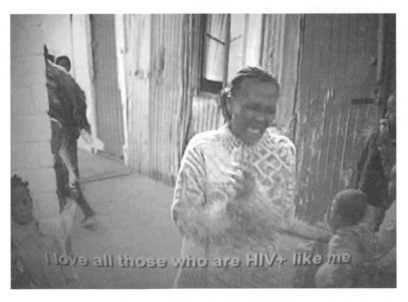

Figure 14.3 HIV activist Queenie Qiza

Beat It! presenters often read letters on-air from viewers that affirmed the motivating messages of the program and the burgeoning existence of the "positive community." For example, in the last episode of the 2000 series, a viewer's letter was read that praised the engaging, empowering aspects of the support group as a collective:

> Your program gives us hope and it motivates us people living with the virus...I want to open a support group so that I can teach other people how to beat HIV. (2000, ep. 12)

Robins (2006, 314) has described how the construction of a "positive community" through the discourses of HIV activists in South Africa has resulted in the "social reintegration and revitalization" of large numbers of HIV-positive people. *Beat It!* attributed similar benefits to open and active membership in the "positive community," and sought to portray active involvement in the community as part of the transformative potential of a positive disclosure. In episode 11 of the 2003 series, support group member Busisiwe Maqungo recounted her initially hopeless reaction to her HIV diagnosis, followed by her revitalization through HIV activism and outreach:

> I just thought my end to life had come. I would just go home and wait until I die. Working for the community is one of the helpful ways—when you are HIV-positive—because I volunteered for TAC and educated people. My life just got easy because I knew I was helping other people living with the virus, and those who don't have it, so they can be protected...I got a job at UWC [University of the Western Cape], where I work with students...I'm like their role model on how to live positively with HIV.

As with disclosure, *Beat It!* presented a positive dimension of HIV by opening support group members to new opportunities. In many instances in the program the transformative, life-sustaining nature of the "positive community" drew comparisons with religious salvation. These comparisons were prevalent in statements about antiretroviral medication and involvement in HIV organizations, primarily TAC. In episode 7 from the 2003 series, footage from an antiretroviral pilot support group included the following statement from one of its male members:

> I become well when I see other people who are HIV-positive. And they are beautiful, as I am beautiful now. They counseled me first...They told me about treatment...I am who I am, I am healthy.

This statement foregrounded the notion of a new, wonderful becoming, and an elevated sense of self and regard for other HIV-positive people as a result of the life-sustaining potential of ARVs.

THE PROMOTION OF "POSITIVE LIVING" IN *BEAT IT!*

Echoing the discursive influence of HIV activist narratives from overseas, *Beat It!*'s participants often framed their advice about "positive living" within pop psychological discourses of self-help and self-love, emphasizing the importance of emotional well-being. In almost every episode of the program, *Beat It!*'s participants were encouraged to ensure that their health was maintained, to "live positively" with HIV rather than to die of AIDS. The "positive lifestyle" the show promoted entailed active care of mind and body: from nutrition and mental health, to exercise, vaccination, procuring early and effective treatment for opportunistic infections, and adhering to antiretroviral treatment. An understanding of the mechanics of HIV itself, its transmission, its symptoms, and its potential treatment, was presented as the core of the "positive lifestyle." One of *Beat It!*'s central themes was therefore the education of its viewers in the physiological properties of the disease, often through the creative use of graphics that demystified its biological workings.

The underlying message of all aspects of "positive living" remained the encouragement of individual assertiveness and action. One support group guest who tested HIV-positive after an abusive relationship told viewers:

> Find out who you are. Stand up for yourself. Do what is best for you. Focus on what you can change—especially your mind and your heart. Change your life to suit yourself, not anyone else. (2005, ep. 6)

This individualism was tempered by the support group dialogue that followed, in which the pursuit of a confident and positive sense of self was situated within a broader community context:

> Jason Wessenaar [presenter]: I think some of these things of self-worth...self-respect, things that you work on as an individual, but also I suppose with support from school, from the community, from neighbors...Maybe we need to find ways in schools...in support groups, or just in the community to find ways to build self-esteem, to help people to feel that they love themselves enough, they have the self worth.

> Sisonke Msimang [women's rights activist and *Beat It!* guest]: We need to think different about our messages, produce messages that are about a whole person, a complete person, a healthy person, mentally, physically and spiritually. And then we'll be on the road to empowerment for both boys and girls.

Mental health was portrayed as a central constituent in the formula for "positive living." In outlining the history of HIV programs created by international development agencies, Nguyen (2005, 127) has explained that first-generation programs followed a "top-down" approach, imposing models for behavior change upon poor world populations in ways that denied agency and negated efficacy. "Second generation" programs, on the other hand, adhered to the principles of GIPA (Greater Involvement of People with AIDS), as outlined by UNAIDS and other international development agencies in the latter half of the nineties. Furthermore, second-generation awareness initiatives were couched in the idioms of "empowerment" and "self-help" initially constructed by North American HIV activists. The evolution of these development discourses thus explains the American flavor of many of *Beat It!*'s lifestyle messages, but especially those regarding mental health. In a telling moment on the show, for example, Justice Edwin Cameron asserted the importance of a positive mindset and overall mental health in living positively with HIV:

> There are five or six million South Africans who are claiming their lives through "positive living," through positive attitudes, and through access to treatment...My life is continuing. I feel blessed...I'm fifty-two years old now, I hope I'm going to reach age eighty...I know this virus is not going to knock me down. (2005, ep. 14)

Also significant about this statement is its construction of an enormous "positive community," inclusive of every HIV-positive South African, collectively involved in the pursuit of a "positive lifestyle." Cameron's statement conveyed a sense of gratitude, an active and energetic engagement with his life, and a repudiation of victimhood. Many other episodes of *Beat It!* emphasized the importance of happiness in the maintenance of overall health and treatment adherence, with an entire episode of the 2005 series devoted to "Mental Health and HIV" (2005, ep. 20).

The role of nutrition in living positively with HIV was another component of *Beat It!*'s "positive lifestyle." However, the program's discussions about nutrition emphasized that a healthy, balanced diet did not have to be expensive, thereby reassuring poorer viewers that they too could live positively with HIV, just like the members of the support group. Some of the program's earliest messages endorsed the role of nutrition and alternative therapies in the treatment of HIV before such claims became the subject of political controversy.[2] Nonetheless, whenever nutrition and alternative therapies were discussed among the support group, the importance of monitoring by allopathic medical professionals was emphasized. For example, in episode 9 of the 2003 series, Anthony Fernandes stated:

> I think it's important for us people who live with HIV and AIDS to monitor ourselves through our doctors as well. You know, we can still fight this disease with good nutrition and a healthy lifestyle.

Support group member, Prudence Mabele, stated shortly thereafter:

> I'm still living a healthy lifestyle, sleeping a lot, eating, relaxing...taking vitamins and homeopathy and aromatherapy, all of those things. But [my CD4 cell count] worries me, I always check when it is the right time.

The importance of eating vegetables was highlighted later in the 2003 series when a documentary insert showed one of the support group members buying food. Images of fruits and vegetables appeared on the screen while support group member Matthew Damane's voiceover stated the importance of a balanced diet.

Beat It! later broadcast an episode that addressed the issue of miracle foods and supplements (2004, ep. 15). Support group member John Vollenhoven recounted how a woman lost her twenty-two year old daughter to AIDS because she fed her daughter only carrots in the belief that they would cure her HIV. "So she died of carrots?" one support group member asked. This episode included support group members' accounts of how their own dietary manias had taken a negative toll on their health. Fernandes explained how he had "panicked" in the wake of his HIV-positive diagnosis, pursuing a severe health diet that entailed consuming copious raw food smoothies that had disrupted the normal functioning of his liver. Busisiwe Maqungo later recounted a short-lived obsession with African potato because "I was so desperate to get my hands on anything that could help me" (2004, ep. 15). *Beat It!*'s frequent portrayal of the mistakes and vices of the support group was a strategy to encourage viewer identification. Treichler has argued that the most effective HIV campaigns are those that embrace difference and highlight complexity (1999, 221). Faithful to these principles, *Beat It!* presented its viewers with a range of behaviors and responses in its attempts to foster broad-based awareness and speak to a diverse viewing public.

Other aspects of physical wellbeing that *Beat It!* emphasized as part of a "positive life-style" included exercise, dental hygiene, vaccinations, and frequent medical check-ups to prevent or treat opportunistic infections. In addition to its focus on mental health, the program devoted episodes to educating poor and disabled viewers on how to access social grants in order to support themselves and their families. An episode from the 2005 series was even devoted to "positive dying"—including information about how to write a will and which funeral policies protected the interests of people who had died of AIDS. The most prominent aspect of the "positive lifestyle," however, was adherence to ARVs, beginning with the drugs that prevent the mother-to-child transmission of HIV.

PREVENTING MOTHER-TO-CHILD TRANSMISSION OF HIV

The struggle to procure ARVs for pregnant women in order to prevent perinatal transmission of HIV was the central mobilizing force in the emergence of South Africa's HIV treatment access movement. TAC's formation was premised on its founders' objective to initiate a campaign for a national PMTCT program (Iliffe 2006, 145). Due to the close-knit ties between TAC leaders and the production staff of the Community Media Trust, PMTCT thus became the primary subject of *Beat It!*'s first series.

The year of South Africa's first democratic elections (1994) coincided with a break-through in HIV treatment, when it was discovered that monotherapy with the ARV drug zido-vudine (AZT) led to dramatic reductions in the rates of HIV transmission from mother-to-child *in utero* (Heywood 2003, 278). In 1998, a clinical trial in Thailand indicated that a short course of AZT, administered from the thirty-sixth week of pregnancy, reduced rates of vertical trans-mission from mother to child. This discovery meant that the cost of prevention of mother-to-child transmission regimens began to fall because it had been shown that a shorter course of treatment was effective in preventing perinatal transmission. It fell further still in 1999, when the HIVNET 012 trial proved that a single dose of the ARV nevirapine reduced perinatal trans-mission (Guay et al. 1999). At this time in South Africa, rising HIV infection rates saw approx-imately 70,000 babies born HIV-positive each year, with a spike in infant mortality attesting to the fatal effects of AIDS (Heywood 2003, 279). The National AIDS Plan of 1994 recognized the initial discoveries around PMTCT, and called for measures to be taken to prevent perinatal transmission. But by 1997, government failure to act on these measures was criticized by an alliance of activists and doctors, who sought to pressure the Department of Health to establish programs of PMTCT. When TAC was formed in December 1998, one of its explicit goals was the establishment of state-run PMTCT programs. TAC met with successive ministers of health Nkosazana Dlamini-Zuma and Manto Tshabalala-Msimang in order to outline these demands, which were initially well received. These discussions ceded joint statements that AZT's cost was a major obstacle to the national PMTCT program, and led TAC to embark on a campaign to lower the prices on essential ARVs through direct pressure on pharmaceutical corporations.

The potential expense of national PMTCT programs plummeted in 1999, when a Ugandan clinical trial proved that a single dose of the cheap antiretroviral nevirapine was also successful in reducing perinatal transmission. With a view toward the establishment of a South African PMTCT program, newly inaugurated Health Minister Tshabalala-Msimang visited

Uganda to evaluate the efficacy of the treatment (Nattrass 2007, 62).[3] At this juncture, HIV activists increased their demands for public access to ARVs, touting the successes of the PMTCT pilot program administered by Médecins Sans Frontières in Cape Town's informal settlement of Khayelitsha (Hodes and Holm 2011).[4] The second episode of *Beat It!*, screened on independent South African network eTV (entertainment television) in October 2000, also heralded the successes of the Khayelitsha pilot PMTCT program. Footage of a young black woman inside her shack was accompanied by an upbeat voiceover that proclaimed: "Phumeza is HIV-positive. She has received AZT which has prevented her from infecting her baby during pregnancy" (2000, ep. 2). The voiceover then noted that former President Nelson Mandela had "called for urgent steps to protect South Africa's children from the HIV/AIDS scourge," and drew on the moral authority of South Africa's iconic political figure to emphasize the imperative of the PMTCT program.

Beat It! focused on the issue of perinatal transmission, particularly in its earlier episodes, as one of the clearest examples of the life-saving properties of ARVs, and of the tragedy and injustice of avoidable infant mortality when government obstructionism barred access to treatment. The testimonies of *Beat It!* support group member Busisiwe Maqungo illustrated this two-pronged approach. As the most popular member of the support group, Maqungo's confessions and assertions led hundreds of viewers to write in and declare their admiration for her. On numerous occasions throughout the series, Maqungo recounted, with pain and anger, the tragedy of her baby's death from AIDS. She believed that had she gained access to PMTCT therapy at a government postnatal clinic, her daughter would have lived:

> I'm still grieving the death of my child…It's haunting me and that's why I get angry when I see children dying. Because when I infected her I didn't know that I was HIV-infected. Let's say that I *did* know I was HIV-infected and I was given nevirapine and she was born HIV-free. Every time I think about it, I cry, and I don't want to cry [she starts to cry]. (2000, ep. 7)

Maqungo's case reflected another aspect of South Africa's HIV policy when, after public access to PMTCT had been mandated by the Constitutional Court, in essence forcing government to roll out PMTCT, she became pregnant again. In a dramatic episode that documented the developments in her PMTCT program adherence, Maqungo explained that she had taken nevirapine during labor and that her baby was given nevirapine syrup. She had also bottle-fed her baby, and footage showed her nursing him with the bottle while she recounted (figure 14.4):

> I don't want to take a chance of baby getting infected through breast milk. He is going to test [for HIV] when he's nine months, he's still six months now. I'm hoping that my baby is going to be negative. (2004, ep. 13)

The episode then broadcast the testing procedure and Maqungo waiting anxiously for its outcome. In one of *Beat It!*'s most dramatic scenes, Maqungo was shown walking down a hospital corridor with her baby in her arms, on the way to fetch her results. Suspenseful music punctuated the footage, which then showed her seated in the doctor's consulting room, awaiting the result of her child's HIV status. When the doctor told her that her baby was HIV-negative, Maqungo shrieked with glee and began to cry, hugging her baby closely. "Oh my god," she said to the doctor, "Thank you very much!" She then turned to her baby and said, "we've got very good news for you, baby [shaking his hand]: you're a very, very healthy baby. I'm so happy!" In a clear

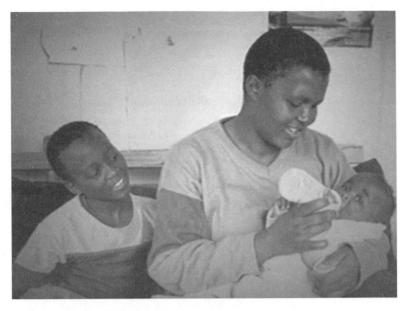

Figure 14.4 Maqungo bottle-feeding her baby

illustration of the efficacy of PMTCT, the doctor responded: "I knew you would be...You've been through the program, you took the medication, so now we know that this program works." Driving the emotive force of the scene even further, the camera focused in slow-motion on a close-up of Maqungo's grateful expression, then cut back to the support group where she was shown with her baby seated on her lap, both smiling broadly (figures 14.5 and 14.6).

The use of AZT in the prevention of perinatal HIV transmission had already been discounted by the Health Minister, who had disregarded extensive scientific evidence regarding

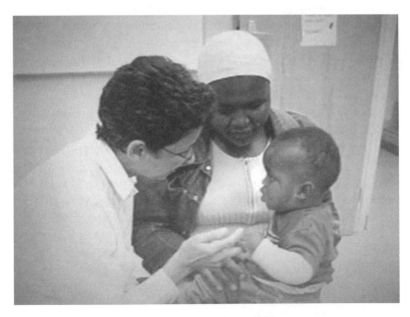

Figure 14.5 Maqungo's grateful face

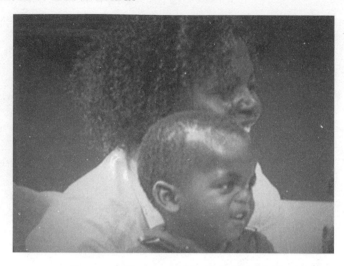

Figure 14.6 Maqungo with her baby on her lap

the drug's efficacy and instead focused on its potential toxicity. In response, the World Health Organization published a review of the evidence, describing it as an "essential drug" for PMTCT and confirming its safety (Nattrass 2007, 62). In 1999, the Medicines Research Council released a study that indicated that a national PMTCT program was cost-effective, and that it would cost less than 1% of the national health budget to implement (Moodley et al 2003, 725 – 735). In spite of this, in mid 2000 the government refused an offer by Boehringer-Ingelheim for a free supply of nevirapine for five years. In July 1999 the South African Intrapartum Nevirapine Trial (SAINT) was launched to establish whether nevirapine was effective in a local context. Its findings were strongly in favor of a national PMTCT program. Despite this, and to the bewilderment of its researchers, the Department of Health reacted with a lack of interest to its initial results (Heywood 2003, 285–6). *Beat It*'s sixth program in the 2000 series, entitled "Free Antiretrovirals for Pregnant Mothers," addressed these issues directly. It documented the events of the International AIDS Conference in Durban 2000, which saw a turning point in South African HIV activist policy from government accommodation to outright opposition. The "Special Report" of the episode, "Mother-to-Child Transmission (MTCT) Prevention Update", broadcast a speech by Adeline Mangcu, a TAC activist as well as member of the *Beat It!* support group. Mangcu stated: "Think about this: a hundred and sixty babies are born HIV-positive *every day* [in South Africa], and the government is saying 'No!' to AZT" (2000, ep. 6). The episode then broadcast a series of images from the PMTCT program at the MSF clinic in Khayelitsha, while the presenter cited a 50 percent reduction rate in perinatal transmission as proof of the program's success. This episode also invoked the medical authority of the doctor working in the Khayelitsha PMTCT clinic, who stated: "I have argued for the expansion of the program on a national scale, but the national Department of Health is still holding back" (2000, ep. 6). After the 2000 IAC, the minister of health convened a meeting with the nine provincial Members of the Executive Committee (MEC), the provinces' most senior political figures working in healthcare. Here it was decided that the government would continue its policy of not using AZT, and that two pilot sites would be established in every province at which nevirapine would be tested for a further two years before a national program of PMTCT would again be considered. The HIV activist and medical communities reacted with frustration and disbelief, and *Beat It!* broadcast numerous interviews with leading HIV medical researchers, all of whom opposed the government's decision.

As far back as 1998, Health Minister Tshabalala-Msimang had couched her opposition to PMTCT in a "discourse of unaffordability" (Nattrass 2005, 39). Following international scientific revelations about PMTCT with AZT, doctors began administering the drug to pregnant women in South African hospitals. The minister soon ordered a stop to this, arguing that the "limited resources" available to the Department of Health were best spent on HIV prevention (Iliffe 2006, 143). Despite the arguments of medical experts and economists that the cost of AZT was cheaper than that of treating pediatric AIDS, the minister remained unswayed (Nattrass 2005, 39; van Niekerk 2005, 153). Nonetheless, it became a popular tactic to oppose the government's refusal to provide HIV medicines by emphasizing the financial benefits of treatment. In a *Beat It!* episode from the first series, the medical authority of renowned HIV experts was invoked to disprove the official line that PMTCT was unaffordable. Dr. Glenda Gray, at Baragwanath Hospital, emphasized the necessity of treatment access and the irrationality of the government's refusal to initiate PMTCT in her statement that: "To give nevirapine, not only is it the right thing to do, it's that you save lots and lots of money. So the government's decision to withhold the life-saving intervention for children makes no coherent, rational sense at all" (2000, ep. 7). Directly after, the episode conveyed the moral imperative of making PMTCT available in an interview with Jackie Schoeman from the Cotlands baby sanctuary in Johannesburg. Schoeman was pictured next to a swinging bench and slide, vital symbols of childhood that contrasted with her disturbing revelations about the deaths from AIDS of the children in her care:

> [W]e've had five deaths in the last week, and it's an extremely painful death for the children...They become very thin so it's painful if you touch them, they have oral thrush and chronic diarrhea so they get dehydrated, and it's normally quite a long, drawn-out process.

The episode then cut directly to images of activists Zackie Achmat and Mark Heywood at the TAC press conference after the Durban International AIDS Conference in July 2000. Achmat announced: "TAC will commence legal proceedings to compel the South African government to act on the findings presented over three weeks ago, and revealed publicly, at this conference, on the efficacy of nevirapine and AZT in the reduction of MTCT" (2000, ep. 7). To prove the misguided nature of the government response and to highlight the recalcitrance of the Health Minister, the episode then juxtaposed snippets from Tshabalala-Msimang's statements at an IAC plenary with those of activists and doctors involved in successful PMTCT programs in the Western Cape:

> Tshabalala-Msimang [addressing the conference]: And in any case, we don't believe that the only way to prevent MTCT is by using ARVs.

> Achmat [interviewed in his office]: The first reason that the government is dragging its feet is that it's found itself in an ideological muddle of whether HIV causes AIDS, and that is completely unacceptable.

> Tshabalala-Msimang [addressing the conference]: You don't have enough resources to buy the drugs. We can't just be jumping on the bandwagon because we've heard that somewhere nevirapine was being administered.

Beat It! chronicled the deterioration in relations between the Department of Health and leading HIV activists. Heywood (2003, 290) described these as having "reached their nadir" after the Department's decision to withhold nevirapine in spite of SAINT's supportive outcomes. This pushed TAC into legal action against the government to demand public access to PMTCT. Shortly thereafter, the Department of Health threatened legal action of its own against the Western Cape Health Department, which began dispensing nevirapine at public clinics in January 2001 despite the Health Minister's instructions for a go-slow on the drug (Heywood 2003, 288).

Beat It!'s seventh episode from the 2000 series countered the government's actions by focusing on the successes of the Western Cape clinics and featuring testimonies describing nevirapine's efficacy from the perspective of clinicians involved in the PMTCT pilot. The episode was dedicated to the memory of three babies whose mothers were all members of the *Beat It!* support group, and who had died of AIDS in the absence of public PMTCT programs. The program's "red noose award," presented with irony to an organization or person who had violated the rights of the HIV-positive community, was delivered by *Beat It!* presenter Sipho Nhlapo to "all those who are holding [up] the introduction Mother-to-Child Transmission Prevention Programme using either AZT or nevirapine" (2000, ep. 7). His statement incorporated many of the arguments in support of public PMTCT: the affordability of the treatment; the promising results of the SAINT trial; and the success of the treatment in other national contexts. The statement also presented access to PMTCT as a human right, pointed to the health minister's unreasonable opposition to AZT and nevirapine, and condemned the indifference of South Africa's political elite to the suffering and death of citizens. This statement was accompanied by a montage of newspaper headlines, articles and cartoons bolstering Nhlapo's critique. He said:

> Preventing the spread of HIV from a mother to child is a basic right [image of the newspaper headline: "State stalls on 'effective' drug: Trials indicate R24 [approximately $3] drug can prevent MTCT infection." So this PMTCT, using either AZT or nevirapine, is approved in many countries...I think its registration should be rushed through immediately [article with a picture of

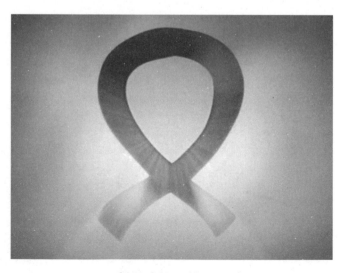

Figure 14.7 Image of the red AIDS ribbon morphing into a noose

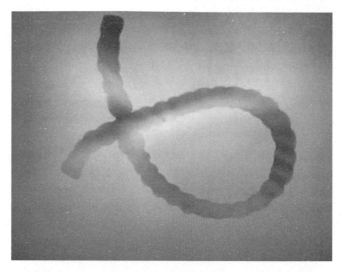

Figure 14.8 Image of the red AIDS ribbon morphing into a noose

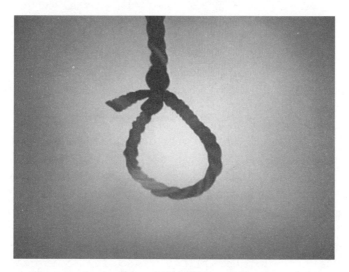

Figure 14.9 Image of the red AIDS ribbon morphing into a noose

Tshabalala-Msimang and the attributed quotation: "don't jump the gun on nevirapine"]. So, if you are a bureaucrat sitting at your desk, protected by a good salary, medical aid and other benefits [image of a cartoon depicting the health minister and President Mbeki "fiddling while Rome is burning"], and are involved in denying the right to life for thousands of kids born with HIV who could otherwise be saved, then you really deserve the noose [image of the red AIDS ribbon morphing into a noose, accompanied by the sounds of a flushing toilet and booing crowd] (Figures 14.7, 14.8, and 14.9). (2000, ep. 7)

The Health Minister's resistance to PMTCT continued into 2001, when the introduction of nevirapine to pilot PMTCT sites was delayed by the Medicines Control Council's failure to register the drug.[5] When it was eventually registered, in April 2001, Tshabalala-Msimang did nothing to implement provincial pilot programs. (Nattrass 2007, 95). On July 17, 2001, TAC again initiated legal action against the minister and all of the provincial ministers of health (with the exception of the Western Cape Minister), by sending a legal letter that queried why the national and provincial ministers of health had not scaled up PMTCT beyond the pilot sites. Tshabalala-Msimang's response reiterated claims about limits in the capacity of the health system and the possibility of drug resistance which had been discounted previously.

Beat It! continued to engage with the PMTCT controversy for the remainder of its first series. The program responded to the doubts cast on PMTCT efficacy and sustainability through frequent assertions of the safety and successes of established programs, holding interviews with doctors, nurses, mothers, and even some high-ranking employees of the Department of Health (including Nono Simelela, chief director of HIV/AIDS, and Fareed Abdullah, chief director of Support Services for the Western Cape Department of Health). The support group also hosted a number of discussions about the imperative of PMTCT programs, including emotive personal testimonies of members whose babies had died of AIDS. Footage taken at PMTCT clinics showed nurses teaching treatment literacy to rooms of attentive mothers, and episodes broadcast copious images of healthy infants and mothers subsequent to successful PMTCT interventions.

On August 21, 2001, TAC, together with Save Our Babies (a coalition of pediatricians and the Children's Rights Centre), filed a constitutional claim against the government for violating the right to health through preventing public access to PMTCT programs. The coalition argued that two pilot sites per province were not enough to meet the growing public need for treatment. These charges were supported by a series of affidavits from experts who attested to the medical, fiscal and legal imperatives of PMTCT (Nattrass 2007, 95; Heywood 2003, 294). Despite abundant evidence to the contrary, the government's case was fought on the basis that PMTCT drugs were unaffordable and unsafe, and that nevirapine spurred HIV resistance and mutation that could have "catastrophic" consequences for public health (Heywood 2003, 296). Doctors who had prescribed the drug outside the pilot sites were accused of acting irresponsibly, and the Western Cape Department of Health was reprimanded for acting against orders to halt provincial PMTCT pending the outcome of the pilot studies. But partial rollouts of PMTCT in the Western Cape and KwaZulu-Natal had produced remarkable successes, discrediting the government's claims about the detrimental effects of the treatment and the alleged difficulties in administering it. Evidence from these pioneering PMTCT sites strengthened TAC's case against the government.

In the weeks prior to the judgment, TAC conducted an intensive mobilization of activists in support of a national program of PMTCT, arranging workshops to explain the details of the case and strengthening alliances with other activist organizations. Mobilization was stepped up in the days before the PMTCT court case judgment, culminating in a mass action march captured by *Beat It!* cameras (although production time and funding dictated that it was screened only in the next series). Protesters carried placards that read: "Stand up for your rights," and images of jog-trotting and banner-waving protestors were accompanied by on-screen text that stated: "Protestors demand the right to prevent mother-to-child-transmission of HIV" (2003, ep. 3). *Beat It!* presenter Nombeko Mpongo, in voiceover, stated: "The Constitutional Court, the highest court in South Africa, has ruled that you have a right to prevent passing on HIV to your child." The episode then depicted the final judgment of July 5, 2002, which rejected the appeal filed by the health minister against the court's findings in favor of TAC. Footage of Judge-President Chaskalson reading the judgment was screened, along with images of TAC's lawyers embracing each other and jubilant activists celebrating outside the court (figures 14.10 and 14.11).

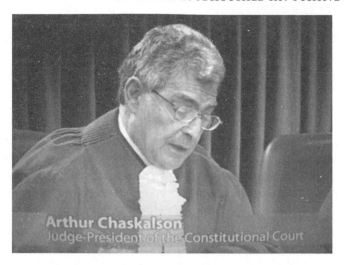

Figure 14.10 Judge-President Chaskalson

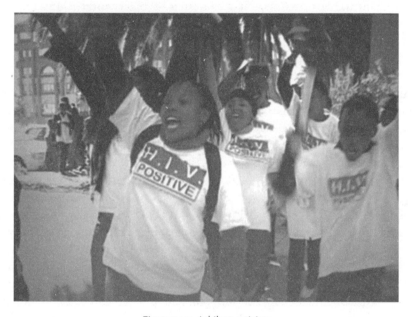

Figure 14.11 Jubilant activists

The judgment found that there was no evidence that nevirapine was unsafe, and ordered the government to remove restrictions on the drug "for the purpose of reducing the risk of MTCT of HIV at public hospitals and clinics" (Heywood 2003, 311–12). By December 2002 TAC had charged the health minister and MEC for Health in Mpumalanga with contempt of court for their joint refusal to endorse PMTCT. Tshabalala-Msimang's failure in this regard was unsurprising. In a notorious South African Broadcasting Corporation news interview on March 24, 2002, a few months prior to the judgment, she was asked by the television presenter: "Will you stand by what the court decides?" The minister of health responded: "No, I think the court and the judiciary must also listen to the regulatory authority, both of this country and the regulatory authority of the US."[6] When asked by her surprised host, "Are you saying 'No'?" Tshabalala-Msimang definitively replied, "I say no. I am saying no" (*Why Must I Die?* 2005).

Beat It! episodes continued to focus on the prevention of mother-to-child transmission of HIV in subsequent series. But portrayals were generally more optimistic than those from the 1999 and 2000 series, which sought to convey the tragedy of avoidable infant deaths from AIDS and the iniquity of the government's obstruction of PMTCT programs. As PMTCT became more widely accessible, *Beat It!* episodes focused on the issue of breast versus bottle-feeding, delving into both the stigmas around bottle-feeding, and its benefits in preventing the transmission of HIV via breast milk. In an attempt to allay the public fears that were sown by Health Minister Tshabalala-Msimang and President Mbeki's public exaggerations of the toxicity of ARVs, however, the program continued to screen interviews with health care workers who attested to the safety of PMTCT regimens, particularly nevirapine.

CONCLUSION

The access battle for PMTCT, documented closely by *Beat It!*, was an early example of the "judicial activism" employed by HIV activist leaders. TAC members sued the government for violating the health rights of South African citizens by obstructing PMTCT programs, and sympathetic media coverage and activism around the court case fueled public support for HIV treatment access. The 2002 judicial victory inspired the HIV activist movement to expand its campaigning objectives, and public access to antiretroviral treatment for all in need became the central goal of the movement.

Beat It! thwarted stigmatizing representations of HIV through normalizing the disease, encouraging disclosure, constructing a strong and welcoming "positive community" and promoting a "positive lifestyle." However, HIV remains heavily stigmatized in South Africa. Health campaigns and treatment literacy initiatives have helped to reduce stigma and discrimination, but HIV-positive people are still feared and persecuted for living openly with the disease (Maughan-Brown 2010, 364–368). True to its reflection of the real experiences of HIV-positive South Africans, and in spite of its messages of openness and positivity, *Beat It!* also portrayed a darker side of the realities of HIV in South Africa. Medical practitioners and other guest experts made frequent statements that challenged the upbeat tone of the program's activists, animating HIV as wily and brutal. HIV was described by different healthcare practitioners as a "clever disease" that attacks the brain, breaks down muscles and drains the body of nutrients. In explaining the severity of recurrent opportunistic infections in the 2004 series (ep, 1) Dr. Nombulelo described HIV as "a steadily worsening disease." Other medical experts conveyed the exceptionalism of HIV that support group members had tried so hard to dispute.

Numerous episodes of *Beat It!* portrayed HIV-related stigma as widespread and tenacious. Informants described the persistence of stigma within families, hospitals, schools, the media, and many other public institutions. This was often cited as the reason that the majority of HIV-positive South Africans keep their status a secret. For instance, in an episode from the 2002 series, a COSATU (Congress of South African Trade Unions) representative explained that, out of a union of over 10,000 workers: "There's just one or two where I know they're happy to disclose in the factory."

One of the last programs of the 2005 series further attested to the continuation of high mortality rates from AIDS. In an interview with Reverend Richard Mthethwa, the head of the All Nations Funeral Parlour in KwaThema, Gauteng, Mthethwa complained that the number of AIDS deaths was overwhelming local burial services. This episode was reminiscent of older, doom-laden documentaries about AIDS because of its footage of coffins, a cemetery, and a child staring at a grave to the accompaniment of melancholic music (2005, ep. 23). Another *Beat It!* episode from the 2005 series mimicked the morbid preoccupations of early AIDS documentaries in South Africa (Hodes 2007) because of its inclusion of gruesome and lingering footage of the somatic ravages of AIDS-related Kaposi's Sarcoma (2005, ep. 7). Such frightening images attested to the pain and suffering caused by HIV-infection, trumping the episode's overall message of hope thanks to ARVs.

Despite its efforts to depict HIV as yet another chronic, manageable illness, escalating mortality levels and persistent stigma remained the South African reality that *Beat It!* was compelled to reflect. But while stigma persisted, the overwhelming tone of the program remained largely optimistic. The support group and the majority of the program's guests focused on empowerment through information, and upliftment through positive belonging and activism. This was perhaps best captured in the show's title and tagline: "Together we can *Beat It!*"

The program's use of the therapeutic tactics of confessional TV talk shows strove to counter the widespread silence that persisted around the HIV pandemic. And in its passionate promotion of the "positive lifestyle," the show sought to win adherents, not only to the activist community, but also to the broader ethos of living positively with HIV. Over the years of broadcast examined in this chapter, *Beat It!* grew into the largest national multimedia HIV education initiative in South Africa. Through its use of new media strategies that portrayed the possibilities of extended survival with HIV, and its galvanizing depictions of the imperatives of ARVs, *Beat It!* played a formative role in documenting and popularizing the struggle for public access to HIV treatments in South Africa.

15

"C'est Le Wake Up! Africa"

TWO CASE STUDIES OF HIV/AIDS

EDUTAINMENT CAMPAIGNS IN

FRANCOPHONE AFRICA

Daniel B. Reed (Indiana University)

SIDA est	AIDS is
SIDA est	AIDS is
SIDA est présent...	AIDS is present
Jolie femme, a-oh	Pretty woman, a-oh
Jolie femme, protège-toi...	Pretty woman, protect yourself

—From "Protège-toi" by Aboutou Roots, Côte d'Ivoire, 1997[1]

In Côte d'Ivoire, where I was living in 1997, artistic responses to the HIV/AIDS pandemic served as periodic visual, verbal, and acoustic reminders of the presence of the disease. Riding on buses, minibuses, or taxis, or walking by open-air restaurants, one might hear one of the most popular songs of that year, Aboutou Roots' "Protège-toi" ("Protect Yourself"). Like so many responses to HIV/AIDS in Francophone Africa, this song wraps a profoundly serious message in an accessible aesthetic package. Clearly, this is a strategic decision; given that one of the goals of much artistic output in this domain is educational, many artists and producers select popular artistic forms through which to communicate their messages (see Okigbo 2010; Stephenson and Davies 1994). Yet, I would suggest that effective educational outreach is but one factor influencing such artistic choices. Consider the case of "Protège-toi." The song begins in a musically pensive mode, centered around the chilling refrain, "SIDA est, SIDA est, SIDA est présent" ("AIDS is present"). But, by the time the song has ended, the listener has arrived at a dance party, as a rollicking beat, punctuated by percussion and a prominent, melodic bass line supports the lyrical warning, "Jolie femme, protège-toi" ("Pretty woman, protect yourself"). The undeniably joyous feel at the song's end implies that, while the tragedy of HIV/AIDS impacts African lives and one must be careful, one cannot let it dampen one's spirits, or "joie de vivre."

As exemplified by "Protège-toi," popular songs on topics related to HIV/AIDS are common in Francophone Africa and are widely circulated in audio and video form. Songs, however, represent just one of many expressive forms employed as responses to HIV/AIDS in Francophone Africa. Cartoons, calendar art, clothing, sculptures, photo essays, radio dramas, television sitcoms, live theater, and poetry all join music as expressive forms that have been used to comment upon, process, and disseminate messages about HIV/AIDS in French-speaking regions of Africa. Many such artistic responses, such as "Protège-toi," are entirely locally generated and produced. A number of other artistic responses, however, have been organized and funded by agencies based abroad, often in the United States. Such initiatives are highly collaborative efforts, involving multiple agencies operating in a transnational network of discourse, organization and funding. UN agencies such as UNESCO, non-governmental organizations (NGOs), health-based organizations, faith-based organizations, research universities, and national governments are just some of the players who join forces in campaigns to combat HIV/AIDS in Francophone Africa using the arts. These campaigns are characterized by their use of multiple artistic forms to disseminate messages related to HIV/AIDS prevention and education.

In this chapter, I will focus attention on these broad-based, internationally organized and funded, multipronged campaigns. These types of initiatives, widespread on the continent (and beyond), are generally labeled "edutainment" campaigns—edutainment being, just as it sounds, a genre of entertainment designed to teach important messages. Edutainment campaigns demonstrate clearly and specifically ways in which "HIV/AIDS...has forced populations to situate themselves within a global system of relationships, knowledge, and health discourse" (Barz and Cohen 2008, 148). Using the arts, these campaigns both localize transnational discourse and globalize local discourse on the topic of HIV/AIDS. Transnational discourses (stemming from funding sources, systems of organization, research agendas and methods, and concepts generated abroad) are translated into local expression (e.g., musical styles, clothing, local languages, local ways of speaking about sensitive issues such as condom use). Meanwhile, local discourse about sexuality and health is understood in terms of international health concepts and is, at times, expressed in internationally recognized symbolic forms (e.g., languages such as French and English, the voices of pop stars) arguably geared toward not just local but also regional and transnational audiences. Undeniable power dynamics are at play in these relationships, as local agencies and artists financially depend on the large budgets of foreign agencies in order to effectively fight the spread of the disease. Along with that funding come foreign-born agendas, concepts, methods and strategies, which impact the ways messages are spread. And yet, the foreign agencies are themselves dependent, for example, on the star power of famous African musicians for the realization of their agendas. For these campaigns, music emerges as a particularly effective means of interweaving local and international discourses and of expressing edutainment campaign messages in emotionally affective, accessible forms. For this and other reasons, music is often the central prong of these multipronged initiatives involving multiple artistic forms.

There have been many campaigns that fit the edutainment characterization in the past two decades in Francophone Africa.[2] In this chapter, I will highlight just two, both of which were based in Abidjan, Côte d'Ivoire. The first, "Chaussez Capote" ("Put on a Condom"), initiated in 1991, is the earliest edutainment campaign in Francophone Africa I have yet encountered. While innovative in many respects, Chaussez Capote was smaller in scale than most of its successors. As such, Chaussez Capote anticipates but lacks some of the general tendencies described above that characterize many later edutainment campaigns. In contrast, "Wake Up! Africa," begun in 1997, brought to full fruition the general patterns associated with such campaigns (including a standard approach to creating content) and thus will receive more attention in the pages that follow. Like the song "Protège-toi," and indeed like many artistic responses to HIV/AIDS in Africa, the messages propagated in these campaigns tended (a) to acknowledge the social and physical trauma of HIV/AIDS; (b) to offer practical education to prevent its spread; and (c) to express the idea that realizing the behavioral changes spelled out in the educational messages can provide not just protection but also hope and resilience. Simply put, these campaigns utilize the arts to educate and offer hope in the face of tragedy.

CASE STUDY ONE: CHAUSSEZ CAPOTE

One of the earliest multipronged, anti-HIV/AIDS initiatives in Francophone Africa, "Chaussez Capote" ("Put on a Condom"), began in 1991 in Abidjan, Côte d'Ivoire. Chaussez Capote was funded and organized by two multinational agencies based abroad: ORSTOM (Office de la Recherche Scientifique et Technique d'Outre-Mer)[3] of France and UNESCO. The stated target audience for Chaussez Capote was "Francophone African youth" (Deniaud n.d.), though it seems to have had little or no impact beyond its home base in Abidjan, and, considering the language it employed, appears to have been designed specifically for an Ivorian audience.

Chaussez Capote, while more modest in scale than most subsequent such initiatives, and apparently only mildly successful, nonetheless can be viewed in hindsight as quite innovative in certain respects. Particularly noteworthy is the way in which the project began. In 1991, researchers involved in the project interviewed forty-eight youths between the ages of fourteen and twenty-five in Abidjan and the smaller city of Dabou, which is located west of Abidjan on the Ivorian coast. In the interviews, the researchers explored strategies for encouraging condom use in this age group (Deniaud 1993a). Information from these interviews was then used to write the lyrics of the campaign's theme song, titled "Jeunesse, Chaussez Capote" ("Youth, Put on a Condom"). This song, performed by Abidjan rap group RapMC, became the title song of a cassette released by the campaign in 1992 (Deniaud n.d.). Joining the title song on the cassette were other songs on the themes of youth, relationships between young couples, contraception, and AIDS. Organizers selected some already well-known songs for the cassette, while others, like the title song, were written specifically for the project. A range of musical styles popular at the time in Côte d'Ivoire was represented on the cassette in order to maximize its appeal. While the title song was in the rap genre, also included were songs in the genres of Congolese soukous, Caribbean zouk, and rock (Deniaud 1993a).

If organizers selected musical styles that they hoped would maximize the audience for their message, they made language decisions accordingly. Côte d'Ivoire is extremely diverse linguistically, with over sixty indigenous languages spoken in the country. The colonial language, French, and an African trade language, Jula, are the most widely spoken languages, and generally are used to communicate across ethnic lines. Nearly all of the national media, meanwhile, is in French. Not surprisingly, then, to reach as many Ivorians as possible, lyrics of the title song, "Jeunesse, Chaussez Capote," were written in French and Jula (Deniaud 1993b). While French and Jula (or closely related Mande languages) are spoken in other West African countries, the specific choice to pair these two particular languages suggests that Ivorian youth were the primary target audience.[4]

Informed by the research conducted at the project's start, the title song's lyrics focused on "technical information on using condoms while also correcting misconceptions, such as the idea that regular condom use may cause sterility" (Deniaud 1993a). Condom use instruction is quite explicit in the lyrics, which describe the kinds of details one might expect to hear in a face-to-face safe sex education program. Misconceptions, such as the ideas that condoms can cause harm and minimize pleasure, are also directly addressed, as in the following excerpt: "Neither the condom nor the lubricant cause harm to the penis or vagina. Having put on the condom, the moment comes to unite yourselves. Exquisite minutes of love and pleasure!" (Deniaud 1993b). The lyrics thus exemplify the general edutainment pattern of offering an educational message instructing listeners in behaviors that can lead to positive, hopeful outcomes.

In August 1992, approximately eight hundred copies of the cassette were distributed at no cost to organizations and businesses frequented by youth (Deniaud n.d. and 1993a). Songs from the cassettes received limited airplay on Ivorian radio and television. François Deniaud claims, however, that this initial release was largely unsuccessful, which he attributes to the small number of copies produced and limited distribution (Deniaud 1993a). In response to this lack of success, in December 1993 organizers produced a second cassette including some "different songs and short recorded messages by popular African singers for local duplication and sale at a subsidized price" (ibid.). Perhaps to soften the pedantic emphasis of the original release and widen the appeal of the campaign, the second release included new "love songs without any reference to illness or condoms" (ibid.). The short, recorded public service announcements on the second release added the star power of three of the most internationally famous Francophone African popular musicians—Papa Wemba of the Congo, Youssou N'Dour of Senegal and Angelique Kidjo of Benin—in order to attract increased attention (ibid.). I have yet to find information, however, evaluating the relative success or failure of this second release.

In addition to the cassette releases, in Spring 1993 Chaussez Capote campaign organizers decided to disseminate their message in a visual form—cloth. The use of clothing as a promotional tool—for example, by campaigning politicians and political parties—is widespread in Africa. In selecting cloth, then, Chaussez Capote organizers were choosing an expressive form widely accepted as a tool for the promotion of important ideas in the African context. Furthermore, this decision was specifically informed by the campaign's initial research project, which found that young people were particularly receptive not just to spoken messages but also to those delivered in visual forms (Deniaud 1993a). The Chaussez Capote cloth (see figure 15.1) features the phrase *entre-nous* (between us) along with various images promoting condom use, including a panther symbolizing a well-known brand of condom and a couple metaphorically representing protective behavior by sheltering themselves under an umbrella. This cloth was eventually ordered by "the National AIDS Committee, a condom social marketing project, and the French agency for development cooperation" (ibid.).

Compared with later edutainment campaigns, such as Wake Up! Africa, Chaussez Capote can be likened to an independent label music release in scale and scope. Apparently it lacked either the budget or the organization (or both) to promote and distribute its message widely. Yet, like independent music releases, Chaussez Capote was homegrown, attempting to base its rhetoric in local ideas generated through research with local youth. Interestingly, though, the musical expression of those local ideas took international forms—rap, Central

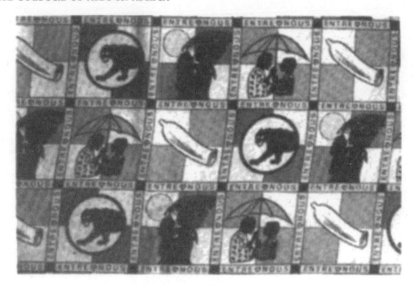

Figure 15.1 Chaussez Capote cloth

African pop, Caribbean dance music—albeit international forms hugely popular in the local context. As is common in edutainment initiatives, the foreign and the local interweave in interesting ways. Funded and organized by foreign agencies, utilizing multiple expressive forms (pop songs, PSAs, and cloth) and employing languages strategically selected to maximize impact, Chaussez Capote centered its campaign on a song mixing education and a hopeful message, and focused on an audience of urban youth. The campaign featured many elements that would be further developed in future edutainment campaigns.

CASE STUDY TWO: WAKE UP! AFRICA

The Wake Up! Africa campaign exemplifies the type of edutainment campaign of which there have been quite a few in Francophone Africa: a regional initiative, it was funded and spearheaded by multiple United States based agencies in collaboration with locally based organizations; it was multifaceted in terms of its use of a variety of popular artistic forms to disseminate is message; its primary target audience was urban youth; and it was educationally focused. The project was administered in Abidjan by the Santé Familiale et Prévention du Sida (SFPS), an organization founded in 1994 by USAID's Regional Economic Development Services Office for West and Central Africa.[5] SFPS's Behavior Change Communication component was charged with carrying out the campaign, which was directed by The Johns Hopkins Bloomberg School of Public Health/Center for Communication Programs (CCP) in partnership with the U.S.-based nonprofit Academy for Educational Development. Though based in Abidjan, the campaign extended its reach not just to Côte d'Ivoire but also initially to Cameroon, Togo, and Burkina Faso, and eventually to other French-speaking African countries. The goal of the Wake Up! campaign was "to motivate listeners to take personal responsibility to prevent the spread of HIV/AIDS by protecting themselves" (Center for Communication Programs 2005b). Central to the campaign was the song "Afrique, lève-toi" ("Wake up, Africa"). In addition to sponsoring audio and video broadcasts of this song on radio and television, the campaign disseminated its message via a major concert performance, television spots, a documentary, posters, pamphlets, and T-shirts.

The utilization of popular artistic forms to disseminate messages is commonly employed by the CCP in similar campaigns around the world. Jane Brown, a CCP employee who worked on the Wake Up! campaign, describes this approach as "entertainment education" or "edutainment" (Brown, p.c.).[6] Brown asserts that edutainment initiatives endeavor "to be entertaining but also engage people to have a better understanding of the health issues that we're trying to address and the behaviors that can be protective or that can be harmful" (ibid.). As Barz and Cohen have written, musical responses to HIV/AIDS in Africa often emerge from "frameworks of health-based knowledge" stemming from previous experiences of internationally funded aid organizations (2008, 152). Wake Up! Africa upheld this pattern, in that it applied strategies developed in previous initiatives by the CCP and its collaborators.

The Song

The centerpiece of the campaign, the song "Afrique, lève-toi" resulted from collaborative efforts between SFPS and Artistes Associé Contre le SIDA (Artists Against AIDS), an international organization of Francophone African musicians united for activism against the pandemic. Inspired by and modeled on the famous 1980s anthem, "We Are the World," which brought together many famous pop musicians from the United States and the United Kingdom to raise funds to combat hunger in famine-stricken Ethiopia, "Afrique, lève-toi" featured more than two dozen of West and Central Africa's biggest stars, including the Democratic Republic of the Congo's Papa Wemba, Tshala Muana and Koffi Olomide, and Côte d'Ivoire's Meiway, Aïcha Koné and Nayanka Bell (Center for Communication Programs 2005a).

Considering that the Wake Up! campaign utilized a variety of artistic media, it is worth considering why they chose a song as the central means of disseminating their message. One need look no further than the liner notes of the CD for an explanation of this decision. In a section subtitled "Why Music?" the liner notes state:

> In Africa, music is a powerful vector of communication. In the traditions of long ago, it was through music that the values of society were transmitted from generation to generation. It is also via music that the community honors its most meritorious citizens, just as it is via music that mediocre persons are punished. Today, there are geographical, cultural and linguistic borders; however, music has no borders. Thus Africa remains sensitive to the language of music. It is in this sense that this project was born, in order to spread through song a message linked to the major problem of AIDS. (SFPS and APS 1997)

Clearly, directors of the campaign recognized the extent to which music in Africa was highly regarded as a communicative tool, particularly for communication regarding social values. As seen below, the lyrics of "Afrique, lève-toi" emphasize a consideration of values as pertains to containing the spread of HIV/AIDS. The notion that music has no borders is reflected in the fact that artists from various countries were brought together to sing this song that, though primarily in French, also transmits its message in several African languages. Thus, given its powerful role throughout history and its effectiveness as a communicative tool in a context still today favoring oral communicative forms, it is not surprising that the campaign chose a song as its primary means of message dissemination.

The CCP determined that songs were particularly effective as forms of edutainment in part because it felt music could affect people in multiple ways simultaneously. As Brown explained, "We try to grab people from an emotional place but also then provide them with the information and strategies for how they can protect themselves" Brown, recalling that songs are central to many CCP edutainment campaigns, continued: "The beauty of a song is that you can play it on the radio, you can play it in nightclubs, at a concert for example. And let's face it, PSA's are nice, but people aren't going to quite remember the PSA the way they're going to remember a song. I think [the song "Afrique, lève-toi"] was the centerpiece [of the campaign] because first of all it enabled us to get a lot of different messages across at the same time, while a PSA might focus on a particular one" (Brown, p.c.). Song, with its emotional affect, its utility as a memory aid, its ability to communicate relatively lengthy text and multiple messages in the form of lyrics, and its portability, renders it a particularly effective tool in edutainment campaigns.

Musically and lyrically, "Afrique, lève-toi" typifies the general approach found in many artistic responses to HIV/AIDS in Africa. While acknowledging the social and physical trauma of HIV/AIDS in Africa, the song's lyrics also encourage listeners to take action to minimize risk (practicing fidelity, using condoms, knowing their HIV status) and to accept people infected with the disease. These messages are delivered over the song's danceable groove, creating an overall effect of a feeling of hope and resilience in the face of catastrophe—again, the common approach in edutainment-driven artistic responses to the disease.

Lyrics and Language

Language choice in popular music, especially in postcolonial contexts, is often strategically motivated (Berger 2003; Reed in press). The French language serves to create a unified audience across national borders of the former French colonies in Africa. Given that the primary audience of the campaign was urban youth in Francophone African countries, it is not surprising that most of the lyrics of "Afrique, lève-toi" are in French. Certain phrases of the song, however, are in African languages such as Lingala and Jula. The incorporation of African languages communicates on two levels: first, in the Democratic Republic of the Congo and Côte d'Ivoire, Lingala and Jula respectively are second only to French in terms of their popular usage. The phrases sung in these languages can reach the Lingala and Jula speakers who might not be fluent in French, and furthermore can be understood by many citizens of each respective country on some level. Secondly, though, the inclusion of indigenous African languages serves to locate the song in Africa, imbuing its message with a sense of African identity that is less effectively communicated via a colonial linguistic code.

The song's central message is obviously that of its title—Wake Up! Africa. Interestingly, this idea is expressed most prominently in a phrase combining French and English: "C'est le Wake up! Africa" (it's the Wake Up! Africa). This phrase serves not only as the song's most prominent refrain, but also simultaneously identifies the campaign itself and its central message; in fact, this phrase is excerpted and used in other contexts outside of the song itself, such as the opening and closing moments of the brief television spots discussed later. In the CCP's terms, "C'est le Wake Up Africa" is a "call to action," which is a central feature of all CCP edutainment campaigns (Brown, p.c.). Brown elaborates, "Sometimes our calls to action are very specific, like, 'go to your nearest health clinic.' This one's a little more vague, but then throughout the song, you get the specifics...So, yes that's the jingle—you want that on everybody's lips— c'est le Wake Up!" Such "jingle"-like usages of this refrain reinforce the sense of its role as both a lyrical theme and a musical motto of the campaign.

That the campaign's lyrical theme, "Wake Up! Africa," is stated in English in this francophone context warrants consideration and can be variously interpreted. Most generally, phrases in English are not uncommon, and in fact can even be popular, in many urban, postcolonial Francophone African contexts. In 1990s Côte d'Ivoire, for example, T-shirts featuring English phrases were common sights. Given the hegemonic dominance of the United States in the economic, military, and cultural spheres, the popularity of expressions in the language of global dominance might be seen as an effort to align oneself with that source of power (and against the former colonial power—France); at the very least, English was widely viewed as "hip" at this moment of Ivorian history.

More specifically, expressing the theme in English can be read as an effort to link this initiative to the transnational movement to combat the spread of HIV/AIDS, whose institutional and economic power is located in the English-speaking world, most significantly in the United States—home of the funding and organizational institutions behind the Wake Up! campaign. Of course, the primary intended audience for the song consisted of French speakers, but organizers might also have selected English to ensure that the motto would be heard and understood by English speakers who might be able to provide further economic assistance. Brown, however, does not recall explicit discussion of this strategy when the campaign was being organized and implemented. She speculates that the "coolness" associated with English in Côte d'Ivoire at the time was the prevailing factor in influencing this decision. Furthermore, Brown describes the strategic and aesthetic impact of such a multi-lingual phrase as having a desired impact: "It makes it stand out a little bit, like 'Wait—that was in French *and* in English!'" Brown concedes, though, that another factor might have been that the lead people on the campaign were Americans, and that much of the campaign's literature and related concepts were likely expressed first in English before being translated into French and African languages (Brown, p.c.).

While the song's central theme is for Africans to wake up, the lyrics also identify *why* Africans must wake up. Exemplifying the first of the common themes found in many artistic responses to HIV/AIDS—especially those that are part of edutainment campaigns—the following passage acknowledges danger and expresses fear. In this moment, the song recognizes the extent of the calamity, attesting to the power of the virus and lamenting the millions who have perished.

Mais où va-tu donc Africa...	But where are you going, Africa
Ta route est pleine de danger...	Your road is full of danger
Ne vois-tu pas ce torrent	Don't you see this torrent
qui murmure les voix des disparus	That murmurs the voices of the disappeared,
Des millions des vies humaines	Of millions of human lives
H.I.V. le roi de virus	H.I.V., the king of viruses
A paralysé la mère nature	Has paralyzed mother nature
Sacrificiées par le SIDA	Sacrificed by AIDS

But, as in so many other artistic responses to HIV/AIDS, this song also offers hope in the face of tragedy, achieved through education and following practical advice. The lyrics transition quickly from a characterization of the hellish nature of the pandemic to the identification of a practical form of salvation—the condom:

Pourtant le monde nous offre le ciel	However, the world offers us heaven
Le préservatif	The condom
Pour ne pas finir au martyr	So that we don't end up as martyrs
D'avoir aimé à la folie...eh...	Who had loved in madness...

After identifying the condom as a solution, the song momentarily transforms into a mini-drama that places the listener in the context of a relationship and the heat of desire. Remembering that the Wake Up! campaign's primary audience was urban youth, it is logical that this portion of the song's message was delivered by two young pop stars, one female and one male—Congo-Kinshasa's Aby Surya and Nick Domby of Burkina Faso. The two stars replicate in song a dialogue between potential lovers about engaging in safe sex. The dialogue begins with these words sung by Surya:

Tu vois je brûle d'envie pour toi	You see I burn with desire for you
Et je veux te donner mon corps	And I want to give you my body
Mais si tu refuses de te protéger	But if you refuse to protect yourself
Je n'irais pas me sacrificier	I will not sacrifice myself

Playing the role of the passion-filled young man, Nick Domby replies:

Regarde-moi dans les yeux	Look me in the eyes
Et dis-moi si tu vois bien	And tell me if you really see
Tout l'amour que j'ai pour toi	All the love I have for you
Car je me protège aussi	Because I also protect myself

Responding to Surya's expression of desire and demand for protection, Domby articulates the idea that choosing to use a condom not only can enable one to safely experience what one desires, but also is, in and of itself, an expression of love. In this mini-drama, Surya and Domby thus represent a model of ideal, responsible behavior in the critical moment when life-saving decisions can be made.

Music

The musical setting of these lyrics accentuates the positive, hopeful outlook of the song's primary message. Unquestionably, "Afrique lève-toi" is a dance song, which in the African context can be understood as a natural choice. The fundamental link between music and dance in Africa is well documented, and dance music genres frequently top the charts in Francophone African countries. Choosing a dance music genre can be understood as a strategic move, an effort to wrap the campaign's message in an accessible and extremely popular artistic package. In the documentary film released by the campaign, Cameroonian musician and Wake Up! participant Manu Dibango states, "It seems that we often listen to messages with our feet" (SFPS and ACS 1998). While the Wake Up! campaign's promotional materials indicate that the song is based on a Congolese rhythm, composer/arranger/keyboardist Al N'Zimbi describes the song as being musically diverse. In the same campaign documentary, N'Zimbi describes the process of creating the song as being one in which he made an effort to incorporate musical elements associated with the genres of each participating musician, especially in the moment of the song when said musician is featured (SFPS and ACS 1998). Even a cursory listen to this song reveals that, while it is united by a repeating refrain, it sounds a bit like a musical journey, almost like a medley of different styles. Jane Brown confirmed that this arrangement is a musical manifestation of the idea of transcending boundaries in an effort to embrace as many people as possible in transmitting and receiving the campaign's message. Brown added that the inclusion of musical styles from across the region metaphorically asserts that, like music, HIV/AIDS also knows no boundaries. Musically, then, this song expresses the notion that as Africans, "we are all really in this together" (Brown, p.c.).

Despite the variety of feels and styles included in the song, the overall effect is one of musical accessibility and a positive, rhythmic groove. Jane Brown describes the song as "very upbeat...I think you can understand the urgency behind it, but it's also somewhat celebratory because [it shows that] people really can do something...and that there's a place that everyone can take action" (Brown, p.c.). Most of the song is in a major key, with the exception of the refrain, "C'est le Wake Up! Africa," whose melody features a minor third, lending the phrase the sense of urgency Brown identifies. This phrase is simple but catchy—clearly designed as a melodic hook—which works like a brief jingle whose role is to be unforgettable in the mind of the listener. If the melody is unforgettable, the hope is that the message will be, too. Musically, then, this song can be compared to "Protège-toi" and many other songs about this topic that emphasize the positive message of hope.

Additional Forms of Wake Up! Message Dissemination

While the song was the centerpiece of the campaign, visual arts were employed as well to disseminate the message. Most prominent were two different iconic images, each featuring a green globe with an enlarged Africa at its center—one with the campaign's title in English and a second more commonly used form including the campaign's title in French. The latter image featured an African continent composed of the smiling faces of the African musicians who contributed to the project (see figure 15.2). Brown asserts that the intent of this image was similar to the motivation to include many musical styles in the song—to demonstrate a sense of connectedness within Africa, and between Africa and the world. Like the musical "call to action," this image was used as a visual symbol of the campaign—on T-shirts, on posters, on the CD cover, and at the beginning of televised forms of outreach including the music video, on the documentary, and the short spots. In the spots, in fact, this image is preceded by a kind of explosion, with debris flying through the air—perhaps akin to what Barz calls a "shout" (2006, 215) that draws attention to and announces the seriousness of the message to follow.

The song, "Afrique, lève-toi" premiered in concert at the opening ceremony of the tenth International Conference on AIDS and STIs in Africa (ICASA), which took place on December 7, 1997, in Abidjan. Present at this event were three sitting presidents: Henri Konan

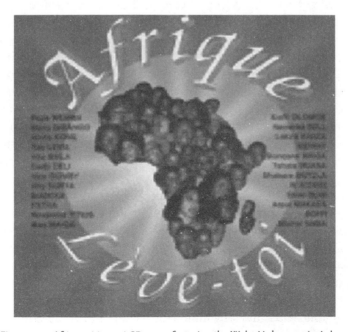

Figure 15.2 Afrique, Lève-toi CD cover featuring the Wake Up! campaign's logo

Bedie of Côte d'Ivoire, Blaise Compaoré of Burkina Faso, and France's Jacques Chirac. The concert featured Papa Wemba, arguably the most internationally recognized of all the musicians who contributed their talents to the song's recording.

Following this kickoff performance, the campaign went into full swing, beginning a process of dissemination that continued actively for at least two years. Mass media, particularly radio and television, was the primary means of dissemination. The song received heavy airplay on national, commercial, and local radio stations in Côte d'Ivoire, Burkina Faso, Togo, and Cameroon (Center for Communication Programs 2005a). The song also became a regional hit, peaking at number 11 on Africa N° 1, a station that broadcasts out of most major Francophone African cities, as well as Paris.

Television was employed extensively to disseminate the message in the form of a music video, television spots featuring pop music stars, and a documentary film about the project. National television stations placed the Wake Up! music video in regular rotation in their music video programming, and also used the video as a transition piece between other types of programming. The brevity of the television spots (thirty to forty seconds each) permitted TV programmers to utilize them in a variety of ways. The spots were frequently aired during prime-time programming, including the moments just before the extremely popular nightly news. Also significant was the inclusion of the spots during television broadcasts of the vastly popular All Africa Cup soccer tournament (Center for Communication Programs 2005a). Featuring several of the stars who sang on the recording, each spot targeted a specific component of the Wake Up! campaign's broader message. For example, Meiwey urged viewers not to abandon people living with AIDS; Nayanka Bell stressed that HIV testing must be a prerequisite to intimate relationships; while Aïcha Kone emphasized fidelity, offering her relationship with her husband as a model to follow. As in the song itself, these spots spotlighted these popular artists—already idealized by large segments of the population—as models to emulate regarding their thoughts and behaviors in relation to HIV/AIDS. As Papa Wemba states in the documentary film, "I think that the message is very well supported and well received by the population if it is artists who try to deliver it" (SFPS and ACS 1998). Each spot closes with the visual and sonic signifiers of the campaign—the artistic logo and the jingle-like refrain from the song—in a clear effort to cement the message in the mind of the viewer.

Nearly two years following the campaign's formal kickoff, SFPS initiated a new stage of the campaign in an effort to further broaden its reach. On December 1, 1999, in conjunction with World AIDS Day, SFPS began supplying NGOs in the four project countries "with copies of the Wake-Up! CD and cassettes, the music video and discussion guides to help groups conduct educational sessions around the song's key themes" (Center for Communication Programs 2005a). NGOs found creative ways of using these materials for educational purposes, as documented in the Johns Hopkins Center for Communications Program's Web site:

> In Togo, a local NGO organized hair and fashion shows for seamstresses and hairdressers. Showcasing the talents of the target audience, Wake Up! was used as the music for the show, and many of the hairstyles and clothes incorporated AIDS prevention themes. In Burkina Faso, Wake Up! was distributed to peer educators working with truckers and commercial sex workers and the song was played in the most popular bars dotting the main highways. In Cameroon, the song was played during intermission at soccer games and handball tournaments, and used in educational sessions at local church groups and colleges. In Côte d'Ivoire, the song and the spots could be heard at local

gas stations and at outreach events in prisons. (Center for Communication Programs 2005a)

Thus, over time SFPS broadened the forms of distribution, as well as the venues in which education related to their campaign occurred. A consistent strategy can be seen throughout this range of initiatives, however. Hairstyles and special printed cloth are, like popular music forms, extremely popular and widespread forms of creative expression in Francophone Africa, and thus are particularly effective means of message dissemination. Prisons and bars frequented by truckers and commercial sex workers represent extensions of the venues for message dissemination beyond that of urban youth populations. But clearly campaign organizers and their NGO affiliates chose venues and populations where the spread of the virus was particularly common.

While there was undeniably great value and logic in extending Wake Up! outreach initiatives to contexts and people considered high-risk, Barz and Cohen worry that such strategies might also have a down side. They note that the edutainment tendency to pinpoint at-risk groups such as prostitutes highlights their moral deficiency and adds "additional levels of social stigma to the disease" (2008, 150). Although television spots such as that featuring Aïcha Kone seem to emphasize that HIV/AIDS is everyone's problem, and the spot featuring Meiway specifically encourages people not to stigmatize people living with the disease, campaign outreach to prisons and sex workers might have reified the very social stigma the campaign sought to dispel. On the other hand, although outreach to high-risk groups is clearly publicized on the CCP's English-language Web site (Center for Communication Programs 2005a), it is possible that the campaign chose not to publicize such efforts on the ground. Organizers might have assumed that the general populace—to whom the campaign delivered mass-mediated messages that endeavored to destigmatize the disease—would remain unaware of the outreach to high-risk groups, and would thus be immune to the potential of increased stigmatization.

CONCLUSION

In her study of performative responses to HIV/AIDS in Mali and South Africa, Louise Bourgault describes entertainment/education or edutainment as a "process of designing and implementing an entertainment program, to increase audience members' knowledge about a social issue, create more favorable attitudes, and bring about a change in their overt behaviors regarding the social issue" (2003, xxv). This description accurately characterizes much of the intent and form of both the Chaussez Capote and Wake Up! Africa campaigns. Unfortunately, I have uncovered no documentation of the extent to which either campaign had the desired outcome of influencing or changing behavior. The CCP's Web site indicates that there has been no formal evaluation of the impact of the Wake Up! campaign, though organizers estimate that an audience of "no smaller than fifty million people may have been exposed to the Wake Up! messages" (Center for Communication Programs 2005a). The audience exposed to Chaussez Capote was surely far smaller, though I have found no evidence of impact studies or estimates.

Bourgault's model, however, only takes us part of the way toward a theoretical understanding of how edutainment campaigns function. Despite the lack of evidence of impact, following Barz, I would assert that both campaigns are best understood as forms of medical intervention (2006a, 222–223). Barz's "positioning of musical interventions within the domain of general care and treatment" (Barz and Cohen 2008, 152) implies that such artistic endeavors will have positive medical outcomes, as has been the case in Uganda (Barz 2006a). That we lack impact data about Chaussez Capote and Wake Up! Africa does not negate the fact that, unquestionably, their intent was to bring about positive medical outcomes. Barz's argument is important in that it helps us understand edutainment not as art *about* a medical problem, but as actual medical practice that can work precisely because HIV/AIDS "is more than a medical crisis"; it is also "a culturally defined and determined social phenomenon" (Barz 2006a, 222). Approaching the pandemic in part as a cultural phenomenon underscores the critical importance of translating foreign-born methods of treatment and educational discourses into local forms of expression, as both Chaussez Capote and Wake Up! Africa attempted to do. Basing interventions on face-to-face research with people in target communities, selecting expressive forms that are popular and considered part of local communicative currency, engaging African artists to deliver unscripted TV spots in their own words—these are just some of the ways in which these campaigns both engaged and contributed to a "culture of AIDS" (Barz 2006a; Barz and Cohen 2008, 152) in Francophone Africa. That many forms of music in Africa are culturally recognized as healing resources only further underscores the value of understanding both the disease and edutainment campaigns in both medical and cultural terms.

To state the obvious, HIV/AIDS edutainment campaigns embody the vast economic inequities between Western nations and those in Africa, inequities that force Africans to engage transnational discourses and foreign organizational structures to effectively address the pandemic. One might question whether edutainment campaigns, furthermore, reify perceptions of Euro-American intellectual and/or moral superiority (cf. Barz and Cohen 2008, 149; Okigbo 2010). Regardless, these campaigns, with good intent, are engaged in work that understands HIV/AIDS as a global problem necessitating a recognition of our shared humanity. By supporting the creation of art that articulates the extent of the calamity of the HIV/AIDS pandemic, identifies behavioral remedies, and expresses hope, HIV/AIDS edutainment campaigns promote the same message found in Aboutou Roots' "Protège-toi": Yes, HIV/AIDS is present, but we must keep dancing.

16

Singing Songs of AIDS in Venda, South Africa

PERFORMANCE, POLLUTION, AND ETHNOMUSICOLOGY IN A NEO-LIBERAL SETTING

Fraser G. McNeill (University of Pretoria)

Deborah James (London School of Economics)

INTRODUCTION

Ethnomusicologists and anthropologists of southern and South Africa have long argued that the composition and performance of songs and dances is integral to affirming or creating identities. Early research, with an apparently more conservative emphasis, highlighted the role of musical performance in configuring fixed social contexts, delineating life-cycle stages, political allegiances, or gender positions. A subsequent generation of scholars, with a more transformative focus, has embraced social theories that account for the emergence of popular forms in the wake of capitalism and industrialization. They have examined how musical performance can transcend social positioning to create new practices and ideas of society and selfhood (Erlmann 1991, 1996; Coplan 1994; James 1999, 2006). The current chapter challenges both of these approaches by providing a critical analysis of musical performance in a context of high HIV/AIDS prevalence: the Venda region of South Africa, whose rich musical tradition was initially made known to the academic community by the writings of John Blacking (1962, 1965, 1967, 1969, 1973).

Our chapter first addresses the use of group performance by female peer educators, who incorporate and adapt specific musical genres into their public promotion of safer sex. Through the strategic combination of songs from the anti-apartheid struggle, Christian churches and "traditional" repertoires, peer educators attempt—with partial success—a symbolic and material transformation of themselves from unemployed rural women to quasi-social workers, fluent in biomedical discourse and thus capable of promotion from voluntary to public sector paid employment. Music is central to this process, not only because it provides an easily accessible and readily understandable medium for the transmission of knowledge, but also because the peer educators claim to "sing about what they cannot talk about" (McNeill 2008).

However, peer educators are not the only people who sing songs about AIDS in the Venda region. In the second half of the chapter, we turn our attention to a musical contribution from a male-dominated solo genre known as *zwilombe* (sing. *tshilombe*). This contrasting case study facilitates a critical appraisal of the peer educators' efforts through a wider ethnographic lens, demonstrating the extent to which Venda men and older (initiated) women frame the educators' actions in terms of a dynamic "folk model" of sexual illness (cf. Good 1994). Following this line of understanding, we show that peer educators—and the biomedical knowledge they tout—have been drawn into and have become the objects of a web of suspicion and blame through which they are labeled as vectors of the virus. As perceived experts in biomedicine, their conspicuous knowledge of contraception (and to a lesser extent abortion) translates through the folk model as an expression of their own intimate experience. They are thought to be acquainted with the regulation of their own reproductive capacities in unnatural and inherently dangerous ways. They are thus thought to be contaminated with blood-bound pollution and are constructed as constituting a threat to fertility that places them at the heart of a perceived crisis of social and sexual reproduction in the region more widely (Comaroff and Comaroff 2004). Both the peer educators and *zwilombe* musicians represent distinctly marginal social groups; both propagate distinct, and partly conflicting, forms of knowledge with the hope of consolidating their prospects of social advancement. Creative musicality is the central process through which this knowledge is transferred to the wider public. As we describe later, these two bodies of somewhat distinct yet partially converging knowledge can be categorized as "biomedical" and "folk" respectively. They represent attempts to secure productive and reproductive capacities to act on the world; but they lead to very different conclusions about how best to avoid disease. Peer educators employ music as a means of asserting new individualized and entrepreneurial strategies of self-advancement into full-time government employment through fluency in biomedicine. *Zwilombe* musicians, in contrast, mobilize their musicality as a means of reacting against new, imposed, and fragmentary forms of (re)production, exchange, and consciousness in order to assert older identities. In doing so, they enunciate a rather different political alignment. Symbolic references to post-apartheid traditionalism are woven into guitar songs designed to restore, and show their singer/composers' allegiance with, collective patriarchal/ ancestral authority over the perceived rise of fragmented individualism.

As a contribution to the emergent discipline of medical ethnomusicology, then, we highlight in this chapter the inherent dangers of privileging songs that are rooted in bioscientific worldviews over those which emerge from folk cosmologies of health and/or sickness. It is only by recognizing the interaction between the intended social effects of these two paradigms and the protagonists who produce and deploy (and are in turn justified) by them, and by seeking to understand some of their *unintended* effects, that we may begin to tease out the complex contexts and processes that give rise to musical performances upon which one approach to medical ethnomusicology might be based. A similar recognition of the reciprocal interrelation between structural forces and local protagonists is necessary in order to understand how ethnomusicology *in general* might be repositioned in the setting of twenty-first century South Africa. How might both the conservative and the transformative approaches to ethnomusicological analysis be reconfigured in a setting of neo-liberal or "millennial" capitalism? Authors have pointed to the way in which the lure of capital accumulation and the promise of prosperity is often experienced by the world's marginal people, instead, as the frustration of increasing economic insecurity and inequality (Comaroff and Comaroff 2000). At the same time, the idea of "neo-liberal governmentality" draws attention to the way such marginal people, excluded from the riches of the few, are subjected to increasingly hegemonic forms of regulation and control—albeit emanating from areas other than the normal ones: that is, other than the organs of the state (Ferguson and Gupta 2002). Despite the apparent pervasiveness and hegemonic character of this global socioeconomic form, we do not assume that its influence determines musical expression. But neither do we insist that individual musicians have sufficient power to counteract it completely: to do so would be to fall into the trap of countering an overly determinist approach by reverting to the familiar narratives of "resistance," or reiterating the "structure vs. agency" debate (Long 2001). Instead, we show how both female peer educators and male guitarists, as musical "brokers" (Barber 1987), produce new forms of identification even as they appear to mediate between old ones.

POST-APARTHEID VENDA: AUTHORITY RETRADITIONALIZED, CULTURE COMMODIFIED

At just over one million in number, Tshivenda-speaking people (*Muvenda* sing., *Vhavenda* plural) constitute only 2.3 percent of the South African population (Statistics South Africa 2003). This minority status is exacerbated by linguistic and geographical factors: Tshivenda is an unusual, and generally incomprehensible language in South Africa since it is not of Nguni origin (like Zulu or Xhosa); rather it is part of the Niger-Congo linguistic cluster that includes Shona in Zimbabwe and Lozi and Zambia. The Venda region—formerly an "independent" homeland under the apartheid regime—is also geographically remote, situated in the northeast of the country, bordering directly with Zimbabwe and the Kruger National Park. The fact that Venda is peripheral to South Africa's centers of power and influence has led to a stereotypical representation of the region and its inhabitants as mystical and highly secretive masters of the occult who possess an extraordinary ability to invoke witchcraft: a conviction that has been reinforced by the recent increase in ritual murders in the area (see McNeill 2007).

Despite this apparent peculiarity, however, the region shares broadly similar socioeconomic and political characteristics with other parts of rural South Africa and, since the official demise of apartheid, has undergone significant political and economic change. In economic terms, a dramatic fall in the number of migrant laborers—and a widespread rise in unemployment in the region more generally—has impoverished many. While a minority engage with criminal livelihoods, a majority in the region are dependent on the extensive welfare handouts of the current "distributional" regime (Seekings and Nattrass 2005), or on funding given by international donors to the plethora of NGOs in the region, which serve to cover a distinctly under-developed reality with a veneer of "development" (cf. for example Southall 2007). In political terms, Venda's incorporation in 1994 into the Northern (later Limpopo) Province under the democratic leadership of the first ANC-led government was preceded by a series of political maneuvers that surprised many commentators. Most significant, perhaps, were the opportunities created for traditional leaders—widely accepted as apartheid stooges in the former Bantustans—to participate in the structures of post-apartheid governance. Reflecting global trends in the growing influence of traditional authority (cf. Oomen 2005, Koelble and Lipuma 2005), post-apartheid South Africa has thus witnessed, especially in the former Bantustans, a significant reinvention of traditional leadership. The policies of "development" alluded to above have often been introduced and implemented in rural areas through—or at least with the approval of—these recently bolstered structures of kingship. Kings, chiefs, and headmen have thus taken a central role in the political economy of the post-apartheid era.

The recent bolstering of traditional leadership in South Africa has been accompanied by broader processes of retraditionalization, through which "culture" and "tradition" have served to legitimize chiefly authority. However this has not promoted harmony in the corridors and courts of traditional power. In Venda, as in other parts of the country, these processes have entailed very publicly re-enacted conflicts between leading royal dynasties, each bent upon establishing itself, in response to government requirements, as the source of Venda's true paramount chief by 2009 (Mufamadi 2004). Such conflicts have exacerbated historical tensions between the rival centers of power and encouraged the implementation of policies that highlight the ANC doctrine of African Renaissance.

Official attempts have been made to increase the number of headmen under a chief (in a ceremony known as *vhuhosi*), and to increase the frequency of female initiation schools under the control of specific royal houses. By reinstating "forgotten" ritual knowledge—from initiation schools that had become largely obsolete—at the core of royal polities, these actions have served to bolster the generational and patriarchal authority not only of traditional leaders, but also of older women as ritual experts. This knowledge, however, comes at a price. "Centers" of tradition have, in the Venda region, been established to provide initiation (as part of a wider process of cultural education including teaching the royal language and training in the arts of healing) in highly rationalized, commoditized ways that invoke the notion of "development." Appropriated by members of younger generations, such as many of those who make up the ranks of HIV/AIDS peer educators, this modularized packaging of knowledge has threatened the legitimacy of traditional authority and its associated sacred discourses. Paradoxically, then, traditional leaders have potential access to significant resources to facilitate development and economic growth for their subjects, but ultimately depend upon the ancestral past for their legitimacy in the current political dispensation. The need to balance these contrasting impulses pervades all of Venda social and political life.

PEER EDUCATION: PROMOTING SAFER SEX THROUGH SONGS

The revival of traditional authority and its associated cultural forms should not, then, blind us to leaders' and followers' new-found zest for securing the future through "development." Simultaneous to the process of traditionalization and the entrenchment of patriarchal authority, rural areas of South Africa have witnessed an unprecedented growth in development-based NGOs and quasi-government bodies devoted to such causes as the eradication of poverty, the promotion of health, and the bolstering of women's rights through anti-rape campaigns. AIDS-related NGOs in particular have flourished, and peer education has been a core pedagogic strategy for many of them. Peer education creates a space in which younger women—mostly through the singing of songs—promote biomedical notions of sexual health and healing. However this space should not be conceptualized simply as a site of "resistance" against the newly entrenched structural forms of authority. It also provides young women with a basis for securing positions of employment in health-related government programs, and as such acts as a potential vehicle for upward mobility among the rural poor. Young women's desire to change the social/sexual health environment is matched by their desire to transcend and move away from it. The same patriarchal sociocultural environment constructs their female bodies as polluted and thus as vectors of the very virus they are charged with eradicating (McNeill 2011).

One setting in which these women have found such opportunities is in the Forum for AIDS Prevention (FAP)[1], a "nonprofit" organization in the Venda region devoted exclusively to HIV/AIDS education and care programs. The FAP has been in operation since the early 1990s and expanded rapidly into a substantial provider of AIDS education in South Africa's Limpopo Province. Co-operating extensively with provincial/local government bodies through such things as securing regular government tenders for the outsourcing of voluntary counselling and testing (VCT) and home-based care (HBC), FAP is "non-governmental" only in the broadest possible sense (see James 2007, 34–5, 41).

Peer educators form the largest and oldest section of the FAP's mostly voluntary work force. Over five hundred in number, and mostly young (between twenty and thirty-five) unmarried women, they are divided into over twenty projects throughout the Limpopo Province and beyond. They are instantly recognizable with their uniform: a bright red skirt, white shirt with red writing, and a bright red bag with "Community against AIDS" printed on the front. As with similar projects discussed by Campbell (2003), FAP volunteers adhere to a strict weekly program that was designed and is monitored by the Project Support Group (PSG) based at the University of Zimbabwe. Theoretically, the projects are rooted in "participatory" approaches to health promotion in which women can allegedly take collective control of their sexual behavior though the development of so-called health-enhancing contexts (cf. Kalipeni et al. 2007). Following PSG guidelines, peer education groups aim to achieve this end though a combination of approaches. At least once a week, they hold "house meetings" during which they split into groups of three or four, and select two homesteads in which they give advice on HIV transmission and treatment, discuss family planning, and distribute condoms. In addition to this, peer educators meet for weekly "ongoing training" that gives them the opportunity to report back on the previous week's activities, to eat together, and to rehearse for Friday public meetings at which they perform the songs discussed later. It is through the weekly repetition of this agenda that project designers intend to empower the volunteers. Volunteers, in turn, are supposed to acquire and transmit heath-enhancing knowledge as well as implement it in their everyday lives, thus becoming positive role models for change (Campbell 2000).

But the seemingly straightforward social processes involved in the acquisition of biomedical "health-enhancing" knowledge belie various complexities involved in its dissemination. The first of these complexities concerns the social origins and modes of livelihood of the educators themselves. Some of them were recruited from beer halls where they engaged in sex work, and others heard of the projects through friends. They volunteer for up to thirty hours a week and receive a small monthly cash stipend in return. Volunteers are encouraged to initiate income-generating activities (IGAs) to supplement this stipend. Although the FAP has reported some success of its members' co-operative efforts farming chickens and making bricks, many of its peer educators nonetheless continue to earn a living through sex work as most loosely defined: that is, they exchange sex for food, money, clothes, phones, etc. with multiple concurrent partners with whom they often maintain long-term transactional relationships (Hunter 2002; Bähre 2002).

The second source of complexity comes from the uneven and disjointed connections between HIV/AIDS education on the one hand and wider discourses that inhibit open, public conversation regarding causes of death on the other. In the Venda region, there is a close connection between knowledge and assumed experience. Thus, in a similar way to that in which peer educators' knowledge of contraception is connected to their assumed experience of it, public displays of knowledge related to death may be equated with the potential implication in fatalities of those doing the display (McNeill 2009). Similar patterns of blame have been reported in southern Africa more widely, binding HIV/AIDS into complex webs of secrecy and suspicion that prohibit its inclusion in open, public conversation (see, for example, Stadler 2003).

The general reluctance to discuss AIDS openly in this region is thus rooted *not* in a widespread "collective denial" of its existence (see, for example, Reid and Walker 2003, Campbell 2003, Lwanda 2003) but rather in the complex relationship between AIDS and causes of death—enmeshed in networks of witchcraft accusations—through which AIDS has been framed as a "sent sickness" (Farmer 1990, cf. Ashforth 2002; 2005). The avoidance of open conversation in this context is employed as a safety precaution, collectively undertaken by individuals to protect them from the constant threat of guilt by association (McNeill 2009). Since, then, peer educators cannot "talk about" AIDS, they "sing about" it instead.

While the justifications behind this assertion are complex, and a full explanation here would lead us away from the main points we wish to pursue, a brief explanation is necessary. In Venda, potentially dangerous knowledge, such as that pertaining to sexual health or death, is conventionally transmitted through the lyrics of songs, generally in highly prescribed ritual contexts, and under the protection of an ancestral hierarchy or a Christian God. Most peer educators have direct experience of this form of communication through their attendance at female initiation, where girls become women by entering into the stratified structures of ritual knowledge, graduating with the socially recognized ability to manage monthly ablutions, and maintain fertility. In this controlled ritual context, stratified by hierarchies of ritual knowledge, the ancestors (though the authority of ritual elders) actively facilitate healthy reproduction, mostly through the performance of initiation songs. Music, in this context, acts as a medium for the complete, safe, transference of ritual knowledge while the songs and dances of initiation represent the desire for continuity in healthy social and sexual reproduction (cf. Blacking 1969; 1973, La Fontaine 1985). By framing AIDS education in songs that are expressed in the same terms as these genres, and that are thus convergent with the current intensification of traditional political power in Venda and with the sacrosanct character of related associations, peer educators seek the relative protection these genres afford in different contexts. In this way they pursue new ends by old means.

The specific ways in which educators employ their musicality, however, result from a combination of individual creativity with the language and practice of modern developmental-style "training." These are deployed in the setting of "workshops," organized in collaboration with various donor agencies, with the aim of refashioning preexisting songs into their current form: intending to form a kind of musical "trap" (Gell 1999). They make simple lyrical and stylistic adjustments with the intention of drawing in the audience. As the audience members attempt to sing along with the educators, they should notice the new lyrics. This, in turn, should theoretically encourage open discussion about their meaning. The educators, as biomedical experts, are trained to step in at this stage of the performance and furnish the audience with authoritative information about HIV/AIDS, before distributing free condoms.

This theory of community engagement has enjoyed only partial success. Educators have succeeded in involving the audience, but only to a very limited extent; the tactic works especially well when a performance is held in a clinic or other female space. But most Friday public meetings are held at beer halls, clinics, or other public spaces, with audiences composed, in a contingent manner, of anyone who happens to be there at the time: schoolchildren, unemployed men, married wives, or the elderly. They can reach over fifty in number or be less than five. The extent of participation varies greatly from week to week, depending on where the performance takes place, the character of the audience, and the choice of songs for that week.

As a result, the public response to peer education songs often leads not to "participation" but to expressions of shock, amusement, discomfort and, occasionally, outright anger.

The songs that we analyze below are taken from a selection of over two hundred peer education songs, recorded over a ten-year period. We present three examples, one from each of the categories used by the educators to describe their songs: "church," "struggle" and "traditional."

DIRAGA (LIT. DRUGS: ANTI RETROVIRAL MEDICATION)

Leader: *Hu shuma diraga maduvha ano,*	We use drugs (ARV), these days,
Hu shuma madarada maduvha Ee, Ahh!	We use drugs, these days, oh!
Chorus: *Diraga maduvha ano, iyo weah!* (x3)	Drugs, these days, oh!
hu shuma madaraga maduvha ano	We use drugs, these days
Leader: *Vha tshi ha-Lufule vha do i wana*	You will get it at Lufule [clinic]
Vha tshi ha-Siloam vha do i wana	You will get it at Siloam [hospital]

This is an adaptation of a very popular choral song used by several mission church groups throughout Venda, of Lutheran and/or Catholic origin. It is usually performed in the Shangaan language, and most versions of it are reportedly sung to celebrate changes in the seasons or significant life-cycle rites of passage such as a christenings or weddings. Not surprisingly, church songs are used by peer educators during ongoing weekly training sessions for opening and closing prayers, and for the blessing of food. Different groups thus bring the songs and melodies from their Sunday worship into the peer education arena. They either present an adaptation they have written themselves, or work in small groups to find alternative lyrics that can encapsulate succinctly biomedical notions of HIV, AIDS, treatment, and prevention. During public performances, however, many people in the audience associate church songs with sacred spaces and see their secularization as blasphemous. This is especially so when peer educators use shock tactics as a means of grabbing attention, as in a popular Zion Christian Church (ZCC) anthem that they have changed from "Jesus is number one!" to "Condom is number one!" The peer educators are acutely aware that such transformations court potential controversy, but they regard controversy as a point in the songs' didactic favor:

> When we are busy singing these songs from church, some people [laughing] can get very cross with us. Even my auntie told me she was not happy about us doing it like this. It's as if we are stealing from them, or laughing at Jesus. But we say "No! They should be blessing us because isn't it that the Bible says 'God is Love,' and how can you love if there is no life?" Really, if people are getting shocked, then we think that is good! They must just get tested and use condoms. (McNeill interview with peer educator, March 2005)

As we suggested above, however, their musical repertoire is not limited to church songs. Peer educators also modify songs that are associated with political activity against apartheid. Struggle or "freedom" songs have recently been described as

> short slogans set to simple melodic phrases, sung *a cappella* (unaccompanied) and repeated over and over in a call and response style. They are created and sung collectively, and frequently modified as politics, attitudes and

circumstances change, and are almost exclusively non-commercial. (Gilbert 2007, 426)

Moreover, struggle songs are "ubiquitous but largely informal and un-professionalised" (ibid., 423) and currently constitute a dominant medium of popular political expression throughout South Africa. Although reference to these songs is scarce in the existing literature on South African music, they are clearly related to the originally Zulu *isicathamiya* genre (Erlmann 1996) and, like it, have their origins in the music of South Africa's ubiquitous mission churches which mutated into the more recognisably African genre of *makwaya* (lit., "choirs") that has stylistic origins in the combination of "southern African singing traditions with Christian hymnody" (Gilbert 2007, 426; James 1999; 2006, 155; Manuel 1988).

These songs, used outside the country during the struggle years to build an ANC identity (Gilbert 2007, 422), remain hugely popular within South Africa. The overt purpose of struggle songs, especially when deployed by ANC structures in exile, was to send out a political message and encourage collective political action (Nowlin 1996). Given the historical context and explicit political critique inherent in this music, it is perhaps not surprising that until the un-banning of the ANC in 1990, they remained illegal, were primarily an oral form, and were only (officially) recorded outside of South Africa. Some recordings, such as Song 2 below, are kept in the archives of Radio Freedom (as the ANC station was known when it was broadcasting from Ethiopia, Zambia, Angola, Tanzania, and Madagascar). Although the purveyors of many genres such as jazz, reggae, gospel, choral, and some traditional music were actively engaged in challenging the policies of segregation, the struggle songs in question were distinct in several ways. Chief among these was the accompanying *toyi toyi* dance that grew to symbolize the preparation for warfare (McGregor 2005). During the apartheid era, the lyrical content of struggle songs was highly politicized and aggressive. The example we provide here, from the Radio Freedom archives, has a threatening message for the political leaders of the Apartheid-era homelands. The chanting comrades exchange Mangosuthu ("Gatsha") Buthelezi, previous head of the KwaZulu homeland, for other leaders of the puppet regimes such as (Patrick) "Mphephu" in Venda and (Lennox) "Sebe" in Ciskei, and prophesize their apocalyptic rendezvous thus:

HEY, WENA GATSHA[2]

Hey wena Gatsha	Hey you, Gatsha
Amasi abekwe elangeni	It's only a matter of time
Sodibanda	We shall meet
Ngebazuka	With a bazooka

Songs of the struggle were outlawed due to regulations over what could, and could not, become popular music. They accompanied illegal political rallies and demonstrations. The recognized experts in leading them were groups of ANC members, especially the youth league and MK soldiers in training, or their commanders such as the late Peter Makoba who championed the "one settler, one bullet" slogan through the genre. The popularity, illegality, and informal character of struggle songs were intrinsically interconnected. They circulated largely in nonstandardized formats and the lyrics changed depending on the leader. The versions aired on Radio Freedom were reinvented in different languages throughout the country, and even their increased standardization after 1990—when record companies such as BMG started making commercial recordings and artists such as Amaqabane, Blondie Makhene, and various African church choirs produced standardized versions with synthesized backing instrumentation—did not substantially alter their character as informal and vernacular conduits for the expression of popular feeling in local settings.

Given that contemporary Venda remains an ANC stronghold, such songs often become part of the entertainment: either at public gatherings during and after local ANC ward meetings when they are sung in praise of old and new comrades, or as part of beer drinking and/or meat-eating repertoires through which men remember the past and comment on the present. They are, however, more widely associated today with general protests, being performed by groups of women presenting a petition to Parliament in anger at the extent of sexual violence in the country, or by civil society groups protesting against police inefficiency in ritual murder cases.

The considerable influence that struggle songs had in the past has thus to some extent been brought into the post-apartheid political arena, where they are used both in praise of and in anger against the ANC-led government. It is in this context that peer educators attempt to harness the power associated with them by utilizing the genre in public performances. As one said:

> [T]he struggle is not yet over. We are still struggling, can't you see? It is not enough that we can vote, but voting is important. My house remains without water and I still cook on a fire at night. Anyway, now AIDS is the enemy, it kills us secretly just like the Boer used to, and we should fight it [AIDS] as we did before with the Boer.

AIDSE

Leader:	AIDSE! (3x)	AIDS!
Chorus:	i ya vhulaya (2x)	It is killing
	i ya vhulaya, e Aidse	It is killing, this AIDS
Leader:	Kha ri luge	Let's get ready
Chorus:	Kha ri luge Afurika,	Let's get ready, Africa
	i thivhele, e Aidse.	To prevent this AIDS.
Leader:	ARV! (3x)	ARV!
Chorus:	i ya dzidzivha (2x)	It knocks out
	i ya dzidzivhadza tshitshili	It knocks out the virus

This song has reportedly had multiple incarnations, and is associated with different activities by various groups. The peer educators mostly recalled it as a funeral song sung by women in the Mphephu era of Bantustan separation, with lyrics that asked "Khosi, Khosi, a ri tambuli?" ("Lord, Lord, are we not suffering enough?"). Others contradicted this explanation and argued that it was a song performed by soldiers in the ANC military wing, Umkhonto We Sizwe (MK), asking God to bless them and their families left behind in South Africa while they underwent training in neighboring countries. In part because of this ambivalent and polysemic character, struggle songs constitute an important aspect of the peer educators' arsenal. The emotion with which they are performed is a stark reminder that freedom is a recent acquisition and that AIDS threatens to destroy it.

In a manner akin to the attempted incorporation of political elements through struggle songs, peer educators also invoke "tradition" (mvelele) as a means to legitimate further the promotion of safer sex. Most strikingly, and of important symbolic value, they open every public performance with the actions of the domba "python dance"—the most emblematic symbol of fertility in female initiation. During this dance, performers shuffle towards the stage, imitating a group if initiates (*vhatei*) undergoing the rites of adulthood. Peer educators also use the *murumba* drum when performing traditional songs, an instrument central to the processes of *vhusha* and *domba* girls' initiation (cf. Blacking 1969).

The potential repertoire available to peer educators is connected to and restricted by the classification of communal Venda music into genres performed by men, women, adults, and children (see Stayt 1931; Blacking 1965, 1967). As mostly young women, peer educators use a combination of *malende* (songs sung by men and women at communal occasions, especially during harvest time and at the homecoming parades of initiates), *vhusha*, *domba* (from the female initiation schools), *tshifase* (a courting dance for teenagers closely related to initiation school songs), and *tshigombela* (young girls/women's entertainment). *Malende, tshigombela,* and *tshifase* have historically been employed extensively to construct and articulate social commentary on contemporary affairs (Kruger 1999) but they are also associated with an idealized, conservative, long-lost past. It is the power associated with this historical perspective that peer educators try to capture when using traditional songs, and it is precisely because of their historical role in channelling social critique behind ancestral protection that they choose to transform them into part of the AIDS education repertoire.

LELE (FEMALE INITIATION SONG)

Chorus: *Iyo lele, lele, lele*
Leader: *Vhatukana havha mmbondolola mmawe*
lu vhonna a tina khaladzi
thi malli khaladzi nnduni mmawe

Be patient, be patient, be patient
These boys are looking at me
they see I don't have a brother
my brother won't marry me

This refers to a brother, who is expected to stop other boys proposing to his sister, as she is not yet ready to be married. There will come a time when he must allow her the freedom to have a boyfriend.

F.A.P. LYRICS

Chorus: *Iyo lele, lele lele*
Leader: *Doropo yo thoma nga nne mmawe*
Ngauri a tho ngo ita nga khondomu mmawe
Zwino khondomu i phesini mmawe

Be patient, be patient, be patient
The drop (gonorrhea) started with me
Because I didn't do it with a condom
Now the condom is in my handbag

Lele is sung, according to the peer educators, in the *musivheto* initiation prior to the *vhusha* school which is entered after the first menstruation. They assert that, in this context, *Lele* urges young girls to ignore the sexual advances of boys. Blacking has, however, recorded a version of it as part of the *ndayo* sessions of the *vhusha* ceremony (1969; cf. McNeill 2007). In the song, the initiates are reminded that their brothers have a duty to protect them against any unwanted attention. But the predicament of the girl is also important; she may marry a young suitor, but she could never marry her over-protective brother. The message to girls here is that there comes a time when they will be in a position to be married and relinquish their brothers' protection, and that too much protection is not always a good thing. Until then, however, they must refrain from intercourse. In the peer educators' version, the social context is transformed and the sexual instruction manipulated to suit the new content. First, there has been an attempt to move the song from a relatively closed, quasi-sacred female initiation ceremony, into a patriarchal public arena. Although, as mentioned earlier, the message is most effectively received in all-female arenas, the intention is to transcend these boundaries and to carry it beyond them to the public at large. Second, the lyrical content is transformed from a sympathetic riddle promoting abstinence to a direct confession of a sexually transmitted infection. The condom is an unambiguously advantageous addition to the average girl's handbag (*pessini*—lit., "in the purse").

For peer educators in Venda, then, the way in which their message is delivered is very important. Specific songs are chosen to be adapted not just for the ease with which lyrical changes might be implemented in them, but also for preexisting symbolism in the song, dance, rhythm, or genre. Perhaps there is an element of pragmatism here in that music is one of the cheapest and easiest ways to pass on information in rural South Africa; but virtue has been made of this necessity. Symbolic association with music of the struggle has immediate and obvious implications, placing peer educators at the center of the contemporary struggle against AIDS while invoking the powerful spirit of a mass agitprop social movement to which many in their audience once belonged. The choice of specific struggle songs is not random; there is deliberate use of praise and funeral songs that seek to elicit emotional responses in those who hear them. Moreover, although church music is perhaps an obvious choice, by replacing "Jesus" with "condom," peer educators make a flagrant attempt at shock tactics in a generally conservative religious environment. Condoms become sacred, worthy of worship and sacrifice with the eventual gift of life over death.

The association with tradition (*mvelele*) thus reveals another important dynamic of the peer educators' intentions. By appropriating specific genres such as *malende, tshifase,* and initiation school music and dance, AIDS education is veiled symbolically in "Vendaness," and assumes the protection of ritual contexts. For the educators and project designers such choices represent an attempt to legitimize the performance.

Peer educators' use of these musical genres to transmit biomedical discourse to the general public can be seen as an attempt to convey AIDS education through a medley of media and, by extension, to transform themselves from a relatively powerless group of young women engaged in immoral transactions into a coherent army of warriors against social injustice, legitimized by reference to traditional ancestral authority. In doing so, they have cobbled together a *bricolage* of historically constituted meanings, presenting them in one coherent performance in which each musical tradition takes on a new significance in the context of AIDS prevention.

The content of the songs is as important as (if not *more* important than) the method of delivery. It demonstrates a sound understanding of both basic biomedical knowledge and the services offered by the government and AIDS related organizations such as the FAP. For a group of unemployed and undereducated women who live close to the poverty line, this knowledge (and the ways in which it is learned and presented) may indeed be experienced as empowering in that it demonstrates significant differences between them and other unemployed women in the area. With regular government contracts for voluntary counselling and testing (VCT) and home-based care (HBC) being implemented by the FAP, this demonstration of knowledge brings them closer to a job "in the government," with all its associated rise in status and economic security. For at least a few, this promise of paid work has been realized. Singing these songs, then, invokes a dual notion of hope: hope that the "nation will not perish" and hope that the singers may benefit from the situation by progressing into employment. It is a public display to their friends and neighbors of their transition from "sitting around doing nothing, waiting on God to help me" into a more respectable, proud, and ultimately employable position of quasi-social worker (see James 2002). To this extent, the songs of peer educators, and their weekly performances, provide spaces for constructing and projecting a distinctly positive identity through which peer educators strive to negotiate positions of power and authority in adverse, unfavorable circumstances (cf. Erlmann 1996, Coplan 1994).

The songs presented above thus represent more than an appropriate mechanism by which peer educators in Venda seek to transfer AIDS-related knowledge. But to what extent do they actually fulfill this primary, pedagogic task? If project designers, advocates of peer education and writers on medical ethnomusicology promote the use of songs as an effective and culturally appropriate process of transferring knowledge, does the evidence from Venda suggest the success of such a strategy?

In a recent analysis of Ugandan performance genres, Barz argues that women's AIDS songs have played a significant role in the country's impressive reduction in HIV transmission rates: both as therapeutic interventions in their own right and as media for AIDS education in remote regions (Barz 2006).[3] It is indeed likely that Venda peer educator songs have been effective in instigating action among some of their listeners. They may have encouraged a pregnant woman to be tested for her child's sake if for no other reason, or convinced a commercial sex worker to manage her occupational hazards by using condoms or reducing the number of sexual partners, and they have certainly sparked conversations about antiretroviral medication and VCT. We must take care, however, in positing a causal connection between people's hearing of the songs and their implementing of the advice contained therein. There is little evidence in the AIDS literature that "accurate" knowledge (whether it be presented in song, text, or radio) leads to behavior change in African populations. As we demonstrate below, the biomedical position can be reinterpreted and/or challenged through its incorporation into conservative, patriarchal folk models of illness in a way that serves to stigmatize further the women who promote it.

ZWILOMBE AND A "FOLK MODEL" OF SEXUAL ILLNESS

The word *zwilombe* (sing. *tshilombe*) is the collective noun for a specific group of male musicians in the Venda region. Defined by Blacking (1965, 28) as "wandering minstrel[s]," they perform with guitars, *dende* (a gourd bow), *tshidzholo* (an elongated zither), and lamellophones or "thumb pianos" (*mbila*). Linguistically, the term *zwilombe* is constructed from the same root as the term for *malombo* rites of affliction (*u lomba*—to fetch something from far away or to borrow from a spirit) and *tshilombe* musicians are thus associated to a significant extent with the hidden world of the dead. As we suggested earlier, these musicians are inherently marginal figures who, like the peer educators, have an investment in conveying specific forms knowledge in the context of a significant post-apartheid retraditionalization of the political economy in Venda. Kruger has elaborated on the ambiguous position of *zwilombe* musicians, suggesting that although they are not recognized as religious or political figures, they are spiritually sanctioned and "consequently present themselves as the voice of ancestral spirits or God" (1999/2000, 22). From this position of relative power, *zwilombe* musicians construct models for and of social reality that constitute

> [a] comprehensive, long-term strategy which attempts to influence the attitude and behavior of people in the promotion of an ordered, supportive social environment...they are prophet-musicians who act on spiritual command...their instruments become "spirit," symbolic extensions of religious authority. (Kruger 1993, 510)

It has been suggested that historically every royal courtyard had a *tshilombe* whose job consisted of entertaining the king and his royal councilors through song and dance. As Kruger (1993) has shown, *zwilombe* believe their talents to be hereditary. However, it would be erroneous to see *zwilombe* as a conservative social institution engaged in the promotion of patriarchal or hereditary structures of political power. Despite the gravitas of their association with ancestral authority, the fact that the songs are articulated by "traveling minstrels"—marginal figures who mostly perform for beer or *folla* (anything that can be smoked) and who often present various locally recognized symptoms of psychological imbalance or "madness" (Kruger 1993, 1999/2000)—has made the genre more liminal than official or canonical. This marginality enables songs and their singers to be openly critical where others would not dare to articulate such criticism.

Tshilombe musicians thus resemble peer educators in one respect: they can "sing about what they cannot talk about." In the setting of the volatile political climate of the independent homeland era, for example, *tshilombe* musicians exploited their peripheral status to make scathing attacks on the violent and corrupt ministers in the Venda government (Kruger 1999/2000, 20):

Ngevhala ndi Vho-Ravele	There is Mr. Ravele, struggling to eat
Vho vhulaya na vhone Vho-Mphephu	He killed Mr. Mphephu
Vha tshi nyaga tshidulo a shangoni la Venda	He was after the presidency of Venda
Ri la ri vhanzhi u zwimbela dzi a talula	Many ate, only one became constipated
Havha Vho-Ravela vhone vho dzhia hetshi	This Mr. Ravele took the position
Tshidulo tsha president P.R. Mphephu	of President P.R. Mphephu
A si zwavho, vho tou renga	It is not yours, you just bought it.
Ndi kwine vha ndzhie	It is better to kill me by ritual murder.

In this way, as spiritually sanctioned social commentators with a desire for an "ordered social environment" and a tendency toward articulating criticism, *tshilombe* musicians write and sing songs on pressing concerns of the day. They perform at beer halls, parties, and other public occasions, moving in similar circles to peer educators but with very different positions in the social and spiritual hierarchy. Where melodies are likely to remain consistent in repeat performances, *tshilombe* lyrics are rarely standardized, but are based on recurring themes and phrases that constitute a core to each song. Such dynamics, Barber (1991) reminds us, lie at the very heart of oral performance throughout the African continent. Their variability, in addition to owing much to a core African oral aesthetic, is also partly due to the pragmatics of remembering lyrics—most songs last at least ten minutes. Moreover, the vast majority of performances are made after significant quantities of beer have been consumed, sometimes adding to the flow of consciousness of lyrical composition and at other times seriously hindering it.

After taking such a central role in constructing and delivering critiques of Bantustan politicians, and of the apartheid system in general, *zwilombe* musicians found themselves in an ambiguous position at the dawn of democracy. While they had seemingly navigated away from endorsing any political associations, they were, as self-confessed voices of the ancestors, moving ever closer to the centers of traditional power (largely under the Mphephu lineage) from which the Bantustan leadership had been constituted. This proximity, combined with "critical distance" (Drewal 1991), explains *zwilombe* musicians' overwhelming feeling of responsibility for securing the healthy reproduction of the Venda nation: as voices of the ancestors they must speak the truth as they see it. Yet even when this truth appears as provocative criticism of traditional leadership, it still marks a strong symbolic connection between the musician and the king. The reinvention of traditional authority in the post-apartheid era, under the democratic leadership of the overwhelmingly popular ANC, thus provided *zwilombe* musicians with a means to reposition themselves vis-à-vis the moral discourse that secures their power to act on the world. With the impact of HIV/AIDS beginning to show in the endless succession of weekend funerals and the increasing crowdedness of cemeteries, they had something else, other than apartheid, to sing about.

The following song, "Zwidzumbe" ("Secrets"), was performed in public for the first time in 2000 by the famous and prolific *tshilombe* Solomon Mathase. At that time, Mathase called it "Ri Tshimbilanayo" ("We Walk With It") and complained through the song that promiscuous women were "carrying AIDS around with them," infecting men and "the sons of the nation." Through the verses, he called for these women to adhere to the laws of "God's country," since now they walk without giving due thanks or deference, causing the nation to perish (*lushaka lu khou fhela*) in the process. This general theme is remarkably similar to a song by *tshilombe* Mmbangiseni Madzivhandila, recorded by Kruger (1993, 348–56), in which promiscuous girls, with an insatiable sexual appetite, are blamed for harboring and spreading HIV.

"Zwidzumbe" illustrates the "folk model" of HIV/AIDS that *zwilombe* musicians have their vested interests in promoting. "Folk models" (Good 1994) or "Indigenous Knowledge Systems" (Liddell et al. 2005) represent "a culture's collective body of accumulated knowledge and wisdom" (ibid., 624). Within this body, "illness representations" in southern Africa have readily incorporated elements of biomedical explanations since the earliest exposure to them. Notions of pollution, infection, bacteria, dirt, etc. have long been common proximate causes of ill health answering the *how?*—while witchcraft and ancestral vengeance generally provide ultimate explanations for the *why?*

In Venda, as in other regions of southern Africa, elements of the biomedical model of AIDS are remarkably similar to the representation of sexual illness in indigenous knowledge systems.[4] Both focus on blood, semen, and sexual transmission. But the folk model leads to a rather different set of conclusions about how disease should be avoided. It has been brought to bear upon, or used to explain, social settings in a way that has yielded gendered and generational patterns of blame. Women—and specifically young women—have been held responsible for generating a buildup of pollution through slack moral practices (cf. Bujra 2000, Baylies 2000) that symbolize a perceived wider neglect of traditional and ancestral authority. In Venda, we can trace this pattern of blame through songs performed by older men. Again, the focus on songs is not arbitrary; the *zwilombe* genre to which we now turn has a history of commentary on such controversial topics.

In this version, recorded in 2005, Mathase shifts between the voices and opinions of many different actors, simulating gossip and social situations in which AIDS is discussed. Through this process, he poses questions and provides answers to construct a complex representation of the ways in which HIV/AIDS is understood by the majority of poor, rural Venda men and older (initiated) women. His performance is a powerful articulation of the extent to which AIDS has been incorporated into the conservative and patriarchal folk model of sexual illness.

ZWIDZUMBE (SECRETS)[5]

(65)	*Houla mudulu, nda ndi sa mufuni zwone,*	That grandchild, I really loved him,
	na u la nwanawanga,	and that other child of mine,
	nda ndi sa mufuni zwone vhone	I really loved him too,
(66)	*mara u pfi o vhulwa nga yenei Aidse*	but they say he was killed by this AIDS
(67)	*vhone, vhopfa uri zwone ndi zwifhio?*	You, what did you hear?
(68)	*U la munwe ari hupfi hai!*	No! He slept with (ate) another woman
	O tou wela	who was unclean after an abortion
(69)	*Munwe ari hai!*	Another said No!
	Thiri o vha a khou pfana	isn't it that he slept with
	na u la musadzi wa vho-Mukenenene?	The wife of Mr. so and so?
(70)	*Nwana wa vho-Mukenenene vhone vha Muthemba*	you know, the child of Mr. So and so
(71)	*ula?*	That one? Do you really trust her?
	ari thiri u tou nga o vha o bvisa thumbu?	Didn't she have an abortion?
(72)	*Munwe ari hai!*	Another said no!
	Thiri o vha a na zwilonda nga nnyoni?	Doesn't she have sores on her vagina?
(73)	*Munwe ari hai!*	Another said no!
	O vha o tou vhifha muvhilini	she was pregnant (lit. ugly in the body)

[Now speaking as a practicing *inyanga* (traditional healer)]

(74)	*Ngoho mara zwone*	Really, but honestly,
	zwa vhukuma ndi zwifhipo?	Which one of these is the truth here?
(75)	*Tshihulwane, o vhuya a dida*	they visited me, the great one,
	na kha nne ari ndi mufhe mushonga	so that I could give them medicine
(76)	*A tshiyo pfana na nwana wa Vho Mukenenene nene*	when he fell in love with that child of Mr. So and so
(77)	*thumbu a yongo fara*	but she could not conceive a child
(78)	*Mulandu ndi zwilonda*	the problem was these vaginal sores
	zwe zwi la zwa we ndi li a 'gokhonya'	they led to her getting 'gokhonya'[6]
(79)	*A vho ngo vhonna na ula*	Didn't you see that one,
	nwana wawe wa u thoma, o mbo di lovha	her first child died
(80)	*O vha o funa o ya hangeni*	she should have consulted
	ha 'vho Nyatshavhungwa'.	Mrs. Nyatshavhungwa[7]
	Thiri na vhala vha a zwikonda?	Isn't it that she can deal with these difficult things?

In this extract, Mathase raises closely related key issues that sketch the parameters of an etiology widely perceived in southern Africa: contraception (*o tou wela*), notions of socially unacceptable promiscuity, and the role of traditional healers in treating conditions such as vaginal sores (*zwilonda*, often leading to the illness known as *gokhonya*). These issues are connected, as the following discussion demonstrates.

Toward the end of the song, Mathase makes an explicit connection between AIDS and the woman who "could not conceive a child": a reference to the use of the contraceptive injection/pill. In his own words (translated from Tshivenda):

When a woman is sleeping with a man, the bloods are not the same. This has not really been a problem unless you were sleeping with a prostitute who had too many mixtures in her blood and could always give you illness. The problem now is that women are using the pills and injections from the doctors...they get them at the clinics...I have seen them trying to hide it. When women use the pills to prevent a pregnancy, she will get pimples and wounds and smelly discharge from her vagina. You know women every month they have their period, now after taking the pill the periods disappear, so where does the dirty blood go?! It gets into their veins, they cannot conceive and they get this AIDS or whatever. Then the man gets inside her without knowing and catches it.

This idea of "mixed" or dirty blood that ought to have been taken out of the female body through the menstrual cycle is widespread. It is linked to notions of pollution, sexual taboos, and social and physical illness throughout southern Africa. For Karanga speakers in the Ndanga and Bikita districts of Zimbabwe, it is known as *svina* (lit., "dirt") and avoidance of it is fundamental to the maintenance of fertility and sexual health. It is thought to be in particular abundance before the first period after a woman gives birth, and thus sex is highly taboo during this time (Aschwanden 1987, 21–23; Ingstad 1990, 33 among Tswana). In Malawi, some traditional practitioners have also conceptualized the symptoms of AIDS as a direct result of female transgression of blood-related sexual taboos (Lwanda 2003). Similar observations have also been made in Botswana (Ingstand 1990; De Bruyn 1992; Heald 2006). In other regions of South Africa women's bodies are also conceptualized as highly suitable places for harboring "dirt." As Leclerc-Madlala (2002) has shown in KwaZulu-Natal, menstrual blood is intrinsically connected to notions of pollution and sexual health. She suggests that this wider complex of meaning has been mobilized to provide non-biomedical explanations for the AIDS epidemic and that "women's promiscuity" (ibid., 91) is widely regarded as being primarily responsible for the unhealthy contamination of blood (cf. Ashforth 2005, 160).

Demonstrating the historical connections made between diseases of the blood, pollution, and the female body in Venda, Stayt comments of conception that

> a child receives its flesh and blood from the mother, and sensory organs and bones from the father...probably because of the respective colours of the menstrual flow and the semen...all illnesses connected with the blood thus come from the mother's side of the family. (1931, 260–61)

For Mathase, then, and reflecting wider regional beliefs, the natural cycles that remove pollution from the female body are central to healthy individual and thus social reproduction. The introduction of methods of contraception such as the pill and the injection put this system in danger by regulating the flow in ways perceived as unnatural that result in the trapping of "dirt." Women who use—or are *suspected* of using—contraception thus harbor dams of dangerous pollution that will eventually make them, and men who come into intimate contact with them, ill.

This sickness can take a variety of forms, such as *zwilonda* (line 72; open genital sores that resemble the third phase of syphilis), *gokhonya* (line 78; also known as *lukuse*, through which a woman's children die in infancy), *tshidzwonyonyo* (a red, burning rash on the genitals similar to thrush), or *tshimbambamba* (through which a woman develops yellow pimples in the genital area that burst during sex and cause a white, smelly discharge similar to gonorrhea).

This complex of sexually transmitted infections is known in TshiVenda as *malwadze dza vhafu-makhadzi*: the illnesses of women. As a blood-borne infection transmitted through sexual intercourse, AIDS has been incorporated easily into the frame. In the same way, at some point in history, syphilis was incorporated as *thusula* and gonorrhea as *doropo*. The ways in which these sexually transmitted infections are explained through the biomedical lexicon render them quite compatible with the so-called "Indigenous Knowledge System" (cf. Liddell et al. 2005).

Like scientific explanations, any folk model is a historically and culturally constituted code of understanding (Good 1994). The ways in which AIDS has been incorporated into Venda etiology, as we have seen, draw consistently from relatively recent, "outside" influences on the model. The contraceptive pill and the injection are available only from clinics that practice "Western" biomedicine. The pills that can terminate a pregnancy are also located behind doors to be dispensed confidentially by doctors in clinics or hospitals. While we have seen that the folk model has absorbed much of the biomedical material, this has not occurred in an arbitrary manner. Rather, it has done so in a way that renders science guilty of encouraging the dangerous buildup of pollution. This is because the peer educators have introduced a corpus of knowledge that competes with the folk model in claiming to hold the key to healthy sexual and social reproduction.

The evidence currently in question raises a final issue that will bring us to a conclusion: the role of *certain* women in facilitating the spread of AIDS and other sexual diseases. In "Zwidzumbe," Mathase sings of the young girl who cannot be trusted (line 70–72). The protagonists in the song's dramatic dialogue are unclear whether this untrustworthiness comes from her having ever been pregnant, from her having aborted a child, from her being diseased with *zwilonda* (genital sores), or from the identity of her current lover. Venda girls' initiation is explicitly concerned with the maintenance of a conservative female sexuality based on systems of gendered and generational authority. This system of authority also exists within a wider patriarchal sphere and thus legitimizes—and is legitimized by—ideal values such as virginity until marriage, appropriate sexual relations and fertility. These values are defined in contrast to "deviant" forms of behavior such as extramarital affairs and promiscuity, which are thought to cause illness and thus disrupt harmonious social interaction. As Hunter (2002) and Wojcicki (2002) have shown, however, sexual networks in South Africa cannot easily be explained in terms of Eurocentric notions of promiscuity or prostitution. Multiple concurrent long-term relationships are common, and not necessarily viewed as socially unacceptable, between older men and younger women. They involve complex transactional negotiations and a degree of commitment from both parties. This commitment is often reinforced through the upkeep of children that may come from the relationship. And yet it remains partial, in that men generally try to limit knowledge of "secret lovers" to a limited circle of trusted friends and relatives. In Venda, this kind of relationship is manifested in the social institution of *farakano*, through which a married man may have several secret lovers *mufarakano* (plural *mafarakoano*) (cf. Van Warmelo 1989, 207). This term is used to distinguish a secret lover from an official wife (*musadzi* or, respectfully, *mufumakadzi*), for whom bride wealth will have been paid and with whom a man seeks to establish a successful homestead (*mudi*, plural *midi*). A wealthy man may have several *mafarakano*, to whom he may propose marriage if the circumstances are favorable. The tensions between *mufarakano* and *mufumakhadzi* are a common theme of popular songs in Venda. Through the improvisation of *malende* lyrics, for example, married women often recall with nostalgia their romantic *mufarakoano* liaisons, but bemoan their husbands' preoccupation with secret lovers outside the homestead. Through the same genre, men congratulate each other on their prowess in managing *mafarakano*, but also warn each other of the potential dangers they present to managing a stable homestead. In this way, the institution of *farakano* is recognized as contradictory by men and women in divergent ways, but is widely accepted as a part of life by both.

In turn, *mufarakano* and *mufumakhadzi* are categorized linguistically and socially in relation to casual girlfriends (*tshifevhe*, plural *zwifevhe*) with whom some men have irregular sexual relations for on-the-spot cash, without maintaining long-term socioeconomic bonds. In Tshivenda, the prefix *mu* signifies human properties, while *tshi* relates to things. *Zwifevhe* offer what has been called "survival sex" (Wojcicki 2002) and in Venda, they work mostly in the vicinity of larger towns such as Thohoyandou, Makhado, and Musina. Many of them are economic migrants from neighboring Zimbabwe, who are *en route* to or from Johannesburg.

The girl that Mathase sings about in "Zwidzumbe" falls out with the socially accepted categories of *mufumakhadzi* and *mufarakano*. Rather, Mathase describes the characteristics of *zwifevhe*. Unlike women who seek to bear children with their lovers, this girl—and those of her ilk—are suspected of using the contraceptive pill or injection to prevent pregnancy. It is also implied that she and others like her are more likely to have had an abortion and failed to have their womb cleaned (*o tou wela*). For Mathase and his peers, she represents a threat to their patriarchal authority to control the world around them: she is a manifestation of their perceived crisis of social and sexual reproduction (Comaroff and Comaroff 2004). As a result, older men and initiated women hold such "deviant" members of society responsible for spreading what they understand to be diseases harbored within the female body (*malwadze dza vhafumakhadzi*), of which HIV/AIDS is one.

While not necessarily a full-time commercial sex worker, the woman in Mathase's song may be occasionally involved in one-off financial transactions for sex. Alternatively, and importantly, she might have been *rumored* to be using the pill or have had an abortion. To re-quote Solomon from above: "The problem now is that women are using the pills and injections from the doctors . . . they get them at the clinics . . . I have seen them trying to hide it." In addition to full- or part-time sex workers who have "always" been bearers of illness, then, there is the more recent category of women using biomedical techniques to regulate their fertility. It is to this recently constructed category that peer educators, with their prolific knowledge of biomedical concepts declared publicly on a weekly basis through songs, are thought to belong. For Mathase and his peers, and for initiated women, it is inconceivable that the peer educators' claims to biomedical knowledge, like ritual experts' claims to ritual knowledge, would *not* be rooted in the familiarity of practice. They are guilty through association, caught in the web that connects knowledge with experience.

CONCLUSION

In this article, by teasing out the complex social contexts and processes that give rise to musical performances, we have illustrated ways in which both conservative and transformative theories about the impact of musical performance may have validity. In order to build on its strengths, medical ethnomusicology, we argue, must be ever mindful of the need to be aware of these complexities, especially if one of the goals of research is to apply new knowledge to benefit health outcomes. In order to take account of such complex contexts, it is also necessary to remind ourselves of the broader national and global settings in which such social processes and identities unfold. If we are to reassess the validity of ethnomusicology's classic approaches for a transitional and post-liberation social order where national political projects interact with market-driven change in often contradictory ways, two possibilities present themselves. On the one hand music might appear as yet another consumer item in the confusing array of means whereby decentered and recentered—but commercialized—identities are created: a means by which fragmented subjects might attempt to assert new individualized and entrepreneurial strategies for self-advancement, as much of the writing on neo-liberalism affirms. On the other hand, we could understand music as a means whereby people react against or resist these newly imposed fragmentary forms of production, exchange and consciousness: a means to assert older identities more in line with traditional or patriarchal authority. In the context of the material presented in this chapter, the peer educators would represent the first case, a *zwilombe* performer such as Solomon Mathase the second.

Seen in one way, both of these cases might appear to dovetail with the imperatives of neo-liberal capitalism in a globalized world. The explanatory value of the neo-liberal model, however, has been too readily and uncritically adopted (see Cooper 2005). An examination of post-apartheid South Africa reveals that the state, both during and after apartheid in different ways, has played a key role, intervening in the process of redistributing wealth—especially, in recent years, through pensions, disability grants, child and support grants. It has constructed a particular kind of welfarist dependency; a "distributional regime" (Seekings and Nattrass 2005, 314). The peer educators' use of musical performance, although apparently serving their own ends as self-promoting individuals in a global marketplace, is ultimately part of a strategy aimed at securing their position in the setting of a health sector in which the state plays a significant role, both as employer and as policy endorser. The *zwilombe* guitarist draws on and derives some of his musical efficacy from the current reinvention of the chiefship and Venda kingship, and hence of patriarchal authority in general: both of which derive from and are legitimized by current state policy. While the reinvention of the chiefship can certainly be seen as linked to neo-liberal-style "decentralizing" and "outsourcing" processes (Koelble and LiPuma 2005), it also embodies a discourse through which the chief or patriarch, as local representative of the state, will ensure the welfare of his subjects/family members rather than setting them loose on the uncertain tides of market-driven change. Such observations would lead us to follow Stefan Ecks in qualifying the use of the model by speaking of "near" rather than "neo-liberalism" (2006).

Overarching structural models are inadequate for explaining social change—and the role of music that accompanies it—in any specific context. This is not only because those models fail to acknowledge the specificities of such a setting and ignore the continuities between such settings and the older social orders which gave birth to them. It is also because they fail to recognize the extent to which specific sets of actors can play a role in shaping responses to these settings. It is too simplistic to assume that whatever strategies individuals deploy merely serve to further broader, overarching political/economic projects. By looking at both peer educator musicians and *zwilombe* guitarists as cultural "brokers" (Barber 1987), we do not deny the importance, pervasiveness, or influence of these broader structures: but we do insist that the values created or affirmed are mediated through local settings and by the groups of people situated within them.

Such brokers traverse the interpretive gap between more easily recognized social categories by interweaving diverse social and cultural threads; by "constructing and managing social contexts, enrolling and juxtaposing a variety of elements" and assuming identities in relation to their strategies of interaction "through a process of 'translation' that permits the negotiation of common meanings and definitions and the mutual enrolment and co-optation into individual and collective objectives and activities" (Latour 2000, cited by Mosse and Lewis 2006, 14). In a setting like that of post-apartheid South Africa, the very process of cultural brokerage continually produces new forms of identification even as it appears to mediate between old ones (James 2011). Both peer educators and *zwilombe* musicians, seemingly facing each other across the apparently unbridgeable divide that separates modernity from dyed-in-the-wool patriarchal tradition, draw on elements and styles of the new social order in creating their identities through musical performance.

17

Interlude
"Let's Get Together"

The following lyrics represent two apparent variants of the same song, recorded roughly three years apart from each other in different regions of Uganda.

Namirembe Post-Test Club (2001)[1]	**TASO Mbarara Drama Group (2004)**[2]
Let's get together / Care for each other	*Let's get together / Care for each other*
Sisters and brothers / Make this world	*Sisters and brothers / Make this world*
* a happy place*	* a happy place*
Love / AIDS cannot win	*Love is so sweet / AIDS cannot win*
It's a duty for you and me	*It's our duty for you and me to play our part*
To play a part / Let's get together	
Let's get together / Care for each other	*Let's get together / Care for each other*
Sisters and brothers / To play a part	*[Sisters and brothers] Sisters and brothers*
	Make this world a happy place
	Love is so sweet / AIDS cannot win
	It's our duty for you and me to play our part
We have a message to the world	*I have a message for the world*
So people die night and day because	*There's people dying night and day*
* of AIDS*	* because of AIDS [Because of AIDS]*
A disease that has no cure	*That has no cure [That has no cure]*
It's a message of prevention and sticking	*It's a message of prevention by*
* to one partner*	* sticking to a partner*
And caring for the sufferers of AIDS	*And caring for the people with AIDS [People with*
	* AIDS]*
African women are suffering	
Jobless widows with orphans	
Having a disease that has no cure	
It's a message to all women and	
* sticking to one partner*	
And caring for their husbands and children	

Let's get together / Care for each other
Sisters and brothers / Make this world
  a happy place
Love / AIDS cannot win
It's a duty for you and me

To play a part / (Spoken) Let us all
  get together
Children, mothers, fathers
And everybody in this world
To fight this deadly disease
I know and I believe
Together we can

Let's get together / Care for each other
[Sisters and brothers] Sisters and brothers
Make this world a happy place
Love is so sweet / AIDS cannot win
It's our duty for you and me to play
  our part
Let's get together / Care for each other

[Sisters and brothers] Sisters and brothers
Make this world a happy place
Love is so sweet / AIDS cannot win
It's our duty for you and me to play our part
Let us think of the beloved ones
Sad for relatives and friends to lose their lives
  [To lose their lives]
Because of AIDS [Because of AIDS]
For precious men and women,
The elders, youths, and children,
Now let us join our hands and save
  the world [And save the world.]
Let's get together / Care for each other
[Sisters and brothers] Sisters and brothers
Make this world a happy place
Love is so sweet / AIDS cannot win
It's our duty for you and me to play our part
Let's get together / Care for each other
Sisters and brothers
Make this world a happy place
Love is so sweet / AIDS cannot win
It's our duty for you and me to play our part
Everybody in this world
Should always fight hard for his life [For his life]
Not to suffer because of AIDS
  [Because of AIDS]
We should work hard for the young ones
Who are the future leaders
Protect them not to be infected with AIDS
Let's get together / Care for each other
[Sisters and brothers] Sisters and brothers
Make this world a happy place
Love is so sweet / AIDS cannot win
It's our duty for you and me to play our part
Let's get together / Care for each other
[Sisters and brothers] Sisters and brothers
Make this world a happy place
Love is so sweet / AIDS cannot win
It's our duty for you and me to play our part

18

Aesthetics and Activism

GIDEON MENDEL AND THE POLITICS OF PHOTOGRAPHING THE HIV/AIDS PANDEMIC IN SOUTH AFRICA

Michael Godby (University of Cape Town)

Former President Thabo Mbeki's intervention in the HIV/AIDS crisis in South Africa, and the angry response of most Western commentators to his initiative, make it clear that, in addition to being a humanitarian catastrophe, the pandemic is a fraught political issue.[1] Although generally hidden by the media's attention to the scale and human experience of the disease, and strenuously denied by biomedical authorities, there remain important points of contention in the understanding of the nature of HIV/AIDS. There is still dispute about the precise relationship between HIV and AIDS; the efficacy of treatment of the different human immunodeficiency viruses; the origin(s) of the disease; how transmission may relate to certain cultural practices; and, perhaps most important, the question of whether AIDS is indeed a single biological entity that can be controlled by specific medical treatment and changes in social behavior, or whether it is a complex socio-cultural phenomenon with biological manifestations. Mbeki's challenge might be identified as an African view of the pandemic were it not for the fact that countries like Botswana are unequivocally committed to biomedical solutions to the catastrophe. But Mbeki's insistence that the alleviation of poverty is an essential part of any campaign against the disease, and his rejection of the "simple superimposition of Western experience on African reality" (Mbeki 2000a and 2000b), typify a widespread resistance to Western solutions foisted on the continent. In this context, the work of the documentary photographer is more than usually fraught. While the imbalance of power between photographer and subject is a problem for documentary photographers at any time, the photographer documenting the HIV/AIDS pandemic in Africa is likely to be identified automatically with the power of Western cultural and economic interests.

Gideon Mendel, a photographer entirely committed to biomedical treatment of the pandemic, has explored the potential of his medium to empower his African subjects in relation to the debates just outlined. Born in Johannesburg in 1959, Mendel started his career with the international agencies Agence France-Presse and Magnum Photos, documenting the political turmoil in South Africa of the 1980s. In 1987, suffering burnout, Mendel withdrew from photographing situations of conflict, focusing instead on recording Yeoville, the rapidly changing suburb where he lived in Johannesburg. In 1988, he documented the several competing commemorations of the 150th anniversary of the Great Trek, the pioneer column that opened up the interior of South Africa for white, Afrikaner settlement. His resulting exhibition, *Beloofde Land* (1989), received mixed responses, although it has since been recognized as a significant moment in the deconstruction and disempowerment of the symbolic vocabulary of Afrikaner Nationalism (Godby 1998).

AESTHETICS AND ACTIVISM

In 1990, Mendel moved to London and joined the agency Network Photographers, which invited him to contribute an essay to the exhibition *Positive Lives*, subsequently published in 1993. Stephen Mayes, managing editor of Network and co-editor of the collection, outlined the themes and issues of the project in his introductory essay as follows: "These photographs show how the whole of society is involved with HIV: its transmission, the provision of care, the support structures, the attitudes and (when the virus strikes closer to home) the emotions. A medical condition has become a social condition, and we are all required to form a response and to accept a responsibility—whether by action, thought, or by simply trying to understand" (Mayes 1993, 14).

At first glance these comments would seem to apply to any documentary project on HIV/AIDS. On second thought, however, it soon becomes clear that they reflect the first-world conditions in England, where the *Positive Lives* project originated. Although, as Mayes indicated, there was an amount of discrimination, particularly in homophobic circles, against people associated with the virus, the general level of tolerance and acceptance in England permitted an extraordinary intimacy in the representation of the disease. Indeed, the very ambition of the project to record emotional states and capture the reality of lived experience reflected a society that had both the will and capability to care for all its citizens. The photographs themselves confirmed the highly developed condition of medical and social care in that country.

In the same year *Positive Lives* was published, Mendel traveled to Zimbabwe and spent ten days photographing at the Matibi Mission Hospital. On his return to London, the photographs were published in *The Independent* newspaper's Saturday magazine supplement. Titled "AIDS: A Challenge to African Health Care," the series included a sequence of photographs taken at the bedside of a dying man. In interviews, Mendel always recalls his own anxiety at photographing a man so near death, but remembers also the command of the doctor in charge at the time: "Come on, man, do your job."[2] The representation of such extreme suffering, as well as the conditions of poverty shown, constituted an entirely different image of AIDS from the one in *Positive Lives*. The photographs portrayed Africa as unable to cope with the scale, the costs, and the social consequences of the pandemic. But these images of HIV/AIDS also differed from standard Western representations in other ways. Unlike the *Positive Lives* project, which was published by English people, of English people, for English people, Mendel's Zimbabwean photographs were made by and for Western media, an arrangement that, in potentially silencing the subjects of the photograph, presented a formidable barrier to communities attempting to take responsibility for their own struggle against the disease.

In 1995, a colleague of Mendel suggested that the Iziko South African National Gallery (ISANG) bring the *Positive Lives* exhibition to Cape Town and add a specially commissioned South African component to the show. This arrangement, sponsored by the Terrence Higgins Trust, has become the model for the *Positive Lives* exhibition to travel the world: with the core collection joined by an exhibition of local work. For the Cape Town exhibition Mendel visited Hlabisa in KwaZulu-Natal, one of the worst hit areas of the country, and presented this new work alongside the original Network show. The following year Mendel won the Eugene Smith Award for Humanistic Photography with a portfolio of his work in South Africa and Zimbabwe and a proposal to extend this work to Zambia and Tanzania; and in 1998 he won first prize in the World Press Awards for his pictures from those four countries. Mendel has returned to South Africa and Zimbabwe several times since (more recently he has worked in Malawi, Uganda, and Mozambique), sometimes piggybacking his AIDS work on other commissions.

In 1998, Mendel published the first version of *A Broken Landscape: HIV and AIDS in Africa*, as a supplement to the photography magazine *Reportage*. In his introduction to the collection he writes: "These photographs show the human dimensions of the epidemic…Beside documenting the lives of families hit by the illness, they look at the work being done by many dedicated local people—some of whom have the disease—to combat the problem through education and care…Among the obstacles they face are lack of education, poor primary health care, the social dislocation caused by migrant labor and women's low position—all of which help to spread the disease" (Mendel 1998).

In these words, Mendel draws attention to the means by which he sought to bridge the gap between himself as a Western photographer with the power to represent his subjects in any way that he chooses, and his subjects, who have little control over the creation of their own image. Typically, photographers in Mendel's situation, impelled by a sense of urgency to communicate both the scale of the pandemic and the human cost, tend to create images of extreme suffering. Such images are, of course, rhetorical. They are designed to mobilize their viewers to take action to assist the subjects of the photographs. But, inevitably, these images are the views of outsiders, well intentioned in their way, but aimed over the heads of their subjects. Such images, it has been argued, effectively confirm the disempowered status of their subjects by assuming that they are incapable of taking any action on their own behalf (Rosler 1990).

Mendel's approach in his first version of *Broken Landscape* was to go beyond documenting the lives of the families hit by the illness and record the work being done to combat the disease through education and care. "In Africa, as elsewhere, people with HIV and AIDS are starting to mobilize, to challenge prejudices and help their communities fight the virus," he noted in his introduction. Photographically, he represented this initiative by extending the range of subject matter from scenes of suffering to images of caregiving—by families, health care specialists and communities—and to education for the prevention of infection. Such photographs subtly changed the image of AIDS in Africa from one of hopeless suffering to one of responsibility and possibility.

In his acknowledgements, Mendel noted that Population Services International helped fund the booklet, and that their affiliates in Africa gave logistical support; he also included a photograph of PSI's work promoting the use of condoms in Johannesburg. The effect of this and other declared relationships with aid agencies is important beyond issues of funding and subject matter. Compared with a photojournalist, a photographer working with aid agencies will have direct access to both patients and aid networks on the ground, will spend considerably more time with these subjects, and can expect a more informed and discriminating readership. These considerations have a profound effect on the nature—and quality—of the images that are made.

This reciprocal relationship with aid agencies continued into Mendel's larger project. Confusingly also called *A Broken Landscape: HIV & AIDS in Africa* (Mendel 2001a), this book was published by Network Photographers in association with ActionAid, a British-based organization directly involved in HIV/AIDS projects in fifteen African and four Asian countries. As a publicity pamphlet issued with the book put it, the organization aimed "to promote absolute control" of the pandemic and "a sustainable quality of life for people living with HIV/AIDS and affected communities." True to this spirit, Mendel's photographs were arranged in short essays that represented the patients and their families over a period of time, thereby showing the people involved in different situations and relationships that obviously suggest more complex identities.

Mendel's concern with an evolving subjectivity, rather than the habitual representation of suffering, extended first to the practice of naming his subjects, which is surprisingly unusual in documentary photography, and then to recording their individual narratives. In an attempt to represent the broader community with which ActionAid was concerned, Mendel also recorded the images and statements of survivors (including parents and orphans), of health workers (both regular nurses and homecare workers), of AIDS educators, sex workers, AIDS support groups, and AIDS activists, amongst others.

Mendel's concerns in his second *Broken Landscape* project epitomize the differences between the genres of news and documentary photography. Where the former is concerned simply with recording an event, the latter may be understood as documenting the experience of people involved in the event. This understanding, that photographic subjects are complex identities that change in different situations and in different relationships, necessarily demands the sustained involvement of the photographer (both intellectually and emotionally) over a period of time; invariably it also demands a similar commitment on the part of the viewer.

Traditionally books have served well as vehicles to facilitate these intense viewing experiences, but increasingly photographers have begun to make use of art galleries for this purpose. Mendel has pursued this option too, exhibiting both his two *Positive Lives* projects and *A Broken Landscape* in the contemplative space of art galleries. When Mendel proposed bringing *A Broken Landscape* to Cape Town in 2001, he intended it as part of a larger program of events, arguing for his exhibition as an opportunity to use the museum as "an arena for a changing installation of photographs and other documentary material that addresses what is going on in Cape Town in the fight against AIDS" (Mendel 2001b). He was referring here to initiatives such as the Western Cape Provincial Health Department's mass program of preventing mother-to-child transmission of HIV; also a trial program of providing antiretrovirals in the informal settlement of Khayelitsha, administered by Médecins Sans Frontières.

In his proposal Mendel spoke of the gallery as a "live documentary space," a venue "not only for displaying work, but also as a place where ideas and experiences are exchanged, with opportunities created for the participation of people living with HIV/AIDS and in fighting the epidemic" (Mendel 2001b). He fulfilled this ambition when, during the term of his exhibition (December 2001—April 2002), a group of women living with HIV/AIDS was brought to the gallery by activist organizations. Drawn from the city's poorest communities, these women produced memory boxes both to pass on memories of themselves to their children and as springboards for engagement with the public. In addition, the gallery space, which is immediately adjacent to Tuinhuis (the official residence of the state president) and close to the Houses of Parliament on Cape Town's Government Avenue, was used regularly as a platform for raising public consciousness about AIDS-related issues.

The exhibition took place at a particularly heated moment in the history of HIV/AIDS activism in South Africa, when the Treatment Action Campaign, having forced major international drug companies to accept the use of generic equivalents in South Africa, then took the government to court to force it to provide antiretrovirals on demand. The exhibition kept pace with these developments, and activists, including Zackie Achmat, chairperson of the Treatment Action Campaign, and Judge Edwin Cameron, used the gallery space both to affirm their demands and to show solidarity.

For his second set of images for the ISANG *Broken Landscape* exhibition, Mendel brought forward an idea he had developed with an HIV/AIDS advocacy group in Mozambique, of having people represent themselves within a frame of gaffer tape he made on the wall, either with their own image or, if for any reason they did not want their identity to be made public, by filling the frame with any object they felt would speak for them. In this exercise, the photographer renounced most of the conventions of formal portraiture but provided a platform for his subjects to speak, both through some symbolic form in the image and, more directly, in text panels adjacent to their image. People living with AIDS, beneficiaries of the Khayelitsha antiretroviral program, AIDS activists, and others made use of this platform and expressed their concerns verbally in a variety of ways.

While some participants simply recounted their own stories, others wrote of the benefits of their treatment or directly attacked government policy on antiretrovirals. Verbal testimony, in the form of narratives, was juxtaposed with letters—one panel took the form of a formal petition to the state president, signed by individuals in the photographs adjacent. As the project developed, Mendel released his subjects, as it were, from the gaffer tape frames and represented them in less constricted portrait formats. At the same time, he attempted to present more of their lives by capturing sequences of action on contact sheets that, like the portraits themselves, he scanned and printed on large format canvas screens. Some of these contact sheets also were accompanied by explanatory text.

Fundamentally, in these works and in a similar portrait essay he made subsequently in Lusikisiki, Mendel was attempting to change the balance of power that exists between photographers and their subjects. While hinted at in *A Broken Landscape*, in his later work Mendel deliberately abandoned the aesthetic criterion on which much of his career as a documentary photographer had been based. Images were printed digitally on canvas screens; control was relinquished to the subjects of his portraits; and text was prioritized over image. These were remarkable steps for a photographer; and yet, paradoxically, Mendel depended on the context of the gallery, and the idea of "art" that it promotes, to introduce these changes.

In his later work for the exhibition, Mendel appeared to aspire to the condition of installation art, an art form that depends not on the traditional aesthetic criteria of discreet visual forms, but on the communication of meaning through the interaction of form with specific systems of signification. In this sense Mendel's work could be compared with Sue Williamson's *From the Inside* (2002), a project that connected the gallery space with the outside world by having particular statements of people living with HIV/AIDS written up as graffiti in public spaces and then reproduced as paired photographs in a gallery. But where artists such as

Williamson depended on the gallery context to create a limited edition commodity, Mendel used the gallery as a vehicle for promoting the visibility of his cause and that of his sponsors, the Treatment Action Campaign and Médecins Sans Frontières amongst others. For Mendel, it did not matter whether he sold any photographs from the ISANG exhibition, because his livelihood depended not on sales but on future commissions that would be forthcoming if public consciousness was raised and political targets were achieved. In so doing he was able to use the contradictory criteria of art, and its ability to endorse simultaneously aesthetic and anti-aesthetic forms, to validate different aspects of his project.

It is a strategy that invites criticism. On the occasion of its exhibition in Johannesburg, Tim Trengrove-Jones condemned Mendel's photographs in *The Broken Landscape* exhibition as "fatally invisible" (through the repetition of well-known imagery of suffering), "inappropriate" and "redundant" (because of the presence of textual testimonies), and as dead as the museum space in which they were displayed (Trengrove-Jones 2002). It is, of course, appropriate for a critic to question the effect of exhibitions of documentary photography on popular consciousness, but it is short-sighted of Trengrove-Jones not to recognize that the images and the texts are in fact part of the same project, and that the photographer, in radically changing his methods of photography, was actively engaging with both his medium of representation and the institutional frameworks within which he is working. By taking his canvas screens out of the gallery context and using them in installations and the march against Parliament, for example, Mendel actually transformed the institutional space of the gallery or museum from a repository of "relics" to an active political platform. Updating the language of the Struggle, which emphasized a sense of urgency in the composition of the image, and promoting distribution of the image through a selected range of media (Weinberg 1991), Mendel's AIDS work demonstrates a similarly partisan approach to co-opting institutions—of the media, new technologies, and even art—that affect, or even determine, one's ability to get the message out.

POSTSCRIPT

Since 2002, significant developments have occurred both in the history of the HIV/AIDS pandemic in South Africa and in Mendel's own work. HIV/AIDS remains, of course, one of the most important issues confronting the country. But the struggles that had characterized the image of the pandemic in the nation's media, against the Pharmaceuticals Manufacturers Association (PMA) to gain access to cheap generic drugs on the one hand, and against the government to provide antiretrovirals through the Public Health Care Service on the other, were won, at least in principle, soon after the ISANG exhibition. In fact, the PMA had dropped its case against the government and the Treatment Action Campaign a few months before Mendel's *Broken Landscape* exhibition opened at the National Gallery in December 2001. In the same year, the government made the antiretroviral drug nevirapine available to prevent mother-to-child transmission. Finally, in November 2003, in large part because of pressure by the TAC ahead of the national elections in April 2004, the government authorized the national rollout of ARVs in the public health care service.

To a great extent, these victories have removed HIV/AIDS from the popular media; the essential work of treatment and care continues largely outside the spotlight of media attention. Mendel himself has continued his coverage of the pandemic, notably in essays on AIDS orphans in Mozambique and documenting the lives of individuals living on potentially life-saving ARVs in the Eastern Cape. But, increasingly, he is working elsewhere, both on the

HIV/AIDS subject in different parts of the world and on new, socially related material. With the passing of time it is possible to see Mendel's HIV/AIDS work in southern Africa as the product of an extraordinary conjunction of events. Mendel's rootedness in South Africa, his history as a committed Struggle photographer, the urgency of the new struggle against HIV/AIDS, his shared project with agencies that were prepared to take on the government and the major pharmaceutical companies and, not least, his connections with the art world in Cape Town, allowed him both to reflect on his practice as a photographer and to develop a unique form of visual argument.

19

A Lady Who is an Akadongo Player

SINGING TRADITIONALLY TO OVERTURN

TRADITIONAL AUTHORITY

Rebekah Emanuel

THE SCENE

A woman sits in the gathering place of the village, playing an *akadongo* (also known as a thumb piano or lamellophone). The people slowly settling themselves around her know that in their area of Uganda, men, and men alone, typically play the *akadongo*. She sings out loud, which again, men only do. She sings, "When you tell them that AIDS is killing everybody / Even me, I am going to die with you, ladies. / I am advising you to abstain from sex and keep yourself safe." Her words urge women to take control over their own sexuality. Her very body, by crossing the musical gender strictures, by standing up and singing as a woman, demonstrates her message. Through a relatively simple act, she is a local revolutionary. This woman's performance, straightforward on the surface, disguises a complex set of tactics and arguments, each carefully attuned to her audience and locale.

The woman's name is Vilimina Nakiranda. She is a farmer in rural Kibaale, Uganda. She wears a traditional green dress, a *gomesi*, which offsets her short soft hair and black eyes—eyes that become lively when she sings or talks. Passing on the red-dirt path, one would not know she was staging a revolution on moral grounds. Her firm step is like that of other sprightly grandmothers, and her hands bear the roughness of raising a hoe above her head and driving it down into the ground for hours in the heat, working to grow sweet potatoes, yams, and cassava. This is the traditional work of a rural village woman. Vilimina dresses as women have dressed for generations. She farms in the way women in her village have farmed for generations. Vilimina sings her songs in the traditional village spaces, using the instruments and rhythms honed over generations in the Busiki district. However Vilimina is not quite acting traditionally. "My names are Vilimina Nakiranda / a lady who is [an] *akadongo* player / from Kibaale in Busiki." Vilimina is from Kibaale in Busiki: this is the essence of her identity, and its traditions are the rhythm of her life. And yet she is a lady. A lady who is an *akadongo* player. In these little changes she makes to traditional performance lies a fully formed, culturally clever, barricade-breaking moral argument about women's proper roles, and saving lives from AIDS.

This chapter unpacks the layers of her song, first explicating the symbols she uses and how they portray gender, AIDS and marginalization as linked societal ills. It shows how she reappropriates these symbols, transforming them from the standard bearers of traditional hierarchy to playful and assertive images of a new sexual order. Second, this chapter turns to unpacking the six arguments she puts forward to convince her audience to change. Third, it examines how she sets the stage for her arguments to be widely accepted. Vilimina uses tradition to undermine and reinvigorate itself: picking traditional settings to make her audience more comfortable and receptive to challenging messages and laying the groundwork for a much larger social movement with her maverick use of tradition to deliver nontraditional messages. When Vilimina exits, an extraordinarily clever (even sneakily revolutionary) message has been left in the hearts of her listeners.

"OMUKAZI OMOTEGUU" ("A MARRIED WOMAN WHO DOES NOT RESPOND TO INSTRUCTION FROM HER HUSBAND"): VILIMINA'S SONG

In order to step inside the circle of Vilimina's audience and understand what she is conveying to fellow villagers, one must listen closely to her song. Her performance opens, as is traditional, with a gracious welcome to the audience. She introduces herself: "My names are Vilimina Nakiranda / a lady who is [an] *akadongo* player / from Kibaale in Busiki." The moment she has introduced herself, Vilimina dives directly into outlining the portrait of a good wife. A good wife is a woman who is understanding, who maintains her friendships, who loves her children, and who can talk with her friends without triggering any problems at home. She is always clean and, Vilimina repeats, she shows love. Vilimina then paints the picture of a good husband as a man who has good manners, loves his wife and children, and is friendly at home. She contrasts these roles with the social reality she sees around her; she asks why women waste time with husbands who are always complaining, and she pleads with couples to stop complaining and stop fighting. Vilimina then sings "Gentlemen why do you fight for leftover[s] / People, the children didn't eat" (Barz 2007, p.c.). She continues with the verses below (Barz 2007, 245–46):

> *We ladies, we used to sit behind the houses*
> *The real truth is we used to cry from behind there*
> *We used to put on only half a gomesi [traditional Ugandan women's dress]*
> *We used to drink water in gourds that were already drunk from*
> *But these days we eat using forks because we are now civilized*
> *We now drink water in cups*
> *We also sit on chairs very well*
> *We even cross one leg and we are happy*
> *I have come to advise you*
> *Stop complaining*
> *Marriage issues are not easy things to discuss openly*
> *The first thing you fight about is washing the trousers*
> *Well, stop fighting*
> *Things are different nowadays*

There are those youth and others who keep fooling around with their bodies
They do not listen to their friends
You, children, you better change your behavior
What I am telling you is very important and may help your family
What makes me sad is that the youth do not listen to advice
When you tell them not to get married to older women they do not listen
When you tell them that AIDS is killing everybody
Even me, I am going to die with you ladies
I am advising you to abstain from sex and keep yourself safe
AIDS came to kill us
I am advising the youth to keep themselves safe
Stop shaming us
These young boys are so difficult to understand
We do not want you to shame us
We women learned the endongo [Lusoga, bowl lyre] some time ago
We women now even play the engalabe [Lusoga, long drum]
We put on the leg rattles
I am very happy. Bye bye, we see you people. I have gone[1]

Gregory Barz, one of the members of her audience and the ethnomusicologist who recorded this song, remembers that while on the look-out for musicians, he had seen her approaching across the red dirt of the village square carrying an *akadongo* and he asked his local musician colleague about her: "[The musician] shrugged his shoulders saying he was also curious because he had never heard [of] a 'lady *akadongo* player'" (Barz 2006a, 41).

As he settled down to listen to her, Barz remembered that several elements seemed remarkable in contrast with other Ugandan performances he had been listening to for the past decade:

> In "Omukazi Omoteguu" Vilimina Nakiranda sings about several dramatic social shifts that have been experienced within women's culture in Kibaale-Busiki. In response to the health crisis brought on by the rapid spread of the HIV virus in this and many of the surrounding villages, women now use music to address other local women publicly and advise the youth of the village—specifically girls—to adopt behavioral changes regarding sexual intercourse. Vilimina's closing sentiment is significant—she suggests that the women of the village have now begun to play *endongo* and *engalabe*, local musical instruments typically played only by men in this region of the country. That women in this region have now co-opted male performance traditions—and have done so in very public arenas—indicates both a significant departure from cultural norms and an assumption of power and authority regarding public health issues. As she accompanied herself on the *akadongo*, Vilimina sang a powerful series of messages in her songs for all present—men and women—in which she outlined ways local women in the villages must fight back against AIDS, reclaim their health, and change their lives. (Barz 2006a, 240)

There is something eye-catching about a woman performing on a traditionally male instrument while simultaneously singing about women claiming control over their own sexuality.

Listening to the words, one wonders if there is something special she is accomplishing through this pairing. By analyzing how she uses older, traditional symbols in new ways, I will suggest that a carefully choreographed series of arguments are put across in a culturally legible way.

WE USED TO CRY FROM BEHIND THERE: VILIMINA'S
REFLECTIVE DISTANCING

When first approaching this song that so clearly challenges the cultural status quo (both in lyrics and in presentation), one must ask: What made Vilimina, a local village woman who works as a subsistence farmer, take the habits and power structures she grew up with, develop a critique of them, and then stand up to sing about it? Vilimina did not describe what thought processes she went through before coming up with this message; yet, based simply on her performance and her background, Vilimina has clearly engaged in what some call "reflective distancing": stepping back from the norms of communal life, evaluating them, and identifying what needs changing.

What made Vilimina develop this critique? Her song itself may provide an answer. The structure and lyrics of her song imply that her critique originated first from a comparison of real gender relations with ideal gender relations, and second from the damage wracked by AIDS.

Vilimina opens her song by describing the ideal wife and husband's loving and harmonious interpersonal relationships. She contrasts this ideal with the concrete difficulties of "the real truth" where women sit behind their houses crying. Her ideal wife and ideal husband are described in directly parallel, egalitarian language. Even their idealized attributes are listed in almost the same order. What makes a woman a good wife also makes a man a good husband: possessing good manners, showing love to family members, and fostering a good home.[2] In reality, however, women and men are not equal; women sit behind the house and cry and drink from gourds that were already used. By making this contrast, Vilimina holds up her community's social norms for examination and steps back from the situation to suggest that current realities should change. She then moves from this reality to describe how gender dynamics are already changing. With these changes, she sings, "we [women] are happy"—highlighting that real improvement can and does occur. This seems not only to be a message for her audience; it is part of what convinced Vilimina herself that something was amiss and needed changing. The stark disparity between the ideal and real seems to be the first origin for Vilimina's songful reflection.

The second origin is the horrors caused by AIDS. After discussing gender, Vilimina moves to call for changes in sexual behavior, citing the devastation of AIDS: "You, children, you better change your behavior…/[because] AIDS is killing everybody." She follows this AIDS message with a second statement of how gender and sexual dynamics are changing, completing the thought. Structurally AIDS is sandwiched between two statements about gender.

Placing the AIDS messages between her comments on gender effectively pairs calls for AIDS action with calls for gender-related social change. The rhythmic line that links Vilimina's opening gender critique with her ensuing AIDS critique is sung "Things are different nowadays," a line that ambiguously refers to both AIDS and changes in gender relations, forcing the audience to realize how much each is tied to the other.

With respect to AIDS, the lyric "things are different nowadays," suggests that the ravages of AIDS are part of what forced Vilimina to think differently and reconsider old sexual standards. She sings, "AIDS is killing everybody" and points to abstinence as an appropriate response. The effects of AIDS seem to motivate Vilimina to reexamine her inherited social standards; she sees a need for change.[3] With respect to gender, the lyric "things are different nowadays," seems to suggest that women are equalizing their roles.[4] If men once expected women to wash the dirty trousers, and would become angry if women resisted, "well, stop fighting / things are different nowadays." The couple should adjust to this and other gender changes. Perhaps these images offer the hope that allows her to see sexual behavior change as a real possibility.

Thus, Vilimina not only steps outside her daily life to formulate new thoughts about women or AIDS, revolutionary in itself; she actually takes two seemingly independent phenomena and links them—creating a broader thesis that gender relations and AIDS deaths are linked.

I Bet You 5,000 Shillings It Will Rain Tomorrow: Enacting Reflective Distancing

However, it would be a shallow analysis to suggest that Vilimina is simply indicating how her own thought process occurred. She is doing more. She is enacting reflective distancing—taking her audience through the very steps with her.

The distinction between describing something in speech and actually doing something through speech was clarified by J. L. Austin in his groundbreaking *How To Do Things With Words* (1975). Austin refers to the act of doing something through speech as a "performative." It is distinct from a simple description or even an assertion because it is not describing something that already exists and giving a true or false account; rather it is making something new occur. One classic example of a performative speech act is the assertion "I bet you 5,000 Shillings it will rain tomorrow." Those words do not describe the occurrence of betting, but actually constitute the betting itself. Saying the words does the act. As we examine "Omukazi Omoteguu" more closely, we will find that performative actions are used repeatedly by Vilimina Nakiranda.

In "Omukazi Omoteguu," Vilimina may well be describing her own process of reflective distancing; yet she is also enacting it performatively with her audience. As she proceeds through the lyrics of her song, she asks her audience to engage in reflective distancing: drawing their imaginations toward what an ideal couple would look like, and then bringing their attention to their own real-life domestic situations. More explicitly, by reexamining their social realities in the context of AIDS' devastation, and in juxtaposition with idealized gender relations, Vilimina forces her audience to distance themselves and ask in their minds what went wrong and what needs to be changed.

WE ALSO SIT ON CHAIRS: MARGINALIZATION AS LINKED TO GENDER AND AIDS

Vilimina's song contains yet another layer. Not only has she observed a link between gender and AIDS problems, but she also connects this understanding with other patterns of societal marginalization, including lack of hygiene, social hierarchies, and economic dependence. Her song suggests that those who join her in reflective distancing may also see that these issues are linked, and that all such marginalization must be reevaluated.

Vilimina's references to uncleanliness, social inferiority, and economic dependence are made in culturally coded language, which may be difficult to unpack for non-local listeners. This section unpacks each reference and how it is used toward the overall argument of the song. The following lines are at the crux of this argument (Barz 2006a, 250):

Gentlemen why do you fight for leftover[s]
People, the children didn't eat
We ladies, we used to sit behind the houses
The real truth is we used to cry from behind there
We used to put on only half a gomesi
We used to drink water in gourds that were already drunk from
But these days we eat using forks because we are now civilized
We now drink water in cups
We also sit on chairs very well
We even cross one leg and we are happy

Cleanliness

The first reference to cleanliness occurs when Vilimina describes the ideal woman, singing "she is always clean." However, the less perfect "real truth" was that women were not only unequal, they were also unclean and of low social standing: "The real truth is we used to cry from behind [the houses]... / We used to drink water in gourds that were already drunk from / But these days we eat using forks because we are now civilized / We now drink water in cups" (Barz 2006a, 250). According to Barz, drinking from gourds already drunk from is a reference to hygiene: men have drunk from the gourds and they have not been cleaned before being used again (Barz 2007a). However nowadays Vilimina tells us that women use forks to eat—rather than the standard practice of using one's fingers, sometimes from a communal serving dish. The use of cups replaces drinking from a communal ladle or gourd. Women's hygiene, and the corresponding risk of infection from daily habits, has improved.

In the Ugandan context, cleanliness is highly relevant in a song about AIDS. Images often portray HIV-positive people as sick, unclean, and spreading contamination. There have been especially strong cultural taboos against sharing food with people living with HIV because of the sense of contamination (Kaleeba and Ray 2002, 243).[5] Through her imagery, Vilimina ties improving equality and cleanliness for women with an improved ability to prevent AIDS.

Social Strata

Vilimina's line "But these days we eat using forks because now we are civilized" does not just refer to hygiene, however. It also refers to social standing. Around Vilimina's community, many Ugandans in higher social strata have appropriated Western, so-called "civilized" eating customs (Barz 2007a). These have become social markers. Ugandans from lower social strata often aim to appropriate these customs in a second iteration, as a mark of their shared "civilized" or upward-looking social status.[6]

Locally, the connection between Westernization and AIDS is a subject of controversy. Many see Western medicine, Western-funded NGOs and other imported innovations as the solution to AIDS (Kaleeba and Ray 2002). Others have argued that Western-inspired changes to gender roles and promiscuity are the causes of the AIDS scourge. Here Vilimina seems to pair becoming "civilized" with upward mobility, increased happiness for women and the possibility of resisting the spread of AIDS.

Economic Dependence

As an introduction to the lyrical section about inequality and cleanliness, Vilimina wails, "Gentlemen why do you fight for leftovers. People, the children didn't eat." Although these lines might seem out of place to non-local ears, Vilimina is actually presenting a searing critique of financial dependence even within the family. Vilimina's description of a father taking seconds before the children have eaten suggests an interaction between poverty and traditional social relations, where the father eats first whether or not adequate food is available. Vilimina also evokes the economic dependence of the woman and her children on the man, where all a woman can do is call on social opprobrium to ask her husband to stop depriving the children of food. Knowledge of the wider social context, where people with AIDS need more expensive, nutritious food (Kaleeba and Ray 2002, 243), shows that this reference links poverty and AIDS as well, suggesting that the actions of men in power may sometimes deprive their dependants of needed resources.

Vilimina references poverty again only a few lines later when singing about women who only put on half a *gomesi*, the very dress she wears as she sings. A *gomesi* is the traditional brilliantly colored Ugandan dress composed of a matching cotton skirt and top with flared shoulders, both tied around the waist with a silk belt. According to different interpretations Ugandan listeners gave, this line might either refer to women who are so poor that they can only afford the skirt of the *gomesi* and must go without the traditional top, or to women who are so poor that they cannot afford the belt, which is made of expensive silk (Barz 2007a). Under either interpretation, Vilimina is referencing women significantly bound by poverty. Contextually, Vilimina connects this portrait of poverty with women's subservience to men: the men who make their children go hungry, whose gourds the women must drink from second, and whose eyes the women must hide their tears from. Far from being mere colorful details, Vilimina has selected her scenes to tie together the issues of gender inequity with cleanliness, social mobility, and economic dependence.

Sexuality

These images crescendo with a potent symbol of how things are changing. Playing with the same imagery of appropriating western traditions, Vilimina sings about how women are now sitting on chairs and even crossing one leg. In addition to referencing rising through social rank as marked by Western traditions,[7] Vilimina powerfully evokes gender dynamics. Traditionally, men sit on stools, while women kneel on the ground with both legs to the side (Barz 2006a, 240). Women are thus always positioned lower than the men. Vilimina says that now women sit on chairs—at the same level as men. They even move their legs apart, crossing one over the other. Sitting at the same level and crossing one's legs are assertions of power as a woman and as a sexual being.

Finally, at the end of the song, Vilimina adds the image that holds it all together. "We women learned the *endongo* [Lusoga, bowl lyre] some time ago / We women now even play the *engalabe* [Lusoga, long drum]." The *endongo* and *engalabe* are instruments that men, and men only, traditionally play. The *engalabe* is a long wooden tube that sticks up between the legs, providing quite a sexual visual image. By verbally appropriating male musical symbols she grants traditional male autonomy to women.

By weaving these images together, Vilimina points out how cleanliness, social class, and economic dependence are intertwined with gender and AIDS. According to Vilimina's song, new gender relations are associated with women drinking from clean, unused cups, being upwardly mobile, and no longer as dependant. These changes allow women to distance themselves from AIDS. Most importantly, women who have power can assert sexual autonomy. Then there are no tears behind the house: "We even cross one leg and we are happy."

Without specific framing and examination, this conceptual linkage is not necessarily obvious. Indeed neither local people nor those in the international community would all automatically connect these phenomena.[8] Vilimina thus voices a specific interpretation of the world around her, arrived at through reflection and a critical evaluation of the status quo.

DRUMS, MENSTRUATION, AND POWER: REAPPROPRIATING SYMBOLS

Vilimina does not use traditional symbols coincidentally or merely to add color. They offer an argument in and of themselves. Far from simply enacting a cultural practice to use images, Vilimina uses symbols when they function as an effective argument in her song and uses explicit definition when it serves better. Indeed, Vilimina uses an explicit definition devoid of any symbols at all in describing the ideal wife and husband: "People, a good understanding husband is always with good manners and he loves the wife / He loves his children / And is friendly at home / because [it] is good at home / [The understanding of a good] husband is now settled" (Barz 2007b). These are lines that say exactly what they mean; they require no independent understanding of specific cultural heritages. Through their near perfect parallelism with the description of the good wife, Vilimina highlights women and men's similarity and equality when they are in their ideal state, only to show how this is broken through her manifold symbols depicting a sad, unequal relationship. The multiplicity of culturally dependant symbols suggests that Vilimina understands the subordination of women as culturally formed. She uses the symbols to ground a cultural critique.

Vilimina uses traditional symbols in her song–but she uses these symbols in striking, even jarring ways. By placing inherited traditions in unusual contexts, she forces the audience to question the validity of the tradition they represent. In fact, Vilimina uses traditional symbols to challenge tradition itself.

Traditions are created and held in place by the force of repetition. They are referenced as sources of authority and as tags of identity. Reappropriating laden symbols is a clever move Vilimina makes that takes advantage of the fact that each symbol is founded on a basic functional object or activity, and that its social meaning is primarily based on context (rather than in the object itself). By shifting the context a symbol can suddenly take on a new meaning—a coding that is often a slyly aggressive commentary on the older, enshrined meaning. Frequently, symbols that used to stand for tradition or authority begin to stand instead for what could be. They wordlessly take on the weight of an implicit argument for change. In its new context, the older image can no longer be taken for granted—it must instead be argued for. Reappropriating symbols forces authority to justify itself. Tradition itself is both undermined—traditions are held in place by repetition and reverence—and yet simultaneously reinvigorated by becoming an important part of a current debate and the focus of renewed attention and renewed, if shifted, practice.

Vilimina's lyrics "We also sit on chairs very well / We even cross one leg and we are happy" evoke an intricate, inherited, social structure—one, as stated earlier, in which men usually sit on stools, and women kneel low to the ground with their knees together. Yet Vilimina's image does not simply take this received reality of sitting and kneeling and reinforce it, or even make a claim based on its authority. Instead, her reference sets the tradition and symbols within the new context of "Westernized" chairs, and shifting domestic sexual politics. Listeners are forced to justify to themselves why women should kneel to seated men. They are confronted with another option, where women and men sit at the same level, both able to cross their legs. In the context of other options, the traditional kneeling must now be argued for, and the dicta of authority given rational justification. Thus, by referencing an established tradition in a new context, Vilimina's symbol becomes the entryway to a new area of thought and discourse.

Moreover, while listening to the song, the audience begins to connect these changes with wider changes in gender and sexual relations. Sitting on a chair becomes associated with sitting in the house, not behind it, and perhaps even drinking out of a cup. The communicated image becomes not one symbol to be reassessed in isolation, but one point in a larger pattern to hold up to scrutiny. This type of symbolic reappropriation is only possible inside an embedded social context. Sitting is, essentially, just sitting. Only in a given cultural context, where sitting on the ground means one rather specific thing, and where sitting on a chair means something completely different, do the particulars of sitting take on symbolic meaning that can be communicated without saying anything else. By recontextualizing them, Vilimina's symbols become word-less arguments, connections between concrete daily actions and more abstract critiques about gender and hierarchy.

This pattern of symbolic reappropriation occurs even more potently when examining Vilimina's references to musical instruments. At the moment of crisis in her song, immediately after singing about the wreckage of AIDS and how people must take control over their sexuality to halt AIDS deaths, Vilimina sings: "We women learned the *endongo* some time ago / We women now even play the *engalabe*." In these references Vilimina evokes a long tradition of gender dynamics around musical instruments in her home in eastern Uganda. Barz, along with others, has researched these gendered musical traditions and notes:

> In many regions of East Africa...specific gender roles are prescribed, inherited, transmitted or adopted for and by men and women in traditional village music-making...Women, for example, are typically discouraged from playing, and in some cases are not allowed to play musical instruments in eastern Uganda. Many men in this area believe that women should never play instruments; men play instruments and women dance. Some men are of the opinion that women should be discouraged from even touching musical instruments, especially drums, or passing near them; they tell women not to sit on drums let alone play a drum. (Barz 2006a, 240)

Barz quotes Ugandan musician Centurio Balikoowa to explain the menstrual origin of these traditions: "Historically women did not have access to many things and they used to not put on those undergarments, so if it was time for that thing [menstruation] and they sat on a drum it was believed that it would spoil the what? The drum. But, over time, this translated into a deeply felt belief" (Barz 2006a, 240). Barz further comments that even now "If [women] do touch a drum, it is considered a social taboo. In fact, even today in many villages in eastern Uganda I have been told that if a woman jumps over an instrument she will become barren, never being able to produce children. Instead of telling women directly not to sit on a drum during times of menstruation due to possible harm to drums caused by leakage, men often times merely tell women that they are not allowed near drums" (ibid.).

Thus, Vilimina's reference to the long *engalabe* drum (played as the long wooden tube sticks up between the legs) and other male instruments does not simply reference the instrument itself, but rather an entire social tradition of gender and power hierarchies, carefully coded in patterned, meaning-imbued behavior. The long drum's meaning was up until now held in place by the force of habit of only men playing the instruments, the taboo surrounding menstruation, and by the force of local power relations. Vilimina does not cite the long drum to either draw on its authority (and thereby bolster her own claims) or to reinforce its traditional (male-controlled) heritage and context, as many might. Rather, she places the symbol in a new context of being played by women, and thereby uses the symbol itself to challenge traditional gender constructions. The image of a woman playing a large, wooden, long-drum sticking up between the legs paints a vivid picture of women in control of a sexual interplay.

The instruments Vilimina sings about thus begin to signify the connection between the various topics of gender, sexuality, agency and AIDS, and also begin to signal an implicit argument that women should assert this agency. Vilimina, by changing the meaning of playing the long drum, indicates that she is challenging these powers. The meaning of playing drums thus becomes a microcosm of larger societal changes.

I now turn to elucidating the specific arguments Vilimina makes in her song to convince her audience to adopt more egalitarian, sexually safer practices.

THE ARGUMENTS

Although her audience members may have settled around her simply because they liked the way her voice rose and fell, Vilimina's song is not merely aimed at pleasing her audience. Instead, she wishes to change her listeners—and in rather intimate respects. Upon inspection, Vilimina's song employs an impressive range of arguments to convince her audience to enact the changes she advocates. In the following section I unpack six of her arguments.

Vilimina packages her message two ways: verbally and performatively. At root, Vilimina's message is that sexual behavior needs to change in order to prevent AIDS; and to change their behavior women must have more control. She puts forward this message verbally through three arguments: (1) Through a means-end argument in which she urges listeners to behave as she prescribes if they want to remain healthy and happy; (2) through a normative argument asserting that her prescriptions are the morally right thing to do; and (3) through an authority-based argument that roots her claim in her personal authority as an HIV-positive woman. Vilimina also proclaims this same message performatively: (4) she models her argument physically, by personally embodying the troubling problem of AIDS deaths and enacting each of three moral steps with her body in the course of her song; (5) she creates a power-based argument by singing her song in public and openly challenging social conventions, thereby demonstrating that women do have the agency to address AIDS; (6) finally, she enacts a pre-figurative argument where she acts out and partially creates the type of society she would like to see.

What I am Telling You is Very Important and May Help Your Family: Vilimina's Verbal Message as a Means-End Argument

Within the words of her song, Vilimina emphasizes how following her directives will achieve something her audience wants. Behavior change, she argues, will prevent AIDS deaths and avoid shame; and assuming more control will make women happier and healthier. I call this approach Vilimina's "means-end" argument.

When Vilimina addresses AIDS, she sings: "There are those youth and others who keep fooling around with their bodies / You, children, you better change your behavior / What I am telling you is very important and may help your family / AIDS is killing everybody / I am advising you to abstain from sex and keep yourself safe" (Barz 2006a, 240). First, these verses clearly embody an instrumental argument for staying alive: AIDS kills; so to avoid AIDS killing you, you must listen and change your behavior. Second, Vilimina makes it clear that by keeping themselves safe, all people, and youth especially, will effectively avoid shaming the collective: "I am advising the youth to keep themselves safe / Stop shaming us." Third, Vilimina paints her changes as a route to happiness. Women cry behind their houses when they are subservient to men, but when women have more power and sit on level with their men "we are happy."

Setting a Moral Tone: Vilimina's Verbal Message as a Normative Argument

As with all means-toward-ends arguments, Vilimina's attempts at persuasion only convince someone who agrees with her goals: if you want to avoid dying of AIDS, you must change your behavior; if you want to avoid shaming your community, you must change your behavior; if a woman wants to be happier, she must work for gender equality. Not everyone agrees with the goals; if one does not, the behavior prescriptions hold no weight. However Vilimina ties these changes to moral prescriptions in an attempt to override simple preference. I call this moral argument her "normative" argument.

Vilimina wails in her song over the reality that determines everything else: the devastation and deaths caused by AIDS. AIDS is "killing everybody"—including herself. Implicit in her argument is the recognition of the essential moral problem of people dying needlessly. Vilimina points out that these deaths are preventable—indeed everyone has the capacity to do something about this problem. Morally, everyone is bound to prevent this horror. From the simple reality of a devastating epidemic of death (the "is") and the capacities to fix it (the "potential") Vilimina's song derives three moral imperatives (three "oughts"):

1. *Everyone ought to prevent AIDS by changing their behavior—personally and collectively.* Vilimina says this in concrete ways, aimed at everyone, through phrases such as "I want you to abstain from sex and keep yourself safe." She also singles out specific groups with more general messages, such as "You, children, you better change your behavior." (A line that comes immediately after criticizing youth who "fool around with their bodies.")

2. *If all people have the ability to either transmit or prevent AIDS, then people must be treated as responsible for this agency.* This claim is closely tied to the third "ought" claim.

3. *The communal structures that block people, and women especially, from acting on their agency to prevent AIDS should be changed.* The expectation that people avoid sex to prevent AIDS requires that people are able to refuse sex, and that the culture around them deems such refusal to be socially acceptable.

When addressing the costs of AIDS, Vilimina locates the solution in women taking on traditionally male sexual autonomy. Notably, this prescription echoes the first part of the song's movement from tearful costs of gender inequality to newly seated equality and happiness. This pairing of problem and answer, however, holds a radical moral argument within it. When Vilimina addresses the ladies, singing "I am advising you to abstain from sex and keep yourself safe," she is not heard neutrally in Vilimina's village circle. In the cultural context it can be hard and culturally proscribed for a woman to refuse to engage in sexual activity with a man. This situation is especially true if she is married to him; or if she is in an informally "kept" relationship with him; or if he might take another wife when he is displeased with her (which can be culturally acceptable, particularly in rural areas); or if she is economically dependent on him and he controls her very ability to eat (Kaleeba and Ray 2002). To refuse sex would be an assertion of more autonomy than is often traditionally accorded women. Thus, the message of sexual abstinence itself, when aimed at women, might raise questions of autonomy in the minds of villagers. Vilimina underlines this question of autonomy in the title of her song. "Omukazi

Omoteguu" means "A married woman who does not respond to instruction from her husband."

Echoing the first empowerment solution given earlier in her song, Vilimina answers the concerns about AIDS with an image-laden demonstration of women's ability to take on sexual and interpersonal autonomy: "We women now even play the *engalabe* [the long drum]" (Barz 2006a, 240). As noted, the prohibition on women playing drums started as a menstrual taboo and has become associated with punitive infertility if a woman dares disobey. Vilimina's line thus turns the tables, causing drum playing by women to become an assertion of sexual and political agency (Barz 2006a, 240). The answer to women not being able to refuse sex, and therefore spreading HIV, sings Vilimina, is for women to stand up and claim the ability to refuse sex.[9] If women have the ability to either spread or prevent AIDS, they must be in control of this agency and societal expectations need to be restructured to recognize this agency.

This claim thus argues for increasingly universal agency. Although the movement toward increased autonomy that Vilimina makes explicit is a claim for women (she mentions how women play men's instruments and sit on seats at men's levels), she also sings about how youth and children need to regulate their sexuality. Implicitly, Vilimina notes that the expectation that they control their sexual behavior necessitates both the autonomy to do so and the social acceptability of exercising this autonomy.

I am Going to Die: Vilimina's Verbal Message as an Authority-Based Argument

In the verbal lyrics of her song, Vilimina is making one further argument: an authority-based argument. She herself is sick with and will die from AIDS. Despite the stigma frequently attached to the virus and disease, she makes the courageous move of sharing this information publicly, singing "AIDS is killing everybody / Even me, I am going to die with you, ladies / I am advising you to abstain from sex and keep yourself safe" (Barz 2006a, 240). In so doing, Vilimina invokes her personal experience as authority, using it to reinforce the strength of her imperatives (behavior change and universal autonomy) as she set them forth in her normative argument.[10]

Being an Argument: Three Performative Acts

Vilimina does not make an argument only by talking about women playing male instruments. She *is* a woman playing a male instrument. What do we, as careful audience members, make of this? Vilimina articulates verbal arguments in her lyrics while enacting performative arguments with her body. I will attempt to explain systematically how Vilimina acts out performative arguments for female autonomy, first by showing how her actions reappropriate the cultural significance of playing and singing to form a new meaning, and second by arguing that the meaning she creates with her actions is best understood as (1) a moral argument, (2) a power argument, and (3) a pre-figurative argument.

As in the examples of verbal reappropriation discussed before, Vilimina does a simple set of actions—she plays a lamellophone and sings out loud. Outside of a cultural context these musical actions are innocent of further meaning. In the cultural context she is in, they usually signify and reinforce a male social role of hierarchical agency. However when Vilimina *as a woman* enters the middle of the village clearing and begins singing out loud and playing the lamellophone, what they stand for changes. By doing them as a woman, she enacts a critique of the traditional meaning and the hierarchy itself. The observer is forced to question traditional gender and power structures by comparing them to other possibilities (enacted before their eyes), and consider their validity in the context of current moral urgencies. This is what Vilimina explained verbally when describing women playing drums; but in playing the lamellophone, she makes the same argument with her body.

The Moral Argument Embodied

Morally, Vilimina is able to make an argument with her body that she also makes verbally with her lyrics. As a known HIV-positive woman who may die shortly, publicly singing and playing a song about AIDS, Vilimina embodies before her audience the moral difficulty of people from their community dying from AIDS. Standing in front of her audience on the packed earth, she physically indicates her potential to address this difficulty by doing AIDS activism in her community. She proceeds to enact the three "oughts"—that of behavior change, asserting women's agency and restructuring society to acknowledge that agency.

With respect to the first "ought"—behavior change—Vilimina does not, and cannot, enact the behavior change of refusing or avoiding sexual encounters in public. However she does show performatively that she has had a change of heart since contracting AIDS, enough to become educated about AIDS and become an activist in her community for such behavior change.

Vilimina addresses the second "ought"—asserting women's agency as individuals capable of addressing AIDS—through a power argument. By composing and singing her song, Vilimina proves that women can actively address the problem of AIDS in their communities. Her audience members, by witnessing her song, are in fact recognizing a woman's ability to do so.

Finally, Vilimina embodies the third "ought"—restructuring the community in light of AIDS and women's abilities to prevent illness—by enacting a pre-figurative argument. By a "pre-figurative" argument, I mean that Vilimina acts out the reality she envisions; her actions and their consequences generate in miniature the broader societal change she advocates. Vilimina creates what she is arguing for by successfully orchestrating a communal event, where people gather to think about AIDS and how to address it, and where people listen to a woman as an authority on AIDS. By listening to her, those gathered include women as a source of authority and recognize their agency, if only for the moment. In the next two sections I will try to unpack exactly how Vilimina's performance embodies the power and the pre-figurative arguments.

The Power Argument

Vilimina embodies the idea that women have the agency to address AIDS in two ways. First, her performance is an assertion of power: she plays and sings aloud, in public, as a woman. Almost any time any person stands up publicly to say something, it is an assertion of power; in Vilimina's social context, this is all the more true. Vilimina is not just humming lyrics about women claiming power—her public singing in itself is actually claiming power.

Second, separate from her specific performance, Vilimina is willing to publicly challenge and redefine communally significant symbols. Taking something that is known throughout the community as representative of the current social order (an order that incidentally places Vilimina rather near the bottom), and simply redefining what the symbol signifies by using it differently, represents an obvious assertion of power. Indeed, audience members may feel uncomfortable, angry, giddy, or incredulous watching her, emotions that underline the force of what she is doing. Vilimina, by sitting at the gathering place of her village, playing male instruments for all to see, and singing for all to hear, powerfully displays her own power to unilaterally initiate symbolic changes in her community.

Vilimina marshals this power not simply for its own sake but to arm her moral arguments in physical form. It is only because she is willing to claim the jurisdiction to play publicly that there is any performative component of her argument at all. Vilimina demonstrates physically the claims that she makes about agency, namely that women can and do—as her audience members see before them—have agency with respect to addressing HIV. Moreover, the audience, simply by their act of witness, recognizes communally that women already have some agency with respect to HIV and AIDS. This act fulfills the second "ought" in Vilimina's normative argument.

Creating the Society She Wishes to See By Being It: The Pre-Figurative Argument

By reconfiguring the social power structure, Vilimina brings both the audience and herself a step closer to the societal re-arrangement she seeks. Asserting the power to change societal symbols, and then acting out that power, she enacts a revolutionary female agency and creates the social rearrangement that she claims is morally necessary ("ought" three). No longer are the main authorities to speak about AIDS male community elders or medical professionals, but rather they now also include HIV-positive women—the stigmatized bottom of the pecking order.

Vilimina is a local visionary in this way. Not only does she reflect on her societal experience, come up with penetrating evaluations, formulate multiple arguments addressing the moral urgencies she identifies, suggest concrete plans, argue for them, and spread the message by song, she also creates the very changes she wishes to see in the world.

By attending to a curious detail we can see that while Vilimina acts out societal change, she envisions even more. If one distinguishes between Vilimina's performative and verbal claims, at least one difference becomes apparent: Vilimina is playing a male instrument, the *akadongo*, and singing aloud. However, verbally she asserts that women sit on chairs, cross their legs, and play the *endongo, engalabe,* and the leg rattles. Barz, an ethnomusicologist who has lived and worked in East Africa for over a decade, noted that he has never, in all of his research, seen a woman playing an *engalabe,* or long drum. Vilimina thus makes verbal claims that go beyond what has already happened in her village to point toward what can happen in the future.

USING TRADITION TO UNDERMINE AND REINVIGORATE ITSELF

While she argues against traditional social norms, Vilimina does not jettison tradition. She instead uses the traditional symbols as an entryway into the topics she debates, reinforcing the importance of tradition. For example, Vilimina chooses traditional drumming to talk about sexual politics. Rather than rejecting the gendered drumming tradition, which she seems to see as oppressive, in favor of a newer symbol, Vilimina specifically chooses drumming because it is replete with cultural meaning. In doing so Vilimina reinforces the significance of drumming and of tradition.

Yet, having opened the discourse, Vilimina promotes values that are notably nontraditional: science-based health messages (safe sexual practices), universal agency, and rationally grounded arguments accessible to all. For example, by singing about women drumming, Vilimina argues for increasingly universal agency. Drumming, seen specifically as a traditional act, becomes the gateway for Vilimina to promote rather nontraditional values.

By engaging traditional symbols, Vilimina thus reinvigorates them, making them pertinent and powerful within a current debate. Drumming is no longer an ossified, rigid tradition, irrelevant to modern life, nor one that has become merely routine; rather drumming becomes a tradition deeply implicated in the current changes with which Vilimina's community is struggling. As community members negotiate how to deal with Vilimina's innovations around drumming, they will simultaneously be grappling with the role of women and the devastation of AIDS in their current society. The tradition, far from being set aside, becomes a new, crucial mode of discourse for the most pressing discussions.

Yet Vilimina's assertions of science-based safe sexual practices, universal agency, and rational argumentation also undermine the power of received structures in favor of new structures. Old meanings of drumming that were once held in place by the power of communal, lived tradition are being unpinned and morphed, old power-relations between men and women are being challenged and altered, arguments that could once be made based on the truth and sanctity of tradition are now being held up against arguments based on universally accessible reason. Vilimina uses tradition as an entry point into creating new discourses, at once revivifying old traditions, and undermining the old power claims held within them. In Vilimina's hands, these changes all function to address the pressing moral imperatives occasioned by AIDS.

PSYCHOLOGY, DISDAIN, AND COMMUNITY: TRADITION AS SELF-AFFIRMATION

No doubt, even a non-Kibaale born audience member will intuit that the changes "Omukazi Omoteguu" proposes can feel a bit threatening. Most people know that no matter how persuasively an argument is made, no matter how well it is performed, many will cast derision on it and dismiss it if they feel it threatens something they care about. The normal, generations-old functioning of daily life, especially in the intimate realms of romantic relationships, is surely something that most of Vilimina's audience cares about. So is not dying—and Vilimina confronts her audience with her own and others' quickly approaching deaths. Many messages are threatening to hear, perhaps none more so than messages of looming death. Thus, even if Vilimina can use six different forms of verbal and performative argumentation, her point is still in peril of not being heard.

Remarkably, Vilimina's use of tradition itself surmounts this hurdle. Modern social psychology helps explain how she effects this. The dismissive defensiveness people feel when something that matters to them is challenged allows people to preserve their fragile sense of self in the face of threatening information. Social psychology research indicates that when presented with threatening arguments, people will discount the argument irrespective of the argument's strength. However, a way of preserving one's sense of self, while simultaneously giving credence to threatening arguments, is also available. If the same threatening argument is given with a self-affirmation (affirming an unrelated aspect of self which the person values and feels confident about) the defensive effect almost completely disappears, and people evaluate the argument based primarily on its strength (Sherman and Cohen 2006, Correll et al. 2004).

Self-affirmations consist of two parts: (1) activating a concept of self other than the threatened one; and (2) making sure that the individual feels confident and unthreatened (affirmed) in this alternate self-concept so that his or her self-integrity can remain unchallenged (Sherman and Cohen 2006). The theory suggests that this sense of security in one's self-integrity allows the threat in the other domain to be viewed objectively, rather than as an attack on the self—therefore defensive responses are no longer as necessary (Sherman and Cohen 2006, 182). Interestingly, self-affirmations also seem to increase memory capacity and ease of recall (ibid.).

A self-affirmation might allow fellow villagers to hear Vilimina's messages openly (and recall them when they are making real life-decisions). I suggest that by using familiar, traditional rhythms, in a familiar village square traditional for music playing, surrounded by friends all listening to Vilimina play a familiar sounding instrument, Vilimina evokes a sense of comfort and of being part of a larger community. This is a very important part of self-identity and creates a sense of being at ease and unthreatened. By using a traditional music medium for her messages, Vilimina creates a self-affirmation.

I was not able to talk with Vilimina's audience members to ask questions about this dynamic, or conduct a controlled psychology experiment. However, others who sing about AIDS to fellow villagers in similarly culturally controversial ways report that with the use of music, their listeners become comfortable and relaxed. Listening to music, audience members feel less isolated and are more conscious of being part of a supportive community. They are less threatened. Without music, their audience is uneasy or uninterested in what they have to say. Members of the Bukato Youth Fellowship who sing about AIDS in Uganda report that "music helps people not to feel isolated. It gives them comfort to stay among us and helps keep them in a positive state" (Barz 2006a, 240). The leader of an AIDS advocacy group in Iganga, Uganda explained that music "helps people to remember certain things, past or future. Now when it comes to the client, it refreshes him, soothes the mind they say, acting as a catharsis, blowing out their inside feelings and in most cases, people can change how they feel" (Barz 2006a, 240). These musicians, and many others from around Uganda, cite the sense of community and comfort that can act as the alternate self-concept in an affirmation; they also cite people's openness to new arguments when listening to traditionally presented music.

By contrast, when the same messages are conveyed through other media, such as radio talk shows or lectures, the audience is less receptive: A member of Bukato Youth fellowship states that with music "they will...realize the danger of AIDS...It has a bigger impact than just using a radio talk show because most people like to listen to music. So once you pass through that channel it gets better" (Barz 2006a, 240). Music does something special to get people ready to listen. Aida Namulinda, a farmer, musician, and community AIDS activist states it even more strongly: "No one will listen to us unless we bring our drums!" (ibid.).

By using traditional musical forms of communication, villagers like those seated around Vilimina's circle under the shade of the village mango tree may feel more comfortable and supported. They are likely to be open to new, challenging ideas such as gender equality and new sexual practices, in a way that they would not be if simply presented with the arguments. Once again we see Vilimina leveraging her tradition to make rather nontraditional points articulate and heard.

BUT THESE DAYS: USING TRADITION TO BUILD A SOCIAL MOVEMENT

Vilimina's points must be heard far and wide to be effective. As she explains in "Omukazi Omoteguu," AIDS is an infectious disease; even a few cases of AIDS can spread exponentially, and even a low percentage of at-risk behavior can keep transmission and death rates high. "What makes me sad is that the youth do not listen to advice...AIDS is killing everybody." Vilimina recognizes that saving lives requires large-scale behavior change—the norms of society must be readjusted on a complete, collective scale. Her maverick use of tradition builds the potential for a strong social movement, capable of widespread change.[11]

Theorists Donatella Della Porta and Mario Diani summarize the hallmarks of a social movement: "Social movements are a distinct social process, consisting of the mechanisms through with actors engaged in collective action...are involved in conflictual relations with clearly identified opponents...are linked by dense informal networks, [and] share a distinctive collective identity" (Della Porta and Diani 2006, 252). By co-opting traditional symbols, Vilimina provides the basis for each one of these prerequisites.

Vilimina's performance embodies all of the elements of conflictual action: it is aimed at a specific social change, namely sexual behavior change and increasing women's domestic agency; and its demands would damage the interests of the established authorities, especially men who traditionally have power over most domestic and sexual matters. Like conflict in many social movements, Vilimina articulates her targets both in political terms (as a move to redefine and change existing societal structures) and in social terms (as an effort to change the ways people think of themselves and interact).

A key element in motivating people to conflictual action (where they would not have been involved or interested before) is providing an interpretive frame (Della Porta and Diani 2006, 252). Many things occur in the world, but only in certain times and places are they identified as specific problems that need to be tackled and changed. Events become issues because people identify them as such. An interpretive frame is a way of capturing the mechanisms that people use to make sense of the world around them in a way that sees patterns, derives meaning, and motivates action. According to Della Porta and Diani, interpretive frames are composed of a diagnostic component, which enables people to recognize certain social occurrences as problems; a prognostic component, which seeks possible strategies to address that identified problem; and a motivational component, which identifies the impetus for acting and helps participants overcome the costs of action.

Providing this interpretive frame is perhaps the most explicit goal of Vilimina's song. She diagnostically helps her audience identify the AIDS epidemic as a problem that faces them, and helps them understand its linkages with gender oppression and marginalization. She prognostically explains that behavior change and social reorganization are the proper responses. Finally, she motivates people to take these steps by warning them of impending death while also using traditional music practices to provide a nonthreatening way to face these risks and opportunities.

The real punch in Vilimina's interpretive frame, however, comes from her mode of delivery: using traditional symbols. Using local traditions such as drumming and sitting on chairs as an entry into a broader argument is especially effective, since it trains participants to see, embedded in daily occurrences and the fabric of their culture, a larger argument that demands certain responses of them. This is exactly the type of interpretation that effective movements must offer to their participants. When Vilimina's audience members go home and consider where to sit, they will see how an abstract issue is imbedded in their daily lives. The opportunities for resistance, sitting on a chair rather than the floor for example, become increasingly obvious and potentially tempting.

The second hallmark of a social movement is a dense informal network—where people who are involved in the same causes know each other through innumerable social connections, but are not all organized by one overseeing body. Vilimina makes use of tradition in a way that leverages preexisting social ties to permit just such a network.

One common feature of successful movements is that they often draw on or co-opt existing networks. Theorist Jo Freeman observes that prerequisites to an active social movement include "a pre-existing communications network...within the social base" and a network that is "*co-optable* to the new ideas" (Freedman 1973, 794). By using traditional musical communication networks in Kibaale, Busiki, Vilimina can co-opt existing networks. In performing her songs in the village much like many male musicians do, she draws on an old tradition of people gathering in village areas to settle down and listen to a musician perform. Barz quotes several activist musicians as pointing out that people will not come to be told messages about what they should do, but they will come if they hear music, since there is a tradition and a network of people that all come to listen when the drums start (Barz 2006a, 240). A network of music appreciators exists, but Vilimina is using them as a network of possible converts. Moreover, because Vilimina does not just use the traditional forms of communication in traditional ways, but makes some eye-catching changes, her performances may be especially intriguing to members both inside and outside of the usual music-appreciators network, attracting a crowd. Thus Vilimina's co-opting of traditional communication mechanisms facilitates the second, key characteristic of a social movement: creating movement networks.

The final, essential requirement for a social movement is a sense of collective identity. The reappropriation of traditional symbols that we have analyzed up to this point functions extremely effectively to catalyze this process of identity formation. When symbols such as the long drum are reappropriated they begin to take on a new, controversial social meaning. The symbols begin to function as a language or code for the arguments being discussed. Those who are conversant with the symbols and aligned in opinion can often suddenly feel they are part of a new club.

The language of reappropriated symbols can allow in-group members to communicate easily with each other, especially on pertinent topics, since the symbols stand for particular movement arguments and frames of interpretation. The image of wives sitting on chairs on the same level as their husbands can be used by people who agree with Vilimina as a shorthand for the larger argument of embedded gender inequality in the daily realities of Busiki life. The symbols can thus be used as abbreviated markers of social and moral argument when used with other people who understand the issues.

Simultaneously, this language of activists' symbols can help identify who is part of the movement and who is not, as many languages do. The sense of shared identity is especially strong when the language functions partially through code—where in order to understand exactly what is being conveyed, some background is necessary. For the uninitiated, codes usually look like symbols and words that are familiar, but in an order or context that does not quite make sense or form any identifiable meaning. Vilimina uses symbols that already have interpersonally acknowledged meanings in her area of Uganda. It is already a local code, yet she encodes a second set of meanings by interacting with these symbols in new ways. To most people, a chair is simply something to sit on, or perhaps something men sit on, but for Vilimina and her audience it also represents male power and domination. The language Vilimina creates thus can function like a code, further serving to create a sense of group identity for those who understand the implicit inequalities that a mere chair highlights. This silent understanding differentiates the conversant group from those who cannot quite catch what all the fuss is about.

In cases where the meaning of Vilimina's symbol is more widely recognizable, using a particular symbolic vocabulary functions as an assertion of power and legitimacy. In Busiki, singing and playing publicly and using all of the traditional forms and nuances of Kibaale musicians is a language to be used by those who have donned the power to proclaim a message. By playing male instruments in the village square, Vilimina asserts that what she has to say is important; regardless of her gender, she has the legitimacy to broadcast a perspective.[12] Her performance can consequently activate a sense of group identity among those watching—as people smile incredulously at friends, thrilled and shocked, or alternately murmur to each other about boundaries that should not be crossed—creating nervously combative alignments. For marginalized members of the group witnessing this performance, Vilimina's assertion of power and legitimacy can be especially heady, transformative, and potentially unifying.

Thus, Vilimina's maverick use of traditional symbols as tools to create and stand for a normative argument seems to lend itself to the final, essential component of social movements: group identity formation. This is the finishing touch to a complex armory of tactics Vilimina uses in her song to create social change. In her "Omukazi Omoteguu" Vilimina not only enacts reflective distancing and then proceeds to lay out her manifold verbal and performative arguments for preventing AIDS and equalizing gender roles, but she also sings her audience into receptiveness, and finally lays the groundwork for it to spread into a social movement.

I AM VERY HAPPY, BYE BYE, WE SEE YOU PEOPLE, I HAVE GONE

Vilimina's finishes her song with a semi-traditional ending, addressing her audience: "I am very happy, bye bye, we see you people, I have gone." As the dying notes of the *akadongo* waver in the air, the audience is left with Vilimina's hallmark flair. Certainly she literally sounds happy to have performed and moves away carrying her *akadongo*; but she also plays upon the traditional song closure, underlining her messages one last time. I am very happy, Vilimina sings at the end, I am happy as an empowered woman who sits on chairs and crosses her legs and is happy. This is how women can be happy. I am gone, Vilimina sings as she moves away, I am gone, I will show you with my body what AIDS will do to me and you, it will kill us and we will be gone. As the *akadongo* notes last in the ears of her hearers, Vilimina moves away, leaving us only her message.

20

"What Shall We Do?"

OLIVER MTUKUDZI'S SONGS ABOUT HIV/AIDS

Jennifer W. Kyker (Eastman School of Music/

University of Rochester)

"Although you may have a granary spilling over with wealth, and a cattle pen bursting with live-stock, without health you are a poor person," sings Oliver Mtukudzi in the song "Mupfumi Ndiani." Since the late 1970s, Mtukudzi has been one of Zimbabwe's most popular musicians, renowned both for his distinctive musical style and for the perceptive social commentary in his lyrics. Mtukudzi's songs about HIV/AIDS constitute a small but important part of his extensive repertory, and have come to play a significant role in the national discourse of AIDS in Zimbabwe. Maurice Vambe has observed that among Zimbabwean musicians, "Mtukudzi has an enviable capacity to produce a discourse…that exists in the domestic sphere, and is seem-ingly not overtly political but occurs within contexts that have political implications" (Vambe 2004, 185). Nowhere is this more apparent than in Mtukudzi's songs about AIDS, where lyrics describing the effects of HIV/AIDS within the private lives of individuals and families call attention to deeply political aspects of the disease, exploring issues such as disclosure, agency, behavior change, and access to treatment.

In 1986, Mtukudzi wrote his first song about HIV/AIDS, "Stay with One Woman," as part of a musical competition organized by the World Health Organization in response to the growing pandemic. Mtukudzi won the competition and traveled to Switzerland to perform the song for an international audience. However, as he described to me, his own understanding of the disease was very limited at the time:

> By then I did not yet have any real knowledge about AIDS, I didn't under-stand. But I did have the information I had been given. So, okay, if there is such a thing as this, then probably "Stay with One Woman" would be

helpful... So I just wrote this in order to be able to compete, thinking, "I really must write something that makes sense about HIV and AIDS, about protecting oneself from AIDS." (Mtukudzi Interview, Jul. 23, 2006)

Upon returning to Zimbabwe, Mtukudzi released a second song, "Ndakuyambira," with the intention of raising local awareness about HIV/AIDS. He has subsequently written several other songs about AIDS and has participated in numerous public health campaigns and HIV prevention initiatives in Zimbabwe. In his songs, Mtukudzi approaches HIV/AIDS from a variety of perspectives, accommodating multiple ways in which Zimbabweans might understand and respond to the disease. In this chapter I discuss four of Mtukudzi's songs about AIDS: "Todii" and "Mabasa," from the 1997 album *Tuku Music*, "Akoromoka Awa" from *Bvuma-Tolerance*, released in 2000, and "Ndakuyambira," composed in the late 1980s and subsequently re-released several times, including its most recent release in 2004 on the album *Collection, 1991–1997*. Together, these songs illustrate Mtukudzi's multifaceted musical portrayal of HIV/AIDS in an environment where issues such as the languaging of HIV/AIDS, the relationship between gender and agency, and even the expression of human emotion have become increasingly politicized and contested.

"WHAT SHALL WE DO?"—THE POLITICS OF HIV/AIDS WITHIN FAMILIES

Mtukudzi's best-known song about HIV/AIDS, "Todii," was released on the album *Tuku Music* in 1997. "Todii" explores the effects of HIV/AIDS within the context of the family, challenging listeners to consider how issues of gender, power, and agency have come to define the politics of transmission and treatment.

TODII	WHAT SHALL WE DO?

Chorus *(in Shona, Ndebele, and English)*
Ho todii? Senzeni?
What shall we do?
Tingadii? Senzenjani?
What shall we do?

Zvinorwadza sei kurera rufu mumaoko?	How painful is it to raise death in your hands?
Ungadii uinawo utachiwanawo?	What shall you do now that you have it, the virus?
Zvinorwadza sei kuchengeta rufu mumaoko?	How painful is it to care for death in your hands?
Ungadii uinawo utachiwanawo?	What shall you do now that you have it, the virus?
Bva zvapabata pamuviri pasina raramo	Now that a pregnancy has taken hold with no future
Ungadii uinawo utachiwanawo?	What shall you do now that you have it, the virus?
Bva zvapatumbuka pamuviri pasina raramo	Now that a pregnancy has germinated with no survival
Ungadii uinawo utachiwanawo?	What shall you do now that you have it, the virus?

Chorus

Zvinorwadza sei kubhinywa newaugere naye?	How painful is it to be raped by the one you live with?
Ungadii uinawo utachiwanawo?	What shall you do now that you have it, the virus?
Zvinorwadza sei kubhinywa neakabvisa pfuma?	How painful is it to be raped by he who married you?[1]
Ungadii uinawo utachiwanawo?	What shall you do now that you have it, the virus?
Achiziva unawo utachiwanawo	Even as he knows that you have it, the virus?
Ungadii uinawo utachiwanawo?	What shall you do now that you have it, the virus?
Endi uchiziva unawo utachiwanawo	And you know that you have it, the virus
Ungadii uinawo utachiwanawo?	What shall you do now that you have it, the virus?

Chorus

Seri kweguva hakuna munamato	Beyond the grave no prayer can reach
Varume tapererwa	Men we have been decimated
Utachiwanawo	The virus
Dondipai mazano	I implore you, give me advice
Ungadii uinawo utachiwanawo?	What shall you do now that you have it, the virus?
Seri kweguva hakuna muteuro	Beyond the grave no prayer can reach[2]
Mambo tapererwa	Lord, we have been decimated
Utachiwanawo	The virus
Dondipai mazano	I implore you, give me advice
Ungadii uinawo utachiwanawo?	What shall you do now that you have it, the virus?

Chorus

In the chorus to "Todii," the question "What shall we do?" is reiterated in all three of Zimbabwe's major languages—Shona, Ndebele, and English—sung in call-and-response fashion by Mtukudzi and his female backing vocalists. This interaction between Mtukudzi and his female vocalists calls attention sonically to the gender dynamics explored in each of the song's verses. Furthermore, as a rhetorical strategy, the insistent repetition of a single question seems intended to provoke listeners to think about how to respond to HIV/AIDS, whether as individuals, families, communities, or a nation. Mtukudzi likewise extends this strategy to the song's verses, in which his backing vocalists respond to each new line he sings with yet another question, "What will you do now that you have it, the virus?"

The use of questions is a common rhetorical strategy in many of Mtukudzi's songs, and it is particularly prominent in his songs about AIDS. The interrogative nature of "Todii" emphasizes the importance of a personal response to HIV/AIDS, encouraging listeners to think critically about the epidemic. In her linguistic analysis of songs from another popular Zimbabwean musician, Thomas Mapfumo, Alice Dadirai Kwaramba has observed that questions "do not propose that the musician is genuinely enquiring...Instead the questions are indirectly highlighting some facts that both the musician and the audience already know, thus encouraging the audience to do something about it" (Kwaramba 1997, 47–48). When I spoke with Mtukudzi, he confirmed that "Todii" expressed a desire to foster dialogue and discussion among his listeners:

> I wrote that song to try and make people talk about it, and hopefully they'll start understanding that this disease really exists, for sure. So okay, well, what are you going to do about it? What would we do, or what should we do, if you hear that your wife is pregnant and HIV positive? What do we do? (Mtukudzi Interview, Jul. 23, 2006)

The repeated use of questions in the lyrics to "Todii" therefore serves the primary function of advocating for discussion as a first step toward taking action in response to the HIV/AIDS epidemic.

Mtukudzi also uses questions, however, to call attention to the complexities of agency and gender within the family, pointing to particular limitations on women's ability to respond to HIV/AIDS within the institution of marriage. In the song's first verse, Mtukudzi asks how it feels to care for death in one's own hands, a rhetorical question intended to highlight the plight of mothers raising children infected with HIV in the absence of adequate treatment options. This verse also draws attention to the predicament facing HIV-positive pregnant women, who must confront the possibility that their children may be born with the disease. In the song's second verse, Mtukudzi further emphasizes the relationship between gender, power, and HIV/AIDS by asking how a woman feels when she is raped by her own husband, even when he knows her to be infected with the virus.[3] In these two verses, Mtukudzi suggests that within the institution of marriage, the ability of women to protect themselves from HIV, or to access treatment for themselves or their children, is severely limited. "Todii" thus illustrates a power dynamic that exists primarily within private, familial contexts, yet has highly political repercussions in the public sphere. It suggests that relationships between gender and agency must be taken into account to determine what might constitute effective prevention or treatment campaigns.

"Todii" was written in the late 1990s, at a time when HIV infection rates were rising dramatically in Zimbabwe, and treatment options were extremely limited. During this time, AIDS was a prevalent theme in songs written by a variety of other artists in both commercial and noncommercial realms. Among other commercial releases during this period, for example, Thomas Mapfumo's song "Mukondombera" ("AIDS"), warned listeners away from promiscuous behavior in order to avoid contracting the disease. Outside of the music industry, participants in a variety of social and religious events also sang about AIDS, performing both newly composed songs and contrafacts pairing new words with preexisting melodies. For example, lyrics to the *jiti*[4] song "Mombe Yeumai" ("The cattle of motherhood") originally tied an individual's death to problems with his mother's bride wealth; these lyrics were later altered to suggest AIDS as a new probable cause of death. In the 1990s, the following contrafact to "Mombe Yeumai" was sung around Zimbabwe:

Mwendamberi ndourayiwa	*Mwendamberi*[5] I shall be killed
Mwendamberi ndourayiwa nemukondombera	*Mwendamberi* I shall be killed by AIDS
Vakomana matipedza	Young men, you've decimated us
Vakomana matipedza nemukondombera	Young men, you've decimated us through AIDS

As HIV/AIDS became more prominent within the Zimbabwean musical landscape, the breadth of ways to portray the disease in musical terms expanded significantly, ranging from songs seeking to reduce stigma and facilitate open discussion to those perpetuating negative stereotypes of the disease. As Maurice Vambe and Aquilina Mawadza observed, many Zimbabwean songs about AIDS during the late 1990s participated in the production of a moral discourse that portrayed women as dangerous vectors of the disease, whose fertility must be regulated through the institution of marriage. This tendency, they argued, stymied HIV-prevention efforts, as an emphasis "on the sexual aspect of AIDS...helped produce a moral language enjoining women to be virtuous when in most cases the women [had] little power to influence certain socio-cultural attitudes engrained in society" (Vambe and Mawadza 2001, 65).

Vambe and Mawadza cited a variety of musicians whose songs they believe to have contributed to this type of discourse on gender and HIV/AIDS, including Thomas Mapfumo, Leonard Zhakata, Clive Malunga, and Busi Ncube, among others. That they did not include Oliver Mtukudzi among these artists suggests that Mtukudzi's music presented an important alternative to the type of discourse that portrays morally loose women as the primary carriers of disease. Indeed, Mtukudzi has long been recognized as a musician with a progressive stance on gender, as illustrated by his participation in a variety of initiatives to promote gender equality in Zimbabwe. As an artist, he has released several songs, including "Tozeza Baba" ("We fear father") and "Nhaka Sandibonde" ("Inheritance is not a reed mat"), which address the emotional and physical abuse of women within the institution of marriage.[6] Mtukudzi also participated as an actor and musician in the feature film *Neria*, produced by Media for Development Trust, which sought to educate viewers about the legal rights of widows. His song "Neria," written as the film's title track, laments the exploitative treatment of widows and encourages women to hold strong in the face of adversity.

Mtukudzi's contributions toward gender equality have been widely recognized in Zimbabwe. Writing in the magazine *Moto*, for example, Percy Zvomuya has observed that "no musician...has continually brought to the fore a pronounced pro-female cause in the same way that Oliver Mtukudzi has done...Mtukudzi has functioned as the dilator of our consciousness and the sensitizer of our conscience where the plight of women is concerned" (Zvomuya 2000, 21). Mtukudzi's progressive approach to gender has influenced how he sings about AIDS, and his songs constitute an alternative to the type of musical discourse, identified by Vambe and Mawadza, which treats women as dangerous carriers of disease and seeks to control their sexuality through marriage. In contrast, Mtukudzi's songs articulate complex relationships between gender and HIV/AIDS, acknowledging limitations on how women are able to exercise their agency. The text of "Todii" is a powerful example of how Mtukudzi has encouraged listeners to think critically about social expectations regarding marital rights and responsibilities in the context of the AIDS epidemic.

Despite Mtukudzi's progressive approach to gender, in the deeply politicized environment surrounding HIV/AIDS in Zimbabwe, his songs about AIDS have been critiqued and contested. In 2004, for example, Tawanda Chisango, an employee of the Southern Africa AIDS Information Dissemination Service (SAfAIDS), published an article identifying "Todii" as an example of a musical discourse that serves to engender a sense of hopelessness and despair for people living with HIV/AIDS:

> Oliver Mtukudzi's song *Todii?/Senzenjani?* (What shall we do?) talks in metaphorical terms about bearing death like a child and how painful it is to know that you have AIDS. This can only bring profound sadness and negative reflections to People Living With AIDS. The song further talks about a baby, carried

in an infected mother's womb, which does not have a chance for survival. This is simply not true. For instance in Africa, in the absence of intervention, rates of Parent to Child Transmission of HIV vary from 15% to 30 without breast-feeding, and reach 30 to 45% with prolonged breastfeeding. (Chisango 2004)

Chisango's criticisms of "Todii" focused both on his perception that Mtukudzi's approach to singing about AIDS could exacerbate feelings of suffering and despondence among people infected with HIV, and on what he saw to be a lack of factual information in this particular song with respect to mother-to-child transmission. Writing several years after "Todii" was released on *Tuku Music* in 1997, Chisango did not adequately contextualize the song as having been composed in an era before mother-to-child prevention campaigns were scaled up in Zimbabwe, beginning in the late 1990s. Even if Chisango had revised his criticisms in order to account for decreasing mother-to-child transmission rates, however, his objection to "Todii," was not simply that the song fails to deliver accurate information about HIV, but that it reproduces a structure of feeling prejudicial to people living with HIV/AIDS. In Chisango's comments, it becomes evident that emotion itself has become politicized in the context of the HIV/AIDS epidemic in Zimbabwe, giving the private and domestic lives portrayed in Mtukudzi's songs highly political and contested resonances in the public sphere.

Perhaps because of the integration of English, Shona, and Ndebele lyrics in its chorus, "Todii" has appealed to a wide audience both in southern African and further abroad, making it one of Mtukudzi's most successful songs internationally. As Deborah Korfmacher has observed, "'Todii' is the most popular song in other African countries in which Tuku [i.e., Mtukudzi] regularly performs, including South Africa, Tanzania, Zambia, and Botswana" (Korfmacher 2001, 37). Mtukudzi's manager, Debbie Metcalfe, has likewise suggested that "Todii" was instrumental in Mtukudzi's rise to international prominence in the late 1990s.[7] Despite the song's success abroad, however, Mtukudzi told me that "Todii" remains much less popular with audiences in Zimbabwe, speculating that this may be due to the stigma still surrounding the disease:

> I am afraid that probably the song didn't serve its purpose...it was never that popular here in Zimbabwe, I don't even understand it. And yet the whole world feels it's a beautiful song. I think probably Zimbabweans understood the song, and probably at that time with the AIDS issue, it was so scary to talk about it, and yet that was why I wrote the song, so that people can talk about these AIDS issues more freely. (Mtukudzi Interview, Jul. 23, 2006)

Mtukudzi intends for his songs to break through the silence surrounding HIV/AIDS in Zimbabwe. Despite attempts to use his position as an artist to address important issues such as gender and personal agency within the context of the epidemic, however, Mtukudzi's songs about AIDS have been accepted only gradually by audiences struggling with stigma and fear.

"NDAKUYAMBIRA"—MUSIC AND BEHAVIOR CHANGE IN HIV PREVENTION WORK

Much like "Todii," "Ndakuyambira" ("I have warned you") met with little enthusiasm after it was first composed in 1988. In an interview with Deborah Korfmacher, Mtukudzi ascribed its lack of popularity to the fact that when he initially began to perform the song, "'people were so arrogant about AIDS. They didn't want to hear it'" (Korfmacher 2001, 36). As Korfmacher observes, however, the song took on a new relevance nine years later, when it "was re-recorded in 1997 on the album *Chinhambwe*, at a time when there was hardly any family left that was not in some way affected by HIV/AIDS. The song became a hit because the issue had become a reality for people" (ibid.). "Ndakuyambira" provides a compelling example of the complex metaphorical imagery Mtukudzi employs to encourage discussion about HIV/AIDS, and to emphasize to his audiences that the disease must be openly acknowledged. It also represents Mtukudzi's most explicit call for behavior change, raising the question of how songs about AIDS contribute to HIV prevention work in Zimbabwe.

NDAKUYAMBIRA	I HAVE WARNED YOU
Hiyo hiyo hiyo hiyo hiyo	Hiyo hiyo hiyo hiyo hiyo
A hiyo huwowo huwowo huwowo wowowo	A hiyo huwowo huwowo huwowo wowowo
Hiyo hiyo hiyo baba ndoenda	Hiyo hiyo hiyo, father I am going
A hiyo huwowo huwowo	A hiyo huwowo huwowo
Hiyo hiyo hiyo baba ndoenda	Hiyo hiyo wowo, father I am going
Shoko rakafamba	The message has traveled
Ndokufamba rikafamba	It has traveled around and around
Ruzivo rwapararira nyika wani	Knowledge has circulated throughout the country
Njere dzapararira ona iwe	Intelligence has circulated throughout, look here
Mave kuziva seri kwesadza kune usavi	You have come to know that relish follows *sadza*[8]
Seri kwemusuva kune usavi mudhara	After each bite of *sadza* there is relish, old man
Ukabata vhunze remoto unetsva	If you touch burning coals you will be burned
Iko kutambira murufuse unetsva	There, playing in the embers, you will be burned
Chorus: Ndakuyambira ndakuyambira ini	*I have warned you, I have warned you*
A hiyo huwowo huwowo huwowo	*A hiyo huwowo huwowo huwowo*
Ndakuyambira ini	*I have warned you*
Hiyo hiyo hiyo baba ndoenda	*Hiyo hiyo hiyo, father I am going*
Chaunonzi rega ndochiri mumaoko	What can be given up is that which is held in the hand
Chaunonzi siya ndochawakapfumbata	What can be left is that which you hold onto
Chikava muropa ndechekufa nacho	Once it is in the blood you will die with it

Chaunonzi rega ndochiri mumaoko iwe	What can be given up is that which is held in the hand
Ukangonzi siya ndokunge wakabvumbata	If you can leave it, then you were holding onto it
Chagodza mutsinga ndechekufa nacho	What has settled in the veins you will die with
Chiri muropa ndechekufa nacho	What is in the blood you will die with
Chiri mutsinga ndechekufa nacho	What is in the veins you will die with
Chorus	Chorus
Ukabata vhunze remoto unetsva	If you touch burning coals you will be burned
Iko kutambira murufuse unetsva	There, playing in the embers, you will be burned
Chorus	Chorus

In the lyrics to "Ndakuyambira," Mtukudzi begins by appealing to audiences to recognize the seriousness of the HIV epidemic, observing that news of the disease has traveled throughout the country and that AIDS can no longer remain hidden or secret. His use of the metaphorical image of eating stiff maize porridge, or *sadza*, accompanied by a side dish of relish emphasizes that AIDS has become as common and familiar as the everyday act of eating; no one can claim to be unaware of the disease. Mtukudzi also elaborates upon the well-known Shona proverb, or *tsumo*: "What can be given up is that which is held in the hand / What is in the blood you will die with." In the context of HIV/AIDS, this traditional proverb acquires a striking meaning. While the phrase "what is in the blood" was originally intended to refer to innate personal characteristics, this imagery assumes an entirely new and more literal significance with respect to a virus such as HIV, which is transmitted through blood and other bodily fluids.[9]

In "Ndakuyambira," Mtukudzi also emphasizes the need for behavior change in response to the HIV/AIDS epidemic. By cautioning listeners against playing with burning embers, Mtukudzi metaphorically reminds them to refrain from engaging in behavior that may place them at risk for contracting HIV. While it is difficult to determine exactly how Mtukudzi's musical messages about HIV/AIDS may engender behavior change among listeners, the extent to which his music has been used in prevention campaigns in Zimbabwe suggests that many institutions and individuals involved in HIV prevention work understand his songs as an important resource in the fight against the disease. Barb Ncube, who has worked for various HIV education and prevention organizations, suggested to me that Mtukudzi's songs encourage behavior change because his music "becomes people's way of living. It makes them continue to think about it, and actually I think that's the beginning of any change system. People start talking, talking a lot about it, thinking, thinking, thinking about it. Then, soon enough, they will start behaving in that direction" (Ncube Interview, Aug. 5, 2006). Public health workers also repeatedly emphasized to me that they perceived Mtukudzi's music to be especially effective in enabling them to target a wide demographic, including both rural and urban populations, and all ages of listeners. Mtukudzi's sustained involvement in HIV-prevention campaigns indicates that the public health sector perceives his music to be an integral component of creating effective initiatives capable of reaching a wide and diverse audience.

Mtukudzi's music, voice, and image have been used in prevention campaigns by a broad spectrum of organizations, including Zimbabwe's major counseling and testing service provider, Population Services International (PSI), the Southern Africa AIDS Information Dissemination Service (SAfAIDS), the International Organization for Migration (IOM), and various branches of the United Nations, such as UNICEF and UNAIDS. As part of large-scale public health campaigns, Mtukudzi's music is one among many resources mobilized in the fight against HIV. In this context, the metaphorical language he employs to sing about the disease plays off of numerous approaches to HIV/AIDS, including more direct messages about safe sex, voluntary counseling and testing, and various other aspects of prevention and treatment. As different types of messages and media interact in HIV prevention campaigns, each acquires multiple layers of significance, complicating their interpretation. Mtukudzi's songs are deeply imbricated in this process, and their meaning has come to be determined both by the sonic and textual qualities inherent to them, and by their inclusion in various HIV prevention initiatives.

Despite the serious nature of Mtukudzi's messages, many of his songs about AIDS are intentionally written to encourage listeners to dance. In the texture of "Ndakuyambira," for example, percussion plays a prominent role, filling the space between interlocking lines played on guitars, bass, and synthesizer. Lines of sung text are interspersed with passages of syncopated vocables, further adding to the song's rhythmic interest. While these musical choices may seem incongruous with the somber content of the song's lyrics, they illustrate Mtukudzi's belief that music plays an important role in easing the emotional burden of those affected by illness and death. As Mtukudzi told me:

> Even right there at a funeral, those *sahwiras* [ritual best friends], they come singing, and acting happy. Because they're trying to neutralize the tension which is there, and the pain which is there. They want to lighten that pain... If you are suffering, song is intended to alleviate your pain. (Mtukudzi Interview, Jul. 23, 2006)

The indigenous term *sahwira* refers to a reciprocal relationship between two families. Traditionally, a family's *sahwira* has the responsibility of aiding them upon the death of one of their members, preparing the body for burial and assisting at the funeral. In addition to this important role during burial rites, a *sahwira* also acts as a trusted counselor, who is perceived to be able to offer objective advice. In his music, Mtukudzi seeks to play the role of a *sahwira* to the nation, counseling and advising his listeners in his songs. Despite the seriousness of the lyrics to "Ndakuyambira," however, Mtukudzi's message is conveyed in a dynamic and energetic musical medium meant to appeal to listeners, to solicit their active involvement through dance, and to relieve them of the emotional tension associated with illness and death.

"MABASA"—THE POWER OF THE HUMAN VOICE

"Mabasa" ("A difficult task"), was released in 1997, almost a decade after "Ndakuyambira." In this song, Mtukudzi engages with a strikingly different musical approach to AIDS, emphasizing the expressive power of the human voice in narrating the effects of HIV/AIDS on Zimbabwean communities.

MABASA	A DIFFICULT TASK
Aiwaiwaiwa, aiwaiwaiwa	Aiwaiwaiwa, aiwaiwaiwa
Ndozviudza aniko?	Whom shall I tell
Kuti paita mabasa pano	That here there is a difficult task?

Chorus

Tumirai mhere kuvakuru kuno kwaita
  mabasa
Ndozviudza aniko?
Kwafukudzika vakuruwe

Vakuruwe
Kwaita mabasa kuno
Aiwaiwaiwa
Kwaita mabasa

Misodzi yapera hapana achachema

Zvakurwadzira mumoyo chinyararire
Chinyararire
Iko kubata maoko hakuchina chiremerera

Kwafumuka uko zvichabatsirei?

Kwafumuka
Hausi uchengeri kusara takararama
  varume
Kana kuri kungwara uko tichavigwa
  naniko?
Nani?

Achachema mumwe ndiani?
Achanyaradza mumwe ndiani?
Achabata maoko mumwe ndiani?
Iwe wafirwa, ini ndafirwa
Zvino achachema mumwe ndianiko?
Vakuruwe
Firo yavako makore ano
Kana ndiyo mhedzisiro yenyika
Achachema mumwe ndiani?
Achanyaradza mumwe ndiani?
Achabata maoko mumwe ndaini?
Nhai vakuruwe vakuruwe
Ho vakuruwe vakuruwe
Inga paita mabasa kuno

Chorus

Pwere dzotungamire
Mushandi wotungamira
Sare chembere neharahwa
Zvino acharinda mumwe ndiani?
Achabata maoko mumwe ndiani?
Achachema mumwe ndiani?

Chorus

Send a cry to the elders, here there is a
  difficult task
Whom shall I tell?
It has become something out in the
  open, oh elders
Oh, ancestors
Here there is a difficult task
Aiwaiwaiwa
Here is a difficult task

Tears have run dry, no longer shall
  anyone cry
That which pains the heart, quietly
Quietly
Even condolences no longer have any
  dignity
They have lost all meaning, what use
  are they?
They have lost their meaning
It is not through intelligence that we
  have survived,
If that is intelligence, then who will
  bury us?
Who?

Who will mourn for whom?
Who will comfort whom?
Who will give condolences to whom?
You are bereaved, I am bereaved
Now who will mourn for whom?
Oh, elders
The deaths that are there these days,
Perhaps it is the end of the world
Who will mourn for whom?
Who will comfort whom?
Who will give condolences to whom?
Look, ancestors, ancestors
Oh, elders, elders
Behold, here there is a difficult task

Chorus

The young lead the way
The worker leads the way
Leaving elderly men and women
Now who will look after whom?
Who will give condolences to whom?
Who will comfort whom?

Iwe wafirwa, ini ndafirwa	Who will give condolences to whom?
Zvino achachema mumwe ndianiko?	Now who will look after whom?
Nhai vakuruwe vakuruwe	Hey, elders, elders
Ho vakuruwe vakuruwe	Oh, elders, elders
Nhai vakuruwe vakuruwe	Hey, elders, elders
Inga paita mabasa pano	Behold, here there is a difficult task

Chorus	**Chorus**
Ha, ndozviudza aniko?	Oh, whom should I tell?
Kuti paita mabasa pano	That here there is a difficult task?
Tumirai mhere kuvakuru kuno kwaita mabasa	Send a cry to the elders, here there is a difficult task
Kwafukudzika vakuruwe	It has become a thing out in the open, elders
Kwaita mabasa kuno	A difficult task has come about here
Kwaita mabasa	Here is a difficult task

In the opening passage of "Mabasa," Mtukudzi emphasizes the qualities of the human voice by singing the interjective *aiwaiwaiwa*, which is used to express the sorrow of successive misfortunes.[10] Interjectives such as *aiwaiwaiwa* can be part of everyday speech; however, they are also markedly similar to mourners' cries for the deceased during funerary rites. This type of verbal utterance thus functions as a metonym for the act of mourning. It proves especially powerful in the texts of songs like "Mabasa," giving music the potential to evoke a strong emotional response among listeners.

The next lines of text, "Whom shall I tell / That here there is a difficult task?" play on the double meaning of the word *mabasa*, which literally means difficult or onerous work, but also refers metaphorically to funerals.[11] In employing this figurative expression, Mtukudzi's lyrics embody the struggle to speak openly about something as difficult and painful as death, especially in instances where AIDS may be involved. The theme of speaking out is carried over into the song's next lines, as Mtukudzi's female backing vocalists sing: "Send a cry unto the elders that here there is a difficult task." In this context, the word *vakuru*, or elders, could alternately be interpreted as ancestral spirits, intimating that the severity of the AIDS epidemic may surpass human capabilities and require assistance from the spiritual realm.[12] The lyrics to "Mabasa," like those of "Ndakuyambira," insist that AIDS can no longer remain hidden, using the word *kwafukudzika* to suggest that AIDS "has been uncovered" in Zimbabwean communities. One listener, Esau Mavindidze, specifically interpreted this line to mean that AIDS "is something that is now just happening, there is no longer any hiding. It's now in the open" (Mavindidze Interview, Oct. 25, 2005). As the backup vocalists sing these lines, Mtukudzi responds by reiterating the phrases "whom shall I tell?" "oh, elders," and "*aiwaiwaiwa*." The opening passage of "Mabasa" thus builds in quick succession upon multiple references to the voiced utterance, insisting on the power of the human voice to ask, inform, cry, sing, and talk about AIDS.

Throughout this passage, Mtukudzi reinforces his message through the style of his vocal delivery. "Mabasa" demonstrates a strikingly different musical approach to the theme of AIDS than "Ndakuyambira," and is performed at a much slower and more contemplative tempo. Here, the voices of Mtukudzi and his backup vocalists are foregrounded within the mix against a relatively sparse and open instrumental texture. The rough, almost raspy timbre of Mtukudzi's voice, and his fluid phrasing of the vowel sounds of interjectives like *aiwaiwaiwa*, draw the listener's attention to the expressive qualities of the human voice in the context of illness and death. Mtukudzi's normally confident voice seems even to quiver or waver at points, as he sings the emotionally charged lines of the song. Both in Mtukudzi's vocal delivery, and in the song's insistent references to vocalization and vocality, "Mabasa" emphasizes the importance of human expression in response to the HIV/AIDS epidemic.

"AKOROMOKA AWA"—THE POLITICS OF NAMING AND DISCLOSURE

Silindiwe Sibanda notes that in "Mabasa," as in "Todii," Mtukudzi sings in the first person, thereby avoiding "the danger of sounding 'preachy' and untouched by the HIV/AIDS epidemic…he includes himself not only among the bereaved, but also among those trying to find a solution to the problem" (Sibanda 2004, 53–54). In addition to singing in the first person, Mtukudzi has also composed one song which directly relates how he and his family have been personally effected by the epidemic. During the 1990s, as the rate of HIV infection rose dramatically in Zimbabwe, Mtukudzi lost seven band members to AIDS within the space of two months. Among them was his younger brother, Rob Mtukudzi. "Akoromoka Awa," written in response to these deaths, was released in 2000 on the album *Bvuma-Tolerance*. Mtukudzi's mother was especially affected by these deaths, having lost not only her own son, but also Mtukudzi's other band members, whom she loved as her own children, according to Mtukudzi. He describes "Akoromoka Awa" as a song intended to encourage his mother to move beyond the despondency and grief she felt after this loss. In openly naming band members who died of HIV-related illnesses, it is a striking example of Mtukudzi's emphasis upon the importance of openness and disclosure.

AKOROMOKA AWA	*SHE HAS FALLEN*
Mhemhe atakwira mukaranga	A cry, this woman has breathed her last breath
Akoromoka awa atakwira mukaranga	She has fallen, this woman has breathed her last
Mhemhe atakwira mukaranga	A cry, this woman has breathed her last breath
Akoromoka awa atakwira mukaranga	She has fallen, this woman has breathed her last
Samere Mutohwa	Samuel Mutohwa
Job Muteswa	Job Muteswa
Rob Mtukudzi	Rob Mtukudzi
Inga ndiNicholas	Behold, it is Nicholas[13]
Vanga ramatipa rorwadza	The wound you have inflicted on us is painful
Misodzi mbokoto	A continuous flow of tears
Aiwa ka rwendo rwacho mazoro	No, this journey is one taken in turns
Zvasarire isu vapenyu	It is left unto us, the living
Isu vapenyu	We, the living

Kufuka nekuwarira	To do all that is left
Tozadza mikombe	We will fulfill our commitments
Zvichida tichazosangana	And if it is willed, we shall meet again
Mhemhe atakwira mukaranga	A cry, this woman has breathed her last
Akoromoka awa atakwira mukaranga	She has fallen, this woman has breathed her last
Mhemhe atakwira mukaranga	A cry, this woman has breathed her last breath
Akoromoka awa atakwira mukaranga	She has fallen, this woman has breathed her last

Mtukudzi is widely appreciated as a master of the Shona language, and the lyrics to "Akoromoka Awa" are highly poetic, representing a linguistic register often referred to as "deep Shona," or *Shona yakadzama*. The complexity of Mtukudzi's lyrics is reinforced by his use of words specific to the Korekore dialect of Shona, spoken in the northern regions of the country where his family originates. While my informants understood "Akoromoka Awa" to be about the AIDS-related deaths of Mtukudzi's brother and other band members, none of them could understand the lyrics to the first verse of the song. In an interview with Mtukudzi, I asked him to clarify the meaning of this verse. As he explained, "*Kutakwira*, that's the last breath when you die. So my mom, when she was broken-hearted, it was like her last breath. But I'm saying now, that's your last breath, but you're alive! You have passed that, that last breath of death, you have already passed that. You have just fallen down. But you can wake up and go again" (Mtukudzi Interview, Jul. 23, 2006). While his audience may not pick up every nuance of the complex and poetic language he uses in songs like "Akoromoka Awa," by singing in deep Shona, Mtukudzi challenges listeners to engage with his music as they seek to decipher his messages. Additionally, the use of deep Shona emphasizes the importance of language itself, calling attention to the lyrics of Mtukudzi's songs, which he considers to be the very foundation of his music.

"Akoromoka Awa" is a deeply personal song, and a moving narrative of the grief and loss Mtukudzi's family experienced as a result of HIV/AIDS. When I asked whether it had been difficult to disclose his brother's AIDS-related death, Mtukudzi replied that during the final days of his illness, Rob had come to accept his HIV-positive status, and encouraged Mtukudzi to speak out on his behalf. Mtukudzi felt that using his own family's story in "Akoromoka Awa" was particularly important, commenting, "I'm not immune. I can also be affected. You see, I wanted people to see that even in our family, as a popular family, that doesn't make us any superior from them. We're just like them. What's affecting them is also affecting us. What's infecting them also can infect us" (Mtukudzi Interview, Jul. 16, 2008).

"Akoromoka Awa" raises an apparent contradiction in Mtukudzi's music, for while he openly identifies his brother and other band members who passed away from AIDS, never in any of his songs does Mtukudzi name the disease itself. This silence is absolute, extending even to indigenous terms for AIDS that feature prominently in other popular songs, such as *mukondombera*, a term that originally meant epidemic or plague. The closest Mtukudzi has come to identifying AIDS is through his use of the word *utachiwana*, a generic term for germ or virus, in the lyrics to "Todii."[14] However, my observation of HIV prevention campaigns in Zimbabwe has suggested that *utachiwana* is rarely used alone to refer to AIDS. Instead, it is regularly modified to *utachiwana hweHIV/AIDS*, or "the HIV/AIDS virus." Mtukudzi's use of the word *utachiwana* thus seems at best an oblique reference to AIDS. Given his strong desire to facilitate discussion and openness about AIDS, why would Mtukudzi choose never to explicitly name the disease in his songs, either in English or in Shona?

In his work on AIDS and music in Uganda, Gregory Barz has illustrated many different local names used to refer to AIDS in song, and suggested that this "languaging" of AIDS can contribute to reducing the stigmatization often associated with the disease. For Barz, the use of such local terminology is one step toward breaking through the "linguistic effort by other communities to assign the virus and disease a nameless, unlabeled status" (Barz 2006a, 111). From this perspective, Mtukudzi's songs, which leave AIDS unnamed, might appear to be retrogressive or even irresponsible, contributing to stigmatization rather than fighting against it. However, I suggest that Mtukudzi's decision not to name AIDS is deliberate and carefully considered. In an environment saturated with public service messages about HIV prevention, testing, and treatment, Mtukudzi's music constitutes an alternative local approach to talking about AIDS.

Mtukudzi's decision not to name AIDS explicitly is part of a conscious strategy to move away from the direct language of public health initiatives designed to combat HIV/AIDS through the dissemination of facts drawn from biomedical models of disease, and toward a more characteristically figurative Shona idiom. His own remarks demonstrate that the absence of a name for AIDS in his songs is a carefully considered choice. His words on the subject are worth quoting at length:

> I feel like, if you were to say HIV and AIDS, it's like you have been sent either by the government or an NGO or someone, saying "Go and talk about AIDS." I want us to discuss our topic in a way that we are talking together, it is a problem we both share... because a person is very sensitive. You can give him good information, but he may fail to accept it. He can refuse it because of the way in which you have spoken... Then it doesn't help at all. (Mtukudzi Interview, Jul. 23, 2006)

Mtukudzi's decision not to name AIDS privileges the figurative above direct language, as is evident in the texts of "Ndakuyambira" and "Mabasa." As Silindiwe Sibanda has observed, by not mentioning AIDS explicitly in his songs, Mtukudzi "is behaving in his song the way people in the community behave, and deliberately uses this mirror behavior to make the point more strongly" (Sibanda 2004, 53). This approach increases his music's appeal to a wide audience, for whom the figurative language used by Mtukudzi is not only accessible and familiar, but also represents a powerful way to bring focus and clarity to a situation of extreme difficulty and distress.

Mtukudzi's involvement in the complex politics of naming and disclosure, however, has likewise been contested. The indirect language he employs has been critiqued by some HIV prevention workers, for whom Mtukudzi's approach to singing about AIDS does not go far enough in terms of combating the epidemic, despite its appeal for listeners. While recognizing Mtukudzi's music to be an important resource in HIV prevention work, for example, Barb Ncube also identifies what she perceives to be limitations on Mtukudzi's ability to enact behavior change, citing the relatively small number of songs he has composed about HIV/AIDS, as well as the indirect language he employs in singing about the disease, as factors that potentially diminish the effectiveness of his messages for listeners. In a conversation about the lyrics of another of Mtukudzi's songs about AIDS, "Handiro Dambudziko," Ncube suggested, "perhaps that's why they're comfortable with his music, because he sings in a way that they relate to and they don't have to be shy about. So, it gets there, but maybe not entirely there. We sing along, it makes it interesting, *'Ongorora, chaita kuti musoro uteme chii?* (Look carefully, what is the cause of your headache?)' You know? Hint, hint, get a test. But we can't go on with hint, hint songs for ever. We need to face it now" (Ncube Interview, Aug. 5, 2006). While it may be tempting to idealize the power of music in the lives of people affected by HIV/AIDS, Ncube's ambivalence about Mtukudzi's songs serves as an important reminder both of the margins of musical efficacy and of the complexity of the relationships between music, culture, and disease.

CONCLUSION

In his work on musical responses to HIV/AIDS in Uganda, Gregory Barz has suggested two ways in which music can be understood as a medical intervention: first, when it encourages medical analysis; and second, when it "takes the form of medical treatment itself" (2006a, 59). While Mtukudzi's songs do not perform a specific pedagogical function by teaching listeners how to use a condom or disseminating biomedical information about the disease, they have significantly contributed to how AIDS is understood in Zimbabwe. Mtukudzi's multifaceted approach challenges listeners to consider the relationship between gender, agency, and HIV/AIDS within a larger social context. Through various musical and textual strategies, Mtukudzi advocates for open discussion and disclosure about HIV/AIDS. Metaphor and other forms of figurative language feature prominently in his approach, heightening the appeal of Mtukudzi's music for audiences familiar with the shared cultural materials upon which he has drawn. His rhetorical strategy, highly reliant on the use of questions and of "deep Shona," serves to engage listeners in a musical dialogue, asking them to think critically about their own decisions and choices in the context of the AIDS epidemic. Through listening practices such as singing, dancing, and commenting upon his songs, audiences likewise contribute to this musical dialogue, shaping its meaning. Mtukudzi's music has thus become an important part of the national discourse of AIDS in Zimbabwe, contributing to local understandings of and responses to the disease. His songs reflect the increasingly important role that music has come to play in the public culture of AIDS in Africa. As Mtukudzi observes, "Song is always in between us and our passion, between us and our suffering and pain. The song is always between us" (Mtukudzi Interview, Jul. 23, 2006).

21

Swahili AIDS Plays

A CHALLENGE TO THE ARISTOTELIAN
THEORY ON TRAGEDY

Aldin K. Mutembei (University of Dar Es Salaam)

INTRODUCTION

HIV and AIDS have penetrated the Kiswahili literary works more than any other socio-medical crisis. If we look into the four major diseases that affect most African societies today (malaria, tuberculosis, cholera, and AIDS), we see that the literary cast on AIDS surpasses the rest by far. This situation notwithstanding, it took about ten years from the onset of HIV in Tanzania for Swahili writers to start giving AIDS its due weight in the literary world. Appearing first in poetry, today AIDS has infiltrated Swahili novels and plays to the extent of becoming a genre on its own right.

In this chapter, I address the emergence of the AIDS theme in Swahili plays. Following Ebrahim Hussein's approach to writing a Swahili play (1983), I argue that, aside from some modifications and additions, the basic framework of Swahili plays on stage has remained that of the ancient Greek philosopher Aristotle. Following this argument, I begin by contextualizing AIDS as a theme in Swahili literature. After providing brief histories of Swahili plays and HIV/AIDS in Tanzania, I examine the role of Tanzanian artists in the government's campaign to address the calamity. I will introduce two Swahili AIDS-themed plays, *Ushuhuda wa Mifupa* (*The Skeleton's Testimony*; H. Njozi 1990) and *Kilio Chetu*[1] (*Our Lament*; MAF 1996), and analyze them using an Aristotelian framework. This framework, I argue, presents several challenges for the portrayal of AIDS within Swahili drama. In the conclusion, besides pointing out similarities between the themes of the mid-1970s and the current theme of AIDS in Swahili literature, I raise questions that will require further research in our understanding of the social ramifications of AIDS.

AIDS AS A THEME IN SWAHILI LITERATURE

Oral literature in the form of songs found its way very early on into the literature on AIDS in Tanzania (Mutembei 2001). Back in 1981–82 in the then West Lake Region (now Kagera), people were singing about a paradox later to be known as AIDS. At that time, sorcery was the scapegoat because the first victims were thought to have been bewitched by evil people who envied their success in business across the Ugandan border (Lwihula et al. 1993). The literature reflecting this misunderstanding of the disease, and the general response of people to the disease's ravages, remained primarily in oral tradition for a long time. The first printed literary works on AIDS can thus be traced mainly to several daily Swahili-language newspapers and monthly bulletins. These include poems in the *Uhuru* and *Mzalendo* Swahili newspapers starting in 1982 (see Mutembei 2009), and poems and short stories printed in *Ijawebonere* and *Rumuli*, local monthly bulletins that published in both the Ruhaya and Swahili languages.

From the early 1980s to around 1990 (with exception of one short story), poetry in the form of songs and verses was the only genre whose creators had the courage to discuss the scourge in a literary form. It took some time for writers of plays, short stories, and novels to see beyond the miserable side of AIDS and instead employ their genres to make important contributions to the awareness and prevention of AIDS.

Merinyo's *Kifo cha AIDS* (*Death from AIDS*, 1988) is probably the earliest printed Swahili short story on AIDS. In this story, which also gives its name to the collection in which it appears, the writer offers an optimistic artistic narrative on death from AIDS. With the exception of this story, there was no written literary work on AIDS in Tanzania. It was as if writers and the general society were still not convinced that AIDS was a reality. HIV continued to spread, however, and the number of deaths from AIDS skyrocketed, triggering the writers' consciousnesses. Likewise, the government was slowly accepting the reality of AIDS and saw the need for a nationwide campaign against the disease.

It was during this early period in 1989 that BASATA—the Tanzanian National Arts Council—launched a campaign in conjunction with the government's move to address HIV/AIDS. The nationwide campaign saw theatrical groups staging plays with AIDS-related themes, based on information from the National AIDS Control Programme (NACP), Ministry of Health, and local medical institutions. Playwrights also contributed to a competition organized by the Arts Council to find the best Swahili play on AIDS. The fact that the Aristotelian-framed play *Ushuhuda wa Mifupa* came out as the winner adds further emphasis to my argument about the structures of Swahili plays, which I will now briefly discuss.

A BRIEF HISTORY OF SWAHILI PLAYS

Several scholars of Swahili literature agree that the contemporary Swahili drama is deeply influenced by Aristotelian dramatic conventions. The renowned playwright Ebrahim Hussein has identified a variety of Swahili plays that have followed an Aristotelian framework (1983). Aristotle's drama framework was introduced in East Africa through English plays during the colonial era.[2] Penina Mlama, herself a famous playwright, argues similarly:

> Drama is a theatrical performance that originated in Europe...[I]t came to
> Tanzania through the British...[A]fter the translation of Shakespeare's plays

into Swahili, there followed plays written in Swahili that brought a great change into the content of the play. (Mlama 1983, 206–215)

This change in Swahili plays of the time can also be seen in the tone of Ebrahim Hussein when he argued: "To write a play following Aristotle's arrangement is one of the crucial methods of writing a play, but not the only one" (1983, 204). Hussein, who had never been fond of rules in the creation of art, urged writers to write their plays following their creative imagination rather than adhering to popular conventions. In the same spirit, Mlama (1983) argued that although Swahili playwrights often followed an Aristotelian structure, they nonetheless attempted to modify the form in order to bring out their own voices.

Mulokozi, another admired Swahili literary scholar, put it vividly when he wrote: "[The] Aristotelian play is one type of these plays, [but] here we discuss it in detail because it has influenced so many writers of Swahili plays" (1996, 193). This influence on Swahili plays is not only in Tanzania. Writing the history of Swahili plays and criticism, Wamitila (2002) also pointed out that Aristotle's *Poetics* has had significant influence in the Swahili plays of both Kenya and Tanzania. Mulokozi explained the form's characteristics in the following way: "Swahili-written plays in particular have copied some of the Western ways of writing a play. Most of these reflect Aristotle's structure by using dialogue, actions, scenes and conflict that is resolved at the end" (1996, 197).

Following the above conventions, Swahili plays entered the world of literature in 1950s. Kiango (1973) states that the first to be written were in Kenya by Graham Hyslop. These included *Afadhali Mchawi* (*Better a Witch*, 1957) and *Mgeni Karibu* (*Visitor You're Welcome*, 1957). Other playwrights such as Kuria (*Nakupenda Lakini* [*I Love You, But . . .*], 1957) and G. Ngugi (*Nimelogwa nisiwe na Mpenzi*, [*I am Condemned to Have No Lover*], 1961) followed suit. After the independence of Tanganyika (1961) and Kenya (1963), most Swahili playwrights either wrote in Kiswahili or had their plays translated into the Swahili language. Such works included *Wakati Ukuta* (*Time [Is a] Wall*) (Hussein 1969), *Kinjektile* (Hussein 1969); *Hatia* (*Guilty*) (Muhando 1972); *Aliyeonja Pepo* (*The Taste of Heaven*) (Topan 1973); *Tambueni haki zetu* (*Recognize Our Rights*) (Muhando 1973); *Mwanzo wa Tufani* (*The Beginning of a Storm*) (Kahigi and Ngemera 1976); *Mkwava wa Uhehe* (*Mkwawa of Heheland*) (Mulokozi 1979); and *Tendehogo* (Semzaba 1980) to mention but a few.

As stated previously, several Swahili playwrights later looked into modifying the Aristotelian structures. This attempt in the late 1960s and early 1970s started with free-verse poems and spread to plays in the mid 1980s. Known among Swahili critics (Kezilahabi 2005, Senkoro 2006) as the "experimentation phase" in Swahili literature, this period also involved the inclusion of traditional cultural elements that had once been confined to oral literature. As HIV/AIDS clobbered the country in early 1980s, these writers were forced to join the rest of the society in bafflement with what was happening in Tanzania.

A BRIEF HISTORY OF HIV/AIDS IN TANZANIA

Tanzania is administratively divided into twenty-six regions. According to the 2002 Population and Housing Census, the country had a population of 34,443,603, the majority of which resided in rural areas. In 1983 it was officially announced that HIV/AIDS had reached Tanzania through the northwest quarter of Kagera Region. This event officially marked the beginning of the AIDS calamity in Tanzania. In less than seven years, AIDS cases had been reported in all twenty-one regions of the mainland.

The Tanzanian government's HIV/AIDS webpage notes that "[e]arly in the epidemic, urban populations and communities located along highways were the most affected. According to the

National AIDS Control Programme (NACP)'s HIV/AIDS/STD Surveillance Report No.11 (1996), however, the epidemic rapidly spread to rural communities, and in 1997 more than 10 percent of women attending antenatal clinics in some rural areas had been found to be HIV infected. The cumulative number AIDS cases as reported from surveillance reports collected by the NACP in Tanzania mainland rose from 25,503 at the end of 1990 to 88,667 in 1996" (www.tanzania. go.tz/hiv_aids.html). The page notes further that "over 80 percent of the reported AIDS cases occurred in young people aged 20–44. However, simulation models estimated that only one out of five AIDS cases is reported. NACP, therefore, estimated that in total about 44,250 cases occurred in 1999 and 600,000 cumulative AIDS cases had occurred from 1983 to 1999" (ibid.).

Several research projects have since studied the HIV trends in Tanzania, with the Kagera AIDS Research Project (KARP, started 1986) the pioneer in this region. The HIV indicator survey of 2003–2004 suggested that the HIV prevalence was 7 percent among adults aged 15–49, with the highest infection levels occurring in urban areas. It was also estimated that there were two million people living with HIV/AIDS in the country, with a similar number of AIDS orphans (UNGASS Tanzania 2005). A World Bank report in 2001, meanwhile, estimated that AIDS was "eroding the expected longevity of productive life from the peak of 52 years in 1988 to 48 years currently" (World Bank 2001, 12–21).

The above situation notwithstanding, a significant recent decline has been reported in both prevalence and incidence of HIV in some regions in Tanzania due to interventions undertaken by the government, various national and international organizations, and research institutions in the country. Multisectorial strategies against the spread of HIV, meanwhile, have also been effective. These strategies included the introduction of a section in every ministry that deals with AIDS in the workplace, and the intensification of campaigns against AIDS in all educational institutions, including primary and secondary school. In schools, AIDS clubs started to mitigate the impact of stigma. In local governments, initiatives included addressing traditions that put women and girls at greater risk. The decline in HIV infections could well be attributed to these widespread changes in sociocultural behavior, though a definitive reason has not yet been determined (Lugalla et al. 2004).

This background of HIV/AIDS in the country of Tanzania has influenced and affected artistic works both written and oral. Written Swahili plays are one such genre of artistic work that discuss the situation of HIV/AIDS in the country, a subject to which I now turn.

SUMMARY OF THE PLAYS

1. *Ushuhuda wa Mifupa (The Skeleton's Testimony)*

This Swahili play was written by Ibrahim Ngozi and published by the Tanzania Arts Council in 1990. The play is constructed as one long scene involving several incidents. It opens with lamentations and crying presented by skeleton characters. The skeletons eventually begin a dialogue that builds up the plot and leads to an interlude presented by a narrator. The characters change into human beings (with no names), and then into real people (with names), as the dialogue continues. The narrator, appearing between episodes, helps connect and comment on the action. As the play develops, the narrator encourages the audience to participate.

Ushuhuda wa Mifupa explains the meaning of HIV, provides theories about its origin, and discusses the way it spreads—both myth and reality—before finally introducing its consequences. The play dramatizes the blame and counter-blame surrounding HIV, offers several cultural reasons for its dissemination, and portrays the economic power and gender relationships that influence its transmission. It examines the risk factors involved, as well as the role of

259

both Western doctors and traditional healers in the fight against AIDS. The play also functions as a historical work that documents the response of the Tanzanian people toward the disease, the stigma that developed toward the infected, and the preventive efforts undertaken to control its spread.

2.   *Kilio Chetu (Our Lament)*

This Swahili play, published by the Tanzania Publishing House in 1996, emerged from my actual field experience in Kagera,[3] and consists of one act organized into six scenes. The first scene introduces the plot to the reader. The play's action starts in the second scene with dialogue between two characters—parents discussing the death of their neighbor's child supposedly due to AIDS. The dialogue develops further to include other parents' comments concerning the behavior of their children. The third and fourth scenes comprise dialogues between children as a kind of "answer" to their parents' laments in the previous scene. The children discuss their plight, complain, and lament in their own way to show the consequences of living a risk-filled life. Scenes five and six offer conclusions in which both parents and children are engaged in dialogue while witnessing the tragic deaths of their loved ones.

Kilio Chetu is a play that voices young people's concerns about not being adequately informed about risk factors facing their lives. It is about communicating AIDS-related issues to youths who are the most vulnerable. The play challenges the silence of parents, the governments, and schools on reproductive health education and sexuality. Young people, meanwhile, lament the cultural impediments they face, as well as the conservative nature of their parents in the face of an AIDS tragedy that threatens to wipe out the young generation.

Both of these plays have been used in secondary schools in Tanzania (grades 9 through 12) as part of the mandatory Swahili literature course. *Ushuhuda wa Mifupa* was in the Swahili syllabus up until 2003–2004. The new syllabus has replaced it with *Kilio Chetu*. Both, in my opinion, operate within the Aristotelian dramatic model. They discuss a serious issue that concerns contemporary society using an artistic language. Can they be seen as staging neo-Aristotelian tragedy? To begin addressing this question, I will examine each play's Aristotelian elements and describe challenges that each poses in contemporary Swahili literature.

EXAMINING THE SWAHILI PLAYS WITHIN ARISTOTLE'S MODEL

Tragedy

The first question that we need to look into is whether or not these plays should be seen as tragedies. Once we ascertain this, we will proceed to examine principles upon which a tragedy acquires its quality. Aristotle defines tragedy as "an imitation of an action that is serious, complete and of a certain magnitude" (Aristotle 2004, http://www.kessinger.net). In a tragedy, emotional incidents arouse fear and pity together, leading to a release achieved by revealing the underlying causes of a problem. This emotional release is what Aristotle called *katharsis*.

These two Swahili plays are both tragedies. They each investigate a lethal syndrome that has turned the world into one of confusion, fear, and pity. They obviously imitate a tragic disorder that shakes both the social and economic fabric of most developing societies. Each of these plays also incorporates the six principles Aristotle considered essential to tragedy, which I now turn to examine.

The first principle, the plot, involves the presentation of a cause-and-effect chain of incidents. Both *Ushuhuda wa Mifupa* and *Kilio Chetu* start their plots moving with a lamentation. In *Ushuhuda wa Mifupa* the lamentation starts slowly, with one character giving way to the second in a dialogue that begins to involve two additional characters. The plot in *Ushuhuda wa Mifupa* outlines a complete story that explains the time before the advent of AIDS, moves to the start of the AIDS crisis (the disbelief and confusion in the beginning), and ends with the current situation (the endless search for a cure). The plot is complete, having a unity of action in which the narrator, Mtambaji, serves to bring together its different parts.

Unlike *Ushuhuda wa Mifupa, Kilio Chetu*'s lament is in the form of a song performed by the narrator, who presents the play's story. Indeed, scene one in *Kilio Chetu* introduces the major conflict that all the following scenes attempt to address, thus creating the unified form. This conflict involves the lack of sexual and reproductive health education among younger populations in most African societies. Set in the form of a flashback, *Kilio Chetu* develops toward a climax with that big issue reverberating through all the incidents that follow in the plot.

The middle section of the plot in both *Ushuhuda wa Mifupa* and *Kilio Chetu*—or "the climax"—should be understood as the series of events that reveal how HIV is spread. It is from the climax that we see the consequences of the characters' actions, that is, the effects of HIV infection. In both plays, these incidents are framed within realistic sociocultural backgrounds, mirroring the conditions for the spread of HIV among youths in Tanzania. What is interesting to note is that, whereas most typical Aristotelian plays have a single climax, the AIDS plays do not. The mode through which HIV spreads from one individual to another necessitates the appearance of multiple climaxes in a single plot.

Likewise, the end of the plot (the "resolution") in both plays is caused by the preceding events. That is, in *Ushuhuda wa Mifupa* the lament of the character Mtani and the explanations given by Mtambaji, the narrator, explain the events that follow from the climax. However, unlike typical Aristotelian plays, these AIDS plays do not have typical resolutions. The ending in AIDS plays does not solve or resolve the problem presented at the beginning (McManus 1999, 2). In these plays therefore, although we see the *desis* (tying) we do not actually see the *lusis* (untying)[4] as suggested by Aristotle. AIDS has caused this deviation.

If these two plays are our standard of analysis, then it is safe to say that AIDS plays by their very nature have complex plots. They not only have catastrophe, but also a "reversal of intention" called *peripeteia* and a "recognition" called *anagnorisis* connected with the catastrophe. Aristotle explains that *peripeteia* "occurs when a character produces an effect opposite to that which he intended to produce" (McManus 1999, 2). Indeed, when the sweet prospect of having a sexual encounter changes to bitterness upon realization that that encounter has resulted in infection, we find a *peripeteical* moment of the play. This sudden shift certainly seems to echo a real-world emotional progression accompanying the revelation that one is HIV-positive.

On the other hand, Aristotle defines *anagnorisis* as "a change from ignorance to knowledge, producing love or hate between the persons destined for good or bad fortune" (ibid.). Some HIV-positive individuals might never know from where they got the virus, but even seropositive individuals who *do* know often enter into an internal state of hatred. For example, in *Kilio Chetu*, the character Suzi reaches the *anagnorisis* moment and says (*Kilio Chetu*, 36):

Kwanini Joti…kwanini Joti afe?	Why Joti…why should Joti die?
Ukimwi?	AIDS?
Na mie Suzi nina mimba, mimba ya Joti.	And I Suzi am pregnant, Joti's pregnancy.
Kishá ina maana na mie nina Ukimwi?	Then it means I also have AIDS?
Maana huambukiza.	Because it is infectious.

As I will argue later, Suzi's recognition and lament is the voice of all teenagers who became infected due to ignorance. By the time they have this knowledge, it is often too late and thus they develop hatred, not necessarily of the people who have infected them, but sometimes of the parents and the overarching society. As Suzi puts it:

Mie kwanza sikujua mambo haya. Mama na Mjomba walijua juu ya mambo haya ya mapenzi. Mjomba alitaka kujaribu kuzuia balaa...Mama hakuwa radhi kuachana na utamaduni wa kale...Naapa kwa Mungu wangu, mimi na Joti tungepata bahati ya kuelimishwa, tusingetumbu. (36)

I for one did not know these things. My mother and uncle knew about love affairs. Uncle wanted to attempt to prevent the agony...but mother was not ready to abandon the old traditions...I pledge to my God, had Joti and I received the opportunity to be educated on this, we wouldn't fall into it.

In *Ushuhuda wa Mifupa*, the plot does not develop to the point of *anagnorisis*. The reason for this more restrained approach might be because of the period in which the play was written. In the late 1980s, less was known about spread of the disease. The biomedical arguments developed toward the climax of the play were still inconclusive in the minds of most people who were caught up in the paradox of the disease. Nobody knew for sure whether those were the answers to all the challenges of the crisis or there was something more to expect. This ambivalence is depicted through the characters in these plays, an item that I now move to discuss.

Specific character traits comprise the second principle in a tragedy: "The protagonist should be renowned and prosperous, so his change of fortune can be from good to bad. This change should come about as the result, not of vice, but of some great error or frailty in character" (McManus 1999, 13). The historical pattern of HIV infection in Tanzania emerged within a once renowned and prosperous people. Although in most cases the rich infect the poor (Makurdi 2009, Donnelly 2006, Mozes 2002), infection can still happen between and among poor communities or rich communities. In other words, HIV transmission has historically moved easily within and beyond social and economic boundaries. Nonetheless, most local writings reflect HIV infection as moving in one direction. In these Swahili plays characters mirror this trend.

Characters who spread the virus in both *Ushuhuda wa Mifupa* and *Kilio Chetu* are depicted as either rich people or people with influential social and political status. These characters are frequently blamed by the entire society; they are seen as making mistakes and causing their own downfall. Aristotle calls this *hamartia* (a character flaw). In tragedy, Aristotle says:

[T]he protagonist will mistakenly bring about his own downfall—not because he is sinful or morally weak, but because he does not know enough...the role of the *hamartia* in tragedy comes not from its moral status but from the inevitability of its consequences. (Aristotle, discussed by Barad 2008)

Indeed, lack of knowledge becomes the "biggest transmitter" of the virus. Some people are not aware of preventive measures against the spread of HIV. Most of them, even if they might be aware of these measures, do not have the necessary power to stop the spread of the infection effectively. These people, too, need knowledge to obtain or use such power to their advantage and survival. This observation brings us into the third and fourth principles of

Aristotle's plot, thought and diction. Thought has been understood by other scholars as "associated with how speeches should reveal character," while diction is a stylistic element of a plot projected through metaphor. Aristotle sees diction as "the expression of the meaning in words" (McManus 1999, 4).

In both plays, AIDS is the major theme from which all other arguments develop. Characters give speeches that not only reveal their social and economic status, but also their understanding, or lack of understanding, of both how HIV spreads and how to prevent or control its spread. The use of metaphors in AIDS literature has been examined by several scholars, including Cecil Farber (1998), Susan Sontag (2001), and Aldin Mutembei (2001). In the Swahili literature, AIDS has assumed more metaphors than any other disease. Table 21.1 shows how metaphors have been used in these two plays.

21.1 AIDS Metaphors

USHUHUDA WA MIFUPA		KILIO CHETU	
Metaphor	**Meaning**	**Metaphor**	**Meaning**
Kupukutika, page 2 *Lit. Fall-off, plummeted*	To die	Dubwana, page 1 *Lit. A giant phantom*	AIDS
Rangi mbili, page 8 *Lit. Two colors*	Antibiotic called Tetracycline	Kupukutika, page 1 *Lit. Fall-off, plummeted*	To die
Spea taya, page 8 *Lit. Spare tire*	Sexual partner	Vikawazoa, page 2 *Lit. To collect*	Killed in large number
Kuumwa na nge, page 8 *Lit. Scorpion bite*	To be infected with STD	Kizuka, page 4 *Lit. Very old person*	A person very sick of AIDS
Maduka, page 11 *Lit. Shops*	To treat one's body as a business (i.e., to engage in transactional sex)	Kakanyaga waya, page 4 *Lit. Stepping on a live electrical cable*	To be infected with HIV To be known that one has AIDS
Slimufiti, page 15 *Lit. Slim fit*	AIDS	Pekupeku, page 16 *Lit. Without wearing anything*	Having sex without using condom
Acha Iniue Dawa Sina, page 15 *Lit. Let it kill me, I have no cure*	AIDS	Kula pipi na ganda lake, page 16 *Lit. To munch a sweet in its cover*	To have sex with a condom
Acha Iniue Dogodogo Siachi, page 15. *Lit. Let it kill me, I can't spare a chick*	AIDS	Mnyonyoe manyoya, page 24 *Lit. Shave him/her*	To have sex
Kununua sanda, page 18 *Lit. To buy a shroud*	To be infected	Kala mizizi ya aina zote, page 32. *Lit. Has eaten roots of all kind*	One has used different medicines/drugs
Gharika, page 19 *Lit. Flood, torrent*	AIDS		

The use of these metaphors not only reveals the characters and their roles in the plays, but also how each character's knowledge about sexuality, AIDS, and the spread of HIV has been constructed. The authors' choices of different expressions for each character, and the meanings of each character's associated dictions, mirrors perfectly the general understanding of AIDS in Tanzanian society at that time.

The common argument that is raised in these two plays revolves around the ignorance of the time. In *Ushuhuda wa Mifupa*, the general ignorance of the epidemic and the mechanics of how the disease spreads stymied its prevention, rather than the social impediments. *Kilio Chetu*, meanwhile, takes us a step further to start examining the details of this ignorance. What we hear in *Kilio Chetu*—and indeed as the title, "our lament," itself suggests—is the active voice and the silent struggle of the young generation trying to crush the outdated pillars of tradition. Anna's song (27) and Suzi's lamentation toward the end of the play (36) are ideal representations of the dilemma of the youth. We turn now to the last two parts of the Aristotelian model suggested.

The musical element is the fifth part of a tragedy. Although Aristotle argues that songs or melody should be recited by a "chorus," most Swahili plays use songs as elements borrowed from oral African tradition. One can see a similarity between the Aristotelian chorus and the African *mtambaji* (storyteller) or *msimulizi* (narrator). Both function as more than just performers of interludes; in the play they "contribute to the unity of the plot."

In *Ushuhuda wa Mifupa*, songs are presented in the form of lamentations, and the fact that the beginning is like the ending gives the play an evocative flashback structure that fits well with its subject. The same scenario is seen in *Kilio Chetu*, where the young generation's lament starts with a song.

The sixth and last part of Aristotle's theory is spectacle. I propose not to discuss this, but instead examine an equally important element in a tragedy called *katharsis*.

A tragedy, according to Aristotle, must end with a "cleansing" (purging) or *katharsis*. Borrowing a medical metaphor, Aristotle used *katharsis* to indicate an emotional release associated with talking about the underlying causes of a problem. The strong emotions of pity and fear reach a point in a play where they need to be released, "to reduce these passions to a healthy, balanced proportion." This release gives "pleasure that is proper to tragedy, apparently meaning the aesthetic pleasure one gets from contemplating the pity and fear..." (McManus 1999, 4). This emotional release often comes upon the public revelation of the underlying problem.

I argue that when voluntary counseling and testing has taken place, affected individuals reach a moment of emotional release after being told their HIV status. It is only after reaching the *katharsis* stage, moreover, that infected individuals might acknowledge their status and start living positive lives. In essence, the innermost conscience has agreed to reconcile with the calamity at this stage. But if this stage is not reached, no matter how intensely a person is counseled, the body will just not "accept" any therapy. So, I would argue, the first therapy is indeed *katharsis*.

In *Kilio Chetu*, Baba Joti accepts the bitter reality that his son has AIDS and says, "Nimekuelewa mtani. Hatuna la kufanya zaidi isipokuwa kumwachia Mungu aamue" ("I have understood. We have nothing more to do except to leave it in the hands of God to decide") (34). This realization is a point of *katharsis*, and is experienced in different ways. For example, when Mjomba (Uncle) boldly explains what Joti is suffering from, Joti's mother wipes away her tears, a gesture that the uncle notices, and comments: "Sasa huu ni ukweli wa kwanza hatuna budi kuukubali, japo unauma" ("Now, this is the first reality that we must accept, albeit painfully") (34). Again, the moment of realization for both Joti's father and the mother that their son has AIDS not only brings an emotional release, but, I argue, marks the end of the tragedy.

I now turn to examine the challenges brought by AIDS plays to the Aristotelian theory of tragedy.

SOME CHALLENGES TO THE THEORY OF TRAGEDY

As mentioned earlier, the Aristotelian protagonist—typically a hero—"should be renowned and prosperous" (Aristotle 2004, 13). However, looking critically at the concept of a hero, we must ask ourselves what it means to be a hero-protagonist in an AIDS play. It is true that most of these main characters are prosperous and renowned. But are they really heroes? Heroes bring on their own downfall because they lack crucial knowledge that is only later revealed to them. This tendency is true up to a certain period of time in the context of AIDS. It was true in the beginning, when knowledge of AIDS was still minimal and mystifying. Given the greater knowledge today, however, one would not expect a hero-protagonist to bring his or her own downfall in the same manner. And yet this is still the case in Swahili AIDS drama. The question then becomes whether such protagonists continue to generate pity in the actual world that inspires these plays.

Aristotle says that the hero in the tragedy falls, "not because he is sinful or morally weak" (2004); yet AIDS plays present the opposite situation. In *Ushuhuda wa Mifupa* for instance, we see the medical figure Meneja Dokoa accepting bribes, treating his patients in an unethical manner, and committing adultery with his female patients. Characters such as Meneja Dokoa in *Ushuhuda wa Mifupa* are viewed by society as both morally weak and sinful. The strong influence of religious institutions in most African societies affects public opinion toward people such as Meneja Dokoa, leading them to see him as a deviant character. He consequently fails to embody the qualities of the Aristotelian protagonist in a typical sense.

In a typical tragedy, the hero falls toward the end. However, in AIDS plays, the calamity necessitates the premature death of such "hero"-protagonists for the play to reach its climax and enter the resolution stage. To be able to see the consequences of AIDS, central characters have to die in the middle of the play, including, in most plays, the protagonist. As a result, other characters such as widows, widowers, and orphans end up exemplifying the impact of the AIDS crisis toward the end of the play. This is contrary to what is expected in a typical tragedy in the Aristotelian sense, where the "hero"-protagonist dies at the end. Should these fallen protagonists still be seen as having the characteristics of a hero?

If we cannot talk of a de facto hero in AIDS plays, can we at least see these plays as creating shadow-heroes? In other words, AIDS has led to the creation of characters that arouse pity—the orphans, widows and widower who remain behind to survive the pain and anguish of the disease and its stigma—yet who also live to tell their stories. These may be HIV-positive individuals who live positive lives. Might these characters be seen as heroes in their own right?

The structure of a tragedy, as Aristotle puts it, has a beginning, a middle, and an end. These parts form one unified entity that creates satisfaction by concluding with a revelation of the play's underlying source of conflict. With AIDS plays however, the last part—the resolution—does not qualify as an ending. With AIDS, the tragic mistake, *hamartia*, cannot be resolved. The fact that there is no cure for AIDS stresses the point that the end of the tragedy cannot resolve the problem that created it in the first place.

Another challenge can be seen when one examines Gustav Freytag's triangle. In his triangle, Freytag indicates only one arrow rising from exposition to climax and another arrow falling from the climax to resolution. At the climax we find the two important elements of crisis and reversal (see figure 21.1). However, HIV infection currently does not allow for reversal. Is there a possibility of having more than one climax in such a scenario?

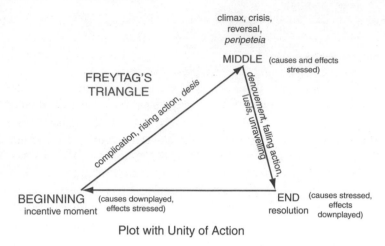

Figure 21.1 Freytag's triangle

CONCLUSION

It might be a poor analogy, but when I look back to the 1970s, I see the *Ujamaa* theme ("collective familyhood") in Swahili literature acting in the same manner that AIDS did in the 1990s. In Tanzania, both literary writers and critics jumped on the bandwagon to start romanticizing about socialism and self-reliance in African societies. Politicians at the time embraced *Ujamaa* as a populist theme. Today, AIDS has become a similarly popular theme among literary writers in Tanzania. In this case, however, there is nothing to romanticize about because AIDS is too tragic to appear glamorous. This situation notwithstanding, there are issues raised in these AIDS plays that attract the attention of any literary critic. One such issue is a rethinking of Aristotle's theory of tragedy.

Following the Aristotelian framework on drama, the Swahili AIDS plays have fashioned representations of people's actions and lives surrounding the AIDS crisis. In so doing, the creation and development of six major parts that make up a tragedy became unavoidable. Of these parts however (plot, character, thought, diction, spectacle, and song), AIDS plays pose a challenge to Aristotle's original framework, particularly regarding plot and character.

As stated earlier, "plot is the soul of a tragedy"; and as it were, what happens in a tragedy depends on the way an "imitation of an action that is complete, whole, and of a certain magnitude" is structured (Aristotle 2004, parts VI–VII). As part of a whole, the ending in AIDS plays does not necessarily make the tragedy come to an end. Suzi's cry in *Kilio Chetu* for instance, comes at the end of the play (36), but signifies the beginning of a tragedy of uncertain magnitude, including the dilemma of infection itself, the future lives of the infected infants, and the general lives of the orphans. The plot in AIDS plays thus becomes as complex as the AIDS crisis, not necessarily following the chronological order of incidents as suggested by Aristotle in constructing a plot.

In building a plot, I have shown for example, that both the reversal of the situation (*peripeteia*) and the recognition (*hamartia*)—which are the most powerful elements in a plot—are different in AIDS plays. But the *peripeteia* is particularly difficult to achieve. Once a person is infected with HIV, there is no reversal situation. Contrary to what is expected in Aristotelian plots, even the gaining of the essential knowledge that was previously lacking—*anagnorisis*—

does not help in resolving the viral crisis in an infected body. The ending, where *katharsis* is expected, is almost impossible to conceptualize in the AIDS tragedy. The dilemma and complex issues that follow the death from AIDS signal the beginning of, or rather a continuation of, tragedy. All these come from actions performed by characters in a play.

Through the two Swahili AIDS plays I have described, I have illustrated that in most cases the vulnerable individuals do not have a chance either to choose or to avoid a crisis. Girls like Suzi in *Kilio Chetu* find themselves in a situation where they are just victims of a patriarchal system. As characters, they do not tally in Aristotle's structure. I have therefore shown that Swahili AIDS plays deviate from the structure of a tragedy as advanced by Aristotle. The question then is: What governs a theory on tragedy? Is it ideal to have general characteristics of a tragedy that should be applicable to any situation? These are some of the issues that demand answers from more elaborate research. That notwithstanding, I have shown in this chapter that Swahili AIDS plays pose basic structural challenges to Aristotle's theory on tragedy.

22

Confronting AIDS Through Popular Music Cultures in Kenya

A STUDY OF PRINCESS JULLY'S "DUNIA MBAYA," JACK NYADUNDO'S "UKIMWI," AND ODUOR ODHIALO'S "NYAKOMOLLO"

Mellitus N. Wanyama and Joseph B. Okong'o

(Moi University, Kenya)

PRINCESS JULLY: "DUNIA MBAYA" ("IT'S A BAD WORLD")

Jully na t'ahero, Jully t'ahero	I truly love Jully, I truly love Jully
Jully na t'ahero chuth, Jully t'ahero	I forever love Jully, I dearly love Jully
Napenda Jully, Napenda Jully	I love Jully, I love Jully
Napenda Jully, Nam'penda sana	I love Jully, I love him dearly
Bwana yangu, Nam'penda sana	My husband, I love him dearly
Bwana yangu, Nam'penda sana	My husband, I love him dearly
Jully na t'ahero, chuth, Jully t'ahero	I truly love Jully, I truly love Jully
Ora ni, t'ahero, ora ni t'ahero	I truly love my mate, I truly love my mate
Ora ni t'ahero chuth, ora ni t'ahero	I forever love my mate, I truly love my mate

An Alice Milly, a nyar gi Naya	I am Alice Milly, daughter of Naya
An nyathi Mika, a nyar g'Okeyo	I am the child of Mika, am the daughter of the Okeyos
An nyar Oyugi, an a'nyar Ochieng	I am the daughter of Oyugi, I am the daughter of Ochieng
Jully t'hero, ora ni t'ahero	I truly love Jully, I truly love Jully
I love Jully, I love you	I love Jully, I love you
Berna manadi, to berna manadi	I am content, yes I am content
Berna manadi, to berna manadi	I am content, yes I am content
Wa dos dwara, to be gin gi pesa	The rich tried to woo me, flaunting their money
Ne' akwero jogo, ni ahero Jully	I refused, I told them, I love Jully
Ahero bet ahero, ahero bet ahero	I just love him, I just love him
Ahero bet ahero, ahero bet ahero	I just love him, I just love him
Jully na t'hero. To mbasna t'ahero	I truly love Jully, I truly love my mate
Wasungu dwara, to gin gi ndege	White men tried to woo me, with their aeroplanes
Ne' akwero jogo, 'I love Jully	But I refused, telling them "I love Jully
No Odiero, I love Jully'	No! White man, I love Jully
I love Jully, I love Jully'	I love Jully, I love Jully"
Wahindi dwara, to gin be gi pesa	Indians tried to woo me, flaunting their riches
N'gatni dwara, to en be gi mali	This man tried to woo me, and he had wealth
Ne' akwero n'gano, 'nina penda Jully	But I refused, telling him, "I love Jully
Ninapenda Jully, ninapenda Jully	I love Jully, I love Jully
Ninapenda Jully, ni bwana yangu'	I love Jully, he is my husband"
Wa dos dwara, to gin be gi moko	The wealthy seek me with their riches
Ja Rusinga dwara, to ni otera	A man from Rusinga promised to take me abroad
Ne akwero n'gano, ana hero Jully	But I refused, telling him I love Jully
Ana hero Jully, anahero Jully	I love Jully, I love Jully
To nene anyiso mama, anahero Jully	I tell you my lady, I love Jully
To nene anyiso daddy, ayudi baba	I told that sugar daddy, "I know your ways"

Anahero Jully, anahero Jully	I love Jully, I love Jully
Wewe mama, wachana sugar daddy	My lady, forget those sugar daddies
Hawa vijana, dunia mbaya	Young people, this is a bad world
Dunia mbaya, dunia mbaya	A bad world, a bad world
Ukimwi iko, kwa maisha yako	AIDS exists, its in our midst
Utakufa mbaya, ugonjwa ya ukimwi	You will die badly from this disease
Dunia mzima, dunia mbaya	The whole world is affected, the world is bad
Dunia mbaya, dunia mbaya	It's a bad world, it's a bad world
Ata Amerika, dunia mbaya	Even in America, it's a bad world
Ata Europa, dunia mbaya	Even in Europe, it's a bad world
Nairobi Kenya, dunia mbaya	Nairobi, Kenya, it's a bad world
Mombasa Kenya, dunia mbaya	Mombasa, Kenya, it's a bad world
Kisumu Kenya, dunia mbaya	Kisumu, Kenya, it's a bad world
Huko bara, dunia mbaya	In the hinterlands, it's a bad world
Ata Awendo Kenya, dunia mbaya	Even in Awendo, it's a bad world
Migori, dunia mbaya	Migori, it's a bad world
Uganda, dunia mbaya	Uganda, it's a bad world
Tanganyika, dunia mbaya	Tanzania, it's a bad world
Ata Amerika, dunia mbaya	Even in America, it's a bad world
Ata swissland, dunia mbaya	Even in Switzerland, it's a bad world
Dunia mbaya, dunia mbaya	It's a bad world, it's a bad world
Dunia mbaya, dunia mbaya	It's a bad world, it's a bad world
Wewe mama, dunia mbaya	Lady, it's a bad world
Kona kona, pia mbaya	Crooked ways are risky too
Mabwana wengi, pia mbaya	Keeping many men is risky too
Wasichana wengi, pia mbaya	Keeping many ladies is risky too
Uzee, wazee, pia mbaya	And elderly people are at risk too
Warembo, warembo, pia mbaya	Keeping many beauties is risky too
Wewe baba, sugardaddy	You old man, sugar daddy
Utakufa mbaya, utakufa mbaya	You will die badly, you will die badly
Utawacha watoto, utawacha bibi	You will leave your children; you will leave your wife
Utakufa mbaya, na bibi yako	You will die badly, so will your wife
Utawacha mama, utawacha gari	You will leave your wife, you will leave your car
Utawacha pesa, utawacha pesa	You will leave your money, you will leave your money
Utawacha bibi, raha wacha nyuma	You will leave your wife, stop this fun

Na gari yako, pia Baba	And your car, Baba
Pia gari, dunia mbaya	And your car, it's a bad world
Dunia mbaya, dunia mbaya	It's a bad world, it's a bad world
Wacha raha, dunia mbaya	Stop having fun, it's a bad world
Utakufa mbaya dunia mbaya	You will die badly, it's a bad world
Utawacha watoto, peke yake	You will leave your children helpless
Wacha watoto, pia mbaya	Leave your children desperate, it's a bad world
Ka chonjo, dunia mbaya	Take care, it's a bad world
Pia gari, dunia mbaya	And your car, it's a bad world

These lyrics, from a recording by Kenyan popular singer Princess Jully, begin as many romantic songs, with the singer professing her love for her husband. This pronouncement is further underlined by her refusal of numerous overtures made to her by other men due to her love for and loyalty to her husband. The song then moves to the whole notion of illicit love, describing relationships and liaisons of all types. The danger of this activity is clearly spelled out: she could be infected with HIV and face certain death, leaving orphans and material possessions behind. The singer has therefore deftly contrasted loyalty and love for one's partner with infidelity. From another perspective, the singer's expression of love and devotion to her husband can be placed within the context of her personal experiences. At the time she composed the song, Princess Jully's husband had just died; and as a widow, naturally, there could have been a number of men trying to approach her for an affair. Consequently, she publicly declared through her song her unwillingness to be solicited because of her undying love for her late husband. The song then becomes a means of fighting back against persistent overtures by other men, while allowing the singer to relate her personal life (through a semi-autobiographical song) to the lives of others in the world with similar situations. It is possible that the narrative of Princess Jully's struggles against these men becomes a parable warning those who, unlike her, might succumb to the wiles of these paramours and end up as AIDS victims. The implication is that one must be careful these days, since one can never tell who is infected with HIV, as well as who is not. Thus the refrain "Dunia Mbaya": the world (life) is hazardous these days.

Princess Jully's use of language offers insight into the nature of her intended audience. The predominant use of Kiswahili (Kenya's national language) makes this message more accessible to the wider community and not just the singer's community (the Luo). English is also employed to dramatize her refusal to engage in love affairs with Europeans who supposedly approached her, thereby adding humor, and also providing an appropriate register for response. Another interesting linguistic aspect of this song is the way it moves easily from one language to another: a form of code switching. In a sense such shifts reflect the ways in which ordinary Kenyans express themselves in practice, normally moving from bits of one language to another. It may not be surprising to find in a conversation a mixture of words or phrases from Kiswahili, English, and Dholuo for example. In a sense, this feature makes the song typical of popular forms, as Karin Barber has stated of African popular culture more generally:

> It is not wholly "traditional"—in the sense given to this term by much Africanist scholarship, that is, purely oral, expressed in exclusively indigenous African languages or images, and coming from or alluding to the precolonial past. On the other hand it is not "elite" or "modern," "westernized"

culture—in the sense of inhabiting a world formed by higher education, full mastery of European languages and representational conventions, defined by its cultural proximity to the metropolitan centres, and addressed to a minority but "international" audience. It is rather defined by its occupation of the zone between these two poles. (Barber 1997, 1)

This description probably partly explains why this song was so popular, because it seemed to capture popular contemporary modes of expression. Humor associated with the singer's Luo accent when she sings in Kiswahili may also have ingratiated this song with the audience. In Kenya, jokes are often made out of the way different ethnic groups express themselves in either English or Kiswahili. Indeed many popular comedies play on stereotypes that represent the peculiar accents and articulation of different ethnicities.

It is arguable that this song belongs to the genre of popular music performed by live bands in night clubs or dance halls. The singer and her band popularized it in such performances, and, as is the case in Kenya, adaptations by other bands helped bring it to the attention of a larger audience in other parts of the country. This song is performed in the typical, highly danceable Luo *benga* style. Apart from live performance, it was also recorded and played in the mass media, with cassettes sold in shops and in the streets. As "club" music, this song carries with it a paradox common in this genre: at one level it is pleasurable to listen to and draws one to the dance floor with its lively beat; yet at another level, it expresses a very serious message. It is as if, in the midst of enticing revelers to enjoy the music, the singer also warns: "you must watch out."

Finally, it is important to mention that the words employed in this song express a theme commonly used in official and informal conversation, on billboards, pamphlets, and so on, warning against behavior that may lead to the spread of HIV/AIDS. What makes the message in this song more unique than these other forms, however, is that it is expressed through music.

JACK NYADUNDO: "UKIMWI HAINA TIBA" ("AIDS HAS NO CURE")

Yawa Nyithindwa, an gi weche miwuoro	Oh our children, I have a woeful message
Jack Nyadundo, Ja Nyahera	I am Jack Nyadundo, from Nyahera
Osiep George wuod Alego	A friend to George son of the Alego people
We apuonjie piny matin	Let me counsel the community a little
Nyithiwa, piny muneno ni	Our children, this world you live in
Piny orumo	Is coming to an end
Magi e ndalo manogoye ngeche	These are the days that were prophesied
Ni jibiro muodo lak	That people will gnash their teeth in pain
Biro nyuomore wede gi wede	Even relatives will marry one another
An omin Tony Nyadundo	I am Tony Nyadundo's elder
Manyicha omako thum moro ka	Who recently performed
Malich, kaparo ni akony piny	Another serious song of advice
Ayaki player	AIDS is a player
Nyako we kelo na	Lady stop seducing me
Gima itin'go akya	I don't know what your body carries
To ka pok o'tieko dwe achiel	Alas before one month is over

To ji adek osetho	Three people have died
Wuod jomoko o'kawo	This son of people grabs
Manyake nyake nyake	Varieties of flesh
All sizes kuja hapa	All sizes usually come here
Shika mimi, manyanga wazi…	Hold me, fair ladies!
Ondiek wuod g'Anyango	Leopard son of Anyango
An Okech nera, ja Kisumu Nyahera	I am Okech your uncle from Kisumu Nyahera
We apuonjie piny matin	Let me counsel the world a little
Wuod g'Alego	Son of Alego
Awuoyo mana e wi ukimwi	I am talking about AIDS
Maradhi ya ukimwi hayana kinga	This affliction has no cure
Kwa hivyo ndugu yangu	So, my brother
Usipo sikiya usio yangu	If you don't heed my counsel
Ninayo towa wakati huu	Which I am now delivering
Utachanganyikiwa hautamini dunia wa	You will crushed by this evil world
Alamo nu nyithiwa, chikuru itu mos	I pray, our children, that you will carefully listen
Ukawye puonjna	To my counsel
Mondo ukalye kata higa achiel	So that you can live even a year longer
Mondo kila n'gato uzingatia, ninayowaambia	So that each person will follow my advice
Mano ayaki mayaka	About AIDS the destroyer
Ukimwi part two	This is part two of my song about AIDS
Yawa winjie duonda	Please listen to my voice
Awuoro mama	I am at a loss
Nyadundo Janyahera amanyo mama	I, Nyadundo from Nyahera, mama
Amanyo nyako adiera	I am searching for the woman who is true
Manyo tama	But I have failed
Amanyo mama	In my search, mama
Bende nene i sunga	Good lady, you must be avoiding me,
Amanyo mama	I am still searching mama
In kanye ha!	Where are you?
Wololo wololo, uwi, uwi, mayie mama	Wololo wololo, uwi, uwi, mayie mama
Mayie denda, ne oketa keta ma aneno	Oh my body, it leads me to
Makne	That which has never been seen before
Donge uwinjo duonda jo dala	Can you hear my voice my people?
Wololo wololo, uwi, uwi	Wololo wololo, uwi, uwi
Mayie tienda, mayie ondin'ga	Oh my body, Oh my back
Mayie gira ni, gira kiki jemna	Oh my penis, penis don't mislead me
Kiki kuodwiya, kiki miya guonyo	Don't embarrass me, don't bring me sores
Kendo i rith n' guta	On my neck
Kendo irith dhoga	And in my mouth

Yawa iketa aneno makne	Oh you lead me to the calamitous
Omiyo Janyahera	That's why I, from Nyahera,
Apuonjo pinyni	Am counseling this community
To moro pok aneno e pinyka	I have never seen such a terrible thing as this
Yawa winji duonda Okello Owuor	Oh heed my words Okello Owuor
Wololo wololo, uwi, uwi	Wololo wololo, uwi, uwi
Mayie mama, mayie Ayaki	Oh mother, Oh AIDS
Yawa Ayaki maya, tinde tieko wa	Oh AIDS the destroyer is ravaging us
Chuo mabecho otieko te	Handsome men it has finished
Nyiri mabeyo olalyie go	It has done away with lovely ladies
Jodongo bende onego,	The elderly it has killed,
Jothum bende otieko te	And the musicians are finished
Jongware bende onego te....	Boda Boda bicyclists it has killed
Donge uwinjo duonda Jo Nyahera	Are you listening to my counsel Nyahera people?
Nyadundo gini oketo a apuonjo piny ngima	Nyadundo I have to warn the whole nation
Wololo wololo, uwi uwi	Wololo, wololo, uwi, uwi
Enyi ndugu zangu mujichunge	Oh my people, take care
Musiamini tho	Don't be a victim
Mujichunge sana	Beware
Ukowapi ukimwi?	What are you AIDS?
Ulitoka wapi ukimwi?	Where did you spring from AIDS?
Hauna ata aibu, uliuwa ndugu yangu,	You respect no one, you killed my brother
Shemeji ukauwa, dada yangu alikufa	Then killed my [brother- or sister-] in-law, my sister died
Sina shangazi, sina babu, sina jirani	I am without an aunt, no grandfather, no neighbor
Tena wanitaka mimi	Now you are out to get me
Yawa iketa aneno maknen	Oh I have seen the unbelievable
Donge uwinjo duonda jo Nyahera	Are you listening to me Nyahera people?
Nyadundo Jack	I, Nyadundo Jack
Apuonjo piny ngima	I am counseling the whole nation
A joji donge i' nena	Georgy, you are my witness
Wololo wololo, uwi, uwi, mayie mama	Wololo wololo, uwi uwi, Mayie mama
Mayie denda, mayie Mayie Ayaki	Oh my body, Oh AIDS
Yawa Ayaki maya, Ayaki tinde tieko piny	Oh AIDS the reaper, AIDS the destroyer
Chwo mabecho otieko te	Handsome men it has finished
Ukimwi haina tiba	AIDS has no cure
Ukimwi haina tiba, Wahindi wana kufa	AIDS has no cure, Indians are dying
Warabu wanakufa, Wazungu wanakufa	Arabs are dying, Europeans are dying

Ulimwengu kote shida	The whole world is afflicted
Yawa pok'na neno makama	Oh I have never before seen such as this
Ndonge uwinjo duonda, Jonyahera	Are you listening to me, Nyahera people?
Wololo, wololo, uwi, uwi	Wololo, wololo, uwi, uwi
Mayie mama	Oh mama,
Manyake wapi sasa	What is the fate of all that tasty meat?
All sizes, all sizes	All sizes, all sizes
Mujichunge sana…	Beware
Wololo, wololo, uwi, uwi, mayie mama	Wololo, wololo, uwi, uwi, Oh mama,
Mayie denda, nyako wuoyi orwako lon'g	Oh my body, Lady, that man is in trousers
To gima otin'go bende akia	But what he is carrying I don't know,
Mach bende Itin'go e lon'g, to	He also carries fire in his trousers,
Bende okowan'gie lon'g	Which does not burn his trousers
Donge uwinjo duonda Jonyahera…	Are you listening to me Nyahera people?
A ndugu zangu mujichunge sana	Oh my friends, take heed
Maradhi ya ukimwi haina tiba	AIDS has no cure
Sisi wanamuziki, watu wengi wanatu dharau	We musicians are despised
Lakini mawaidha tunawapatia, ni mzuri sana	Yet we give you wise counsel
Wanamuziki wengi wameaga dunia kwa sababu	Many musicians have even died because of
Ya usharati, raha haina mwisho	Adultery, merrymaking has no end
Munaona kwenye magazeti, kwenye radio	You see this in the newspapers, and on radio
Lakini ebu mushike mawaidha ninayowapatia	But please take my counsel seriously
Kwamba ukimwi haina tiba	That AIDS has no cure

This song and the next one (by Oduor Odhialo) belong to a genre of Luo music called *ohangla*. The genre is conventionally performed with a prescribed set of instruments centered around a group of seven or eight drums; these drums are arranged on the ground and played in succession by a single drummer using drumsticks. Other percussive instruments (such as shakers), wind instruments (such as the horn), and string instruments (including the one-stringed fiddle, *orutu*) accompany the drummer. More recently, the electronic keyboard and mouth organ have also been introduced, demonstrating the dynamic nature of the genre: musicians regularly make creative changes in relation to audience response, influences from other musics, attempts to create more appealing songs, and the type of occasion and subject that the song addresses. A soloist (and sometimes a chorus) accompanies the instruments. *Ohangla* is dance music and is therefore performed in a vibrant manner, creating a lively atmosphere and drawing the audience to take to the floor. It is performed in a variety of places and events, including clubs, funerals, weddings, and political gatherings among others.

The song above is a lamentation that addresses the catastrophe resulting from the HIV pandemic and warns against behavior that could lead to infection. The singer therefore sings in the typical Luo lamentation voice which involves a crooning tone and interjections typical of traditional Luo lamentation: "*Wololo, wololo, uwi, uwi, mayie mama.*" The result is a somber mood that befits the purpose of a song whose subject is death.

In a sense, lamentation in this genre is apt because there are allegations that *ohangla* was originally performed during funerals, especially during the burial of an elder. On such occasions music would provide the opportunity for singers to comment and reflect on serious and sensitive issues relating to the community, including matters of sexuality.

The first lines of this song are spoken rather than sung. This is typical of African musical performance where vocal parts may oscillate between speech and song. At one level this approach provides variety, and at another it creates a dramatic sense by animating the rendition. Scholars have also remarked on the close link between African languages and music, and the ease with which speech can move into song and vice versa (Nketia 1974, Agawu 2003, Wanyama 2009). Indeed, in Dholuo (the Luo language) there are no distinct words for poetry and song (i.e., that which is sung) respectively. Instead, a single word (often translated as "song") stands for both, and in performance, poetry can be sung or chanted. But this particular song also hints at rap and other contemporary forms that play between speech and song, by including in the text some lyrics from the popular Kenyan hip hop song "Juala" by Circute and Joel (Wanyama 2007). Jack Nyadundo appropriates lines from the chorus of "Juala" into "Ukimwi Haina Tiba" by singing: "*Manyake, Nyake, Nyake, all sizes...*" meaning, lots of meat, in all sizes. In the context the song by Circute and Joel, *Manyake* means the breasts of a lady. This becomes clear when they sing:

All sizes	All sizes
Kama prizes	Like prizes
Kama ballon zina maji	Like balloons they have water
Juala ndo wahitaji	What you need is "juala" [condom]

This means that women's breasts are available in all sizes, some are like balloons filled with water, and so all that a man needs is to be protected when having sex with any woman he admires (ibid.). In the context of "Ukimwi haina tiba," meaning "AIDS has no cure," Nyadundo, like Circute and Joel, dramatically underlines the kind of freewheeling sexual behavior that puts one at risk of contracting HIV. In contrast, while Nyadundo's main point is to caution people about the dangers of promiscuity, which includes the likelihood of getting HIV infection, Circute and Joel focus on promotion of condom use. In the context of Nyadundo's song, the symbolism of "Juala" is also apt, for the term is a *sheng* (Swahili slang) word for meat. Just as there are varieties of meat (beef, pork, chicken, mutton, and so on) there are also lots of potential women for men (who are voracious) to select. The only danger is one might not know who is infected and who is not. But the term as used in this context can also be a reference to the biblical "lust of the flesh" which is identified in the Bible as ephemeral and eventually leading to some kind of self-destruction. One also notices the underlying gender bias of this symbolism, for it seems to suggest that there are lots of women waiting to ensnare men and that it is the former who infect the latter and not *vice versa*. However, there is an attempt by the musician to correct this implied imbalance by poetically remarking later in the song (in lines addressing a lady):

Mayie denda, nyako wuoyi orwako lon'g	O my body, lady, that man is in trousers
To gima otin'go bende akia, mach bende	But what he is carrying I don't know, he also carries fire
Itin'go e lon'g, to	In his trousers,
Bende okowan'gie lon'g	Which does not burn his trousers

These lines warn women that they cannot judge men by outside appearance alone; i.e., that one cannot know who is infected and who is not by merely looking at a person's physical appearance. Fire here is a metaphor for the potential threat that a man can spread through unprotected sex. It does not refer to the burning sensation associated with other STDs. In this case, it expresses the ravaging power of the HIV/AIDS pandemic.

ODUOR ODHIALO: "NYAK'OMOLLO" ("A SONG IN HONOR OF OMOLLO'S DAUGHTER")

Yii yii Ayaki mayaka	Yii yii AIDS the destroyer
Ayaki mayaka	AIDS the destroyer
Ayaki maya baba na	AIDS took my father from me
Mama bende i mayoya	And took my mother from me too
Nyathina bende aonge go	I have lost my child too
Nyamera bende aonge go	I have lost my sister too
To baba bende i mayo a	And you have taken my father too
Baba bende aonge go	I have lost my father
Owadwa bende aonge go	My brother is gone too
Nikech Ayaki mayaka	Because of AIDS the malevolent one
Yii yii Ayaki mayaka	Yii Yii AIDS the destroyer
Adongo min Anyango aonge mor	Adongo mother of Anyango I am grieving
Amolo min Atieno aonge mor	Amolo mother of Atieno I am grieving
Ulimwengu sina raha	I have no happiness in this world
Duniani sina raha	I have no happiness in this world
Wenzangu sina raha	My people I am grieving
Ndugu zangu sina raha	My brothers I am grieving
Kwa sababu ya Ukimwi	Because of AIDS
Nieleze Maradhi ya Ukimwi yalitoka wapi?	Tell me, where did this pestilence come from?
Ukimwi ulitoka wapi?	AIDS where did you spring from?
Uliuwa Baba yangu	You killed my father
Ukauwa mama yangu	Then you killed my mother
Na dada yangu ukauwa	My sister too
Kaka yangu ukauwa	And my cousin
Mtoto yangu pia sina	I have also lost my child
Kwa sababu ya ukimwi	Because of AIDS
Yii yii Ayaki mayaka	Yii yii AIDS the destroyer
We mondo amos Ja Ugenya...	Let me greet the man from Ugenya
Yii yii Ayaki mayaka	Yii yii AIDS the destroyer

Dhano to mana le	Man is just mortal
Le, le to mana le	Mortal, mortal, just mortal
Ayaki mayaka	AIDS the destroyer
Gini Njawo piny	It is ravaging the world
Ukimwi njawo piny	AIDS is ravaging the world
Mayaka terowa	The destroyer is wiping us
Nyiri mabecho 'nego te	It has killed all the lovely girls
Sianda madongo olal go	It has done away with all the big buttocks
To wang'i yom ikwadhe piny	Just show off your lovely face
Nyako wek sungori	Lady stop boasting
Mera wek sungori	My friend stop boasting
Wuoyi wek sungori	Young man don't boast
Keep you dendi	Take care of your body
Mama keep you dendi	Mama take care of your body
Mera keep you dendi	My friend take care of your body
Owadwa keep you dendi	Brother take care your body
Ayaki luoro piny	AIDS is traversing the world
To gino njawo wa	And it is ravaging us
To gini tieko wa	And it is ravaging us
Nyako wek ting'o na	Lady stop carrying yourself around
Nyamera wek suso na	My sister stop swaggering before me
Atoti wek kelo na	Atoti, stop tempting me
Nyathini wek yiengo na	Baby stop shaking your hips for me
Obera wek ting'o na	Lovely one stop prancing around me
Omiyo wek kelo na	And don't try me
Baby wek yiengo na	Baby stop shaking them for me
Nyiri mabecho aneno te	I have seen all the lovely ladies
Nyiri mabecho aneno te	I have seen all the lovely ladies
Sianda madongo amulo ka	I have fondled all the big buttocks
To wang'i yom aneno gi	I know you have a lovely face
To wiyi isuko mama na	And your hair is well done my lady
Omiyo wek ting'o na	So stop trying me
Baby wek yiengo na	Baby stop shaking your hips for me
Atoti wek kelo na	Atoti don't try me
Nyathini wek ting'o na	Girl stop carrying yourself around me
Nyako gimi ting'o bende akya	I don't even know what you are carrying
Abende gima ting'o ikya	And you don't know what I am carrying
Kendo akya ni iting'o ang'o	And I don't know what you are carrying
Mama wek sungori	Mama stop carrying yourself around
Gini mako piny ngima…	This thing is all over the world
I iii iii yii yii yii mayaka	I iii iii yii yii the destroyer
Yii yii mamana	Yii yii my mama
Ndugu zangu chunguzeni	Brothers beware
Warembo chunguzeni	Ladies beware
Vijana chunguzeni	Young people beware
Dunia tinde mbaya	The world is now at risk

Dunia tinde mbaya	The world is now at risk
Odhialo chunga sana	Odhialo be aware
Ogada chunga sana	Ogada beware
Ja k'Obodo chunga sana	Ja k'Obodo beware
Ja k'Omolo chunga sana	Ja k'Omolo beware
Odhis chunga sana	Odhis beware
Mama chunga sana	Mama beware
Ja Ugunja chunga sana	Ja Ugunja beware
Baba chunga sana	Baba Beware
Dunia tinde mbaya	The world is now a risky place
Ayaki luoro piny	Ayaki is traversing the earth
Mayaka tieko wa	The destroyer is finishing us
Nairobi otieko te	Nairobi it has ravaged
To gini tinde luoro piny	And this thing is spreading afar
To Kenya ngima oluoro te	In Kenya it has spread afar
Nairobi ochando wa	In Nairobi it is wreaking havoc
Ayaki Mayaka	AIDS the destroyer
Nairobi Kayole	In Nairobi Kayole
Ayaki mayaka	AIDS is ravaging
Kibera dala	In Kibera my home
Ayaki mayaka	AIDS is ravaging
Ngomongo pacho	In Ngomongo my home
Ayaki mayaka	AIDS is ravaging
Kaloleni dala	In Kaloleni my home
Ayaki mayaka	AIDS is ravaging
I iii iii yii yii yii mayaka	I iii iii yii yii the destroyer
Yii yii mama na	Yii yii my mama
Adongo min Anyango	Adongo mother of Anyango
Alewe piny koda ngoma	I am obsessed with music
Amolo min Atieno a	Amolo mother of Atieno
kwamo e piny koda waya	I am possessed by music
Kisumo Kisumo, Kisumo Kisumo	Kisumu Kisumu, Kisumu Kisumu
Kisumo dalawa	Kisumu our home
Kisumu dala gi Baba	Home of my fathers
Pacho dala gi mama na	Home of my mother
Pacho dala k'Oginga	Home to the Ogingas
Kisumo dala k'Oginga	Home to the Ogingas
K'Ondele to Kisumo	In Kondele within Kisumu
Nyawita Kisumo	Nyawita in Kisumu
Manyatta Kisumo	Manyatta in Kisumu
Obunga Kisumo	Obunga in Kisumu
Nyalenda Kisumo	Nyalenda in Kisumu
Otonglo Kisumo	Otonglo in Kisumu
Rabango Kisumo	Rabango in Kisumu
K'Odiaga dala Kisumo	Kodiaga in Kisumu

Pandya Kisumo	Pandya in Kisumu
Dunga Kisumo	Dunga in Kisumu
Mamboleo Kisumo	Mamboleo in Kisumu
Rafiki chunga sana	Friend take care
Osiepna chunga sana	Friend take care
A' Judi chunga sana	Judy take care
Mama chunga sana	Mama take care
Dunia tinde mbaya	The world is bad
Gini luoro piny	This thing is ravaging the world

The singer, Oduor K'Odhialo, sings in a typical Luo lament voice that includes a vibrato. This sound lends a sense of emotion appropriate to his subject—the havoc wrought by HIV/AIDS. The Luo lament form also includes a repetitive chorus at various intervals, normally serving as an opening phrase for each section of the song while also intensifying the feeling of sorrow:

I iii iii yii yii yii mayaka   I iii iii yii yii the destroyer

By employing this traditional form, which is also performed in dirges, the performer creates a funereal atmosphere that draws his audience to the tragic circumstances surrounding the spread of HIV. This approach frames the message in such a way that those listening to it realize that what Odhialo is expressing is an extremely serious matter.

The singer also plays on the Luo word for the disease when he uses the phrase "Ayaki Mayaka" "Ayaki," translated literally, means "I sweep you away" or "I waste you." The word "Mayaka," which stands for "the sweeper" or "the waster," has also become one of the main Luo terms for AIDS. Thus, a rough rendering of the phrase in English would be "I sweep you, the sweeper" or "I waste you, the waster," or, perhaps more fluidly, "I am the sweeper/waster who sweeps/wastes you." This wordplay vividly expresses the nature of HIV/AIDS, whose symptoms frequently include the gradual and irreversible loss of weight. In addition, the singer uses the rhythmic texture of this phrase to enhance the refrain after mentioning particular locations that have been ravaged by the disease:

Nairobi ochando wa	In Nairobi it is wreaking havoc
Ayaki Mayaka	AIDS the sweeper/waster
Nairobi Kayole	In Nairobi, Kayole estate
Ayaki mayaka	AIDS is sweeping

In the typical nature of a dirge, the song recounts those people "close" to the musician who have succumbed to the disease. This list of names implies that everybody is either "infected" or "affected" by the ravages of HIV/AIDS. Thus nobody can ignore its effects.

Odhialo switches to Kiswahili from time to time, and sometimes directly translates what he sings in Dholuo into Kiswahili. This illustrates that the performer intends to reach out to a broader audience (possibly at a national level) and does not confine himself to a local one (i.e., the Luo community). Such a linguistic choice may further be a direct result of the patrons that come to listen to his music performance, an indicator that he appeals to a multiethnic community. At one point the singer even dabbles in English, using the phrases:

Omera keep you dendi	My friend take care of your body
Owadwa keep you dendi	brother take care your body

While this moment adds humor in the sense that Odhialo deliberately mixes Dholuo words with English words (code-mixing), it foregrounds the essential message, which is to take care of one's body and avoid being infected with HIV/AIDS.

We also notice the repetition of lines that helps to emphasize the message, as well as to contribute to and enhance the rhythm of the song. In addition, repetition of lines is a particularly suitable device in a lament, for it creates a feeling of persistent complaint. There is a sense in which we can also regard repetition as embodying the continuous havoc caused by the disease.

While performing this song, it is clear that the musician maintains links with his audience by mentioning people by name: this kind of greeting/acknowledgement is common in Luo musical performance where the musician takes note of those patrons (or friends) who are present. In this particular case, by mentioning their names, he also shows his concern about their health and vulnerability in the face of the rampant HIV/AIDS:

Odhialo chunga sana	Odhialo be aware
Ogada chunga sana	Ogada beware
Ja k'Obodo chunga sana	Ja k'Obodo beware
Ja k'Omolo chunga sana	Ja k'Omolo beware
Odhis chunga sana	Odhis beware
Mama chunga sana	Mama beware
Ja Ugunja chunga sana	Ja Ugunja beware

This kind of direct address moves the song from the general to the specific, making it clear that the danger of contracting this disease is a reality and can happen to real persons including "you" and "me"; that is why the singer even reminds himself to "take care":

Odhialo chunga sana	Odhialo beware

The performer also plays around with discourses of "desire," drawing our attention to the subject of the body, beauty, and sexuality. Odhialo seems to make us aware that physical beauty that draws a man to a woman can be deceptive, for she may be (in reality) infected. Thus he dramatizes the need for caution and skepticism with regard to outward beauty and sexual attraction—a necessary precaution in this era of HIV/AIDS:

Nyako wek ting'o na	Lady stop carrying yourself around
Nyamera wek suso na	My sister stop swaggering before me
Atoti wek kelo na	Atoti, stop tempting me
Nyathini wek yiengo na	Baby stop shaking your hips for me
Obera wek ting'o na	Lovely one stop prancing around me
Omiyo wek kelo na	And don't try me
Baby wek yiengo na	Baby stop shaking them for me
Nyiri mabecho aneno te	I have seen all the lovely ladies
Sianda madongo amulo ka	I have fondled all the big buttocks

To wang'i yom aneno gi	I know you have a lovely face
To wiyi isuko mama na	And your hair is well done my lady
Omiyo wek ting'o na	So stop trying me
Baby wek yiengo na	Baby stop shaking your hips for me
Atoti wek kelo na	Atoti don't try me
Nyathini wek ting'o na	Girl stop carrying yourself around me
Nyako gimi ting'o bende akya	I don't even know what you are carrying
Abende gima ting'o ikya	And you don't know what I am carrying

The final section of this song contains what may be called a kind of mapping of the extensive spread of the disease, penetrating all the familiar places in Nairobi and Kisumu (for example). The effect of this rhythmic recounting of places is that of an onward march or movement (infection) spreading around; a sinister and worrying situation that calls for an urgent and immediate remedy.

CONCLUSION

It is evident from the analysis and discussion of the three songs in this study that with the onset of the HIV/AIDS pandemic, contemporary popular music in Kenya, while still concerned with the subject of sexuality through the exploration of bodies and desire, has had to confront this theme within the context of the dangers posed by HIV/AIDS. This chapter demonstrates that far from encouraging promiscuity, as some discourses seem to suggest, popular musicians have been actively involved in spreading the message of HIV/AIDS awareness and prevention through their music.

23

Interlude
Grassroots Organizing and
Celebrity Campaigns

THE ARTS AND AIDS ACTIVISM IN MOROCCO

Jeffrey Callen

With a relatively low infection rate[1] and a strong taboo against open discussions of sexuality, AIDS has until recently been relegated to the margins of social discourse in Morocco. In the arts, the subject of AIDS is rarely broached. However, AIDS activists have realized that connecting their work to the arts is a powerful tool in raising awareness, particularly among youth. AIDS activism began in Morocco in 1988 (two years after the first reported case of AIDS) with the formation of Association de Lutte contre le Sida (ALCS). In its early years, the ALCS made little use of the arts in its education and organizational work. Recognizing the importance of outreach to youth, however, it set up a single stand at the premier edition of the Festival Gnaoua et Musiques du Monde in 1998. That festival, held each June in the coastal city of Essaouira, quickly became a cultural phenomenon and the most popular musical event of the year among Moroccan youth. ALCS expanded its presence at the festival and found that its work there was a major boon to AIDS awareness and to the visibility of ALCS. Among the additional perks was an increase in funding from international NGOs, such as the United Nations Population Fund. ALCS expanded its outreach to youth at cultural events and, when I attended a festival of alternative music in Casablanca in 2002, ALCS was there, handing out pamphlets and red ribbons. In 2005, with the support of King Mohammed VI, ALCS dramatically increased its visibility with a two-week campaign known as Sidaction, which included the participation of the country's major radio and television networks. Sidaction included a six-hour telethon that was broadcast on the major television and radio networks and featured celebrities from

Morocco—such as comedian Gad Elmaleh and singer Naima Samih—and the Middle East, including singer Walid Taoufik (Lebanon) and actor Yahia Fakhrani (Egypt). The telethon, which raised 13.1 million dirhams (approximately $1.7 million), also revealed the fractures in AIDS work in Morocco as three prominent organizations refused to participate, stating that they refused to be the "puppets" of ALCS (Rhanem 2005).

In the last few years, the use of celebrities from the world of entertainment to raise public awareness of HIV/AIDS has become an integral component of AIDS work in Morocco. ALCS, with the support of the state, has continued to stage Sidaction telethons, but the primary focus of its work remains grassroots organizing and education work. A newer organization, Ruban Rouge, bases its educational work on the participation of celebrity entertainers in publicity campaigns. Founded in 2001, Ruban Rouge attempts to get people talking about AIDS in order to remove the stigma carried by an AIDS infection. Simo Ben Bachir, president of Ruban Rouge, feels that the use of superstars from around the world is the most effective means of getting the message out to youth: "Young people, especially teenagers are influenced by their superstars...when a doctor does a lecture on AIDS here, nobody cares but when it is a star, everybody listens." A number of Moroccan celebrities have endorsed the work of Ruban Rouge, but the group's greatest success has been its work with popular Lebanese singer Haifa Wehbe, who toured Morocco in support of the organization's effort. Ben Bachir declared the tour a success because Wehbe talked to the media about her support of Ruban Rouge and helped break the silence about AIDS. "Our goal is that people talk about AIDS!" Ben Bachir maintains that the lack of attention to AIDS in the arts is because Moroccan artists do not lead but "follow what happens on the ground" (Bachir E-mail, Nov. 10, 2008).

The Moroccan government's recently increased emphasis on AIDS prevention and treatment also included calling on celebrities and artists to contribute to the effort. On World AIDS Day in December 2008, the Moroccan Ministries of Health and Culture announced the inauguration of a new communication campaign to raise public awareness of HIV/AIDS that included the participation of well-known artists and entertainers. The Minister of Culture announced that the government would provide support to any artist who participates in the fight against AIDS. This official message was accompanied by the signing of the Artists' AIDS Pact by a significant number of artists who pledged to raise awareness of AIDS, to fight discrimination against those living with HIV, and to include the issue of AIDS in cultural events. Prominent musician and actor Younes Megri, a pop star in Morocco since the 1970s, stated that artists can play a key role in helping the public understand the problem and prevent the spread of the disease: "Artists can reach out to people and help get the message across" (Touahri 2008). However, despite the promised government patronage, few artists have turned their attention to HIV/AIDS. Ben Bachir of Ruban Rouge may be right: Moroccan artists may not address HIV/AIDS, a taboo subject, until it has become a more accepted part of the national discourse.

24

Siphithemba—We Give Hope

SONG AND RESILIENCE IN A SOUTH AFRICAN ZULU HIV/AIDS STRUGGLE

Austin Chinagorom Okigbo (Williams College)

BACKGROUND: SIPHITHEMBA CHORAL MUSIC PERFORMANCE AS A FORM OF COMMUNITY AND STRUGGLE EXPERIENCE

The rich and vibrant choral tradition of South Africa cannot be overstated. In the Greater-Durban area of KwaZulu-Natal where I conducted research, one could readily find a large number of choirs in the townships, including gospel choirs, Afro-jazz vocal groups, and large church- and community-based choirs. In the Township of Umlazi, where I worked with several church and community choirs, it is not unusual to see choir members shuttling between choir rehearsals on a given evening. Because people tend to belong to various ensembles at the same time, church and community choirs are careful in scheduling their rehearsal times so as not to conflict with the rehearsal times of other groups in the same section of the township. As a result, there is an abundance of music being produced every day by trained composers and amateurs alike, including elaborate choral pieces, gospel arrangements, operas, a huge collection of *amakorasi* (gospel choruses), and Western classical works.[1]

Thus one can argue that choral singing functions as a significant form of community experience among black South Africans. It is a means of articulating and expressing various dimensions of communal experience, including conflicts, relationships, economic development or poverty, sickness and disease, and social responsibility. According to Beverly Parker, professor of music at the University of KwaZulu-Natal, choral music can be seen as representing a South African, and specifically Zulu, quality of life: it is used to "address issues that affect them and to sustain [them] in times of conflict and struggles" (1997).

The role for music was particularly evident in anti-apartheid struggles, during which music concerts and choral competitions became vessels for quiet communal protest. A performance of Felix Mendelssohn's "Be Not Afraid" from *Elijah*, for example, might be prefaced with a short message emphasizing the song's relation to a collective struggle experience (Detterbeck 2002, 150). In some instances, choral arrangers and directors created Zulu protest songs that interpolated themes of resistance into gospel chorus song texts (Detterbeck 2002, Matshikiza 2000). For example, choirs composed largely of black South Africans were known to perform the song "iJerusalem izwe lethu" ("Jerusalem is our land") as "iSouth Africa izwe lethu" ("South Africa is our land").

In 1996 former President Nelson Mandela declared HIV/AIDS the next struggle, thus triggering a new symbolic and artistic connection between current events and the earlier anti-apartheid struggle. This sentiment now permeates many of the facets of the AIDS discourse in South Africa, including the use of music. Veteran choral conductor Joshua Radebe, for example, noted in an interview that composers in the post-apartheid period are now encouraged to adapt songs to address HIV/AIDS in a manner similar to that of the anti-apartheid struggles (Radebe Interview 2007). Many newly composed songs thus continue to express community experience, reflecting a shared sense of HIV/AIDS as a threat that must be overcome through a concerted communal approach.

The choral ensemble that I will focus on in this chapter, Siphithemba, started at the McCord mission hospital in Durban. Siphithemba's membership consists of HIV-positive young men and women who are engaged in individual and collective struggle against HIV/AIDS. Some, in addition to being positive, have lost loved ones—significant others, brothers and sisters, and friends—to the virus. Others have family members still living with the virus. Members bring their personal experiences to the ensemble, where they articulate and combine these experiences into a singular community ethos. As they struggle individually with the virus, they provide support to one another both within the context of musical performance and in extra-musical activities. In short, Siphithemba's members function as surrogate family to one another as they deal with the effects of the virus: sickness, social stigma, unemployment, and even the need for mutual aid. I argue that their communal approach to dealing with the exigencies of the disease is indicative of an attitude of resilience in the face of the perceived odds of living with HIV/AIDS. Through their musical production, also communally realized, individual members draw from personal experiences and contribute to bits of the lyrics of songs. In performance, these assembled songs are rendered by the whole group: mostly in antiphonal styles with integrated dance. Siphithemba's approach to music making thus remains consistent with choral singing among the Zulu as a significant form of community experience. More broadly, the group's experience reflects the communality of music making in Africa, in which individuals who live a corporate life, or share common values and/or life experiences, use music making both as a form of social intercourse, and for rendering a community ethos in performance (Nketia 1974, 21).

I draw my description here from my interactions with the choir and its members in musical and extra-musical contexts between 2006 and 2007. These experiences provided me significant opportunity to not only immerse myself in their world so as to observe their processes of musical composition and performance, but also to appreciate how the spirituality of their communal music-making translates into their interaction with one another and with the larger society. In these instances, they manifest a strong sense of hope and determination to beat the odds of living with HIV/AIDS.

MCCORD HOSPITAL AND THE BIRTH OF SIPHITHEMBA CHOIR

McCord Hospital in Durban, KwaZulu-Natal was among the first medical providers to offer HIV care and treatment in South Africa beginning in 1996 (Holst Interview 2007; Thomas

Interview 2007; see also www.mccord.org.za). The Sinikithemba Clinic, which is the HIV/AIDS care and treatment center at the hospital, provides "comprehensive care for patients with HIV and their families...including pediatric care, as well as psychosocial and spiritual support to patients and their families" (www.mccord.org.za). Dr. Helga Holst, the medical superintendent at the hospital, noted that the progressive initiative that made this kind of care possible is in line with the same spiritual and humane concern that motivated the missionary Dr. James McCord to found the hospital in 1909 as a medical mission to the Zulu (Holst Interview 2007). According to James Cochrane, "a church that takes preferential option for the health of the person is a church faithful to the healing and wholeness implied by the Latin word *salus*, from which we derive 'salvation'" (2006, 18). In South Africa, as in several other African countries, Christian missionaries are known to have brought health care systems with them as part of the evangelization project. Today, the healthcare infrastructure in sub-Saharan Africa is still largely that erected by missionaries and faith-based institutions both during and after the colonial period (Arhap 2006, 121). McCord Hospital's initiative at providing a comprehensive palliative, psychosocial, and spiritual care to HIV/AIDS patients at the Sinikithemba Clinic must therefore be viewed in the light the missionary project.

By 1996 an estimated 70 percent of medical admissions at McCord hospital were HIV related. At that time, scientists were yet to disseminate antiretroviral treatment widely. But the HIV/AIDS situation in South Africa was already reaching an alarming rate. Doctors and staff could only render minimal medical help to the patients. In the absence of any significant medical help, HIV-positive persons also had to bear the burden of stigma of the disease. The progressive leadership understood that alternative help in the form of spiritual counseling and social support networks could be useful in helping patients cope with the emotional and material burdens associated with being HIV-positive. Thus in 1997 the Sinikithemba (Zulu for "we give hope" or "give us hope") Support Group was founded under the leadership of Mrs. Nonhlanhla Mhlongo, a medical social worker charged with the responsibility of providing hospice services to terminally ill patients at the hospital.

The Sinikithemba AIDS clinic at the hospital was named after the support group, since it was partly an outgrowth of the group and was targeted mainly at members of the support group. The name Sinikithemba denotes the spirituality of hope that has guided the operation of the hospital since its inception. But according to Nomusa Mpanza, it is also a reflection of the hope that people living with HIV/AIDS received from their participation in the support group and clinic (Mpanza Interview 2007). For those living with HIV and AIDS, the group and the clinic served as a source of hope as well as a space for nurturing faith, hope, and determination to live. By 1999, the support group comprised over five hundred HIV-positive members, who met once a week to engage in praise worship, prayer, Bible reading, the sharing of experiences, and mutual encouragement (Thomas Interview 2007). Members could speak freely about how they were coping with their sicknesses, and about the burden of social stigma that they experienced in the form of rejections by family and the society at large. Part of the responsibility of the support group was also to attend the funerals of deceased members and provide support to affected families. When a member was sick, other members from his or her area of residence also went in small groups to visit and to encourage him or her. The support group thus functioned also as a mechanism for looking out for one another, especially in circumstances where HIV-positive individuals had been deserted by friends and relatives.

Most of the members of the support group were not meaningfully employed (some for lack of skills). Many of those who *were* employed risked losing their jobs. Zinhle Thabethe, a member of the Siphithemba choir, lost her job when a fellow employee accessed her office cabinet without her permission, read her diagnosis result and revealed her status to her employers (Hainsworth 2006). As a result, the majority of the support group members had no incomes. Lack of a strong financial base resulted in deficient nutritional habits that were inimical to their immune systems, resulting in opportunistic infections such as tuberculosis, pneumonia, and meningitis. But Mrs. Mhlongo, who coordinated the support group, believed that while HIV-positive persons are still strong, they could be productive and able to earn some living by themselves. She used the opportunity of the support group meetings to encourage members in need to look inwards and figure out any talents or skills they might have that might benefit their economic conditions. According to her:

> We've got people who are HIV-positive, and who have no income...What we are trying to inculcate to people is that they have to work and not beg. Because of their status they shouldn't go around begging; instead they should give something in return. (Mhlongo Interview 2007)

It was during one such meeting that an older member who had skill in beadwork offered to teach others how to make beads. The woman used to make and market beadworks to tourists by the beaches of Durban; but her health deteriorated and she developed severe arthritic pain, which made it difficult for her to handle the beading tools and needles. Mrs. Mhlongo procured funds to the tune of about R300.00 (roughly U.S. $40) to purchase the required materials for initiating the project. In a short time the beadworks grew into a major skill-acquisition project, which generated proceeds and allowed members to earn some form of living. As the project expanded, the parking lot of the Hope Building became a space for training members in sewing and knitting, in addition to beadworks. Staff from a local art program was brought in to teach support group members how to make mosaics. Other skills that were taught included woodworks and wood burning; and even a computer literacy program was introduced. About half the proceeds from these projects went to the individuals who produced the artwork, while half was saved in a fund meant to support treatment for sick members.

It was in the context of the income-generating projects that the Sinikithemba choir was born. All choir members speak passionately about the times when they hummed hymn tunes and sang gospel choruses while working at their projects. Members joined freely in the songs, each to a vocal part in which he or she felt comfortable, and found that their voices blended harmoniously. Some members testified about times when passersby on McCord Street stopped to listen to the sonorous singing of the group as they worked at their projects. According to Mhlongo, "the group sang so well, and sometimes we even shed tears" (Mhlongo Interview 2007). Asked why they shed tears sometimes, she explained that the songs they sang were sometimes emotional because they spoke to their individual experiences of being HIV-positive and being rejected by friends and families. But their singing was not always melancholic. Group members Nomusa and Phakamile attest to other instances when their songs were upbeat, especially when they sang Zulu folk songs and gospel tunes that spoke of courage in the face of adversity. From an interview with Nomusa, the moment that changed everything came in early 1998, when the group members finished their work for the day and spent several more hours singing and dancing. In her own words, "it was like we all went crazy that day, and everybody was watching us. So Nonhlanhla [Mhlongo] suggested maybe we should form a choir" (Nomusa Interview 2007). Thus at Mrs. Mhlongo's suggestion, more than forty individuals in the support group created the Sinikithemba Choir, and began to perform at hospital events. The formation of the choir thus transformed the initial support group into tri-functional entity as HIV/AIDS Support Group, micro-economic project, and choral ensemble.

SINIKITHEMBA OVERSEAS TOURS AND CONTINUED GROWTH

In 2002, Church World Service leaders from the United States visited Durban with the intent of entering into partnership programs with McCord Hospital on HIV/AIDS.[2] During the visit, the leaders were thrilled at the resilience and exuberance that the choir members showed in their musical performance. As a result, the Service pledged to send Tim Janis, a gospel artist from the United States, to come and work with the ensemble. Janis visited Durban the same year, held a benefit concert with the choir at the Durban City Hall, and recorded the album *A Thousand Summers* with both the Sinikithemba Choir and the Imilonji KaNtu choral ensemble. All of the proceeds from the sale of the CD recording were donated toward the funding of "African-run HIV/AIDS treatment and education projects" (Janis, 2002). In December 2002 the Sinikithemba Choir traveled to the United States on a tour sponsored by the Church World Service; they performed in churches and schools in the New York and Boston areas raising awareness about HIV/AIDS, while raising funds to provide antiretroviral treatments for support group members. During this first trip to the United States, the group impressed Dr. Bruce Walker, director of the Center for AIDS Research (CFAR) at the Massachusetts General Hospital, a professor at the Harvard Medical School, and a scientist involved with the CD4/Viral Load research project, which uses McCord Hospital and St. Mary's Hospital in Marianhill outside of Durban as test sites. Walker arranged for the choir to return to the United States in February 2003 for the 10th Conference on Retroviruses and Opportunistic Infections in Boston. Since then, the Sinikithemba Choir has toured the United States on a regular basis, visiting schools and churches in New York, Boston, Philadelphia, Washington DC, Hollywood, Chicago, and Indianapolis. During these trips they have been presented with significant and symbolic gifts, including a replica of the Liberty Bell in Philadelphia, in recognition of their musical contribution to humanity in the circumstances of HIV/AIDS. The choir has also toured the United Kingdom with Elton John. Back home in South Africa, the group members continue to raise their voices in educating and mobilizing communities against the menace of the disease through their songs, participating in hospital, community, and church social-action events as well as AIDS education and treatment-action campaigns. The group also has made three CD recordings and been the subject of several film documentaries.

In early 2006 the management of McCord Hospital determined that the choir had grown and become strong enough to function independently of the hospital. Thus the choir separated and the group was renamed Siphithemba, which in Zulu also means "We Give Hope." The group's new name was not very different from the original one; but it continued to echo the message of hope that the choir members bring to their audience through their music.

SIPHITHEMBA AS A COMMUNITY OF MUTUAL SUPPORT

As group members struggle individually with the exigencies of HIV/AIDS, the choir space comprises a bastion of hope and epitome of positive experience. Hence a strong sense of community characterizes the inner operations of Siphithemba. Members describe supporting one another in good and in bad times; in the celebration of occasions of life and death. An example is the *umsebenzi* (unveiling ritual)[3] that I attended one Saturday with the choir members at Sizwe's family home in Nyoni, a rural town about 130 kilometers north of Durban.

The event marked the unveiling of the tombs of Sizwe's grandmother and two siblings, all of whom had died around two years earlier. The *umsebenzi* was a two-day-long event that had started on Friday with the ritual slaughtering of three goats, one for each of the diseased, and culminated with the slaughtering of two cows on Saturday for a feast in which all the members of Sizwe's family and their village neighbors and friends participated. I had driven with Phakamile, Nomusa, and Nokthula on Saturday morning. Some of the men had gone with Sizwe on Friday afternoon to help slaughter the animals and to run the chores in preparation for Saturday. Most of us joined with Sizwe's family to help with some chores; I even got the duty of *ukuqoba*, cutting of the braid meat, a duty always reserved for an adult male in a gender-mixed environment. Later on Phakamile and Nomusa told me that Sizwe's family and people in attendance had praised Sizwe for his friends whose presence had contributed so much to the event. They even commented on my presence, my feeling at home among them, and my interest in taking a role in the ceremony. In effect the sense of family that the choir shared in being there for one another not only helped to shape the strong social identity of the group, but also helped members to renegotiate their relationships with their own families, who became more open toward them as a result and came to appreciate their human capabilities in spite of their HIV-positive status.

The act of being there for one another was also a useful support mechanism for members who had to disclose their status to their families. For example, the entire choir rallied round two sisters, Wicky and Phakamile Shabane, by traveling with them to their home in Highflats, a rural town of KwaZulu-Natal, and providing them a support system as they disclosed their status to their family. Status disclosure has been recognized in HIV/AIDS discourse as about the most difficult thing that people living with HIV/AIDS (PLWAs) have to deal with. For this reason PLWAs are encouraged to receive counseling before disclosure, and often are encouraged to find a "safe space and right moment" (Ntsimane 2006, 12–13) to disclose. For the members of Siphithemba, especially the two sisters Wicky and Phakamile, their safe space and right moment came particularly in the presence of choir members who functioned as surrogate family to one another, and who were in the struggle together.

THE MUSIC OF SIPHITHEMBA

The history and organization of Siphithemba can be characterized by the sense of community that allows its members to work and forge their experiences together in the HIV/AIDS struggle. Their success hinges mainly on their strong belief that God is with them to strengthen and to guide their efforts, as well as their hope and their determination to beat the perceived odds of being HIV-positive. While this form of hope and resilience is clearly evident in extra-musical contexts, the content of their music bears out their sense of community in the most significant way.

Song Genres: Composition and Adaptation

The process of song composition in Siphithemba exemplifies the group's communal ethos. With some songs, individuals have the opportunity to relate their own experiences in music and combine them with those of other members. There are also quite a number of songs that are composed by individuals, including several each by Phumulani and Sizwe, and one by Phakamile. These latter songs often come out of individual contemplative experience and are often characterized by a mixture of melancholy and hope; they speak, however, to the experiences and imaginations of all. An example of one such song is Phumulani's "Kulukhuni Ezweni" ("It's Hard in this World").

Kulukhuni 'madoda	It's hard men
Kulukhuni ezweni	It's hard in this world
Kulukhuni 'madoda	It's hard men
Oh kulukhuni	Oh it's hard
Kutheni na?	What is it?
Kutheni na, Thixo Somandla?	What is it, Father God?
We maZulu hlomani	Zulus be armed
We maZulu hlomani	Zulus be armed
Hayi hayi, we maZulu hlomani	Hayi hayi Zulus be armed
Siyahamba madoda	We're going men
Siyahamba siy'ekhaya ezulwini	We're going home to heaven
Kumnandi kunokuthula	It's nice and peaceful
Hayi kunokuthula	Hayi it is peaceful
Ekhaya lakho Baba	At your home Father
Ekhaya lakho Baba akufiwa	At your home Father there is no death
Ngifisa' ukuwubona	I wish to see [it]
Lombuso wezulu lakho	Your heavenly kingdom

This song presents a type of soliloquy, with the singer first appealing to men who share the difficulties that come with being HIV-positive in society; then holding a conversation with God that questions the reason for the scourge of the disease; rallying his compatriots to rise up and fight in a sudden outburst of energy and resilience; and ending with hope and a vision of spiritual triumph over earthly ordeals in the heavenly kingdom. One sees in the song a paradoxical relationship between the temporal and the spiritual order: the former full of trials and the latter as an escape. Yet the singer also shows a willingness and determination to engage in a struggle that must transform this temporal order into a state of survival, peace and tranquility, probably similar to that anticipated in the bliss of God's abode. Again this contemplative experience is not unique to Phumulani; rather, it is one with which other Siphithemba members easily identify.

A lot of Siphithemba's other songs are group composed. Based on information gathered from Phumulani and Xolani (another group member), and based on my observation of the choir at rehearsal sessions, group composition can happen in three ways: First, members can adapt, rearrange, and insert new messages into preexisting tunes, allowing then to "connect with what they already know" (Xolani Interview 2007). In a second, less common form of group composition, a new theme and textual message is hammered into a melody that has been made up and harmonized by the group through humming. These themes are often created out of individual experiences as well as issues members know that affect their community. Anybody who is present would be free to add to this message until a fully composed piece emerges. A third avenue the group takes for composition is to begin with a theme and let anybody write something about it based on personal and community experience; from there the choir integrates everybody's contributions into a single song. I will elaborate further, especially on the first two of these approaches.

This process of musical composition reiterates what scholars have long noted about African music as communally generated and performed (Henderson 1995, 136; Burnim 2006,

59; Nketia 1974, 21–34; Stone 2005, 64–67). The communality of the compositional process also shows that individual experience and effort can only engage with the struggle when joined with those experiences of other members of the community.

Adaptation of Preexisting Songs

The practice of adapting preexisting gospel songs follows similar processes of individual and collective effort. Sometimes choir members will make melodic and formal alterations to a song; but more frequently they will alter the text, substituting experiences from the community for the original lyrics. An example of one such song is "Izizwe Mazihlome" ("The Nation Must Arm"), adapted by Phumulani, Sizwe and Xolani. The song was originally composed by Obed Shangase, who had recorded it with the three some years earlier. The A section of the song is left completely intact, with the occasional substitution of *uSomandla* (God Almighty) for *uJesu* (Jesus). The name substitution dates to the group's performance at the 2003 10th Conference on Retroviruses and Opportunistic Infections in Boston, when one of the scientists—probably one of the organizers—came backstage to warn the choir against singing about Jesus in its performance. In Section B, *amakholwa* (Christians) is replaced entirely with *Izizwe* (the Nation), and *sathane* (devil) is replaced with *isifo* (disease or sickness). Sections C and C1 involve slight musical alterations along with textual quotations from choir's original numbers "You've Got to Know Your Status" and "Siyaphela Isizwe seNkosi" ("The Nation of the Lord is Dying"). The song ends with a recapitulation of section B.

A. Nguyelo uJeso (or Usomandla)	This is Jesus
Owayekhona ekuqaleni	Who was there in the beginning
Kuse nguye namhlanje	He is still here even now
B. Call: Izizwe mazihlome bo [*Improvisation*]	The nation must arm
Response: Izizwe azihlome nasi isifo sihlasele	The nation must arm for the disease attacking us
C: Izizwe mazihlome bo [*Improvisation*]	The nation must arm
R: Izizwe azihlome nalubhubhane luhlasele	The nation must arm for the disease attacking us
R: Izizwe azihlome naligciwane lihlasele	The nation must arm for the disease attacking us
C: Zingahlomi ngezibhamu [*Improvisation*]	They mustn't arm with guns
R: Zihlome ngolwazi lokuvikele ubhubhane	But with knowledge of disease prevention
C. Soli: Abstain	Abstain
Choir: Zihlome ngolwazi lokuvikele ubhubhane	Arm with knowledge of disease prevention
Soli: Be faithful	Be faithful
Choir: Zihlome ngolwazi lokuvikele ubhubhane	Arm with knowledge of disease prevention
Soli: Condomize	Condomize
Choir: Zihlome ngolwazi lokuvikele ubhubhane	Arm with knowledge of disease prevention
Soli: Vaccine	Vaccine

Choir: Zihlome ngolwazi lokuvikele ubhubhane	Arm with knowledge of disease prevention
C1. Soli S/A: Uma ufakijazi uzosinda	If you use condom you will be safe
Choir: Zihlome ngolwazi lokuvikele ubhubhane	Arm with knowledge of disease prevention
S/A Call: Uma ufakijazi uzophepha	If you use condom you'll be safe
Choir: Zihlome ngolwazi lokuvikele ubhubhane	Arm with knowledge of disease prevention
B. C: Izizwe mazihlome bo [*Improvisation*]	The nation must arm
R: Izizwe azihlome nasi isifo sihlasele	The nation must arm for the disease attacking us
C: Izizwe mazihlome bo [*Improvisation*]	The nation must arm
R: Izizwe azihlome nalubhubhane luhlasele	The nation must arm for the disease attacking us
R: Izizwe azihlome naligciwane lihlasele	The nation must arm for the disease attacking us
C: Zingahlomi ngezibhamu [*Improvisation*]	They mustn't arm with guns
R: Zihlome ngolwazi lokuvikele ubhubhane	Arm with knowledge of disease prevention

The choir's adaptation of this song leaves a feeling of discontinuity between the Christological message of the A section and the theme of militancy and struggle in the other sections. This seeming contradiction is nonetheless consistent with the original song's theme of struggle, and its call for faith in Jesus as a tool for fighting the devil. The same faith is evident here, but now the enemy is HIV. The choir's use of traditional and adapted gospel songs (in addition to its references to their original numbers) thus aims to connect local audiences with its messages through the use of a recognizable and meaningful musical form.

Siphithemba Song Themes

The thematic motives chosen for Siphithemba's songs reveal the group's consciousness about dealing with HIV/AIDS as a form of warfare, the collective effort required to wage the war, and what attitudes must go with it.

Songs on Struggle and Militarism

Siphithemba has appropriated Mandela's "next struggle" framework for its songs on HIV (Ndungane 2003, 58). They also contribute to HIV/AIDS discourse in South Africa by composing and performing some songs that are imbued with a strong sense of urgency and militancy. At least three of Siphithemba's songs have explicit references to arming and bearing of arms: "Kulukhuni Ezweni" ("It's Hard in this World"), "Izizwe Mazihlome" ("The Nation Must Arm"), and "Ikhalaphi" ("Where is the Cry From?"). At least one addresses fighting and victory ("Siyaphela Isizwe seNkosi" ["The Nation of the Lord is Dying"]); and "Nkonyane Kandaba" ("Royal Sons") is an actual battlefield song.[4] Of all of these, three take the form of gospel songs, while two are preexisting Zulu traditional songs. The gospel songs mostly urge arming with knowledge as a weapon for defeating HIV/AIDS; the traditional songs, however, especially "Nkonyane Kandaba," make explicit reference to actual battlefield experience.

Siphithemba's adaptation of "Nkonyane Kandaba" illustrates the linking of apartheid struggles with the current fight against HIV/AIDS in a subtle way:

Wathinta thina, wathinta abangasekufa	You've touched us who die no more
Safa saphenduka, saphenduk'injebomvu	We die and we return [angry] like the red dog
Solo: We Nkhonyane kandaba	Oh, you royal sons
Chorus: Kwanyakaza umkhomto	The spears are moving
we nkonyane kandaba	Oh, you royal sons

The song depicts a people who have been wounded in battle, but who return stronger and braver, ready to reengage the enemy with a determination to win the battle. In the musical and movie *Sarafina*, set against the backdrop of the 1976 Soweto students' uprising, Mbogeni Ngema inserted it as an interlude connecting one student's injurious encounter with South African police and the student movement's retaliation in an open street battle in Soweto. In a similar manner, Phumulani, the choir conductor, introduced the song at the 10th Conference on Retroviruses and Opportunistic Infections in Boston, after another member had given testimony of her battle with AIDS, thus signifying Siphithemba's determination to live and to defeat the virus in spite of its menace in their lives.

Faith and Hope

The name Siphithemba ("We Give Hope") addresses the faith and hope that the choir and its members bear. As already shown, this attitude was nurtured at the Sinkithemba AIDS clinic of McCord Hospital. All members of the choir express their faith and trust in God as the foundation of their struggle with the virus. In their music, themes of faith and hope are reflected in various ways. Sometimes a song begins with a seeming sense of despair (as illustrated above in "Kulukhuni Ezweni"), followed by a sudden surge in hope, and trust in what God is about to do. Hope, in this case, looks beyond temporary relief to the ultimate peace and tranquility of God's kingdom. An example of this emotional contour can be found in the song "Ngizohamba" ("I Am Going") as adapted by Phumulani:

Ngizohamba, ngiyekhaya	I am going, I am going home
Ngiyolungisa indawo	I shall be okay in that place
Ngoba ekhaya likaBaba	Because at [my] Father's house
Kunezindlu eziningi	There are many houses
Rhythm change with dance	
Call/Response: Maningakhathazeki	Do not worry
Kholwani uBaba	Believe in (my) Father
Izinhliziyo zenu mazingakhathazeki	Your hearts should not worry
Izinhliziyo zenu zingakkathazeki	Your hearts should not worry

An eschatological vision therefore mitigates the feeling of despair, while instilling faith and a sense of hope in God's love and care.

The messages of hope and faith in this and other songs are not meant for the singers alone. They are also meant to bring hope to their audience. The HIV/AIDS pandemic has created an unprecedented form of depression especially in South Africa's black community, comparable only to that experienced under apartheid. According to Mandla Mdabe, a minister in the Methodist Church and HIV/AIDS counselor at the Prince Mshiyeni Hospital at Umlazi, it is hard to see any family or individual who has not been affected by AIDS directly or indirectly (Mdabe Interview 2007). Thus the choir members aim to share their collective perspective with their audience and community: living by faith and hope in God, they suggest, will offer the ultimate answer to the problem.

On Behavior Change

The need for behavior change as a major preventive tool against the spread of HIV/AIDS has become a dominant theme in the current HIV/AIDS discourse. For Siphithemba, however, preventive measures begin with people knowing their status. Thus, in their song "You've Got to Know Your Status" by Phumulani, the choir urges people to know their HIV serostatus and respond accordingly by striving to stay negative if they are negative, or think positively if they are positive.

KNOW YOUR STATUS by Phumulani

A. *You've go to know your status*
'Cause we know our status
You've got to know your status
'Cause we know our status
You've got to know your status
We all know our status

B. *If you're negative, stay negative*
If you're positive, think positive
Abstain
Be faithful
Condomize

C. *[Soprano voice]: Take your medicine*
Choir: Even if you're feeling better
Noma usuzizwa uphila [Even if you're feeling better]

The first section of the song recommends testing, while the second section prescribes the ABC formula as a necessary follow-up to knowing one's status. The third section takes up the issue of treatment; in actual performance, however, various voices overlay the melody with phrases from the A and B sections: "you've got to know your status," "abstain," "be faithful," and "condomize." Siphithemba's conviction that preventive measures begin with knowledge of one's status is borne out in the members' crusade for comprehensive testing in their communities. In interviews, Phumulani, Phakamile, Nomusa and others each testified to having successfully persuaded their family members and friends to test and to seek help from appropriate places.

The case of South Africa is exacerbated however by devastating poverty inherited from decades of apartheid and economic marginalization of Africans in part through the migrant labor system (Meadows 2003, 154). In my experience living in South Africa while conducting this research, I have seen that the migrant labor system is yet to vanish completely amid the progress by the ANC-led government in human and economic development. Even in the Catholic Pastoral Center where I lived as I conducted this research, almost all the black male and female service staff lived in single rooms in the center without their partners and children. They did not have enough time during the month to travel long distances to the rural areas to visit their families, so they remained in the center during their brief 1-1/2 to 2 days off per fortnight. In addition to the migrant workers who are exposed to the dangers of indulging in behaviors inimical to their health, the wives, husbands, and teenage children they leave at home are all in similar danger. Many young people in South Africa grow up without proper parental supervision, more often than not due to parents being away from their families. The situation has been worsened by the massive post-1994 influx of rural South Africans into urban areas in the hope of making a better living. But often people do not get the better life in the city that they dream about. The cities tend to teem with migrant sex workers alongside domestic workers and service laborers (PACSA 2004). There are therefore huge adverse consequences emanating from dangerous lifestyles. The above situation is succinctly captured in Siphithemba's traditional song "Isiyalo" ("Advice"):

A. Call: Asikho isiyalo la izalwakhona,	There's no advice whence she comes
Resp: Asikh' isiyalo la izalwakhona.	There's no advice whence she comes
Chorus: Iphum' ekhaya igqoke kahle	She comes from home well-dressed
Ifike ngalena kwendaba,	She comes across the hill
Ekumule idilozi ilibeke phansi	She strips pants and puts it down
Thubhobho i-game.	For a twenty-cent game
Asikh' isiyalo la izalwakhona	There's no advice whence she comes

B. (*call improvisations with same response*)	
Call: Ayivumi ngishela kwaMasondo ayivumi	She KwaMasondo rejects my proposal
Resp: Ngishela kwaMasondo ayivumi	I propose to KwaMasondo but she refuses
Call: Le'ntombi yenzani?	What is the young lady doing?
Resp: Ngishela kwaMasondo ayivumi	I propose to KwaMasondo but she refuses

In this song KwaMasondo has no parental guidance from her home and blames her reckless sexual behavior on a lack of sage advice. Section B highlights the fact that indulging in this lifestyle is also responsible for many single-parent families in South Africa. One wonders why this girl rejects the marriage proposal. Probably because she believes she will make a better living out of the "twenty-cent game" (prostitution) and having multiple partners than by settling with a single man.

On Stigma and Denialism

Denialism manifests itself at individual and public levels of policymaking (for the latter, see Nattrass 2007). The denialism that I am concerned with here—and as far as Siphithemba's music is concerned—takes place at the local level. Siphithemba members are in agreement that denialism stems from crass ignorance: ignorance of one's status, and what I call a pathological entrenchment in the myths about HIV/AIDS. These myths in turn fuel a sense of stigma that confounds containment of the virus. The choir's call for people to know their status thus becomes a call against living in denial of the reality of the disease. Unfortunately many South Africans seem to see testing largely for its penchant to produce a positive result, rather than about striving to stay negative as the choir's song suggests. My conversations with several young people in the course of this research reinforce the significance of status anxiety in the fear to test. The danger inherent in this form of anxiety is perpetual anxiety: stress, depression, and despair particularly with persons who may have lost intimate partners and close relatives to the virus. For this reason the use of verse from St. John's gospel 8:32: "You shall know the truth, and the truth shall make you free," has become a mainstay against HIV/AIDS denialism in church quarters. Rev. Mandla Mdabe drums it hard during most of his motivational talks at HIV/AIDS workshops.[5] The Cape Town Anglican Archbishop Njongonkulu Ndungane, meanwhile, asserted that "to accept less than knowing [our status and] our partner's status is to risk our suicide" (2003, 61). Although Siphithemba has no song that incorporates John 8:32, some other groups have produced songs that speak strongly about this phenomenon of stress resulting from refusal to know one's status. A theater group from Clermont, which is also based at the St. Clement Catholic Church, incorporates songs and dance in their theatre productions designed for HIV/AIDS education. One of their songs makes explicit use of this biblical verse thus:

> *The Truth shall set you free*
> *Know your HIV status now*
> *Be free from stress, go for blood test*
> *So that you could know your status*

On another level, denialism in South Africa is fueled by a common attitude of men who tend to believe that HIV is a woman's problem, as well as some "culturally related" form of myth that HIV/AIDS is caused by witchcraft.[6] From their own experiences, Siphithemba members understand the dangers inherent in this form of denial. Some of the women in the group tell their personal stories about how, upon learning about their HIV-positive status through prenatal testing, they were deserted by their male partners who denied having anything to do with their being infected. Many of these men likely ended up putting other women at risk by this act of recklessness. Such concerns also explain why many of the choir members have embarked on persuading family members and relatives—and successfully so—to know their status by testing.

As far as denialism comes out of ignorance—that of refusal to know one's status, as well as ignorance arising from myths about HIV/AIDS—so it also breeds forms of stigma built on ignorance. Two types of stigma are particularly important to discuss here: that PLWAs are positive because they are sinners, and that PLWAs are weak and coffin-bound and cannot live productive lives. The first form of stigma arises from the myth that HIV/AIDS is a curse from God as punishment for the sins of people. Consequently those known to be HIV-positive have had to bear the extra burden of being considered victims of their own immorality.

The act of looking at PLWAs as coffin-bound, meanwhile, is largely based on pictures of bedridden, terminally ill patients that are commonly seen in the media. Siphithemba members have defied this picture by becoming role models for a positive lifestyle. For them, positive living meant taking their treatment seriously, being economically self-reliant, and engaging in industry. The opportunity to tour North America and Europe has also helped them to dispel the fears that people have of them as bound to imminent death or as unproductive. In fact it has even earned them envy and jealousy from people who have moralistic attitudes toward them. It was in response to this attitude that Sizwe wrote the song "Sizwile Ukuthi" ("We Hear That"):

Sizwile ukuthi thina bayasizonda	We hear that they hate us
Kudumizwe lonke	It is all over the world
Ukuthi thina sizenza ncono	That we have pride
Soprano: Higher, higher, oh we are going	Higher, higher, oh we are going
Alto: Sinqamu lamazwe thina	We go all places
Refrain: We are going, going higher and higher	We are going, going higher and higher
Trio: Bayosala abanomona	We leave the jealous
Basala bekhuluma izindaba zabantu	We leave them talking about us
Refrain: We are going, going higher and higher	We are going, going higher and higher
Sop Solo: Bonke labantu (improvisation)	All of them
Refrain: Bayazithanda izindaba	Love news [gossiping]
Bayazikhuluma izindaba	They are gossiping

Clearly this song shows the extent to which Siphithemba fights against being stigmatized. The song is a response to those who look down upon them because of their status; but it is also a celebration of their achievements amid the perceived odds of living with HIV and AIDS. Thus the song becomes an expression of pride, and another example of their effort to articulate the sense of resilience in performance.

SUMMARY AND CONCLUSION

In this chapter I have attempted to link Siphithemba to the culture of singing and the role of the church in human struggles in South Africa. Yet Siphithemba must be understood as having a distinctive mode of existence and operation, which is shaped by members' common experience of HIV/AIDS. As a community engaged in a struggle against the disease, Siphithemba's members succinctly appropriate the struggle discourse that still informs the political landscape of South Africa and its social productions, and give it new meaning within the context of HIV/AIDS. The choir's musical engagement with HIV/AIDS can be construed as what Gregory Barz has characterized as "singing for life" (Barz 2006a). When its members sing for life, they give hope of life to themselves, as well as to the world that has continued to witness the onslaught of the AIDS epidemic. As the struggle continues, their fervent hope for a future global conquering of the virus will not be swayed.

25

Young and Wise in Accra, Ghana

A MUSICAL RESPONSE TO AIDS

Angela Scharfenberger (Indiana University)

Many ethnographers have written about the ways oral narratives serve as a primary venue for the transmission of important social messages in African expressive traditions. Through choral performances, the Young and Wise Inspirational Choir in Accra, Ghana communicates messages regarding the prevention of HIV and AIDS. The choir's aesthetic choices reflect a tradition of personal and social expression through oral narratives, while integrating common Ghanaian music genres, including popular music and church choir traditions, and their performances carry both the weight and appeal of those genres. I will describe the social context of performance by the Young and Wise Inspirational Choir in this chapter, while also examining the role of the ethnographer as an advocate in ethnomusicological fieldwork and writing. How are scholars accountable to those with whom we work? How do we use the resources available to us to promote the efforts of our consultants? Such inquiries are not new to the discipline of ethnomusicology (Alviso 2003, Seeger 2008), yet I hope that the particularities of my brief fieldwork encounter with the Young and Wise Inspirational Choir will offer a new lens through which to address these concerns.

On July 26, 2006, I documented a performance of the Young and Wise Inspirational Choir, and conducted an informal interview with the group following the performance. I argue that my integral role as the ethnographer in this study is to support the goals of the ensemble through whatever means I can: in this case, by writing a chapter in a scholarly volume. As Gregory Barz stated in his work with people singing about HIV and AIDS in Uganda, "faced with the dilemma of representation, I choose to embrace ethnography, not only because I can write, but for my partnership and solidarity with the individuals detailed in this study, I have to write" (Barz 2006, 2). While ethnographic writing is imperfect, I argue that it is one possible means of highlighting communicative performance as it affects people and their choices in local arenas.

My case study, based on brief fieldwork with the members of the Young and Wise Inspirational Choir, introduces a dialogue examining the role of the ethnographer as an advocate. I wish for the voices of the members of the choir to speak through this chapter; by presenting their songs, and contextualizing their message I also hope to, in Barz's words, work in solidarity with them.

MEDICAL ETHNOMUSICOLOGY

Gregory Barz's *Singing for Life* examines the phenomenon of musical responses to AIDS in Uganda through lyrical analysis, ethnographic description, and lengthy excerpts from interviews. Barz argues that these grassroots musical responses to AIDS have been partly responsible for the remarkable decline in the overall HIV infection rate in Uganda. He further contextualizes these performances in the humanity of the people with whom he has worked, emphasizing their impoverished living conditions as well as their extraordinary personal stories. Barz's book helped significantly to advance the subfield of medical ethnomusicology, and challenged scholars to document grassroots AIDS musical responses as meaningful, effective ways of addressing the disease (Barz 2006a).

In so doing, Barz joined a growing advocacy movement among the current generation of ethnomusicologists, as expressed by Ricardo Alviso:

> I would argue that the purpose of research should be toward some end that will benefit humanity, including the people we take from—a concept many call *reciprocity*. Anything less only serves to perpetuate unequal relationships and cultural hegemony. Too often, ethnomusicologists acknowledge and analyze the issues faced by the people they work with, yet downplay a responsibility to help them. (2003, 96)

I endeavor to work from this starting point of advocacy, extending out from a performance in the ethnographic moment to consider the influences and consequences of such a performance fully. Further, it is my hope that by contextualizing these performances in the historical and social background of the AIDS epidemic and in AIDS awareness campaigns in Ghana, I can offer a meaningful perspective on the nature of HIV/AIDS advocacy in a region of Africa that lies outside the area of greatest prevalence.

AIDS IN GHANA

In 2006, the year that I visited Ghana, UNAIDS reported that among Ghanaian adults, an estimated 300,000 people were HIV-positive, with a national prevalence rate of 2.3 percent. Approximately 25,000 Ghanaian children were living with HIV. The highest rates were in the eastern region of the country and the lowest rates were in the northern area. Among youth, ages 15–24, 52 percent of males and 32 percent of females reported using condoms; this was about average for other countries in West Africa (UNAIDS 2006). When I again accessed UNAIDS information in 2009, many of the Ghanaian statistics had declined, indicating a 1.9 percent prevalence rate for adults, 260,000 living with HIV/AIDS, and 17,000 children living with the disease (UNAIDS 2009). Young women (aged 15–24) accounted for 1.3 percent of the 260,000 adults living with HIV/AIDS, while young men accounted for .4 percent (UNAIDS 2009).

Of course, there are several ways to interpret such AIDS statistics. Some scholars suggest that these figures are low, particularly regarding HIV prevalence rates. Nonetheless, in comparison with countries such as Lesotho and Zimbabwe, which have much higher prevalence rates, even a possible underestimation in Ghana creates a less dire portrait. I do not minimize the impact of HIV and AIDS on those Ghanaians and their family members who struggle every day. However, this comparison to other African countries, especially some of those represented in this volume, leads to important distinctions in social commentary about, and responses to, the disease as exemplified by the performance choices of the Young and Wise Inspirational Choir.

From my brief experience with the Choir, I saw no evidence that HIV/AIDS had affected members' lives directly. Instead, the choice to perform music about HIV and AIDS appeared to be motivated by their association with Planned Parenthood of Ghana (perhaps in part due to the financial and material resources available to them through that association), and their desire to insert themselves in a trend of national HIV/AIDS awareness campaigns in Ghana that were extremely popular at the time of my fieldwork. Performing music with HIV/AIDS social commentary thus became simultaneously a means of plugging into a longstanding oral tradition in Ghana, a motivation for associating with a modestly funded international organization (through the International Federation of Planned Parenthood [IFPP]), and a way of aligning themselves with Ghanaian popular stars and their videos, with the hope of securing such fame and fortune for themselves. In the sections that follow, I illustrate how the Young and Wise Inspirational Choir accessed these different streams and influences through their music, and the ways that these connections informed their decisions within the composition process. I will then discuss the role of the ethnographer and examine how advocacy might play a role in the ethnographer's work.

AIDS CAMPAIGNS IN GHANA

Ghanaian folklorist Kwesi Yankah has written extensively on the forms of public communication in Ghanaian politics, arts, and media. In an article examining the oral rhetoric surrounding taboo topics such as sexual decisions and sexually transmitted diseases, Yankah argues that messages regarding taboo subjects cannot be addressed openly due to the cultural stigma surrounding disease (2004, 196). Messages that cannot be spoken can, however, be interwoven into song lyrics or enacted through theater, video, and other imagery. John Lwanda, in an examination of music and AIDS in Malawi, argued further that current popular music practices must be considered within a historical continuum of "vibrant orality"—which links modern forms of music performance to early oral poets and historians (2005). Oral traditions such as spontaneous songs and nighttime storytelling once served to educate young and old through moral lessons and mockery in Ghana. By 2006, however, public media such as billboards, music, TV ads, and music videos had joined these other forms of public education. During my fieldwork, for example, billboards with AIDS prevention messages were common, particularly in urban areas such as Legon, near the University of Ghana, that attracted young people.

In Ghana, young people are likely to learn about AIDS through one of these modern forms of "vibrant orality." As early as 1992, John Hopkins University and the Ghana Ministry of Health "used popular highlife music and concert parties during [a] family planning campaign" with apparent success (Amu 2001, 94). The partnership's campaign theme song, "Awo dodo," by S. K. Oppong became a national hit (ibid.). According to one 1997 study, moreover, "TV/Radio" was the second most common way that Ghanaian "street children" (who were largely adolescents) learned about AIDS (Apt and Blavo 1997). When considered as part of the continuum of vibrant orality, it is clear that such forms of communication as music and music videos are often the most effective means of reaching Ghanain youth.

By the turn of the twenty-first century, the use of entertainment to communicate messages on health issues "had become commonplace within the Ghanaian culture" (Amu 2001, 92). A collaboration between several Ghanaian organizations, including the Ghana Ministry of Health, and Johns Hopkins University produced the campaign, "Stop AIDS/Love Life" (Johns Hopkins Bloomberg School of Public Health 2009). This campaign was launched in 2001 with the release of a hiplife music video that involved the "All Stars of Ghana." Amu described the genre of the video as positioned in the "highlife-hiplife-rap vein"; the use of the music video medium as well as hiplife and rap styles indicates strategic choices in communication media that resonated with young people (Amu 2001, 95). According to the Johns Hopkins Web site, condom sales from Ghana's largest manufacturer increased significantly following the release of this video, "jump[ing] from an average of 2.7 million every six months to a record 6.6 million in the six months ending June 1, 2001, illustrating an increase of 144 percent" (Johns Hopkins University Bloomberg School Of Public Health 2009). These statistics illustrate that campaigns involving music videos and other forms of "vibrant orality" that appeal to Ghanaian youth are indeed an effective mode not only of communicating to young people, but also in inspiring changes in behavior. Further, embedding such messages in songs and images shows consistency with cultural taboos against speaking about disease publicly (Yankah 2004).

PLANNED PARENTHOOD OF GHANA (PPAG)

In July 2006, I became acquainted with the Young and Wise Inspirational Choir through Michael Tagoe, a theater major at the University of Ghana's School of Performing Arts in Legon. A soft-spoken man in his early twenties, Tagoe was a peer educator at the Young and Wise center in Laterbiokorshie, in the greater Accra region. Five Young and Wise centers opened across the country, sponsored by the Planned Parenthood Association of Ghana (PPAG) (which in turn was financially supported largely through the IFPP). PPAG has been active in Ghana since 1967, and in 2001 initiated a program to focus its services on youth. This decision was aligned with the IFPP Vision 2000 Strategic Plan, which included the directive to "provide quality SRH (sexual and reproductive health) services to young adults" (Planned Parenthood Association of Ghana 2006).

These Young and Wise centers were comprehensive facilities for the distribution of information and services related to sexual and reproductive health. The Laterbiokorshie center, for example, was a well-kept compound consisting of several buildings and a large cobblestone courtyard. Within the compound were a recreation room, computer lab, library, and a confidential health clinic with inexpensive condoms on every counter. A primary strategy of these Young and Wise centers was to develop programs that appealed to the local youth. The center was welcoming, with a large TV for watching movies and football matches, and it had a computer room modeled after a Ghanaian Internet cafe. All of these elements represented PPAG strategic decisions intended to make the center inviting to young people.

As part of their programs, the center sponsored several performance groups, including an Inspirational Choir, a women's choir, a Drama Group, and a "Culture Group."[1] Churches and other organizations invited these performance groups to their functions to educate their members on sexual and reproductive health through songs, dance, and drama.

The Inspirational Choir consisted of approximately fifteen youths, ages 14–20. A young man directed the choir; while he was clearly the leader, it appeared to be an informal arrangement. Another young man accompanied the choir on a small Casio keyboard with a synthesized drum track; this was the sole instrumental accompaniment. The group's songs were written almost entirely in English, while a few were sung in Twi, the most commonly spoken indigenous language in Ghana. The members of this group, unlike some of their counterparts in other African countries, did not self-identify as being HIV-positive or as having AIDS. Nor did their songs or activities reveal personal experiences with people who were HIV-positive. When I questioned them regarding what influenced their song lyrics, their answers were ambiguous; their ideas did not seem to have a specific source of inspiration. One member simply stated that ideas came to him and he put them on paper.

INTERTEXTUALITY IN THE SONG COMPOSITION PROCESS

In the emerging scholarly dialogue on music and AIDS in Africa, the concept of intertextuality is a useful analytical tool. Richard Bauman addressed this concept through the framework of genre. To Bauman, genre appears as "a set of conventional guidelines for dealing with recurrent communicative exigencies" (2000, 85). The transference of the guidelines of one genre onto another genre is a means for performers to index that genre, bringing into a performance that genre's contexts and norms. In this example, the Young and Wise Inspirational Choir blended two genres: popular hiplife music and Ghanaian Christian choral traditions. By drawing on these two genres, choir members maximized the delivery of their message.

In an assessment of Ghanaian popular music, African music scholar John Collins has outlined significant generational factors, which are determined by sonic characteristics. The *highlife* genre, which was widely popular between the 1930s and the 1970s, consisted of guitars, polyrhythmic bell and clapping patterns characteristic of traditional drum ensembles (and still widely used in Ghanaian popular music), and lyrics in Twi. Highlife gradually declined in popularity, and gave way to new genres that Collins describes as *techno-pop* styles, including hiplife (2002, 69). *Hiplife* features songs composed in "vernacular language" (2002, 71), particularly the sections in which the lyrical delivery is in spoken word or chant style, accompanied by drum machines and synthesizers. Collins argues that these language conventions and electronic sounds give hiplife its "distinctive up-to-date stamp" (2002, 71).

Ghanaian church music also engages several idiomatic musical performance characteristics. Ghanaian Christian choral traditions are characterized by short phrases of call and response; this is common to both Ghanaian traditional religious practices and African American gospel traditions. A high-pitched female vocalist performs the call, and the choral response utilizes three- or four-part harmony.

The Young and Wise Inspirational Choir incorporated stylistic features of both Ghanaian Christian choral traditions and hiplife into the song "HIV Is Real." The song begins with a keyboardist playing block chords to the reggae rhythm of a drum machine. A solo female singer, meanwhile, engages a vocal delivery style often heard in Ghanaian churches, singing in a high register with a nasal tone. As is common in Ghanaian churches, the choir responds to the soloist during the chorus with rich vocal harmonies. "HIV Is Real" also features a hiplife middle section, with a rapping female vocalist, followed by a characteristically hiplife gruff male voice. As the male soloist raps and increases in volume, other members of the choir raise the energy to a peak with shouts of encouragement:

HIV
Is killing us
If we don't do something
We will die
Do you know what is alive?

Why don't we
Rise up now
As we fight,
Then that is
Young and wise
We just want to do

HIV is spreading is so fast
Rise and fly, fly to the last
Cause a life is sustained
So make no mistake
'Cause HIV is real

TWI RAP SECTION

Yareε no kye wo a	If the disease catches you
εte se AIDS sε owuo.	AIDS looks like death
HIV yareε emu yε duro	HIV disease is heavy
εkye wo a	If it catches you
εsε wo ara, efiri wo ara	It's up to you, you are to blame
Amanfɔ,	(My) countrymen
Yareε bɔne bi aba	A bad sickness has come
Na yεfrε no AIDS	That is called AIDS
εre kum amanfoɔ	It is killing citizens
Obia bɔ no ho ban	You should protect yourself
Ɔntwie ne ho mfiri adwambɔ	You should pull yourself away from promiscuity
Yoose kondoms	Use condoms
Sε AIDS kye wo a	If AIDS gets you
Na efiri wo ara	Then you are to blame
Nua, bra Young and Wise	Brother/Sister, come to Young and Wise

There is significance in the group's choice to use Twi or English in different parts of the songs. The choral English sections were sung to a catchy, light-hearted melody, utilizing a narrative form referencing a non-specific "we." The Twi hiplife section, in contrast, used a more direct, imperative linguistic mode. Rather than a third-person narrative, the Twi section addressed "you." During this section, moreover, the language became more explicit with phrases such as "yoose kondoms" ("use condoms") or "εte se AIDS sε awuo" ("AIDS looks like death").

The song combines a communal, hand-clapping church hymn style with the hiplife-chanting soloist in order to signify each of those genres. The group's combination of Ghanaian Christian choral traditions and hiplife styles encourages the participation of young audiences who are familiar with these genres. By adopting a reggae beat, the Choir accesses a genre that is popular with their audiences. With the frequent repetition of the chorus, audiences can join in the response singing. And with the formula of the hiplife rap section, group members can build the performance energy through shouts of encouragement. All of these elements were adopted with the intent of encouraging audience participation in the performance. In accordance with Ghanaian performance aesthetics, audience participation is key for the expression of messages in performance, including ideas about HIV prevention. The Young and Wise Inspirational Choir was aware of Ghanaian media initiatives addressing HIV and AIDS; the choir director expressed to me the hope that they would be able to record these songs and "launch an album." Members of the group recognized that singing about AIDS was a hot topic in Ghana at the time, and hoped that by channeling their talent and creativity in this particular musical direction, they might have increased opportunity for success.

GLOBAL IMAGINATION

Anthropologists John and Jean Comaroff have argued that scholarly discussions of globalization and modernity must consider the agency of local actors as active decision makers. "HIV Is Real," in its demonstration of multiple musical influences, illustrates the ways in which these lines between the local and global "shift as processes of engagements take their course" (Comaroff and Comaroff 1992, 97). Arjun Appadurai acknowledged the relevance of this globalized reality in terms of local civil organizations situated internationally, such as the Young and Wise's relationship with Planned Parenthood:

> As the imagination as a social force itself works across national lines to produce locality as a spatial fact and as a sensibility, we see the beginnings of social forms without either the predatory mobility of unregulated capital or the predatory stability of many states. (2000, 6)

The members of the Young and Wise Inspirational Choir made musical choices that maximized their message in a modern world. Through creative performative decisions that appealed to their generation, they imagined an aesthetic that they enjoyed themselves, while hoping that such an aesthetic would also be more broadly marketable.

The Choir aligned their music with a larger scheme of development and AIDS awareness campaigns, such as the aforementioned Stop AIDS/Love Life campaign, which was widely broadcasted in Ghana at that time. The members of the group told me that they just "wrote down what they thought of," yet they were clearly hoping to receive the attention that other AIDS awareness songs had garnered. Their ambition to produce an album, they noted, was only "waiting on some funds." They were aware of the significance and the relevance of their songs and hoped that singing such messages would also be a means of achieving fame and fortune. In other words, they *imagined* that singing about HIV/AIDS would be their golden opportunity.

TRANSFORMATION THROUGH METAPHORS

How does the performance of the Inspirational Choir effect change in the world? How does it influence the members of the choir themselves? I suggest that the incorporation of metaphor is an essential element in transformation. Gregory Barz also recognized the power of metaphor to empower performers. Barz found that Ugandan musicians could mask concepts about HIV/ AIDS through metaphors of insects, animals, and nature. According to Barz, "[t]his linguistic technique often presents an opportunity for a singer to talk openly—albeit behind a transparent linguistic veil—about health-related issues" (2006a, 132).

I argue that the use of metaphor by the Young and Wise Inspirational Choir activates a similar process. The act of vocalizing certain ideas, particularly in repetition, can be personally transformative for both the performers and the audience. As words are sung and heard repeatedly, their message becomes more powerful.

For example, in the song "We Are True," the Choir uses the metaphor of a journey to describe the reality of someone who is HIV-positive. This metaphor empowers the everyday decision that adolescents face in protecting themselves against HIV by comparing them with the meaningful decisions along an epic journey. It is a warning not to be tempted by the daily trials of the storm, to remain "true," by choosing appropriate sexual behavior. Through this metaphor, the choir members inspire themselves, as well as those around them, to stay "true," to make good decisions:

> It's like a day (journey)
> That's never ceased to end
> But finally you are here
> And we know that you will tell a story some day
>
> Through the storm
> Through the night
> Many, many trials
> And temptations
> In all these things,
>
> We are true, we are true, we are true

This case study illustrates the ways in which local actors—in this case the members of the Young and Wise Inspirational Choir—ultimately make decisions about the communication of messages that are both acceptable and accessible to their audiences. The choir is situated at the confluence of media initiatives such as the "Stop AIDS/Love Life" campaign, the aesthetics of the Christian choir tradition, and hiplife music: a meeting of both genre and moral positioning. This process creates an "intertextual gap" (Bauman 2000, 86)—between the hiplife and church choir genres—which creates an opportunity for the choir members to express themselves creatively and to insert their current interests and motives. By juxtaposing the two genres, the Inspirational Choir creates a bridge between two entities that have at times been at odds: Planned Parenthood and conservative Christian denominations. Ghanaian youth steeped in the cultural practice of "vibrant orality" engage with multiple strands of oral tradition to actively comment on a social problem in Ghana. In the end, their means is an acceptable one in their community where they are invited to perform for HIV/AIDS education events.

CONCLUSION

Since the time of my fieldwork, foreign funding has continued to play a significant role in the prevention of HIV and AIDS in Ghana, particularly regarding sexual and reproductive health services for young people. According to the Planned Parenthood of Ghana website, the International Federation of Planned Parenthood remains its main funding source, but it also draws from several additional sources on the national and international levels, including the African Youth Alliance, the Danish International Development Agency, the Ghana AIDS Commission, USAID, and UNICEF (Planned Parenthood Association of Ghana 2009). Other organizations have invested in short-term projects; for example, Johns Hopkins University was a major contributor to and co-designer of the Stop AIDS/Love Life national campaign. And in 2009, the NGO Japan International Cooperation Agency (JICA) completed a four-year project with the Ghana AIDS Commission (GAC), implemented by the PPAG (Planned Parenthood Association of Ghana 2009). JICA's project focused on a methodology, Behaviour Change Communication, defined as "information dissemination through mass and interpersonal communication" (Planned Parenthood Association of Ghana 2009). PPAG, as the implementing agency for these programs, continues to support youth performance groups such as the Inspirational Choir in order to fulfill its mission to develop communications with the greatest potential to reach and impact young people.

To that end, many of the activities of the PPAG have increasingly focused on music, performing arts, and verbal arts. One news site highlighted a Young and Wise singing competition in the eastern region of Ghana in which choirs from post-secondary schools focused on the theme, "Promoting Positive Lifestyles for Young People" (GNA 2004a). These competitions occurred in regions across the country, with the winners going on to compete nationally. All participating schools received prizes from the PPAG, and the school officials used the competition as an opportunity to remind youth that abstinence was the only "sure means" of protection; officials also reminded adults to support young people in making good decisions. Similarly, another article highlighted a secondary school debate competition in Cape Coast, on the theme, "Adolescent Reproductive Health and Poverty Alleviation," as part of a "Young and Wise week" anniversary (GNA 2004b). These competitions are a cornerstone of the PPAG's methodology to actively engage young people and collaborate with local schools.

PPAG's Young and Wise also engaged the Inspirational Youth Choir associated with the Kwame Nkruma University of Science and Technology (KNUST) in Kumasi to assist its efforts. Formed in 1993, the popular choir continued to grow to a membership of fifty youth. In their collaborations with the PPAG, the Kumasi-based Inspirational Choir wrote at least two songs: "AIDS Is Real" and "Young and Wise." The songs, similar to those performed by the Laterbiorkorshie Young and Wise Inspirational Choir, blended a variety of stylistic features. Interestingly, their songs drew on both traditional Ghanaian rhythms—such as the popular drum and dance recreation style, *kpanlogo*, utilizing the associated bell and clapping pattern— and hiplife, and its characteristic vocal delivery and song structure.

The music videos accompanying these songs were posted on YouTube in 2007, featuring flashy videography with modern stylistic elements and framing, such as panning shots across the musicians and nature settings, "freeze framing" on singers to enhance the emotive power of key lyrics, and the presentation of written lyrics or images on the screen (Youtube 2009). They also engaged another approach to intertextuality by drawing on signifiers of both traditional and modern Ghanaian life. A group of women in modern outfits performed a choreographed dance next to an ensemble of men playing traditional drums. Young men wearing the ritual *kente* cloth slung over their shoulders, as would be common attire for chiefs and elders during ceremonies and special occasions, sang next to young men in Western clothes. By drawing on traditional and modern clothing and music styles, the choir members situated themselves firmly in both. While highlighting a connection to tradition and the past, they also exhibited a modern flair that connected them with the future. Further, they exemplified a "vibrant orality"—tapping into this hybrid medium to communicate their message to an ever-widening audience via Internet sites such as YouTube.

As ethnomusicologist-advocates, our role is to support the efforts of those with whom we are privileged to work. Gregory Barz has suggested that the challenge is to find ways to walk with our consultants and colleagues and to support them in the ways that are most helpful to them. Perhaps, as Elaine Lawless has argued, we can support them through a collaborative ethnographic process (1993). Or as Ricardo Alviso has stated, our support can come through "reciprocity"—giving back to the communities with whom we work (2003). Or, as the Young and Wise Inspirational Choir director suggested to me, and following in the footsteps of many ethnomusicologists before me, perhaps we should help our consultants make an album, such as Paul Berliner's *Soul of Mbira* with Zimbabwean *mbira* players (1978) or Anthony Seeger's *Indian Music: Suya Vocal Art* (2008). In the case of short-term research, and with a group not directly affected by AIDS, the appropriate choice of advocacy has been a challenging one for me. Is the act of being present, paying attention, and being an active witness to a group's efforts by writing about them in acceptable academic venues an effective form of advocacy? I am not always convinced of the impact of scholarly activities. Yet, faced with the limitations of both my fieldwork and resources in this situation, I have resigned myself to this outcome. I chose to reflect on my research with the Young and Wise Inspirational Choir through an academic paper, presented at two national scholarly conferences (Society for Ethnomusicology 2008 and the African Studies Association 2008), which gave me the opportunity to contribute to this volume. It is my hope that through the act of writing, I have highlighted a modern African expressive form, given voice to a growing number of people responding to AIDS in creative, grassroots venues, and continued the dialogue on the meaning of advocacy in the work of future generations of ethnomusicologists.

26

Singing as Social Order

THE EXPRESSIVE ECONOMY OF HIV/AIDS

IN MBARARA, UGANDA

Judah M. Cohen (Indiana University)

MBARARA, UGANDA, JULY 28, 2004

I arrived at the regional branch of The AIDS Support Organization (TASO) around 9 A.M., prepared to view and videotape a performance of the drama group with which I had been working for the previous month. I almost immediately ran into Grace,[1] a member of the group, who was sitting in the canteen just inside the entrance. Her condition had worsened. It seems she had come down with a cold the previous day and was developing laryngitis when I saw her. I reminded her that I was leaving in a few days, and our farewell conversation included writing our information down in each other's notebooks; it seems everyone carried small notebooks around to record their thoughts, write down their schedules, and keep the details of their lives in order. As we ended our discussion, Grace said: "Pray for me: I will be starting ARVs very soon." I told her I would.

I went a few feet down the hall into the day center, a medium-sized multipurpose room, where two drama group members and a few others were waiting for the rest of the group to arrive. Clara, another member, came over and hugged me. In my halting Runyankore, I told her it was good to see her. Several people laughed at my awkwardness with the language, but the exchange certainly broke the ice for those who had been eyeing me with uncertainty. It was good I came, I was told, since TASO's national client representatives were soon to arrive. The drama group would perform during the representatives' presentation to the clientele, and afterward the group would (I thought) perform again in the courtyard out back. I situated myself in the rear corner of the day center to prepare. More members of the group arrived, as did an increasing number of TASO clients. Benches were arranged in rows to accommodate them.

At 9:30 A.M., the first part of the presentation began. Clara gave a long prelude and introduced a man and a woman as TASO's client representatives. The female representative led a long discussion with the clients about the latest developments within TASO; seeing me in the room, the woman also graciously provided a running English translation. Clients voiced their concerns and held extensive discussion about the use and meaning of the antiretroviral drugs that were being expected imminently. Several asked how TASO clients would be chosen to receive the drugs, with particular emphasis on the fairness of the process.

While the national TASO representatives continued the dialogue, more clients continued to come into the room. Additional benches had to be carried in from outside, ultimately seating a crowd of over eighty. People of all sorts were present: people well-dressed and people in rags; men and women carrying walking sticks; young and old; clients with energy to spare, and those lying emaciated on mats in the back. As the meeting went on, I realized the room also doubled as a waiting space: every few minutes an attendant would come in and call a name, and that person would stand up and leave the room for counseling or treatment. Every forty to fifty minutes, meanwhile, a nurse entered with a stack of charts and read off the names of twelve to fifteen people, all of whom would rise from their seats and leave through the doors. The representatives and other speakers were clearly comfortable with this kind of traffic, which involved nearly constant motion throughout the room. As spaces opened up on the benches, members of the drama group and others cajoled people to slide down so others just entering could sit down easily at the ends.

As the discussion with the client representatives began to wind up, I saw a little blond *muzungu* (Caucasian, in this case American) girl lean into the room's front door, then another girl, and then a *muzungu* man and a woman who appeared to be a couple. They eventually disappeared from the forward door, then reemerged through the rear door of the day center. The girls nestled among the clients in the rear benches, while the man, with a still camera, took photos.

Once the discussion with the client representatives had ended, the drama group assembled in the front of the room. The members went through a few of their choral songs, and then sang their "folk song"—a dramatized parable, several months in preparation, urging a program of education, socialization and attitude change toward living with HIV. A female member of the group stepped forward and continued the presentation with a personal testimony recounting her infection with HIV, and her subsequent decision to live positively—a delivery that itself was suspended for a few moments by another long recitation of chart names.

I operated my video camera throughout the performance, hoping I had obtained the correct permissions and trying all along to clarify with the clients around me my intentions to tape *only* the drama group. My actions had the potential to stir discontent, since some people felt coming to TASO still carried a stigma. A misdirected videocamera had the potential of revealing identities that did not want to be revealed, especially given TASO's policy of anonymity. I did my best to keep the camera's lens trained on the front, and to turn the camera off when the drama group was not performing.

After the singing ended, the *muzungu* family left quickly; I could hear them congratulating the drama group members at the front in American English. While the other attendees dispersed, a prominent member of the drama group escorted the family to a Toyota Land Cruiser in front of the building, exchanging kind words, and then eventually receiving a calling card from the man. I later found out that the male visitor was a physician from San Francisco who, a year ago, had chosen that group member as one of a handful of people to be supported on ARVs with funds from the American-based Family Treatment Fund (http://familytreatmentfund.ucsf.edu). Thanks to the ARVs, the recipient told me shortly afterward, he had gone from weighing 62kg a year earlier to 72kg—a dramatic improvement in a place where few still had access to the drugs. He described himself as having been "very weak" before taking the ARVs. I told him he looked much stronger.

After the meeting, I walked out to the back courtyard to join the drama group. The members' second "performance" turned out to be a private meeting with the visiting client representatives. While they had generally remained quiet within the day center conversation, the drama group representatives saw this time as an opportunity to address their own concerns, which they hoped the TASO representatives would subsequently take to the national board. The female representative, in her opening remarks, reiterated the importance of the drama group to TASO's mission (an assertion she repeated in English for me), implying the importance of attending to the members' needs. A local administrator also attended, openly encouraging the group members to speak freely. In response, the drama group members brought up several concerns. The van the organization owned to drive the group to performances was too small, one claimed: it could only carry seventeen passengers while the group numbered twenty-five.[2] Members only received 50,000 Ugandan shillings (about $28) per month for transportation to the TASO Centre, noted another; but the rising costs of hired cabs and boda-boda (motorbike driver) fares meant the sum no longer sufficed for many. Other regions' drama group members, some had heard, had greater allocations for their travel.

Group members also used the forum to air more immediate health and lifestyle concerns. Several expressed frustration about the delayed arrival of ARVs to the area, and their necessarily selective distribution: who would get them first? they asked. A female drama group member asked TASO to help support her children's school fees, and wanted the Centre to offer more child-centered programs. One man spoke eloquently, almost entirely in English, about how his decision to purchase his own ARVs had caused him to go broke before TASO offered to employ him as the drama group's second director. Budget cuts the following year, however, had again left him out of a job and threatened his ability to continue treatment. (He wondered out loud: Might those cuts also have prevented Mbarara from winning the national TASO drama group competition for a second straight year?) Throughout the conversation, the drama group members made sure that an English speaker could sit next to me and translate the proceedings.

The national client representatives listened patiently and earnestly, and responded with respect. While the drama group members seemed to express a great deal of frustration, they seemed to understand the client representatives' answers. The nearly two hours devoted to drama group concerns, however, underlined both the importance of the group to TASO, and the privilege the members felt as the organization's public messengers to the community. After the second session ended, around 2 p.m., both representatives came up to me, introduced themselves, and presented me with requests. One wanted to write a book about how she and her family had been affected by AIDS, and she wanted to know if I, as a writer, could help her. I gave her my information and said I would see what I could do. The other representative asked if I would like to see the music group at his own TASO chapter. I said I did, but that I was leaving in a few days; hopefully, we would keep in touch.

AIDS DRAMA GROUPS

Through its ability to address struggles with HIV/AIDS in Africa through music, dance, and theater, the drama group has gained status among scholars and aid workers as a crucial instrument for disseminating information about HIV, for suggesting behavior change, and for promoting tolerance and inclusion of PLWAs (Gausset 2001, 515–516). Yet the frequent decisions of NGOs to incorporate drama groups into their AIDS campaign models as purveyors of local culture (often in the "edutainment" model) offers a particularly evocative commentary on the global implications of anti-AIDS initiatives. Drama groups, after all, came into being as a kind of African mediation with the West in the first place (Frank 1995). Initially employed to ameliorate local concerns and modify traditional practices, drama groups provided a means for defining modernization and self-actualization from pre-independence times. Scholarship on the topic tends toward two complementary narratives that illustrate drama groups' continued mediation between Africa and the West. African historians tend to view drama groups as part of a continuum of theatrical protest and problem solving dating back to the 1930s (Odhiambo 2008, 41–46); European writers, in contrast, tend to characterize the contemporary drama group scene as emerging from the worldwide "Theater for Development" movement, which came into its own as a form of social action and educational uplift during the 1970s (Epskamp 2006). As Marion Frank notes, these narratives appeared to coexist in local dramatic productions aimed at social betterment decades before the arrival of AIDS: used to rouse villagers to air their grievances, campaign for political causes, call for civic projects, or resolve local conflicts. In post-1986 Uganda, however, a lingering wariness about public political activity, combined with an immediate need to address public health concerns, caused drama group productions to shift their focus to health issues, with a particular emphasis on AIDS—creating a subgenre Frank calls "Campaign Theater." Often supported by Western-funded NGOs, such productions gained reputations as hybrids of European and African theatrical production values. Drama groups would disseminate socio-medical information gleaned from biomedical research studies and frequently present under the moniker of "theater"; but simultaneously, those who engaged in Campaign Theater in Uganda employed African folklore and symbolism, relied heavily on local musical styles, and favored a communal approach to creative input, all of which could be coded as "African" traits. After 1989, drama groups increasingly became an organized force in AIDS education campaigns—observed locally as a meaningful form of anti-AIDS mobilization and supported internationally as effectively communicating key messages about the virus (Frank 1995, 17–18). Campaign organizers regularly looked to drama groups as instruments for education, voices for the HIV-positive community, international public relations ambassadors, and popular targets for NGO-based funding.[3] By the time of my fieldwork in Uganda in 2004, consequently, drama groups had become a prominent part of the AIDS-related landscape.

I argue in this chapter that in part because of its high visibility, the drama group's mediation of local, regional, national, and international HIV/AIDS discourses offers a glimpse of the complex realities and tensions its members must face as actors within a global, multiply manifested web of campaigns—tensions also borne from the form's own history as a point of active negotiation between Africa and the West. These issues are themselves dramatized in the group's presentations, which present local variations of larger social, political, cultural, and health-related issues facilitated by global action against HIV. TASO Mbarara's group show, as a case study, illustrates how drama group performances negotiate a thick network of AIDS-related discourses, while allowing individual performers to negotiate their own stakes in the ideological and medical battle over HIV/AIDS. Taking the role of visible activists, the performers themselves incorporate their drama group activities into larger patterns of resource-acquisition, meaningful action, and self-representation as "people living positively."

THE LANDSCAPE OF HIV/AIDS IN UGANDA

Ethnographic studies of AIDS in severely afflicted regions have shown, in Paul Farmer's words, that "patterns of risk and disease distribution, social responses to AIDS, and prospectives for the near future are all illuminated by a mode of analysis that links the ethnographically observed to historically given social and economic structures" (Farmer 2006[1992], 253; see also Setel 1999, and Fassin 2007). Understanding HIV/AIDS in Ugandan society therefore benefits from exploring the country's position within the networks of global economic, religious, medical, and political discourse that have shaped it over time. These networks have embedded AIDS deeply into the country's cultural fabric since the late 1980s, aided by Uganda's relative stability since 1986, its openness to outside intervention, its population of health professionals already skilled in Western medicine, and the government's early active mobilization against the virus. Scores if not hundreds of AIDS-related NGOs, aided by government sanction and international funds, have arisen to address different aspects of the disease throughout the country.[4] By the time of my field research in 2004, the country's two most prominent daily newspapers, *The Monitor* and *The New Vision*, regularly covered topics related to HIV/AIDS. Condoms with brand names such as Protector and Lifeguard were marketed openly on billboards, storefronts and grocery stores. Other graphic depictions, meanwhile, reinforced a model embodied by the flow of international assistance, with AIDS-related information and resources moving from the cities to the rural areas in attempts to save villagers from the epidemic (see figure 26.1).

Western medical organizations found Uganda's openness to international intervention amenable to research, and universities and international health organizations set up a number of research partnerships there in the late 1980s, resuting in several significant early studies of HIV (Epstein 2007). Ugandans' own early name for the disease—*silimu*, or the slimming disease—also reflected one of many attempts to give to assign a local referent alongside international terms, allowing the population to understand the virus as they experienced it (see Barz 2006, 109–146 for more examples). The rapid introduction of Western HIV/AIDS

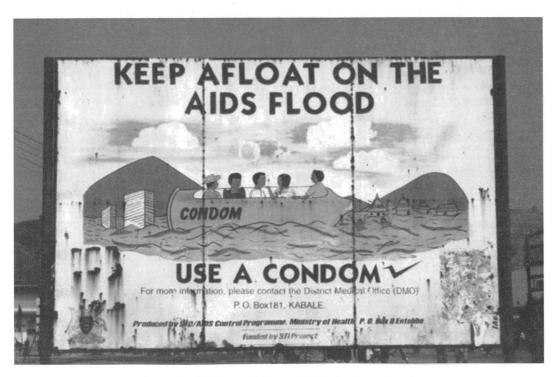

Figure 26.1 AIDS-Related billboard, Kabale, Southwest Uganda

medical conventions into Uganda, however, also galvanized local opposition through a network of traditional herbalists (known also as "African healers," or more derisively as "witch doctors"). Claiming local cures for HIV that did not have the same "side effects" as modern medicine—a claim that invoked the country's colonial past—herbalists took their wares directly to the population by establishing prominent "AIDS herbal research centres" on the main roads of many towns.

Connected to medical developments, performance and creative expression played an important role in the ways Ugandans addresed issues associated with HIV/AIDS. The power of words, sound, dance, and image afforded performers the opportunity to address competing discourses about the disease, and to weigh publicly the advantages and disadvantages each discourse had to offer. Performers' choices could differ from locality to locality, parsing each HIV/AIDS-based landscape to provide residents and organizations with a context for addressing their own personal and communal concerns.

THE LANDSCAPE OF HIV/AIDS IN MBARARA

Mbarara, a small city of about 70,000 residents in southwest Uganda, offers a health profile substantially different from the other urban settings commonly presented in HIV/AIDS literature. Although largely described in travel books as a transit stop, the city contains Uganda's second medical school—founded in 1989 as part of the Mbarara University of Science and Technology (MUST)[5]—and a medical compound, the Mbarara University Teaching Hospital (MUTH), that includes an AIDS clinic. Most research projects on HIV/AIDS in Uganda partnered with the more prominent Makerere University in Kampala. Mbarara, however, had developed its own place in the medical literature as a center for "rural" HIV/AIDS studies, due to its relatively easy access to a large village-based population.[6]

The small medical community in Mbarara reflected a balance between local and global knowledge. Most MUTH medical students came from middle-class families around Kampala and had significant experience traveling and learning outside Uganda. Attending physicians also maintained an international presence: a small cadre of Cuban doctors served on the staff of the hospital as part of an exchange program, joining medical workers from the United States, Germany, the United Kingdom, India, and elsewhere, most of whom came for short periods. MUTH had also become a center for international medical training, research, and service: the Primary Care/Social Medicine program at New York City's Montefiore Medical Center regularly sent residents to MUTH, and the University of California at San Francisco's Medical School had set up a research center in the area.[7] Other medical personnel arrived through connections with smaller medical advocacy organizations, such as Doctors for Global Health.

In addition to the medical complex, the town itself supported numerous AIDS-related initiatives in 2004. The AIDS Support Organization (TASO) and The AIDS Information Centre (AIC), both well-funded and widely known Ugandan NGOs, had established regional branches in Mbarara in 1989 and circa 1993 respectively;[8] and a mobile branch of Hospice Africa Uganda (founded in 1998) provided palliative care to HIV/AIDS and cancer patients in the surrounding villages.[9] Numerous smaller organizations and demographically focused support groups such as NACWOLA (The National Community of Women Living with HIV/AIDS in Uganda) and Youth Alive also operated chapters in the area, relying on peer-based outlets to address its target populations' HIV/AIDS concerns.[10] On the main road on the opposite side of town, meanwhile, a prominent "AIDS Herbal Research Centre" took up the lower floor of a multistory building, offering "traditional African" remedies administered along the lines of Uganda's National

Council of Traditional Healers and Herbalists Associations (another NGO). During trips to town, meanwhile, I frequently passed a parked vehicle from THETA, an organization created "to build in-depth relationships between traditional health practitioners, biomedical health workers, and local communities based on mutual respect, openness and trust";[11] I did not, however, encounter or observe any of its programs in the course of my research.[12]

Religious organizations increasingly intertwined with this landscape of health- and information-based HIV/AIDS organizations. Since its colonial days, Baptist, Anglican, Catholic, and other missionaries had operated in the area; and by the early twenty-first century these groups had all developed sizeable congregations that catered to the needs of various communities (including HIV/AIDS assistance).[13] More recent independent and evangelical movements had fast become a significant force as well: in 2004 the independent Texas-based "Mission to the Ankole" (founded 1997) operated the area's most reliable Internet café in the back of its storefront ministry, turning its technological resources into a gentle proselytizing force.[14] Multi-day tent meetings, meanwhile, complete with amplified Christian contemporary music and American-style charismatic preaching, had become commonplace throughout the region to the point of constituting the most significant public musical events in town.[15]

Christian networks also become a central means by which HIV/AIDS aid and information arrived in Mbarara: the region's only biomedicine-based AIDS clinic, located on the university grounds, came into existence largely with funding by the American Southern Baptist Church in partnership with the Ugandan government. The American physicians directing the clinic served on the Baptist International Mission Board, and those treated at the clinic were actively missionized as part of their follow-up home care.[16] Similarly, a Christian minister (who was also a pre-med student at MUST) often accompanied hospice visits, offering patients salvation along with other medical services; and local hospice newsletters frequently included Christian religious exhortations.[17] International religious organizations thus integrated deeply into a good portion of health-based, cultural, and technological resources within the region. Residents frequently had little choice but to engage those resources within the context of specific, transformative Christian discourses and moral agendas.

The resulting dynamic landscape presented a range of contrasting forces that replicated local/global concerns in the area. Amid a large-scale public presence of HIV/AIDS in Mbarara, individuals took action that often involved shifting alignments, allegiances, and expectations in a competitive marketplace. Such issues resonated in the choice to join a drama group.

THE TASO MBARARA DRAMA GROUP

I came to know of three local AIDS-related drama groups in Mbarara: one supported by TASO, one convened through the AIDS Information Centre across town, and one sponsored by the local chapter of NACWOLA. These three groups seemed to coexist peacefully, and perhaps even synergetically: members of the TASO drama group had told me of their involvement with drama groups from other organizations, often in leadership capacities. While I focus on a single group here, therefore, I acknowledge its presence within a network of city-based drama groups, each of which advocated for an associated but different HIV/AIDS-related agenda (see also Jamil and Muriisa 2004, 22).

The TASO Mbarara group, founded about 1992, served as a vessel for localizing the messages of the nationally situated NGO. Like many of TASO's drama groups, TASO Mbarara's drama group originally seemed to function as a grassroots activity for the clients at the organization's local day care centers (TASO Uganda Limited 2002, 22).[18] The localized drama group model, however, eventually transformed into a major component of TASO's outreach and funding campaigns. In 2003, TASO successfully applied for a multiyear grant from the U.S.-based Rockefeller Foundation to regulate, train, and further mobilize its drama groups. When I arrived in Mbarara in July 2004, the project's impact was apparent: the branch's drama group held regular rehearsals with a music "master," played institutionally owned instruments (which I will discuss later), had its own van for transportation to presentations, and planned its annual show according to an agenda dictated by the national organization. National TASO materials, meanwhile, prominently displayed photographs of drama groups in performance, whether alone or welcoming visiting dignitaries. Upon my arrival, the group's administrative director also told me with great pride that I would be working with the reigning champions of TASO's first national Drama Group Festival (also funded by the grant), which took place in November 2003; perhaps, with my expertise in music, I could help them defend their title (Fieldnotes, July 7, 2004).

In summer 2004, the TASO Mbarara drama group numbered about twenty to twenty-five members, with people seemingly joining based on interest and availability. Rehearsing about four to five hours per week, the ensemble honed a two-and-a-half hour long show for afternoon presentations to local schools and villages. This presentation would serve as TASO's public face both regionally and internationally, offering local audiences information, advice, encouragement, and entertainment; providing funders with a scale of effectiveness; and giving performers an extended opportunity to develop roles as vital communal authorities. In doing so, group members gained experience in traversing the networks of power that supported the ensemble, and, not incidentally, valued these networks as routes to obtaining desired treatment.

The Presentation

National TASO instructed its drama groups to organize its 2004/2005 presentations around the theme "ART [Anti-Retroviral Therapy] in TASO: A combination of ART and Positive Living is the way forward." Based on the anticipated introduction of antiretroviral drugs through the recently ratified American PEPFAR program, the new directive set TASO's drama groups to work publicizing the theme through theatrical, musical, and dance-based formats. Only a couple members of the Mbarara drama group took ARV regimens by that point; to the other performers, these drugs largely represented abstract hope for the future. Thus, the drama group largely had to rely on information supplied by TASO itself to craft its artistic message; and they did so with the open knowledge that the drugs would be made available only for a select few.

Honed under the tutelage of a hired music master, TASO's presentation comprised a spectrum of discrete sections, each presented according to particular conventions: a series of multipart choral songs, frequently performed in white shirts, khaki pants or skirts, and khaki vests featuring an AIDS red ribbon or TASO insignia pin; a half-hour skit performed in costumes that reflected an array of character types and social classes; a personal testimony, usually rehearsed and polished; a question-and-answer session, usually led by the administrative director; a "traditional" narrative song with a khaki-clad chorus backing costumed actors; and a closing "traditional dance" that the group's director ascribed to the Acholi people of North Uganda, performed in stylized, festive traditional dress. Together, these elements presented a palette of discourses that spoke broadly to East African identity, and to the Ugandan regional experience in particular. Both presenters and audiences experienced these disparate pieces as a single event, typically announced in order at the start of a presentation, that moved smoothly from one section to the next with minimal technical explanation.

Performances at villages and secondary schools played somewhat differently from each other—with the latter incorporating more English, holding a somewhat more didactic tone, and providing more conservative responses to questions about sexual behavior.[19] The content, however, remained generally consistent. Choral songs seemed heavily influenced by church (*kwaya*) styles, both musically and in the sense of community such styles fostered (Barz 2006); the music made occasional nods to Afropop arrangements, whether implied or explicit;[20] and the group's lyrics offered generic messages to "Fight AIDS," to treat PLWAs with respect, to assert everyone's susceptibility to HIV regardless of social standing, and to "get tested" for the virus as a social responsibility. Other songs, including a choral arrangement of Philly Lutaaya's 1989 "Alone"—performed with hands on hearts—reflected the history of HIV activism within Uganda (see Zaritsky 1990). In essence, these songs introduced listeners and performers to standardized international health messages, intentionally translated for local consumption in order to begin a meaningful conversation about HIV.

The year's prescribed message, however, received its strongest musical manifestation in the "folk song." Always performed in the local language, the folk song aimed to dramatize the journey of an HIV-positive person from ignorance to knowledge, educating friends and neighbors in the process. By modeling this behavior, the presenters hoped, audiences would shift similarly. In the case of ARVs, the group crafted the following story-in-song: A woman tells her friends that she is not feeling well, and believes she received a lingering illness from her husband. The husband appears, explaining that his ailments (presented as twitching and scratching) appeared after he and his friends stole and slaughtered a cow for food: they felt they had been the victims of some sort of retaliatory spell. The group decides to call a witch doctor (who appears in gross caricature). The witch doctor intones a chant (adopted by the chorus), takes out animal furs, shakes shells together, gives the afflicted family a potion, and scores the backs of their necks. When the ritual ends, the chorus surrounding the action takes over, warning against this approach, and exhorting all people to get tested for HIV so they can be treated with ARVs when they become available. In the end, everyone dances, symbolically showing ARVs coursing through their bodies. Aimed to dismiss superstition in the rural farming areas (further emphasized by the straw hats worn by two of the main characters) in favor of NGO-introduced, Western-funded, testing and treatment, this presentation continued to resemble in spirit the tableau offered by the older billboard in figure 26.1.

Local political forces frequently amplified the significance of these messages. When the drama group arrived at a village in the adjoining Bushenyi district to give its presentation, for example, the director received information that the regional chairman had planned to schedule a visit. Toward the end of the first song, the chairman walked in with his entourage. The attendees in the packed community hall rose while he entered, shook my hand and the hand of the musical director, and found a seat in the front of the room. After the drama group's song finished, the local minister effectively marked a new start of the event, leading the first verse of the Ugandan national anthem, and then offering a prayer praising the drama group's mission. After the drama group sang a couple more songs, the chairman stood up, temporarily halted the procedings, and delivered a forty-minute oration promoting Ugandan President Yoweri Museveni's ABC anti-AIDS program.[21] Shortly after the drama group's presentation resumed, the chairman left. Group members expressed familiarity with this kind of occurrence; on the trip back to Mbarara that evening, they bemusedly critiqued the chairman's speech while recognizing their own power to attract this level of attention to their performances (Fieldnotes,

July 10, 2004). In so doing, they styled themselves as empowered participants in the political scene.

Instruments to Represent The Nation

At least one hour of each drama group rehearsal I attended involved the preparation of an instrumental ensemble piece—a required element on the syllabus of the National Drama Group competition held each November. Performed on locally made "traditional" instruments that were usually too bulky to bring to regular presentations, the piece highlighted several issues the drama group faced in negotiating the symbolic landscape of social and medical knowledge. While the music theoretically represented an integration of African discourse into the group's HIV/AIDS activism, for example, many of the drama group members appeared to have little initial experience with the instruments. Comments offered during communal instruction further illustrated the complex layering developed by the group members in bringing Ugandan and pan-African identity to HIV/AIDS education.

Gregory Barz's description of musical instruments in Uganda (2004, esp. 78–85) exemplifies the general practice of African music scholars to privilege indigenous terms over English terms evocative of colonial history. Calling an instrument a "tube fiddle" rather than an *endingidi*, for example, invokes a lens of Western domination that can be seen as discouraging concerns with the worldviews of local populations. The drama group's instrumental experience, however, reflected a somewhat more complicated relationship with the idea of "African" instruments. In my own travels around Mbarara town and limited observations of the countryside, I found only drums in regular use; and heard none of the "traditional" instruments described in textbooks. Those instruments appeared only in craft shops, presumably for sale to visitors. Musical tastes in Mbarara instead tended to revolve more around an urban aesthetic: electronic stereos, keyboards, and amplified instruments, especially at advertised (largely Christian) music concerts. While drama group members appeared to come to traditional instruments with little prior knowledge, however, they endorsed them as objects of communal history and identity. Such issues sustained even with the drums: when I asked the group's most facile drummer where he learned to play, hoping he might tell me of his apprenticeship to a local drum master, he replied that he learned by observing drummers at his church; and the *engalabe* [elongated] drum, described elsewhere in this volume as a male instrument (see Emanuel), was frequently played by a female member of the group without any comment. The ensemble's use of African instruments thus assumed a reintroduced mark of identity by instilling a sense of culture that differed from mass media-oriented local practices (not to mention fiscal practicality: African instruments, the director told me, were significantly less expensive than equivalent Western instruments).

These instruments helped reconfigure the local/global relations of the drama group's HIV/AIDS activism. At my first rehearsal with the ensemble, the hired music master (who wore a FUBU sweatshirt that day) took me on a public tour through the instruments by their English names—which he also used with the drama group members—and compared them to their Western equivalents. The *xylophone* was "made of wood but we still include it in metallic percussion." A *thumb piano* was "like a regular piano in the West, but much more simply constructed." And the *adungus* (which the music instructor called "harps") were "the type mentioned in the Bible that King David used to play. This," he said, "is the original. It was African" (Fieldnotes, July 13, 2004). The tube fiddle and pan pipes had similar explanations. All these instruments, noted the music instructor, played according to a pentatonic scale symbolizing a relationship with African identity, which "we maintain...as a part of our culture." As the instructor progressively taught the instrumental composition via parts on large sheets of paper posted to the walls, he maintained these connections: indicating the instrumentation with the notations XY (xylophone), TP (thumb piano), Ad (adungu), TF (tube fiddle) and PP (pan pipes), and indicating pitches according to the Western scale: d ("do"), r ("re"), m ("mi"), s ("sol"), and l ("la").

The means by which these instruments created a sonic texture, moreover, had its own vocabulary rooted in colonial African music pedagogy. At one point in the composition, two xylophones played complementary melodies that the music master described as "African counterpoint," while the harps/adungus played a line that he called "basso ostinato," the pan-pipers played an interlocking pattern, and the other instruments filled in similarly. The music master wrote out these melodies using a version of John Curwen's Tonic Sol-Fa notation (1872; see figure 26.2), and they remained on the wall of the day center between rehearsals for other clients to see.[22] As rehearsals progressed, and the instructor moved through different sections of the piece, he highlighted characteristic instrumental interactions through English terms such as "Imitation/Interrupted," "Direct Imitation led by Pan Pipes," and "Modified Silences/Fragmentation," even as he gave the rest of his lesson in Runyankore (Fieldnotes, July 20, 2004). This form of hybrid instrumental instruction mapped onto the drama group members' existing understanding of global AIDS networks, bridging local sound, "Africanness," and communal history with their identities as Ugandans living with HIV/AIDS. Just as with the medical knowledge they addressed, however, the drama group members connected with that sense of Africanness less through trajectories of indigenous practice than through a representation of African tradition framed in Western-centered language and notation.

Global Reaches

The drama group's performances did not constitute the only way for performers to situate themselves within the larger HIV/AIDS ecology. Even admission to the group often required a previous connection to international health care and aid funding pathways. TASO drama group members often joined the ensemble either as privileged clients who also took other positions of leadership within the community, or as participants interested in taking a more active role within the organization (and within anti-AIDS initiatives more generally). When not rehearsing, some of the group members helped counsel clients at the center and others led TASO education programs. Whether as members of the group or in other TASO capacities, everyone in the drama group had become quite knowledgeable about the latest developments in AIDS treatment, and consequently situated themselves optimally to benefit from such knowledge. Their dual visibility as communal and artistic leaders afforded them attention elsewhere in the community as well: during the highly anticipated daylong visit by the two client representatives of the

Figure 26.2 "Tune" Notation

Original composition, TASO Mbarara, July 2004
"Xylophone I " and "Xylophone 2" parts only.
"Thumb Piano/Adungu" and "Pan Pipe/Tube Fiddle" parts not shown.

xy1: | •d:d•m | s•s:s•m | d•m:r•d | $\overline{l:l:l}$ | x•l:l/ | s•s:s•d | m•m:r•r | $\overline{d:d:d}$ |

xy2: :d:d:l_1 | $s_1:s_1:s_1:d$ | $s_1:s_1:s_1:d$ | $\overline{l_1:l_1:l_1}$ | [x]:l_1:l_1:d | $s_1:s_1:s_1:d$ | $s_1:m:s_1:s_1$ | $\overline{d:d:d}$ |

national TASO board I described at the start of this essay, the drama group received more private discussion time than the general clientele. Group members thus valued their dramatic and musical skills as more than an opportunity to become well-regarded emissaries of anti-AIDS efforts; they often developed these skills in tandem with increasing organizational privilege, making them potentially eligible for insider access to the international resources TASO had received from donors and institutional partnerships.

Such privilege also extended well beyond local representation. As described earlier, TASO's annual reports and other publicity materials commonly included photography of drama groups welcoming visiting dignitaries to Uganda, producing both important international cultural meeting spaces and compelling media images. Drama group members thus had ample evidence of their performances' significance on a broader stage. Some—especially those who had been involved with multiple drama groups—consequently began to explore ways to use the drama group format as a means of attracting attention and funds from abroad. Toward the end of my fieldwork, for example, one enterprising member of the TASO drama group asked me privately if I could connect her with funding to start a drama group within the Ugandan military.[23] Others saw their drama group participation as a way to spread messages directly to countries that provided financial and medical resources supporting Uganda's AIDS infrastructure: I received several member requests to bring the TASO Mbarara drama group to the United States (a nearly impossible proposition, I discovered, due to American customs restrictions on PLWAs at the time). Throughout, the drama group members saw their own potential as facilitators of international discourse through their participation—an attribute that had attracted me to them, after all—in effect aiming to meet the intentions of international health initiatives from the grassroots up.

Members from both within and outside the group also acknowledged my presence and interest as proof of the drama group's success at initiating international discussions about HIV/AIDS. At the start of one secondary school presentation, the group's director made sure to introduce me in English as a "visitor from the United States: a professor of music from New York University [who is here] to see what it is we do and how people respond," thus confirming the significance of the presentation beyond the information itself (Fieldnotes, July 16, 2004). Explicit introductions from the group were not always necessary, however. Toward the end of a different secondary school presentation, one of the school's headmasters thanked the group, and then commented that my interest showed that someone from outside Uganda was concerned about Ugandans. Perhaps in response to an editorial in the national paper a couple days earlier, the headmaster then asked me if I would respond to the "rumor" that AIDS was started by white people to destroy black Africans. My answer—that HIV/AIDS was a disease of blood, not skin color—seemed to meet with approbation from the drama group and led to further conversations with students after the talk (one of whom asserted that African medicine was not being given a chance in the face of Western medicine) (Fieldnotes, July 22, 2004). These instances, repeated with other observers from abroad, connected the drama group's undertaking to real, living representatives of the countries encouraging and funding the group's activity—while sometimes also reactivating key nodes of cultural confrontation between Africa and the West.

My presence also helped mediate international HIV/AIDS discourses in the opposite direction, updating the status of one drama group member's leadership role to the American organization that supported his ARV regimen. Shortly after I returned to the United States, one of my housemates from the Mbarara medical compound, who had arrived to work on a project sponsored by the University of California at San Francisco, contacted me with a request for a copy of my videotape from the group's July 28 day center performance. The American doctor I had noticed observing the drama group performance that day had also remembered me, and viewed my tape as a way to document this group member's vitality to those who had funded him. Participation in the ensemble, according to these parameters, would be used to provide a stark illustration of the drugs' positive effects and consequently reflect on the significance and success of the funders' investments. After several E-mail exchanges, the director of the TASO Mbarara day center gave permission for me to send the tape, and I shipped it over in time for the event. These experiences once again reinforced the meaning of drama group participation: not only in spreading awareness of HIV/AIDS in Uganda, but in creating reciprocal images of hope within an international medical, financial, and social landscape of HIV/AIDS advocacy.[24]

CONCLUSION

Steven Robins has noted that "HIV/AIDS activism...has...contributed toward new forms of health citizenship that are concerned with both rights-based struggles and creating collectively shared meanings of the extreme experiences of illness and stigmatization of individual AIDS sufferers" (Robins 2006, 320). While Robins's comments refer to South African PLWAs, they also offer an important context for understanding how the TASO Mbarara Drama Group created and reinforced international discourses of shared meaning through performance, while allowing its members to assert a collective form of "health citizenship" resulting from their status as performers and public emissaries. Through rehearsals, presentations, and publicity materials, the music, drama, and dance formulations enacted by the ensemble became understood as crucial agents for disseminating information about HIV/AIDS locally. Ugandan audiences, as a result, came to recognize their personal health choices within a specifically delineated constellation of local, national, historical, and international frameworks; and the drama group members themselves gained a privileged sense of status as the people who both formulated and benefitted from those frameworks. In Mbarara, the TASO Drama Group presentation represented another reality in understanding the way those infected by the virus told of the AIDS epidemic in their country. Performances hooked into a broad historical web of economic flows, advocacy, health-based treatment, religious ideology, and social and cultural hierarchy that itself drew out of decades-long development-based encounters between Africa and "the West." Performance in this context thus became more than a "therapy," or simply a way to alleviate pain or a sense of stigma. Instead, the drama group's actions served an important role in reasserting locally the coherence and flow of internationally informed healthcare. Using the performative arts to instill in their audiences a sense of community, the drama group's members urged "fellow Ugandans" to make health choices according to a larger field of awareness necessitated by HIV. In doing so, they situated themselves as globally active figures within a vast, complex, and deeply competitive world of HIV/AIDS advocacy.

27

"I'm a Rich Man, How Can I Die?"

CIRCUS PERFORMANCE AS A MEANS OF HIV/AIDS EDUCATION IN ETHIOPIA

Leah Niederstadt (Wheaton College)

INTRODUCTION

In 2002, a circus play entitled *Mekabir Kofari* (*The Grave Digger*) premiered at the National Theatre in Addis Ababa, Ethiopia.[1] Written by Aweke Emiru, then director of Circus Addis Ababa,[2] the performance combined drama, song, dance, and circus skills with a narrative that explored a number of issues related to HIV/AIDS, including modes of transmission and social stigma. Although the topic was serious, the performance managed to convey Ethiopia and its people—particularly children and youth—as aware of, and willing, ready, and able to address the challenges faced by their society. The vibrant costumes, upbeat music, and overall message that HIV/AIDS can be overcome if people are educated about and unite to fight the pandemic also helped to convey a positive image of contemporary Ethiopia. This image is quite at odds with the popular imagination in which Ethiopia is most often associated with images of war, famine, Rastafarianism, and charity concerts such as 1985's Live Aid. Less recognized, however, are efforts to address a range of social challenges, including the development of a circus movement that is the largest on the African continent.

Although circus as a form of performance was nearly unknown when the first troupe was established in Ethiopia in 1991, dozens of circuses now operate throughout the country, and several Ethiopian troupes have performed throughout Africa, Asia, Europe, and North America. From the beginning, expatriate and Ethiopian administrative and artistic staff combined circus skills such as juggling and contortion with indigenous forms of dance, song, and costuming, coupling these spectacles with messages about social challenges such as HIV/ AIDS. They conceived of the country's circus movement as a moral endeavor, one that allowed them to celebrate Ethiopian national identity with an emphasis on ethnic diversity, and to educate the public about a variety of issues. Circus was also seen as a means of empowering the country's youngest citizens, as the performers in Ethiopian troupes are largely children and youth, not adults. As a result, circus in Ethiopia gained a unique form and purpose within the cultural landscape of the region, serving as a creative space for new voices to express themselves on central issues related to development and economic and social equality.

This chapter, based on more than a decade of fieldwork, explores the ways in which the Ethiopian circus movement particularly addresses the HIV/AIDS pandemic (figure 27.1).[3] I begin with an introduction and historical overview of the circus movement in Ethiopia, as well as the country's HIV/AIDS profile; I will then explore several key performances to illustrate how Ethiopian circuses attempt to educate their audiences about HIV/AIDS. In effect, Ethiopian circus performances provide two types of educational messages. First, they reinforce federal, regional, and state government rhetoric about the importance of ethnic diversity in the construction of a national Ethiopian identity. In doing so, they help teach Ethiopians about their country's diversity, recognizing and celebrating it as a key component of national identity.[4] Second, circus shows provide information about a range of health and development issues, and suggest how specific challenges can be resolved. HIV/AIDS has increasingly become a focus of circus performances, due to both the growing number of Ethiopians impacted by HIV/AIDS, and the willingness of non-governmental organizations (NGOs) and government agencies to fund projects that provide educational information about HIV/AIDS.

Circuses comprise a prominent part of contemporary urban Ethiopian culture, remaining vibrant even in the face of limited funding, conflicting donor demands, high staff turnover, and asylum claims made by performers when touring overseas.[5] Several times in

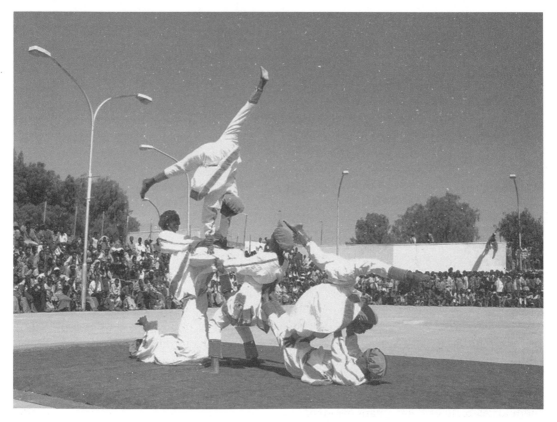

Figure 27.1 Members of Circus Dire Dawa performing a pyramid-building routine. Jijiga, Ethiopia. Leah Niederstadt

the past decade, it seemed possible that the circus movement would collapse, yet troupes continue to function throughout the country and new circuses are still founded. Although it is difficult to estimate how many currently operate, given how quickly troupes may shut down due to funding constraints, approximate twenty-five circuses currently exist at any one time in Ethiopia. More than a dozen of these are members of an umbrella organization called Circus in Ethiopia, which I shall discuss further. The movement's endurance as a whole, and its continual support from both indigenous and foreign donors, suggests the central role circus now holds as a form of theatre for development in Ethiopia.[6]

CREATING AN ETHIOPIAN CIRCUS

Perhaps surprisingly, circuses can be found elsewhere in Africa. Circus troupes—in a wide range of forms and with varying objectives—operate in Burkina Faso, Cameroon, Kenya, Mali, South Africa, and Uganda and indigenous acrobatic troupes have long performed throughout North Africa. Via its Cirque du Monde project, Cirque du Soleil supports circus programs throughout Francophone West Africa and it was once a key donor to the Ethiopian circus movement. Although they are unmistakably circuses, Ethiopian troupes maintain their own constellation of practices. First, with very few exceptions, Ethiopian circus performers are all children and youth who were, until recently, compensated for their participation, although they have never been considered salaried employees.[7] Second, animals are not part of their performances, although not due to concern for animal rights, as several troupes have tried and failed to train monkeys, but rather due to the cost of supporting circus animals. Third, Ethiopian circuses do not use high-wire or tightrope acts or the flying trapeze, and although two troupes have stationary trapezes, they usually only perform on them in their purpose-built performance spaces due to transportion and safety issues.[8] In addition, performances rarely incorporate what Westerners might think of as clowns, although clowning or joking behavior is very common, often incorporated into performances by stock characters, including an *ibd sew* (lit., "crazy person"), an old man or woman who exemplifies either the backward "old ways" or the traditional wisdom of rural culture, or an uneducated individual who usually plays the fool.[9] It is important to note that Ethiopian circus shows typically occur outdoors, not in a circus hall or tent. They are also free of charge to the public. Both factors are key to the popularity of circus throughout Ethiopia because free admission encourages large audiences, which enables the didactic messages to reach more people, while performing in publicly accessible spaces allows for numerous spectators to gather (figure 27.1).

As in many other troupes around the world, Ethiopian circus artistic directors utilize indigenous folktales, music, song, dance, and clothing as a means of making their circus "authentically Ethiopian." In doing so, they have much in common with the Moscow and the Chinese State circuses, which use their national identity as a marketing tool and a means of providing thematic cohesion within performances abroad. In Ethiopia, however, circuses also use costumes, dance, music, song, and props as markers of ethnic identity directed to their *Ethiopian* spectators.[10] Ethnic identity is thus highlighted and celebrated through Ethiopian circus performances. Especially when performed in Ethiopia, moreover, circus shows are didactic. Educational messages about HIV/AIDS prevention or land-mine safety, for example, are either woven into a show's overall storyline, thus transforming it into a full-length circus morality play, or they are presented as short public service announcement-style skits either before or after the performance of circus skills (figure 27.2).[11]

The importance of circus in the fight against HIV/AIDs

It has been over couple of decades since the first HIV/AIDs case was detected in Ethiopia. During this period, the disease has adversely affected the health, economy and other social aspects of the society. Hundreds of thousands have died while many others became orphans due to the pandemic. In addition, quite a number of children are forced to lead their life on the streets.

Many factors are attributed for the spread. Poverty, harmful traditional practices and unemployment are some of the factors. Lack of open discussions and absence of all rounded public involvement in the fight against the disease have also aggravated the spread of the pandemic.

The youth, the productive section of the society, is hardly affected by the disease. The reason for their vulnerability is the fact that they are eager to having sex. The activities under taken in the society also invited them to involve in such affairs which may lead them to making unsafe sex. There is no trend of dialogue between the youth and their family in our society, which again blocks the sharing of experiences with each other.

To address these problems, various governmental and non-governmental institutions are trying their level best. Among these organizations Circus in Ethiopia (CIE) takes the leading position. CIE has been making relentless effort to alleviate this problem in addition to promoting the art, circus, among the society.

27

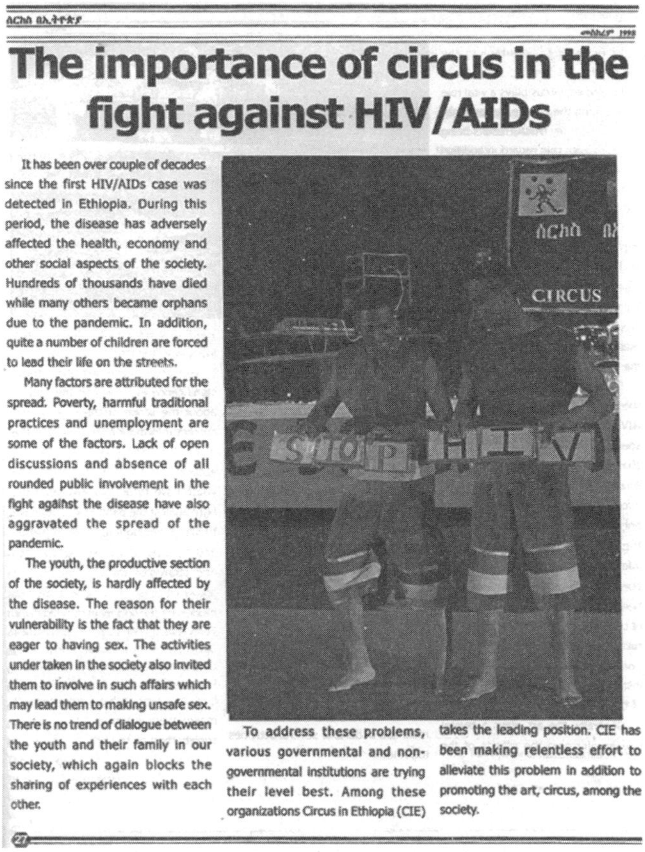

Figure 27.2 Page from *Circus in Ethiopia* showing two jugglers performing with H-I-V "bricks"

In this regard, circus performance in Ethiopia is similar to other forms of theatre for development found on the African continent (Kerr 2002, Marlin-Curiel 2004, Abah 2006). In relation to HIV/AIDS and performance, in particular, Louise M. Bourgault (2003) and Jane Plastow (2004) have shown how theatrical practices, whether indigenous or imported, are utilized to address social, economic and/or political issues of importance to local, regional, and national communities. In the Ethiopian context, however, circus performance might also be considered a form of "theatre of necessity" (Irobi 2006, 34), with HIV/AIDS education as a key focus. This is especially true of the past seven to eight years when donor restrictions on funding increased and available funds decreased, due to the global economic crisis; didactic performances have proven to be one of the few areas international and local NGOs have been willing to fund.

Ethiopian circus began to take shape in 1990, as Ethiopia's socialist regime, known as the Derg, was failing. Although permission for foreigners to live in Ethiopia was restricted during the Derg, a significant number of expatriates lived and worked in the country, employed by NGOs, various United Nations agencies, and private international schools. Two of these foreigners founded what is now Circus Addis Ababa, Ethiopia's first circus troupe, in 1991. Andy Goldman, an American, then worked for the North American Conference on Ethiopian Jewry (NACOEJ) while French-Canadian Marc LaChance worked for the local International Community School.[12] Through expatriate channels, Goldman asked LaChance, an amateur juggler, to perform for the many children under his care. So successful was LaChance's performance that he began teaching the children basic circus skills and developing a show for their families.

In May 1991, however, most of the Ethiopian Jews were airlifted to Israel and LaChance was left a ringleader without a circus. The same month, the socialist regime fell and a transitional government, led by current Prime Minister Meles Zenawi, took power. In the period that followed, LaChance began teaching neighborhood children how to juggle, balance broomsticks on their chins and foreheads, and walk across a low balance beam. Several months later, the children performed on a soccer field near Bole International Airport to a crowd of several hundred—a surprising number of spectators given that no one in Addis Ababa had ever seen a performance quite like it. Consequently, circus staff, both expatriate and Ethiopian, began to conceive of the circus as a means of engaging children and youth in what amounted to an after-school activity. Elmar Brunner, a German schoolteacher and circus performer and trainer, argues that this was a primary factor in the growth of the movement, as circus met the "desire of many children...to be occupied in a useful manner" (Brunner 1998, 61). It actively engaged and challenged them, taught them new skills, and increased their social status. This result is what LaChance had hoped for, as he believed that teaching children to juggle, build pyramids, or turn a cartwheel would build participants' self-esteem and their hope for the future (see figures 27.3 and 27.4). "By far the greatest success can be seen in the lives of the children. They have enormous talent and have reached surprising levels of expertise. Every day they are setting new and higher standards for their peers, the next generation" (LaChance, quoted in LaChance and Soler 1995, 22).

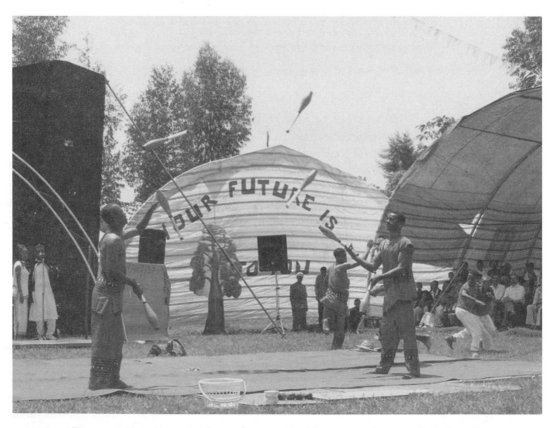

Figure 27.3 Circus Jimma jugglers performing with clubs. Jimma, Ethiopia. Leah Niederstadt

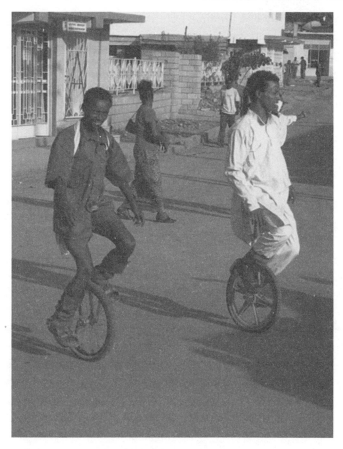

Figure 27.4 Unicycle riders during the 10th anniversary circus parade for Circus Tigrai. Mekelle, Ethiopia. Leah Niederstadt

To support their initial endeavor, Goldman and LaChance relied on contacts within the expatriate community based in Addis Ababa. LaChance's status as French-Canadian also helped them garner support from the Montreal-based Cirque du Soleil, including costumes, equipment, funding, and training. In response to early interest from international NGOs, the circus soon began involving *godana tadaderi* (street children) and emphasized that the organization was helping children who lived on the streets, not just the many impoverished children who already worked on the streets (LaChance and Soler 1995).[13] Circus training was considered a means of providing street children with skills that could be used to entertain passersby, thus moving them away from begging *for* coins to *earning* coins by performing.

The circuses have always retained a link—albeit a nominal one—to *godana tadaderi*, as performances regularly feature storylines centered on the lives of street children. Assisted by Goldman, who supported the circus movement as a consultant and fundraiser, LaChance and other circus staff members soon came to focus on educating, empowering, and caring for their performers and on developing circus as a means of educating the Ethiopian public. Circus Addis Ababa quickly received donations from organizations such as UNICEF, the International Committee of the Red Cross, the Ethiopian Committee of the Red Cross, and Novib (Dutch Oxfam).

In 1993, the circus movement became officially recognized by the Ethiopian government when the Circus in Ethiopia umbrella organization began functioning as a legally registered

NGO.[14] The organization provided funding, training, and administrative support for troupes throughout the country, particularly among its member groups. Of these circuses, five are identified as main branch troupes; eight others are considered associate members.[15] Today, all staff members of the umbrella organization and individual troupes are Ethiopians, with college-educated men holding most of the senior administrative positions throughout the Circus in Ethiopia organization.[16] Most troupe directors, artistic directors, and trainers are former performers and/or have a background in gymnastics or the martial arts; and the majority of performers and staff are boys or men in their early twenties. The dearth of girls and women involved in the Ethiopian circus movement has, however, proved problematic. Troupes have long struggled to meet a common request from international donors that at least one-third of their participants be female, in order to support efforts on the part of NGOs and the Ethiopian federal government to provide opportunities for girls and young women. Several years ago, many circuses attempted to ameliorate the situation by offering positions as trainers to top female performers; however, few remain employed in these positions today.

With the exception of Circus Tigrai, which receives significant support from the Tigrai regional state government and the Tigrai Development Association and which raises funds through several associated business activities, main branch troupes receive most of their operating funds, supplies, organizational support, and other resources through Circus in Ethiopia.[17] Performers and administrative and artistic staff attend training sessions sponsored by the umbrella organization on topics that have included HIV/AIDS education, child welfare, the rights of women and children, and workplace health and safety. Circus in Ethiopia also provides troupes with technical support and materials, which have included professional gymnastics mats and computers. Finally, performers and staff from all five troupes have travelled internationally on tours and training sessions organized through Circus in Ethiopia.

Ethiopian circus performers and staff range in age from five to twenty-five years, with most in their teens; and they claim affiliation to a variety of ethnic groups. The large majority identify with the culture of Ethiopia's northern Christian highlands and as practicing Ethiopian Orthodox Christians, although a number of current performers in troupes in Dire Dawa, Jimma, and Tigrai are Muslim. The overwhelming majority come from impoverished families. Aside from sharing a similar socioeconomic background, performers and local troupe staff actively participate in and identify with urban youth culture, with its emphasis on Ethiopian and Western hip hop and pop music and conspicuous consumption of the latest fashions and hairstyles.

HIV/AIDS IN ETHIOPIA

In the past, consistent and reliable data about the HIV/AIDS pandemic in Ethiopia was difficult to obtain due to the challenges of collecting such data in a predominantly rural, geographically diverse country in which mistrust of local, regional, and national governments remains high and in which religious and social mores against discussing birth control, family planning, sex, and the HIV/AIDS pandemic are deeply ingrained. That said, however, some basic statistics are clear, and efforts to document the spread of HIV/AIDS, as well as efforts to combat it, are increasingly successful. Worldwide, Ethiopia consistently ranks among the top-ten nations with regard to the number of people living with HIV/AIDS, with a 2007 estimate of close to one million (UNAIDS 2008). Nationally, Ethiopia's HIV prevalence rate is estimated at 6.6 percent (compared with rates of more than 30 percent in other sub-Saharan African nations), with the rural rate of infection (3.7 percent) significantly lower than the urban rate (nearly 14 percent) (WHO African Region: Ethiopia [2009]). The rate of infection is, however, still increasing, especially in rural areas where the majority of the population lives (UNAIDS 2005, 28). At the same time, efforts on the part of Ethiopia's government and civil society seem to have had a measurable positive impact—albeit a limited one—on HIV/AIDS prevention and control. For example, since the mid-1990s, the rate of infection among pregnant women in Ethiopia's urban centers has averaged 12 percent; but among pregnant women in Addis Ababa, it dropped from 24 percent in 1995 to 11 percent in 2003 (UNAIDS 2004b, 33). Unfortunately, the country's economic woes meant that less than 1 percent of these women had access to the medication that would prevent mother-to-child transmission of the virus (UNAIDS 2004b, 91), as the cost of such drugs was prohibitive. Although antiretroviral drugs are now advertised and publicly available in Ethiopia's large urban centers, few except the wealthy can afford them unless through programs sponsored by the Ethiopian federal government or international NGOs. The country also faces a significant challenge in caring for the more than 1.2 million children and youth who have been orphaned due to HIV/AIDS (WHO African Region: Ethiopia [2009]).

Efforts to educate the Ethiopian public about HIV/AIDS have been diverse, ranging from the development, implementation, and coordination of government policies at the local, regional, and national level to the founding of HIV/AIDS clubs in schools. Government-coordinated efforts are led by HAPCO, the HIV/AIDS Prevention and Control Office, which maintains local branches in most cities; HAPCO offices in the regional state capitals have often sponsored or helped to coordinate performances by local circus troupes. Other efforts have included dramas and talk shows on Ethiopian National Television and several radio stations. Various theatrical companies, both government sponsored and private, have mounted HIV/AIDS-related drama and comedy performances, and Ethiopia's only contemporary dance company, Adugna Community Dance Theatre Company, has incorporated HIV/AIDS education into its work, particularly its social education projects.[18] Various government agencies, at the local, regional, and federal levels, and indigenous and international NGOs have also sponsored billboards that are erected along roads throughout Ethiopia. These billboards regularly include both images and text (often in the local vernacular), and address a variety of issues from transmission and prevention to combating stigma (figure 27.5). In many ways, the country's HIV/AIDS challenge has also become a key factor underlying the proliferation of circuses throughout Ethiopia, as many saw circus performance as another means of disseminating information to and educating the public about the pandemic.

CIRCUS AS A MEANS OF HIV/AIDS EDUCATION

In Ethiopia, circus performances begin ubiquitously with music, either played by a live circus band or via a CD/tape player hooked up to portable speakers. The music, which ranges from traditional songs in various Ethiopian languages to contemporary Ethiopian and American popular music, helps attract and entertain an audience using a familiar and often comfortable idiom. During pre- and post-show musical interludes, audience members can participate in the performance by presenting gifts (money or personal items) or nonmaterial recognition in the form of hugs and kisses, or by dancing alongside the singer or musician they favor.[19] Though not openly didactic, the musical interludes enable the circuses to establish an easily demarcated physical and temporal space for celebrating ethnic diversity and the urban youth culture with which most performers and staff, and many members of their audiences, identify.

Following the opening set of musical performances, spectators are presented with either a full-length circus morality play that incorporates educational messages into its narrative, or a performance of circus skills that is preceded or followed by didactic skits. As mentioned

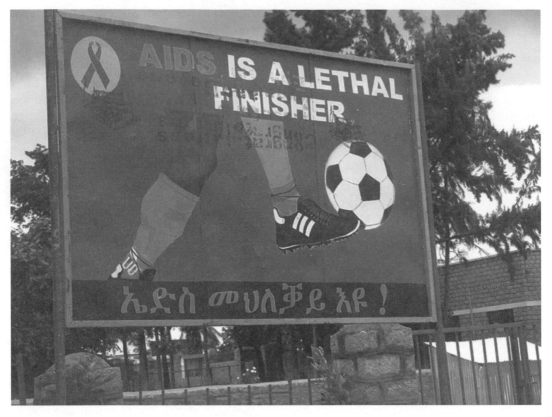

Figure 27.5 HIV/AIDS educational billboard. Tigrai Regional State, Ethiopia. Leah Niederstadt

earlier, these formats can address a range of social challenges, but HIV/AIDS is a key focus of circus performances and provides for rich narrative opportunities due to the following: the multiple means of transmission, many of which are addressed in circus shows; the various forms of social stigma that must be exhibited and challenged; and the need to explain condom use and the importance of testing. As I shall now explore, Ethiopia's circus troupes take different approaches in how they address HIV/AIDS, but many efforts are coordinated by the Circus in Ethiopia organization.

Ethiopian Orthodox Monk as HIV/AIDS Educator

In 2001, Circus Dire Dawa held a performance at a private Catholic school in Dire Dawa, which, like Addis Ababa, is a city administration controlled by the federal government. The show itself was entitled *Selam* (Peace) and represented a conflict between two families—one rich and of noble birth; the other, subsistence farmers—intended to allegorize the relationship between Ethiopia and Eritrea.[20]

Before the performance of *Selam*, however, the circus offered an HIV/AIDS education message in the form of a short skit. A Circus Dire Dawa acrobat strode out on stage dressed as a *moksay*, an Ethiopian Orthodox monk. He wore a black, long-haired wig, a flowing gown dyed saffron yellow and tied with a belt, and a long, beaded necklace, all of which visually referenced the style of clothing, accessories, and hair associated with Ethiopian Orthodox monks. He strode back and forth in front of the audience—comprised of primary school children and their teachers—haranguing them to abstain from sex before marriage, to remain faithful to their spouses, and to follow the teachings of the church in order to avoid HIV/AIDS. When I asked why he was dressed as a monk, I was told that the audience would listen to and understand the message because of the role played by religious leaders in pre-scribing moral behavior and advising people how to live good, Christian lives. A monk was also considered an appropriate character to present an HIV/AIDS educational message in a Catholic school because the overwhelming majority of the students and staff were Christians, either Catholic or Ethiopian Orthodox. Given the important role the church plays in the lives of Ethiopian Orthodox Christians, the decision to have a respected religious elder convey an educational message about HIV/AIDS was both clever and unsurprising, although I person-ally found the "monk" to be somewhat intimidating, as did many of the younger children in the audience, who occasionally flinched in response to his tirade.

Circus Jimma: Condom Use

In May 2003, Circus Jimma inaugurated its outdoor amphitheatre, the first space in Ethiopia purpose-built for circus performance. As part of the weeklong festivities, Circus Jimma held several public shows that incorporated different educational messages and highlighted the skills of the troupe. Among these messages was information about HIV/AIDS prevention provided via two juggling acts, one of which used hats and condoms as props. The hat-juggling act involved three jugglers, a flute-playing acrobat, and the stock character of a rich person, who, in this case, was an older teenage boy (or young man) wearing the latest imported fashions but also conveying a positive message: the importance of condom use. The placement of a clearly rich individual was a role reversal for the typical narrative of an Ethiopian circus play or skit; the rich are usually depicted as greedy exploiters of the poor and weak. As Circus Jimma staff rec-ognized, however, those who can afford to wear the latest styles in clothing, accessories, and hairstyles are often admired and envied by young urban Ethiopians. So, the placement of a rich, youthful protagonist was a calculated and successful decision that introduced a role model for emulation: not only for the clothing he wore, but also for the knowledge he possessed and the behavior he exemplified.

Following some standard hat-juggling, the three jugglers engaged the young flute-player in conversation as the fashionable young man walked onstage. He proceeded to chat casually with the hat jugglers, and the conversation led to discussion about girls and sex. The young man then explained the importance of wearing a condom whenever engaging in sexual activity and pulled out of his jacket pocket a string of immediately identifiable *Hiwot* (Life) Trust brand condoms (figure 27.6). Each juggler received a couple of condoms, packaged in white wrappers with red and black writing, and one of them was given the remainder of the string of condoms, with which he began to run offstage as the act neared its conclusion. This juggler stopped, however, and turned back to face the crowd holding the packet of condoms in one hand and, with a questioning look on his face, pointing at his groin with the other. The trendily attired older character nodded in agreement, much to the laugher of the audience. The performance thus made it clear exactly where one was to use the condom, although not how to put one on. It also reinforced the idea that even rich "cool guys" use condoms and protect themselves (and the girls and women with whom they have sex), contrary to the popular belief that they do not care about the risk of contracting HIV/AIDS or about other people.

The second juggling act also involved stock characters: another fashionably dressed young man and an *ibd sew*, or crazy person. In this act, however, the young man is not worthy of emulation; he is a *duriyay* (gangster), who is not educated about HIV/AIDS and

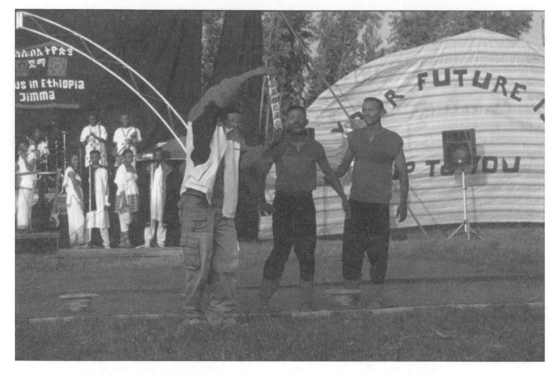

Figure 27.6 Circus Jimma hat-juggling act. Jimma, Ethiopia. Leah Niederstadt

does not protect himself, as his behavior and comments clearly indicated. The *duriyay* strutted haughtily around the stage while the *ibd sew*, whose mental state and social status were indicated by his dirty, torn clothing and the assortment of objects he carried, loudly commented that the "cool guy" was at high risk for catching HIV and developing AIDS. In this instance, the gangster lifestyle exhibited by the young male character was disparaged, while the social outcast was shown to be the voice of reason, thus reinforcing the fact that while some guys look "cool," not all of them really are. Both acts were part of a broader show that placed children and youth in positions of power as educators and voices of reason in what was portrayed as a contemporary urban society focused on materialism and pleasure. Such themes—youth empowerment, disparagement of the rich, and the need for a unified effort to combat social challenges, and to develop Ethiopia—resonate in circus performances throughout the country.

Circus Debre Birhan: Girls' Education/Early Marriage

The domestic work required of girls and women and its impact on their educational attainment are just two manifestations of their lower social status throughout Ethiopia. In rural areas in particular, girls and young women face a number of threats unique to the more conservative environment in which they live compared with their urban peers. These include early marriage, marriage by abduction, female genital mutilation, and other traditional practices that have been labeled harmful by the Ethiopian federal government and condemned by many local and international NGOs. Ethiopia's circuses address many of these issues in their performances, often accompanied by an educational message about HIV/AIDS. In 2005, troupes in Addis Ababa, Debre Birhan, and Dire Dawa all mounted shows that addressed the theme of early marriage or marriage by abduction, and included discussions of HIV/AIDS. Six to eight performances were held by each troupe and were viewed by thousands of Ethiopians in cities, towns, and small villages throughout the country.

In February 2005, Circus Debre Birhan, an associate member of Circus in Ethiopia, performed a full-length circus play for an audience that included senior administrators from the organization, other circus directors, local community members, and, most importantly to Circus Debre Birhan's director Henok Teklu Asheger, leaders from several *kebele*, or neighborhood associations, from nearby rural farming communities. The play combined several of the challenges facing rural Ethiopia, including the importance of girl's education, problems associated with early marriage or marriage by abduction, and HIV/AIDS. The storyline was as follows: a young girl named Shoayay leaves home one morning to attend school after having a conversation with her mother about how much she enjoys her studies and hopes to continue them as she gets older. During a break from class, she and her friends sit and talk about their lives and hopes for the future. While the girl's friends braid each other's hair and talk about the possibility of marriage and family, the heroine studies and comments on how important it is for girls to be educated. Two farmers come onstage, one explaining that he would like to marry Shoayay but that she will not agree to be with him because he does not have nice clothes or good manners. Shoayay returns home and attends to her chores, including the collection of water from a nearby river. While returning home, she walks by the two men who violently break the clay water container on her back, resulting in screams of surprise, then laughter, from the audience. As the girl cowers, crying that she wants to be allowed to go to school, a woman walks into the scene and the two men run off. The next scene opens with the two men meeting up with other subsistence farmers. Shoayay, several friends, and an *azmari* (traditional musician) walk by the men and the farmers kidnap the girl whose friends run off to tell her family. Shoayay's parents are later approached by one of the abductors, who is pretending to help resolve the situation with the assistance of a *shemagale*, a male elder who helps to arrange marriages, or, in the case of abduction, compensation for the victim's family. Marriage by abduction, followed by rape, is still common in many parts of rural Ethiopia, even in the highlands near the capital Addis Ababa. Our heroine is not, however, immediately raped, as the farmer who instigated her kidnapping does not want to hurt her, despite his nefarious friend's encouragement to make her "fully" his wife. The farmer's dialogue made it clear that he could not afford the cost of a wedding or setting up a household, so he resorted to marriage by abduction and chose a girl who he admired for her good behavior and beauty.

This circus play incorporated stock characters of an *azmari*, a *shemagale*, subsistence farmers, and an elderly couple, who play the girl's parents and whose confusion over HIV/AIDS causes great laughter among the audience. HIV/AIDS itself, meanwhile, is portrayed as something monstrous and unfamiliar and depicted by several young acrobats. They are dressed in skin-tight, neon-colored bodysuits that render them alien, almost insect-like in appearance. At one point, they create a pyramid in the shape of a chair, which the father thinks is a throne. When he tries to sit on it, however, the acrobats move and he falls off, much to his embarrassment, to his wife's concern, and to the laughter of the audience. The play also makes it clear that HIV can lead to AIDS as, while in their chair formation, the acrobats hold up small placards that read H-I-V, in English, and that, when flipped over, spell AIDS in Amharic (figures 27.7 and 27.8).

Thanks to the help of the *azmeri*, who does not approve of marriage by abduction and who discovers Shoayay's location in a remote one-room house, the heroine is freed before she has been sexually assaulted and returns home to her mother, who dries her tears. Shockingly to me as the foreign observer who expected the girl's family to report the abduction to the police,

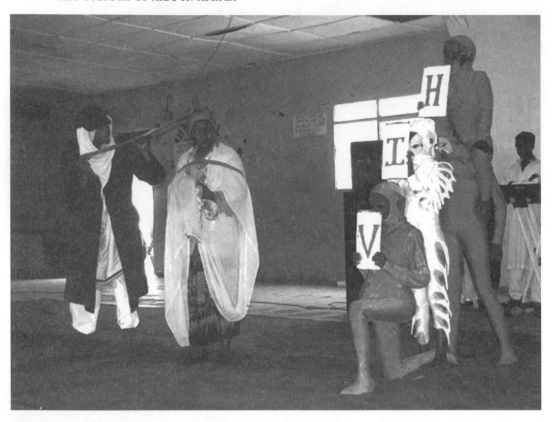

Figure 27.7 Circus Debre Birhan performers demonstrating that HIV becomes AIDS. Debre Birhan, Ethiopia. Leah Niederstadt

the play concludes with the girl and her parents reuniting with the two farmers who abducted her, all nodding in agreement that (1) marriage by abduction is wrong; (2) it can lead to HIV; and (3) girls should be educated. In commenting about this circus play, Circus Debre Birhan director Henok Teklu Asheger deemed it a huge success:

> It was really good for them to see the show. I was watching their faces and they were like this [He then made a serious, but interested face while nodding] so they understood the show. They are farmers; they are our target audience for this show. So it was really a good performance. (Asheger Interview, Feb. 27, 2005)

Through this performance, Circus Debre Birhan's performers met their goal of educating their audience—about the rights of girls and women, about the problems of early marriage and marriage by abduction, about the importance of education, and about the dangers of HIV/AIDS—while also entertaining it.[21] This combination of education and entertainment is a key factor in the popularity of circus performance in Ethiopia. Although the link between girls' education, early marriage, marriage by abduction, and HIV/AIDS was not explicitly spelled out, the messages were clear to the members of the audience with whom I spoke. Staff members of the Circus in Ethiopia organization who attended the show were also full of praise for the play's narrative, although slightly more critical of how circus skills were integrated into it.

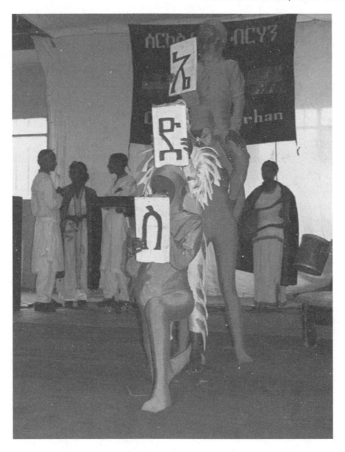

Figure 27.8 Circus Debre Birhan performers demonstrating that HIV becomes AIDS. Debre Birhan, Ethiopia. Leah Niederstadt

CIRCUS ADDIS ABABA AND CIRCUS DIRE DAWA: HIV/AIDS

As mentioned in the introduction to this chapter, in 2002 Circus Addis Ababa premiered a full-length circus play entitled: *Mekabir Kofari* (*The Grave Digger*): *A Circus Ethiopia Play about HIV/AIDS.* Its entire focus was HIV/AIDS education. In the show, a grave digger and his colleague become rich because so many people are dying from AIDS. The troupe members illustrate behaviors leading to HIV/AIDS, including reusing razorblades, engaging in unprotected sex, and contact with a used hypodermic needle. Street children serve as the protagonists of *Mekabir Kofari*: although clearly poor and ignored or abused by the wealthy people who walk by them, they are not portrayed as marginal to urban Ethiopian society but rather as integral actors within it: streetwise, hard-working children and youth who form makeshift families and forge strong alliances to protect themselves. Circus in Ethiopia recognizes them—literally and figuratively—as the future of the country.

The play opens with a song about the spread of the virus throughout local communities, cities, Ethiopia, and the wider world; fire is used as a metaphor for how quickly and destructively the HIV virus spreads. Then, the grave digger and his colleague, the *trumbanefi* (a horn player who announces important news, including deaths), meet and discuss how many people are dying from AIDS. Following a tumbling routine, the scene opens on a family in which the mother worries about the spread of HIV and the father denies the virus's existence, pointing out that they are both healthy and fine, as are their children. Following a song about how children are dying from AIDS, the family's daughter Rahel returns home from the hospital where she works as a nurse. Rahel expresses concern that she pricked herself with a needle that had been used to check her brother Efrem's blood; she is worried that he is HIV-positive. Her father's response is that "family blood is not dangerous." The *trumbanefi* sounds his horn and the family learns that Rahel's friend Hadas has died of AIDS. Rahel's father refuses to attend the funeral, which is considered a huge insult in Ethiopia.

The next series of scenes open with the performers singing a song about *hibret* (unity) and the importance of joining together to fight HIV/AIDS. The narrative shifts to a focus on *godana tadaderi* (street children), particularly the *listro* (shoeshine boys) and the girls selling snacks. While the shoeshine boys complain about the decline in business, the girls comment that everyone should carry a condom but that no one listens to them when they make such suggestions. When the *listro* respond, "Well, that's their problem," the girls reply, "No, it's a problem for ALL of us." A male customer stops for a shoeshine with a girlfriend and when offered a condom as change, he refuses it. The *listro* then comments that the customer should take and use the condom because he is often seen with different women; his girlfriend then leaves him.

The scene shifts back to Rahel and her family who receive the bad news that Efrem, a truck driver, is dying. Another transition leads us to the grave digger and the *trumbanefi* who comment on how many more people are dying; they then turn to face the audience and state that even if someone looks healthy, she or he can be infected. They urge everyone to get an HIV test. The *godana tadaderi* sing a song about the increase in deaths and ask, "Who is responsible for this? Who will be responsible for this?" They ask the grave digger how many people he has buried that day; and after being admonished for not greeting him properly before asking questions, they learn that he has bought condoms. His colleague, the *trumbanefi*, then asks, "Why? You cannot eat them." The grave digger responds that that condoms help protect men and women from HIV and other sexually transmitted diseases, and the street children praise him for using a condom.

Another shift in scene returns us to Rahel's family where her father is cutting the corns on his feet with a used razor blade. The street children tell him that he should always use a new razor blade, but he ignores them. His daughter returns home and is horrified to find that he used the blade with which she had shaved her legs and cut herself. The children sing a reprise of the song about people dying. Rahel and her family talk about Efrem's death, but the father refuses to accept that Efrem died of AIDS. He orders Rahel to leave the house because she insists on acknowledging how her brother died. Rahel's mother says, "The virus is going round and round. Don't deny it any longer!" Rahel and her mother agree that education is key to preventing the spread of the disease. A series of songs then discusses HIV/AIDS awareness, the need to use condoms, and government and NGO efforts to address the pandemic through advertisements, informative public meetings, and television and radio programming.

The *listro* hold a meeting to decide how they can help to address the HIV/AIDS pandemic. They agree that if a customer shows that he is carrying a condom, he will receive a 50 percent discount on a shoeshine. They also decide to stock condoms and educational pamphlets in their shoeshine boxes and to allow organizations like DKT Ethiopia, an NGO that works on HIV/AIDS prevention and family planning, to advertise on their boxes. The *listro* and girls selling snacks also proclaim that even though they are children, they have a right to an education and to speak freely about HIV/AIDS and its impact on their lives.

A return to Rahel's family shows that everyone except the father and granddaughter Pusto has died of AIDS. Pusto is told that she must now beg to support herself and her grandfather, and the street children comment that many families are hiding behind their children instead of acknowledging how AIDS has destroyed their families. A gang of *duriyay* (gangsters) enters the narrative, talking about the money they have extorted from their neighbors, drinking, chewing *chat* (a stimulant leaf), and visiting prostitutes. To save money, they decide to rape a female student or a servant girl; and when one of them suggests using a condom, the others shout "No!" in unison. The street children and the grave digger, seeing the assault in progress, attack the *duriyay* and prevent them from raping the girl.

The grave digger and *trumbanefi* meet again to share their latest news. They have become visibly wealthy and work is easier than ever as the bodies are now so thin: "I only have to dig a grave fifty centimetres down, instead of a meter." They carry mobile phones (at a time when the wait for a SIM card was more than a year), wear expensive, ready-made suits, and refer to their brand-new Land Cruisers, which then sold for more than $100,000 given the federal tax on imported cars. While most Ethiopians live in one- or two-room homes in shared compounds, the grave digger and *trumbanefi* brag that their houses are so big that they have a spare room for each leg and arm, plus a fifth room in which to rest their head. The conversation shifts, however, as the two men comment on the deaths in Rahel's family, and note how her daughter Pusto is now alone on the streets following the death of her grandfather. They resolve to find and care for her. Pusto finally appears sitting under a leaky umbrella in the rain, crying "Do not repeat the mistakes of my family. Who will protect me?" The play closes with the entire circus troupe singing the *hibret* (unity) song and urging the audience to join in the fight against HIV/AIDS.

Mekabir Kofari was a success at every level. The show attracted huge crowds and played to audiences that ranged from *godana tadaderi* to NGO workers, and from ambassadors to local government officials; Ethiopians from every socioeconomic class attended, as did a diverse representation of the capital's expatriate community. The audience reaction to the show—both in terms of its messages and its artistic achievement as a circus performance—was extremely positive. A Dutch NGO awarded Circus in Ethiopia funding to create similar HIV/AIDS circus plays to be performed by each main branch troupe, including Circus Addis Ababa. The funding covered the cost of writing scripts, developing music, stage sets, and costumes, advertising, and other related expenses.

Circus Addis Ababa's second HIV/AIDS-oriented show was called *The Hero*. Also written by Aweke Emiru, the play told the story of a *listro* who tries to prevent his sister from becoming the mistress of a rich man. Throughout the show, characters referred to neighborhoods within Addis Ababa, the rapid growth in private colleges and universities (which few circus performers can afford to attend), and the latest fashions in clothing and hairstyles then popular in the Ethiopian capital. These local references were included to resonate with the audience and caused exclamations of surprise and much laughter among the spectators. The hero, of course, is the shoeshine boy whose efforts prove that children and youth can make a difference, and that education and empowerment, particularly of children and women, are crucial to the fight against HIV/AIDS.

Aweke Emiru then traveled to Dire Dawa where he rewrote the script for that city's local circus troupe: this time reflecting places, practices, and trends associated with Ethiopia's second-largest city. Circus Dire Dawa's version was called *I'm A Rich Man. How Can I Die?* Their circus morality play soundly answered this question through its depiction of the rich man's activities, including adultery, bribery, infidelity, greed, public drunkenness, promiscuity, and the seduction of the *listro*'s sister. The show demonstrated the increasing wealth of the rich man and the *listro's* sister through a series of costume changes that mirrored the latest fashions arriving in *Taiwan*, Dire Dawa's market for imported goods and tailor-made clothing. Although his clothing did not change markedly, as he was rich from the start, the rich man's stomach became larger as the play continued, demonstrating his greed and his ability to eat more than he needed to survive. Meanwhile, the shoeshine boy's sister progresses from wearing torn and dirty trousers, a T-shirt, and broken flip-flops to an imported tracksuit and sneakers, and eventually ready-made jeans, a silk-like red shirt, sandals, and a broad-brimmed hat, all of which were the height of current fashion. Although rudimentary, the play's set echoed the places community members might see as they walked through Dire Dawa's streets, including a café, a *suq* (small roadside shop), and a *bunna bait*, or bar/brothel, above which a sign reads *YeAIDS mirt* (Best quality AIDS).

Eventually, the rich man realizes he is HIV-positive. None of his money can save him. Bribes to his doctor prove useless and, at the time, antiretroviral drugs were not widely available in Ethiopia, so he could not buy medicine to slow the progress of the disease. The rich man develops AIDS and becomes visibly sicker, as evidenced by the worsening condition of his clothing, his slimmer physique, and his slumping body posture. He loses his wealth and status and must face the fact that he has "killed" his wife and his mistress, the *listro's* sister, who laments that if only she had listened to her brother she would not be infected with HIV and be facing certain death. The *listro* mourns the impending death of his sister but resolves to protect himself, his friends, and others from facing the same fate. Once again, children and youth are presented as powerful individuals in contemporary Ethiopian society and the importance of education and unity in the fight against HIV/AIDS are clearly illustrated.

CONCLUSION

Ethiopian circuses have increasingly attempted to address the HIV/AIDS pandemic in their performances and in their other activities. In September 2005, in cooperation with HAPCO, the Circus in Ethiopia organization published a magazine that served as both a circus newsletter and a means of disseminating information about HIV/AIDS; the Amharic text on the cover clearly indicates the cooperative effort (figure 27.9). Articles in the magazine presented the history of the circus movement, its organizational structure and budget, and a profile of Martha Estifanos, a young woman living with HIV/AIDS. Another article titled "The importance of circus in the fight against HIV/AIDS" (see figure 27.2) claims that Circus in Ethiopia has taken "the leading position" in the fight against HIV/AIDS (*Circus in Ethiopia* 2005, 27). It also argues that circus is an effective means of HIV/AIDS education because it breaks the silence about the pandemic, combines education with entertainment, addresses misconceptions about transmission and prevention, and combats stigma (*Circus in Ethiopia* 2005, 28). While it is clear that no single NGO or government agency can really claim to have taken "the leading position" in the fight against HIV/AIDS, Circus in Ethiopia has played an important role in educating the Ethiopian public about HIV/AIDS during the post-socialist period.

In early 2001, I met with Metmku Yohannes, an Ethiopian lawyer who then served as executive director of Circus in Ethiopia. In discussing the organization's various activities, Metmku commented that Circus Addis Ababa's current show included "scripts, songs, all kinds of expression...for disseminating info and education to the public about HIV/AIDS. [It] was performed well and the messaging part was very well received!" He continued by exclaiming that the show's theme was so important that the troupe would soon be "at the Dutch

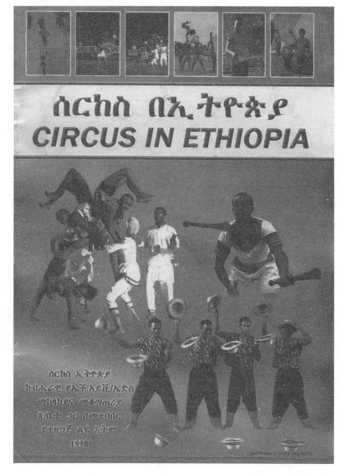

Figure 27.9 Cover of *Circus in Ethiopia* (September 2005)

Embassy...performing the AIDS messages, even for them" (Yohannes Interview, Apr. 11, 2001). Although only a year and a half into my research, I knew then how significant his statement was. Previously, most performances for foreign audiences (and certainly all shows aimed at foreigners that I had thus far seen) had not overtly addressed the contemporary social challenges facing Ethiopia. Even the positive messages about ethnic diversity were often lost on *ferengi* (non-Ethiopians) who do not recognize the difference between Amharic, Konso, or Gurage songs, dances, and costumes, let alone the other ethnic and cultural references found in many Ethiopian circus morality plays. For the most part, shows performed primarily for foreigners consisted almost solely of circus acts and musical performance, with the occasional H-I-V brick juggling act (see figure 27.2) thrown in; this was true of performances at home and while abroad on tour.

Yet, the last decade has seen a shift in focus on the part of Ethiopian circus troupes to incorporate HIV/AIDS education into their public performances whenever possible. As a form of free entertainment combining indigenous performative practices with acrobatics, juggling, and other circus skills, circus performances reach large audiences that can then be targeted with a variety of didactic messages, including those on HIV/AIDS. Circus in Ethiopia's ability to reach hundreds, if not thousands, of spectators at one time is especially important given the high

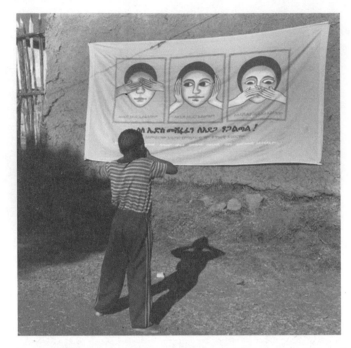

Figure 27.10 Circus Debre Birhan performer imitating an HIV/AIDS education banner. Rosa Verhoeve

rates of illiteracy in Ethiopia, particularly among the rural and urban poor, girls, and women, and the relatively limited access most peri-urban and rural Ethiopians have to traditional news media outlets. Circus performances are also not hindered by a lack of electricity or an appropriate stage; most main branch troupes travel with generators and can perform on any flat surface, as long as a crowd can gather. Although it remains to be seen how effective such performances are in terms of their educational messages, it is clear from watching people attending an Ethiopian circus show that their attention is rapt and that they do follow the narrative, whether about land-mine safety or HIV/AIDS.[22] The information provided, albeit often simplistic, is (nearly always) accurate and educational and is often conveyed with a sense of humor that engages the audience, even on topics that are serious or rarely discussed in public or in the home.

Given the recent spate of natural disasters impacting the global community, international donor agencies working in Ethiopia increasingly demand proof that their funds are used to bring about demonstrable, positive change. They have also begun to require that organizations receiving these funds are above reproach, and that the funds are used—in the case of the circuses—solely for public performances, leaving circus administrators struggling to meet their operating costs and continue performing. In addition, a new, draconian federal law governing indigenous NGOs in Ethiopia has made it difficult for many organizations to restructure to meet the new restrictions, including the demand that they raise the majority of their funding in Ethiopia, as opposed to receiving donations from international NGOs. In part driven by these factors, fundamental changes are occurring to the ways in which Ethiopian circus troupes operate. Circus performances remain didactic, however, and they are still conceived of as a means of educating Ethiopians and presenting—to borrow a phrase from a review of a 1998 circus performance in Australia—"an other Ethiopia," one in which people see, hear, and speak about issues (figure 27.10) that concern them, especially with regard to HIV/AIDS (Bishop and Bishop 1998).

28

Interlude
Interview With VOLSET Youth
Drama Group

Interviewers: Gregory Barz and Vincent Wandera

Do you thing music has played a role in the prevention and control of HIV in your community?*

First of all through music, there is some message you can spread to people. So, in that music, sometimes the sick, we teach them how to be patient, not to fear, [because] some of them [want to] commit suicide. Through music there is [a] message telling them you should not go commit suicide because, it's not good, it won't go away.

Do you remember a time when music was used to convey to someone who is maybe going to take a suicide?

I think it was 1999. When we were having our drama group, somebody got that disease and was going to commit suicide. But after getting our songs he said, "No, I've turned back, I won't do that." Because when you get that disease it is not like you are going to die, you are free to be with your friends, not commit suicide.

Is there another one with another role that music has played?

Some days we go into many villages. So one day we went in a village. We performed our drama and our singing in that village. But we found a man there who said, "For me, I have my HIV. I'm going to spread it to other people." After we sang our songs, our drama, he told his friend he was not going to do the things that I told you.

* VOLSET = Voluntary Service Trust Team located in the Luwero District, Uganda. Interview on August 6, 2001.

As youth, what do you feel when you sing about AIDS or HIV?

When we talk about HIV, you feel bad because you can find a friend of yours suffering without school fees, without anything.

We have no funds to give to the orphans. We feel, I don't know how you can express it, but we feel sorry for them, because me as youth, we have nothing we can do to help. So I feel scared, and me, I learn not to do such, because leaving my children behind suffering is a very bad thing.

Our music and drama can help those people who are suffering from AIDS, who are losing power, because they are going to die. They have AIDS, but through those songs, they can get comfort, and they can protect themselves, although they are not going to be healed.

How can you defend yourself using the music? Supposing I wanted to infect you. How can you fight back?

Sir, let me say if someone wants to infect me, so I leave him. I tell him come to what? To our drama presentation where we shall meet.

How can this eventually change a life?

In some songs there are some scary words that are true. If the song comes to me, and says, "by doing such and such you might get AIDS," I may lose my interest in sex. If a listener is an old man and has children, he might think, "If I die I leave my children orphans," and some of them will get AIDS.

Now, who is your main target group?

We mostly target youth because those older people, whether they've got or not, they're about to die. But, these youth, they will be the government of tomorrow. So, we have to teach them that you don't have to do this and that to get AIDS, in order not to die, because if the youth die, we will not have any government for tomorrow.

What AIDS preventive measures are available locally in your community? And is music part of the preventive measures?

Music is part of preventative care, because when you present, people learn, and they get the message, and the prevention is promoted.

What other preventive measures are viable in our community?

Dramas, drama. Okay we promote dramas to people and give them condoms.

And we have meetings, community meetings whereby we call trained members from far away to help us teach the community about AIDS. So those people who have come will also go and tell the people who have remained at home about what they have learned.

29

Kwaito and the Culture
of AIDS in South Africa

Gavin Steingo (Columbia University)

The standard fool's guide to kwaito celebrates it as "new" music that is global,
intertextual, hybrid—call it what you will—with streams that include house,
disco/bubblegum, rap and reggae, and so on.

—Bhekezizwe Peterson (2003)

A polluting person is always wrong.

—Susan Sontag, *AIDS and Its Metaphors* (1988)

APPLYING FOR AIDS

In 2006, I entered a club in downtown Johannesburg where I was met by two friends. One of them—an immigrant from East Africa—asked me: "Why are you here? Are you applying for AIDS?" He was asking, of course, if the purpose of my visit on that night was to meet a woman. (And it was meant as a rhetorical question—what else could I have been doing there?) I soon found that his question ("Are you applying for AIDS?") was a common one and that meeting a woman and taking her home implied to many men in the club precisely such an application. Aside from the fact that the act of meeting women was seen as inextricably tied to possible HIV infection, it is significant that courting women also means *applying* for AIDS. In a city where at least half the people one might meet in a nightclub have come from far and wide in search for work, the language of applying (and sometimes being "accepted") has entered the very texture of thought. One thing is clear: Johannesburg is a city that offers potential work and pleasure for people from all over Africa; but when you apply for the good life, you apply for its dark underside, too.

It would be a mistake, of course, to understand questions such as the one described uncritically. Considering that the club is located in downtown Johannesburg, it is reasonable to assume that most of people there that night knew about HIV/AIDS and also how to protect themselves against contracting the disease. The "question" I was asked can therefore be interpreted in the following dialectical way: on the one hand, I was being warned (he may just have well have said: "Be careful! Wear a condom!"); and on the other hand, I was being engaged in a kind of playful masculine discourse, a "guys' thing," a specific type of performativity of whose precise meanings I was at that point not fully aware.

I LIKE TO ENJOY MYSELF

Almost no one who attends nightclubs in Johannesburg drives home sober. Road accidents are common and are reported without alarm. Johannesburg roads have other problems, too. The only way for most black workers to get around is on unreliable and often overloaded minibus "taxis" that are often involved in fatal accidents. It is not uncommon on any given day to be told by someone that his/her brother or sister has died in an "accident." Details are very seldom provided and questions hardly ever asked ("How many people were involved? Where were they going?"). Shula Marks and Neil Andersson argue that it is "the acceptance of accident as normal that marks the violent nature of the society" in South Africa (1990, 44). "Accident" is a word so fatal that to pronounce it seems like a death sentence.

In 2006 a friend of mine drove home late one night with a passenger and was involved in an accident. The passenger died, and my friend was in the hospital for several months. Like many (im)migrants in Johannesburg, Peter lives alone, far from his family.[1] Although we have never spoken about it, it is almost certain that he simply got on a bus one day and arrived in Johannesburg with one suitcase, speaking no Zulu or Sotho, and only broken English. Peter and his friends go out about five nights a week (often until well after 4 A.M.) and leave for work early the next morning. They spend a fortune on alcohol (and always insist on buying drinks for friends and friends of friends), and many of them drive home drunk and exhausted. The explanation for this reckless kind of behavior is simple and was given to me without hesitation by Peter: "I like to enjoy myself."

AIDS, poverty, crime. Johannesburg is in many ways a devastated city. But it is also a city seething with late night pleasures, speed, excitement, and dreams. Achille Mbembe argues that "Johannesburg became a central site not only for the birth of the modern in Africa, but for the entanglement of the modern and the African—the African modern." Inhabitants of Johannesburg, Mbembe tells us, express a "mania for wealth, for the sensational and the ephemeral, for appearances" (see Mbembe 2004, 376). It is the inhabitants of these "modern African" urban spaces that I am most interested in.

KWAITO, HIV/AIDS, SEXUALITY

In this chapter, I examine the triangular relationship between sexuality, HIV/AIDS, and popular music in urban South Africa. I focus on the musical genre known as kwaito, which can be roughly summarized as a form of electronic dance music that emerged together with South Africa's democracy in the early 1990s.[2] Kwaito music is not overtly political and is generally thought of as music-to-move-to. Kwaito is party music, and—if we are to believe the common party line—presents and represents the celebration of the newly free youth. Kwaito music and the constellation of other social aspects that make up kwaito "kulcha" more generally are situated at the apex of several struggles. Appearing in tandem with the demise of apartheid, kwaito music became the soundtrack of liberation as well as other struggles still to be fought: poverty, crime, unemployment, and HIV/AIDS.

Much scholarly research on kwaito focuses on the genre's emergence alongside the democracy of 1994. It is important, however, to focus on how the 1980s "prepared" the youth for democracy; that is to say, rather than understanding 1994 only as a radical break from the past (which, of course, in some sense it was), we need to also tease out the continuities. One of the major anti-apartheid strategies among youth in the 1980s was to be "ungovernable." The Young Lions of the ANC Youth League advocated organized but disruptive strikes and marches on the one hand, and complete chaos and unruliness on the other. "Liberation before Education" was the slogan of the times (see van der Vliet 2001, 154.). As Steve Mokwena observes about the 1980s: "*All* forms of control were challenged. Some argue that it was the strategy of 'ungovernability,' preached by sections of the political movement, which is directly responsible for the breakdown of control in the townships" (Mokwena 1992, 30–51).

It is often argued that the politics of disruption did not fully prepare the youth for life after the struggle. Many of the young lions and lionesses who boycotted and burned schools, who were involved in criminal activities, and who refused to listen to or believe anything the Nationalist government (or their own parents) said, are today described as the "lost generation." In many ways, the struggle did not prepare the youth for leading a nation. They are lost. The future is now in the hands of their children.

Importantly, it was precisely this "ungovernable" generation that celebrated the new freedoms of the democratic era, with their favorite music genre—kwaito—as the soundtrack. Because of the sensitive political issues deeply embedded in this generation, struggling against HIV/AIDS proved problematic. In the early 1990s (just as kwaito was taking off) dealing with the problems of HIV/AIDS took a back seat to the struggle for immanent political freedom. Moreover, the strategy of conscious disorganization in townships made productive mobilization against HIV/AIDS very difficult. In the late 1980s, anti-apartheid groups dismissed AIDS education attempts by the white government as "racist propaganda" (see van der Vliet 2001, 155). Black activists—understandably suspicious of any activity whatsoever by the Nationalist government—held that the promotion of condoms by the state was merely an attempt to decrease birth rates among the black population. AIDS was an acronym, many said, for "Afrikaner Invention to Deprive us of Sex" (ibid.). A deep suspicion thus arose of all AIDS "authorities," and this suspicion has remained throughout the first decade of the twenty-first century. A 2003 article in *Y Mag* titled "Condom Wise?" quoted a teenage boy saying: "I think there's a conspiracy to kill off the black nation and put AIDS in condoms" (Kamaldien 2003, 36).

Such ideas—which cannot simply be dismissed as uninformed or ignorant—have no doubt been encouraged by uneven and ambiguous state responses to the AIDS epidemic. Former President Mbeki's infamous public statements about the disease and the more recent Jacob Zuma "shower" scandal[3] are well known, and need not be rehashed here. What I want to emphasize, however, is the inconsistency of messages about HIV/AIDS that reach the youth. We would do well to observe, moreover, that in "the same year that apartheid formally ended in Pretoria, the groundwork for what some have called 'global apartheid' was finalized in Washington, DC" (Sitze 2004, 773). 1994 saw the end of apartheid and the simultaneous establishment of the power of perinatal AZT treatment (ibid.). Only a few years later the World Trade

Organization (WTO) codified a number of clauses relating to Trade-Related Aspects of Intellectual Property Rights (TRIPs) which effectively kept treatment in the hands of several multinational pharmaceuticals. As Adam Sitze comments:

> Not to be outdone where cruel mismanagement is concerned, the World Bank and the International Monetary Fund (IMF), acting with their signature incompetence, responded to HIV/AIDS, not only by adding fuel to the fire, but also, during the late 1990s, by accusing Africans of arson. As scores of analysts have shown, it is no accident that the states which implemented structural adjustment plans in the 1980s were the same ones that found themselves most unable to respond effectively to the spread of HIV/AIDS in the 1990s. (2004, 773)

In sum, South Africa's transition into a liberal democratic state was paralleled by both the onset of the HIV/AIDS epidemic and the establishment of global and local neo-liberal policies (including so-called "structural readjustment").

In the following sections, I will explore the intricate lines of flight that link kwaito with HIV/AIDS and sexuality. Kwaito moved over temporal borders, from the struggle for political freedom, to the struggle over HIV/AIDS. How has a genre—that is almost always referred to as "apolitical"—moved people, moved with people, and been moved by people?[4] What is the relationship between popular music and sexual activity? These are some of the questions I will attempt to answer.

KWAITO AND RAPE?

One of the major contributors to the AIDS epidemic in South Africa is rape. A politically free, but economically disenfranchised youth without opportunity finds itself in a desperate situation. The celebratory ethos of democratic South Africa was, therefore, tainted from the start. The joy of political freedom and the serious partying that ensued in 1994 were, in many ways, made of sand. "After 1994," writes Liz McGregor, "the fervour once channeled into politics went into partying. Years of youth lost to struggle were now reclaimed on the streets of Soweto in giant bashes." (McGregor 2005, 95). We should not forget, however, that this specific brand of neo-liberal freedom has an underside. As Kenny, one of McGregor's main informants said: "The music would go on and on. [There is no doubt that kwaito would have been played at such parties.] Sometimes there would be fights when people were getting drunk. Some people would start shooting. I've seen people who tried to force girls into their cars during one of these street bashes" (cited in McGregor 2005, 95). A common story in South Africa (or rather, a common story told about South Africa): mad parties turn into ugly affairs that end in fights and lead to sexual violence.

The question that must concern us here, however, is the following: what role, exactly, does kwaito play at such parties, and what role (if any) does kwaito have in sexual violence? In this section I examine masculinities, music, and rape as a way of addressing a major cause of HIV infection in South Africa.

Like all other forms of popular music, kwaito has come under fire from journalists and scholars. The most trenchant criticism of kwaito came from cultural studies scholars Sarah Nuttall and Cheryl-Ann Michael. In their brief editorial introduction to part three, "Sound," in the collection *Senses of Culture*, Nuttall and Michael write about Simon Stephens' chapter on kwaito:

> Stephens shows that jackrolling, or gang rape, is frequently accompanied, or primed, by the playing of this music [i.e., kwaito]—as if the acting out of certain masculinities needs a soundtrack. Here is a culture of drugging by music—where no moral or ethical consequences can stake a claim. Sounds works as a narcotic. (2000, 215)

Before entering into the more difficult issues raised in the above quote, I would like to trace Stephens's argument. How does Stephens "show" that gang rape is primed by kwaito? In his chapter, simply titled "Kwaito," Stephens dwells at length on the topic of misogyny and sexism in kwaito (in terms of lyrics, dance styles, dress, etc.) (Stephens 2000). However, Stephens only devotes a very small section to the topic of rape. Having stated that he has long been aware of the "misogynist dimensions of kwaito," Stephens reflects that after attending a concert by kwaito group Boom Shaka he "began to wonder whether kwaito music was a reflection or manifestation of sexual crime" (Stephens 2000, 265). After stating that kwaito has "misogynist dimensions," Stephens lets his mind wonder (and wander): what is the relationship between kwaito and sexual crime? Stephens then fails to mention kwaito again for the next page and a half, during which time he elaborates on the topic of gang rape. Although Simon Stephens has done nothing to establish the relationship between kwaito and sexual crime, he seems to think that it is both relevant and appropriate to devote well over a page to the topic of gang rape (Stephens 2000, 265–266). Even more peculiar is Nuttall and Michael's reading of Stephens' essay. They assert that Stephens "shows" that jackrolling is primed by "this music"—even though he does no such thing.[5] I do not suggest that rapists do not listen to kwaito; I do not even suggest that kwaito does not "prime" sexual violence. I am only saying that Stephens does not "show" this. He does not try to. He simply makes several sexual innuendos and leaves it at that.

One the other hand, ethnographer Kate Wood suggests a more direct link between kwaito and criminality (including rape). She argues that "the pursuit of hedonism (including the sexual variety), celebrated in the often crude lyrics of contemporary *kwaito* music, was an important part of the freedoms imputed to the criminal lifestyles on the fringes of which many men lived" (Wood 2005, 313). Wood further notes that during one alcohol-motivated group rape, the assailants sang a kwaito song (Wood 2005, 309). In personal correspondence, Dr. Wood told me further that "Among the young men [she] lived and worked with, the consumption of kwaito was strongly linked to the consumption of alcohol (and women . . .), especially in the specific space of the shebeen [club]" (Wood E-mail, Aug. 21, 2006).

I would like to examine each of these claims in turn.

1. [T]he pursuit of hedonism (including the sexual variety), celebrated in the often crude lyrics of contemporary kwaito music, was an important part of the freedoms imputed to the criminal lifestyles on the fringes of which many men lived.

Kwaito is often described as a music genre and popular culture phenomenon associated with hedonism. "Hedonism" (and its twin "pleasure") is a term so commonly used in discussions of kwaito that it deserves closer analysis. Ethnomusicologist David Coplan, for example, sees kwaito as a dance form (as opposed to a song form) that accepts the youth's "pleasure principle as a valid replacement for the now painfully passé politicized ideology of social sacrifice" (2005, 21). As I have mentioned, kwaito is often thought of as music for the youth "after the struggle," a music of jubilation and ecstatic partying. Notably, this "jubilation" is also often characterized as chaotic, disorganized, pleasurable, and dangerous. However, to say that "freedom [has been] imputed to...criminal lifestyles" is, strictly speaking, untrue. Democratic freedom in South Africa does not extend to criminal lifestyles. While it is true that oppression by police has slackened (through both corruption and different systems of governance) since the end of the apartheid regime in the 1980s, people are not "free" to lead criminal lifestyles. In fact, South African jails are today fuller than ever. According to Kelly Gillespie:

> [S]ince 1994, the year of South Africa's non-racial elections, there has been a 60 percent *growth* in prison population. South Africa has consistently remained within the world's top ten countries with the highest rates of incarceration, and it is by far the most aggressive incarcerator on the African continent, with some of its prisons 300 percent overcrowded, and large prison-building projects currently underway. (2008, 70, emphasis in the original)

Furthermore, while it may be true that kwaito lyrics occasionally celebrate "criminal lifestyles," this is actually seldom the case. A quick listen to a number of kwaito artists (from Mandoza and Trompies, to Zola and Mzekezeke) illustrates that the lyrics of kwaito address many issues, the minority of which deal with criminal lifestyles. Although some (certainly not most) kwaito fans are involved in crime in some way, kwaito musicians have for years been encouraging listeners to distance themselves from criminal activity. The important kwaito musician and producer Arthur told a journalist for *The Guardian*:

> [Kwaito] shouldn't be perceived as gangster music, 'cos then that way we're just not gonna get anywhere...It has to be something we have to forget about, honestly speaking...Kwaito is clean and we have to keep fighting to keep it clean...'cos it was not meant to hurt other people's feelings. It's supposed to be about rejoicing about who you are as a South African. (Lusk 2003, 45)

The ambivalence in Arthur's words is clearly audible: "it *was not meant to* hurt other people's feelings. It's *supposed to be* about..." And the reason for this ambivalence is clear. Arthur's comments were made shortly after his brother, Makhendlas (who was also a kwaito musician), shot someone at a concert. Perhaps Makhendlas, like Arthur, felt shame and hatred toward criminality—shortly after the shooting incident, Makhendlas committed suicide. Nonetheless, Arthur's intentions are clear: we've got to keep kwaito clean.

In conclusion, we may say that kwaito's relationship to criminality and the alleged "freedom" of criminals is both complex and equivocal. Most kwaito musicians deplore crime. Also, the fantasy of a "criminal lifestyle" (which finds itself in many genres globally, the best known being gangsta rap) is clearly based on the historical imagination. The fascination with criminality—both organized crime and smaller time muggings—goes back at least to the craze in 1950s South Africa for American mob movies (for more on this matter, see Nixon 1994). Crime and gangs are nothing new in South Africa, and they are certainly not a consequence of kwaito. Furthermore, it is a mistake to simply conflate "gangsta" semiotics with real crime. Certainly, the relationship between performance praxis and everyday lived experience is not one of simple correspondence.

 2. During one alcohol-motivated group rape, the assailants sang a kwaito song.
What does this fact mean? Does it mean that (as Nuttall and Michael would have us believe) kwaito is a drug, a narcotic that impairs listeners and perhaps even coerces them to rape women?

Does it mean that men enjoy singing kwaito when they rape women? Does it mean that kwaito is somehow connected to rape, is rape's natural soundtrack, that the rhythm of kwaito is the rhythm of rape?

Two preliminary points should be made. First, we are not told what song the assailants sang. Were the lyrics of the song somehow about rape? Without knowing what song was sung, our analysis must by necessity be limited. Second, we are told that the assailants *sang* the kwaito song. This is significant, since it is usually the grooving beat of kwaito tunes that is glimpsed with a suspicious eye. Surely singing a kwaito song without the rhythmic backing (that is, the rhythm track, complete with synthesized drum and bass loops) is less likely to induce—like a narcotic—some kind of sexual psychosis (if we are to believe, that is, that this music produces such an effect)?

Having raised these two points, the main question again is: what is the exact relationship between kwaito and sexual crime, aside from this one empirical example (in which kwaito is explicitly and literally linked to rape)? Do rapists particularly like kwaito? Was the song that was sung simply a popular song at the time? Is it not possible that rapists, like almost all other non-rapist black South Africans, like a good kwaito tune?

These questions point to a more general level of inquiry and to another question that Stephens has already asked: does kwaito (or any form of popular music, we might add) reflect or manifest sexual violence? This question can, however, be read in two ways. First, given that kwaito does one or the other, does it reflect *or* does it manifest sexual violence? Second, does kwaito do any reflection or manifesting of sexual crime whatsoever? I have consistently attempted to evade this question since I believe that the terms are too simple. Instead, I have turned to a close reading of Stephens, and Nuttall and Michael to see how their various arguments are constructed. Let us leave this point hanging; it is doubtful that we will come to any clear or simple answer.

3. *[T]he consumption of kwaito [is] strongly linked to the consumption of alcohol (and women...), especially in the specific space of the shebeen.*

The above statement was made in a personal correspondence with Kate Wood, and so I will not subject it to careful scrutiny. However, I would like to make a few points, to raise a few questions. First, in nightclubs around the world alcohol, music, and the search for sexual or romantic partners are intimately connected. Kwaito is no exception. What can possibly be meant by the parenthetical remark that women are "consumed" in the shebeen? I doubt that Wood is saying that sexual activity literally takes place in the public space of the shebeen. More probably, Wood means that women are consumed by the "male gaze," that the shebeen is a "meat market," to use a rather vulgar international expression.

Moreover, Wood adds that "chill-out/smoking time" (that is, time that is still social, but on a smaller, more intimate level) "was strictly reggae-time." Like many international venues (including clubs and raves in places like New York and London), harder grooving, more danceable music is heard in rowdier spaces (in the present case, the shebeen), while slower and more "chill" music is heard in smaller and more intimate spaces (hence the "chill-out room" at many raves and parties in South Africa and abroad). Kwaito, again, is no exception.

Wood told me (as an interesting aside) that "[American rapper] Tupac [Shakur]'s song 'Dear Mama' was for quite different reasons a particular hit among the group of young men I hung out with, who constantly wished to pay tribute to their mothers' heroism" (2006, p.c.). Again, we see a much more complex and textured picture of South African listeners, a picture that is not easily reducible to stereotypical (and racist) ideas of black menaces.

We should also be careful not to forget the agency of women. Although women's agency in kwaito is highly contestable, Angela Impey argues that "kwaito has offered women a new kind of agency in self-representation in post-Apartheid South Africa...like Madonna, kwaito female artists have learned to effectively navigate within a repressive discourse to create liberatory musical images" (2001, 47–48). We need to only note the success of kwaito stars such as Lebo Mathosa and Thandiswa to illustrate that within kwaito culture women are not passive observers. Gauging from my own experiences, women in Johannesburg clubs such as the Horror Café, the (now defunct) Rhino Bar, and the News Café in Rosebank seem more comfortable with their bodies and their sexualities than do women in Western Europe or America. In general, young black South African women exude confidence. This is not to say that South African women are not subject to crime and violence. The point is rather that South African women do engage with problems actively on a day-to-day basis, resisting, enjoying, suffering, and living the South African landscape as participants, mothers, sisters, wives, girlfriends, and friends. The slogan of times past has not yet been forgotten: "If you strike a woman, you have struck a rock" (see DeShazer 1994).

TELEOLOGY, REPETITION COMPULSION, AND AESTHETICS OF SLOWNESS

There are two musical characteristics that fans and critics of kwaito often comment on. One: kwaito has a strong and insistent beat. Two: kwaito is slow. Both of these characteristics can be traced to kwaito's origin in House music. An oft-told legend holds that in the late 1980s a House DJ put a track on at a slower speed than he had intended. The crowd loved it, and kwaito was born. In the 1980s, South African black urban youth listened to a variety of local and international genres, the most popular of which were bubblegum (that is, South African disco music performed by artists such as Brenda Fassie, Yvonne Chaka Chaka, and Chicco Twala), South African jazz, gospel, international pop (including singers such as Michael Jackson), and House. Kwaito emerged near the end of the 1980s and gained popularity rapidly as South Africa plummeted toward its first democratic election in 1994. Between the years 1992 and 1998, House remained popular but lost some of its fan base to kwaito. Between the years 1994 and 1999, kwaito and gospel were the two most popular music genres in South Africa. In the last few years, however, kwaito has declined in popularity (especially in urban centers such as Johannesburg and Cape Town), and House has re-emerged as the most popular genre at clubs.

In many ways, kwaito is the same as House, although kwaito is slower and at times has more lyrics. That is to say, aside from tempo, kwaito is rhythmically identical to House. Significantly, the two most commonly commented upon musical characteristics of kwaito (insistent beat and slowness) often enter into the thinking (and perhaps feeling) of sexuality. The steady and somewhat static pulse of kwaito is so often invoked in discussions of the genre's sexiness or raunchiness. Cultural theorist and kwaito admirer Bhekezizwe Peterson writes in a section titled "Shake your arse and your mind will follow?" that "the most frequent social and aesthetic dismissal of kwaito is that it is mindless, repetitive music that caters to the lowest banal and sensual denominator." Yet, as he goes on to point out: "For the record, as dance music kwaito is unashamedly committed to setting down irresistible beats" (Peterson 2003, 203). Similarly, commenting on Lara Allen's observations that the music of the early top kwaito groups "was generally dominated by an unyielding, pounding bass beat that was marginally mediated by other cyclically repeated rhythmic modules,"[6] Coplan writes that kwaito "expressed and embodied the new sound for the post-struggle young black lions and lionesses: a prideful, even predatory roar of pleasure hunting" (2005, 15). In both of these characterizations, rhythm is equated with pleasure and sexuality. It should not surprise us, moreover, that many important South African culture brokers have perpetuated these characterizations. For example, a fashion spread in *Y Mag* (which, incidentally, displays a large picture of kwaito musician Zola on one page) features several black people at a kwaito bash doing what the magazine refers to as a "primal dance." The caption on the first page reads: "Ymag salutes 'the dance,' the primal human ritual signifying love, life, lust, death, celebration" (*Y Mag*, Oct/Nov 2002: 68–80).

This idea comes, no doubt, from the common correlation of (especially masculine) sexuality and virility with rhythmic pounding. Ethnographer and popular music scholar Stephen Amico illustrates, for example, that in a New York gay subculture dancing to House music is a hyper-masculine performance, often equated to a workout (see Amico 2001). He explains, moreover, that the historical linkage in Western thought of women with all that is bodily cannot be applied to this specific New York subculture. Instead, rhythm and body together constitute a specific form of virility and masculinity, even within the sphere of a gay scene.

Thus, while kwaito is coded as masculine, it is a specific type of masculinity. Not quite a feminine masculinity, but an othered masculinity, a *racialized* (marked) masculinity that constitutes both hegemony and subalternity. Kwaito's pulse often automatically leads to a pathologizing of black male sexuality (which in the case of House would probably be marked as pervert-queer). The a(nti)teleogical *drive* of kwaito music can thus be sharply contrasted with the hallmark of Western masculinity, the key term in Western phallogocentricism: teleology. If there is any truth at all in Susan McClary's (in)famous claim that Beethoven's music mirrors Western masculine sexuality in that it is goal-directed—and often violently so, toward orgasm, toward cadence—then kwaito implies a different type of masculine sexuality altogether. Unlike the teleological yearning of Western masculinity, kwaito is seen (rather neurotically, I believe) as the manifestation of a particular neurosis that can only be called repetition-compulsion. Kwaito, and the kind of sexuality that it is often reputed to prime, goes nowhere. Kwaito is rhythmical pounding without vision, without a future.

What of kwaito's slowness? The connection between tempo and sexuality is not often explicit. However, tempo is often described by kwaito fans as an important factor in bodily engagement with music. As I found in recent field research in Johannesburg (May–July 2007), kwaito has lost popularity partly because people feel that it is too slow and is thus difficult to dance to. In a way that deserves further exploration, the bumping and grinding type dancing that often happens in clubs in Johannesburg is often set against a preferred tempo. It is as though bodies felt a need to slow down in the mid-1990s, only to speed up once more as the euphoria of the golden years of democracy dwindled away.

Further ethnographic research may yield additional insights into the sexual connotations of slowness. At this point in my research, only one aspect is clear: tempo is inextricably linked to the production of sweat. Because it is slow, dancing to kwaito means less perspiration. I found, however, that club-goers enjoy the perspiration induced by fast House music (and this reminds us of Amico's observation that in New York dancing to House music is compared to a workout). It seems that sweating is viewed as bodily expression, an embodied reaction to music. As such, sweat is the involuntary outpouring of the body that emerges only in relationship to music. Sweat is often seen as attractive—as a sign that the body is alive and well, not to mention moist and lubricated. Instead of repressing the body's natural reaction to physical engagement with music, it seems that House music fans revel in the force of pushing one's body beyond its normal capacity.

Kwaito, unlike House, is based on a more suave or "chill" aesthetic. Commenting on kwaito's slowness (compared to House), kwaito musician Thandiswa says: "It's because black people don't like to really sweat, you know? You just wanna move enough to style, not enough to get sweaty, just enough to look cool" (quoted in Lusk 2003, 43).[7] I suggest that the correlation of kwaito with *no* sweat could be mobilized as a counterargument against critics of kwaito. Far from being mindless or "drugged," people who dance to kwaito *regulate* their bodies in self-conscious ways.

While I am not ready to draw an explicit connection between HIV/AIDS and the tempo of kwaito music, I point out here merely that tempo is intimately related to the workings of the body, its natural functions, and its porousness. Because constructions of the body often emphasize zones of permeability (see Butler 1993), the correlation of House with sweat, and kwaito with no sweat, has potentially important ramifications for future studies of South African sexuality and music.

LANGUAGE AND CONTAMINATION

As I hope to have shown in the preceding sections, kwaito, rape, sexuality, and HIV/AIDS are all integral parts of contemporary South African urban experience. In the beginning of this chapter, I suggested that the concept of "applying for AIDS" implied that the language of application and work has invaded every inch of the domain of South African life. The reverse is also true: AIDS (and its ramifications) is ubiquitous in South Africa and has infected the entire structure of feeling. Ultimately, several discourses constantly collide into each other: work, AIDS, crime, politics, music, and accidents create a rich repertoire from which "kwaito-speakers" can draw.[8]

As the linguistic equivalent of kwaito music, kwaito-speak is "rich in sound symbolism, antomasia, synecdoche, onomatopoeia and metonym" (Satyo 2001, 141). Moreover, kwaito "specializes in subverting the meanings of words." There are at least twenty different vernacular terms for the acronym "HIV," many of which are extremely inventive.

Sizwe Satyo observes the following names for HIV in South Africa (Satyo 2008):[9]

1. *Ngamagama amathathu*—It's three words

2. *Umasithathu*—Ms. three words

3. *1–2–3* (because of the three letters in "HIV")

4. *Ngu-Hilda, Ivy, Veronica* (note the initial consonants)

As can be seen, the three-ness of the acronym "HIV" has been linguistically exploited by kwaito-speakers. In fact, Tessa Dowling observes that in South Africa HIV (and AIDS) may be referred to by "any popular group or organization with three letters in its acronym" (see Dowling 2007). Dowling has noticed that AIDS is referred to as iANC (African National Congress) and iPAC (Pan African Congress) by both Xhosa and Zulu speakers.[10] Through this imaginative act of signification, the leading political party (ANC) and its rival (PAC) are both referenced in discussions of AIDS. While the use of the terms ANC and PAC in this context is limited to the fact that both are three-letter acronyms, a kind of residual meaning carries through that opens the way for further signifying processes. In this way, discourses of HIV/AIDS and politics are brought together by unlikely means.

Dowling also observes that AIDS is sometimes referred to by the name of a famous kwaito group: iTKZ.[11] In the case of the group, TKZee is an acronym for the three members:

Tokollo, Kabelo, and Zwai. While Dowling is quick to point out that the reason people refer to AIDS as TKZee is "not because the group members have HIV/AIDS or even sing about the illness," but "because TKZ [*sic*] has three letters in its acronym," it is likely that even the improvised and somewhat coincidental coupling produces the inspiration for further creative signification, such as the reinterpretation of TKZee's lyrics as implicitly being about HIV/AIDS.

The crucial point is that talk about HIV/AIDS and talk about music (kwaito) intersect at every turn. It should not be surprising to us, then, HIV/AIDS discourse is also deeply entangled with other risk behaviors. In the beginning of this essay I suggested that accidents are an integral part of South African lived experience. Jean and John Comaroff suggest that accidents are part of a more general tendency in many post-colonies, namely the tendency toward "casino capitalism": "the ethos of neoliberalism that favors speculation, play, and gambling over virtuous labor as a source of wealth" (Comaroff and Comaroff 2006, 14). Within South African risk society, AIDS is at times referred to as iLotto. In this sense, AIDS is conceived of as both risky and based on a certain amount of chance. In other words, one might "apply for AIDS," or take a chance *by* applying for AIDS.

In sum, *language* connects various aspects of lived experience in South Africa in often unforeseen ways. It would be worthwhile to note, moreover, that a link between HIV/AIDS and kwaito is often constructed in a far more profound—yet inexplicit—way (than through a mere reference to TKZee). This connection can be roughly summarized as the *metaphor of contamination*. As has been pointed out by many historians of medicine, medical discourse is often replete with rich culturally situated metaphors. Susan Sontag observes that within the history of medical discourse the body has often been viewed as a fortress and that AIDS is often thought of as a type of pollutant that invades or contaminates the body-structure (Sontag 1988, 8–17). The conceptual connection between viral contamination and the invasion of foreign, alien, or simply "other" bodies into the polis has long been noted. After suggesting that "'[p]lague' is the principal metaphor by which the AIDS epidemic is understood," Sontag writes that one "feature of the usual script for plague" is that it "comes from elsewhere" (ibid., 44–47). In general, there is a "link between imagining disease and imagining foreignness. It lies perhaps in the very concept of wrong, which is archaically identical with the non-us, the alien" (ibid., 48). More specifically, the alterity of AIDS is often coded "African." As Sontag asserts:

> The subliminal connection made to notions about a primitive past and the many hypotheses that have been fielded about possible transmission from animals (a disease of green monkeys? African swine fever?) cannot help but activate a familiar set of stereotypes about animality, sexual license, and blacks. (52)

Thus, ex-Foreign Minister (during the apartheid regime) Pik Botho expressed his fear in this way: "The terrorists are now coming to us with a weapon more terrible than Marxism: AIDS" (cited in Sontag 1988, 62). Moreover, in Western thought a connection has often been made between medical contagion (or contamination) and African music. While contemporary South Africa is ruled by the black majority, conservative (and even racist) ideologies still prevail, even within the black population. The common dismissals of kwaito suggest that this form of music, like AIDS, threatens to invade and destroy society from within.

Moreover, there is ironic fear that kwaito contaminates because *you cannot help but enjoy it*. Many parents in South Africa discourage their children from listening to kwaito because of the negative connotations of kwaito culture more generally (which include uninhibited sexuality, AIDS, and in some cases, crime).[12] The common fear that (popular) music "seduces"[13] listeners goes back at least to Kant who, in his third *Critique*, complained that:

> [M]usic has a certain lack of urbanity about it. For, depending mainly on the character of its instruments, it extends its influence (on the neighborhood) farther than people wish, and so, as it were, imposes itself on others and hence impairs the freedom of those outside of the musical party. (1987, 200)

Kant continues by comparing music to an odor that spreads far and more specifically to someone "who pulls his perfumed handkerchief from his pocket [and] gives all those next to and around him a treat whether they want it or not, and compels them, if they want to breathe, to enjoy at the same time" (ibid.). Ultimately Kant will call music disgusting (*eckel*) because music forces the listener to enjoy it (see Derrida 1981, 3–25). While AIDS is certainly not thought of as an enjoyable illness, it is nonetheless connected to unbridled enjoyment, since AIDS is transmitted primarily through sex. Both AIDS and music, then, have a perverse relationship to pleasure.

In sum, kwaito, AIDS, and politics cross cognitive domains through the use of metaphor. Issues such as contamination and pleasure contaminate the very fabric of language and thought. Ultimately, signifying on kwaito and AIDS is as contaminating as AIDS itself.

KWAITO THINKING POSITIVE

In this section I turn away from sexuality and sexual violence and examine how kwaito artists have engaged problems of HIV/AIDS in explicit, and often constructive, ways. In the early days of kwaito, politicians were concerned about the negative impact that this form of popular music might have on the youth. President Thabo Mbeki famously called kwaito "a distraction" from real political issues. However, as I have shown elsewhere, politicians soon realized that winning an election campaign without the support of kwaito musicians (and, more importantly, those musicians' fans) would be impossible (see Steingo 2007). Almost overnight, Mbeki seemed to have forgotten about his prior concerns and the African National Congress (ANC) began hiring kwaito musicians to play at its rallies.

It is common for people in South Africa to say that kwaito musicians are more powerful than politicians (see Steingo 2007). And indeed, in a certain sense they are. Kwaito musician, actor, and activist Zola has far more influence over the way the youth think than does President Mbeki. Although stated somewhat ironically, "Zola for president" is a phrase on many people's lips (Owen 2006).

In the following, I present two case studies of kwaito personalities who have explicitly addressed issues of HIV/AIDS in post-apartheid South Africa.

I: Zola

> Kwaito kids are made from hunger, abuse, no father, violence and guns. Now as adults we must change the game for the better. Now we must change everything we are made from.
>
> —Zola[14]

Named after the particularly rough and poor area from which he hails, Zola (born Bongi Dhlamini) came to fame through his role as a gangster, Papa Action, on the immensely popular

TV show *Yizo Yizo 2*. Yet his fame from *Yizo Yizo 2* was double-fold: in addition to acting on the show, Zola also sang the hit song, "Ghetto Fabulous," on the show's soundtrack. Zola was already a celebrity when he released his first album, *Umdlwembe*, which went platinum three times in less than a year.[15] In addition to *Yizo Yizo 2*, Zola has acted in two films: alongside Taye Diggs in *Drum* (2004) and as a suave but ruthless gangster in the Academy Award winning *Tsotsi* (2006).

In 2003, Zola launched his own TV show on SABC 1, which has been consistently popular since. In addition to all these achievements, Zola has been involved in many social investment programs, such his partnership with Cell C which resulted in a cell phone plan through which a percentage of the profit from each call is given to AIDS orphanages. Most notably, for this chapter, however, is Zola's sustained work in the HIV/AIDS activism. As a spokesperson for the South African youth, Zola has offered his ideas on HIV/AIDS in Africa in many different forums. In December 2005, for example, he delivered a speech at the Gauteng Health Department's workshop on a new government document highlighting issues of HIV/AIDS; more recently, he joined the UNESCO Artists 4 Life campaign. Particularly significant was his appointment (November 2006) as UNICEF Goodwill Ambassador at the African Development Forum. UNICEF Deputy Executive Director Rima Sala said of the kwaito star:

> Zola is a young leader who is giving all his creative talents to advocate for transformation in society—to draw the public's attention to the terrible impact of HIV/AIDS, female genital mutilation, and poverty of young people on this continent. His efforts continue to inspire many people, especially the youth. His personal story in overcoming poverty in Soweto to become one of Africa's budding young superstars gives hope to millions of youth in Africa who are in a similar situation.[16]

Although he is a zealous AIDS activist, Zola does not see HIV/AIDS as the only problem that Africa faces. He commonly addresses HIV/AIDS in the context of a set of interrelated problems that cannot be addressed separately. Without denying the link between HIV and AIDS, Zola does seem to see the problem of AIDS as related (either directly or not) to poverty (although, at least to my knowledge, he is not particularly concerned with female genital mutilation, as Rima Sala would have us think). In fact, Zola links AIDS not only to other forms of suffering, but also to pleasurable and even righteous aspects of life. As he says: "Today, love is the struggle—with that comes sex, comes AIDS, comes abuse. So ours is a journey of self-identification that is nothing like what the older generation experienced" (quoted in Jooma 2003).

A full analysis of Zola's politics and ethics would require an additional chapter. Here, I would like to briefly touch on some of the more important aspects. Zola's politics are, in fact, very difficult to theorize. This is because, in many ways, Zola advocates what at first-sight looks like standard liberal democratic values that valorize individual hard work and success. Zola consistently urges poor black South Africans to pursue entrepreneurial endeavors, and he seldom (if ever) expresses interest in large-scale political mobilization. Although Zola is very critical of the African National Congress's lack of social welfare and public health projects, he is nonetheless absent at worker's strikes and other similar *organized* struggles.

A good example of Zola's "individualized" politics is his performance at the Johannesburg Live Earth concert in July 2007.[17] Zola, unlike many of the musicians performing at Live Earth concerts around the world, essentially halted the music at one point and launched into a speech. Although he began by ironizing the petit-bourgeois makeup of the audience, proclaiming that to most attendees "townships" were still merely tourist destinations, his rhetoric quickly become indistinguishable from the rather trite discourse of Live Earth advocates. Focusing on domestic spaces and individual efforts to use less energy by switching off lights and using cars less, Zola's discourse effectively repressed structural inequality and advocated the idea that individual acts of environmental kindness are the key to conserving our living (live) earth. Of course, Zola knew who he was talking to, and his mode of rhetoric was somewhat adjusted accordingly. However, in general Zola is more concerned with individual dreams and hopes than he is with structural inequality.

I argue, however, that focusing exclusively on Zola's *politics* obscures other dimensions of lived experience in the South African landscape. As Timothy Rommen has recently pointed out, discussions of politics and power often leave out the *ethical* dimension that is very important in lives of many people throughout the world (see Rommen 2007). Moreover, Foucauldian-based political analysis often amounts to something of a tautology, since the conception of power as inherently productive implies that "there is simply nothing else either this side of [power] or beyond it" (Baudrillard 1987, 39). As a religious Christian, Zola is interested in ethics and spirituality as well as politics, and in this way he introduces difference into analyses where politics has become a totalizing term, "the last term, the irreducible web, the last tale that can be told" (ibid., 42). Seen this way, it would be short-sighted to think that Zola's ethical convictions are the product of some "false-consciousness," that Zola has displaced material struggle by turning to some metaphysical realm. In fact, Zola's politics and ethics are closely related and are used in tandem strategically.

The relative independence of the ethical and the political can also be understood in relation to processes of globalization. As Arjun Appadurai famously argued, in the twentieth century the "work of the imagination" is not a bourgeois pastime or form of escapism for the oppressed (Appadurai 1996). The imagination—which in Zola's case is saturated with religious experience and knowledge—can be used to mobilize people in many ways. Moreover, Appadurai urges us to acknowledge that cultural activity is not always in the service of politics. The challenge, then, is to think of the ethical (or cultural) as related to politics, but as having relative autonomy in the sense that ethical action is not always reducible to political action.

Zola explains his use of the number seven as follows:[18]

> And why I wear a seven on my neck every day, is based on a simple fact that if you follow your Bible right, you'll see that God works around the number seven. The alphabet itself, *G* for god is the seventh letter of the alphabet. The Israelites circled Jericho seven times and the walls crumbled. Christ is killed on the sixth day and the first day he rests on his grave is the seventh day. God creates Earth and Man and then he rests on the seventh day. So we wear a seven as a form of respect and a tribute to what God has given to us.[19]

Reflecting on his religious beliefs, Zola says: "my struggle...is a very political one and a very spiritual one." Seen this way, although Zola asserts that "everything around us is guided and protected by God, otherwise I would have died at birth," he does not believe that humans lack agency. Zola is certainly a historical agent, especially when we understand agency not as some autonomous form of subjectivity. "People are agents," writes Michael Lambek, "insofar as they choose to subject themselves, to perform and conform accordingly, to accept responsibility, and to acknowledge their commitments" (Lambek 2002, 38). Clearly, Zola has accepted ethical responsibility by acknowledging his commitments to poverty, crime, and HIV/AIDS in South Africa.

Moreover, there is an explicitly Afrocentric twist to Zola's faith. "And we strongly believe," he proclaims, "in one verse in the Revelations that says behold for a powerful nation shall rise in the South" (quoted in *Sharp Sharp*, 2003). Zola's Afrocentric exegesis thus positions the Bible as both a spiritual and political text. Zola subjects himself to Biblical injunctions, but always through imaginative interpretive acts wherein a dialogical encounter is staged between the theological and subjective.

In order to understand local responses to the AIDS pandemic, it is important to critique normative political or medical analyses. As I hope to have shown, while Zola is neither a political activist nor a "health worker" in any sense, his unique brand of Afrocentric religious and ethical conviction has made an important contribution to South Africa's fight against AIDS. Most striking, perhaps, are the multiple registers in which Zola attacks HIV/AIDS: at concerts and on TV, for UNESCO and for local government, to South African audiences and to the global media, in the language of politics and in the language of theology, as a poet and as a prophet.

II: Khabzela and Yfm

Fana Khaba, or Khabzela as he was most often called, was one of South Africa's best-loved celebrities until his death of an AIDS-related illness in January 2004.[20] The central question that journalists and scholars have asked about Khabzela is why he (publicly) refused antiretroviral treatment. In a blurb that appears on the front cover of Liz McGregor's book about Khabzela (McGregor 2005), AIDS activist Edwin Cameron refers to "the choices and circumstances that caused this talented and visionary young man to die, when he could have had life."

Khabzela's life and work presents a poignant example of the ambiguities, uncertainties, and tragedies of life and AIDS in post-apartheid South Africa. Why did Khabzela refuse ARVs? Can we be sure that he *should* have chosen ARVs? Is choosing ARVs, as Cameron and McGregor would have us believe, simply a matter of choosing life over death? And, most important for this chapter, how did Khabzela's role as a DJ and cultural broker of kwaito impact his choices about treatment? How did Khabzela's choices about treatment impact the kwaito generation?

Born into a very poor family in Soweto, Khabzela gained some fame early on as a DJ on Soweto Community Radio. However, his real rise to fame came from his DJ work at Yfm.[21] Started in 1997, by 2001 Yfm had become the biggest regional radio station in South Africa with an average of 1.5 million listeners per week. The success of Yfm, particularly during the station's early years, is largely attributable to Khabzela. Together with its official publication, *Y Mag*, and website, YWorld, Yfm, as of this writing, is one of the most important institutions in South Africa. In a study done by the South African government, Yfm DJs were included among the top five most influential people in the country. As Yfm DJ Oskido says: "Yfm is the first radio station created by and conceived for the black youth. It is not a community radio station. It is the mirror, both festive and lucid, of the new generation. Here people talk about everything that concerns them or that challenges them in the townships: violence, drugs, AIDS. It plays the music they like, deep house, R&B, hip-hop, and of course, Kwaito" (cited in Servant 2002). When no other radio station was prepared to play kwaito, Yfm stepped up. In fact, the first song ever aired on the station was the kwaito song "Makeba" by Bongo Maffin. Khabzela was there, from the beginning, promoting kwaito against all odds. It is perhaps not unreasonable, then, that Yfm claims to "own" kwaito.[22] As Yfm DJ Greg Maloka put it: "We made kwaito and kwaito made us" (quoted in McGregor 2005, 108).

Yfm also became a serious forum for the discussion of pressing issues. As station founder Dirk Hartford says: "Yfm's first pamphlet read: 'Sex, drugs and kwaito.' What made Yfm unique was that there was real dialogue about these issues" (McGregor 2005, 110). Hartford, then, does not deny that kwaito is caught up with sex, drugs, and music, but he believes that the best way to move into the future is to engage such issues in a constructive and dialogic way. Thus, on the topic of rape, Hartford suggests:

> The majority of young girls' first experience of sex in South Africa isn't consensual. Most are forced into it. The whole youth culture is like that…The situation out there is horrific. We knew that. But how do you talk about these things? How do you introduce them in a way people can identify with? (McGregor 2005, 110)

As a white male who grew up during apartheid, Hartford is one of a very few who have constructively engaged with the problems facing most black South Africans. Fully aware of authoritarian "education," Hartford and his colleagues at Yfm opened a forum for dialogic and multivocal expression. Khabzela was at the forefront of Yfm's initiative. As one of the most popular DJs at Yfm, Khabzela coined the phrase "Positive Youth of Gauteng" (McGregor 2005, 114). Not only did Khabzela support small entrepreneurial endeavors, but he also tackled the problem of crime head-on by talking live on radio with inmates. Khabzela tried to understand the suffering of prisoners and also warn would-be criminal listeners of their possible fate. Khabzela's "positive" messages also had to do with racial politics. Refusing to speak in English on air, he promoted a specific brand of post-apartheid African affirmation.

Khabzela: activist, icon, hero. It is also worth pointing out that this remarkable man was not only Afrocentric, but he was also a devout Jehovah's Witness. And, indeed, his politics was often informed by his deep religiosity and spirituality.[23] In addition to these rather contradictory tendencies embodied in a single man, Khabzela was known to be a real womanizer. Obsessed with clothes and fast cars, the young superstar was the man of many young ladies' dreams.

In 2003 Khabzela tested positive for HIV. At this point he made a courageous decision—he announced his status on air. The responses to his announcement were overwhelming, and for the most part very positive. Here is a sample: "We are all saddened by what has happened. You are a big asset to our nation. Wish all the high profile peoples in our country can disclose their status like you." "By revealing your status you have already beaten the virus…I hope other people can be as brave as you have been." "Khaba, you are my role model. Without you on the air I'm nothing…You're one of God's sweetest angels." "Just know that the public is one hundred and one percent behind you. You have already made a statement—I decided to get tested today! Thanks for giving me the courage. I only realized now how real HIV/AIDS is. Live on Khaba!" (McGregor 2005, 158). These responses were not exceptions. The "public" was behind him.

At this point Yfm made a plan to become the first radio station hosted by an HIV-positive presenter on the topic of HIV/AIDS. The very meaning of "positivity" was thus shaded with ambiguity: the positive youth of Gauteng. When you are no longer (HIV) negative you are forced to be (think) positive. McGregor writes that it "was at this point that Fana [i.e., Khabzela] made a decision that transformed his life from one that was a huge and valiant success against all the odds to one that was tragedy" (159). After taking ARVs for only a brief period, Khabzela stopped. He refused to rest, and became depressed and agitated. Most people expected the DJ to take his ARVs judiciously and return to work in a few weeks. But this did not happen and Khabzela seemed doomed to self-destruction.

Essentially, McGregor was unable to understand why Khabzela refused to "choose life." She offers several explanations, many of which are not convincing, and none of which could possibly be complete. She suggests, for example, that for a man "who had fought so hard for power and control over his own life," being treated for HIV would have "required a temporary surrender of his independence, a reversion to an infantile state" (160). On the other hand, she suggests that Khabzela may have been "flattered by his new wave of courtiers," and that he regained power through sickness as people began "fawning over him" (161). Counselors Masi Makhalemele and Angie Diale worked with Khabzela for six months, but eventually gave up. Referring to Khabzela's resistance to counseling and treatment, Makhalemele said: "He was so rude. He didn't want to listen. If he would just have listened, he'd have been okay. This was an angry man. It was as if there was something black inside his heart... He knew he had done so much wrong. He had infected so many girls" (quoted in McGregor 2005, 165). Was Khabzela's resistance to Western medicine due to anger and guilt? Possibly, but Greg Maloka—a long-time friend and colleague of Khabzela's—offers a different interpretation. Maloka believed that part of Khabzela's problem was his schizophrenic subjectivity: "There was a Christian force and a traditional African force. [Khabzela] believed in both. He believed both had a place in his heart and in his life. And if they worked together, they would help settle his soul. And unfortunately, when he got ill, these forces went to war with each other" (quoted in McGregor 2005, 170).[24] Ultimately, however, Dirk Hartford's response to Khabzela's demise was probably the most honest: even in retrospect, thought Hartford, he could not fully explain what happened to Khabzela, and why (ibid., 167).

Conflicting belief systems, humiliation, and fear of dependence were probably factors that effected Khabzela's last years. My own interpretation—an interpretation that is partial, at best—resembles McGregor's suggestion that Khabzela refused treatment because he feared losing his dependence. Or, to put it another way, he was *self-determined*, even until death. In trying to understand Khabzela's struggles with HIV, I turn to Kathy Acker's article "The Gift of Disease" (1997). Written shortly before her death (due to cancer), Acker's article may suggest a new way of thinking about our beloved icon, Khabzela.

> I realised that if I remained in the hands of conventional medicine, I would soon be dead, rather than diseased, meat. For conventional medicine was reducing me, quickly, to a body that was only material, to a body without hope and so, without will, to a puppet who, separated by fear from her imagination and vision, would do whatever she was told.

> My search for a way to defeat cancer now became a search for life and death that were meaningful. Not for the life presented by conventional medicine, a life in which one's meaning or self was totally dependent upon the words and actions of another person, even of a doctor. I had already learned one thing, though I didn't at the time know it: that I live as I believe, that belief is equal to the body.

Less than a year before her death, Acker wrote in the last sentence of her article:

> I no longer have cancer. To heal in oneself is to begin to heal the self which is always whole.

Having lived through apartheid and having finally found his place in South Africa, Africa, and, indeed, the world, Khabzela affirmed the right to die. More precisely, he affirmed the right to choose death over life. The important point is that it was a *choice*, and that in choosing *to die* Khabzela had made a decision about how he wished to live his last years. For, while death is a state, dying is a living activity.

Khabzela's negative attitude to his HIV-positive status had the peculiar effect of challenging the very idea of what it means to be positive. If *being* positive (through infection) can easily be fought by *acting* positive (through the right treatment), why did Khabzela react negatively to his positive status? Are the poles of positivity and negativity so unequivocally established that we can simply plot life decisions on some Cartesian axis? Did not Khabzela, in some way, author a new positivity by inverting the poles of the positive-negative axis? I would argue that in deciding not to accept medical treatment, Khabzela had redrawn the cartography of life-paths.

In a certain sense, the debate around Khabzela is reminiscent of age-old attempts to establish unequivocal binary axes of pleasure/pain, and positive/negative. Perhaps unsurprisingly, it was one of the fathers of suspicion—Sigmund Freud himself—who tackled the problem of the pleasure principle head-on by deriving the concept of the "death drive." The death drive was largely invented in order to explain the paradox of primary masochism. How, Freud asked, does one explain intentional suffering? If the psyche is ruled by the pleasure principle (that is, if the psyche is always striving for pleasure), then the striving for pain (unpleasure) can only be the striving for unpleasure *as* pleasure. Acknowledging, tentatively, the "truth" of masochism, we may ask of Khabzela: how did he "derive enjoyment *precisely there where he suffer[ed]*" (Laplanche 1976, 104)? Under the rule of a perverse Pleasure Principle, did Khabzela paradoxically choose unpleasure-pleasure? And how is such a choice possible? I would argue that we need to destabalize our inherited Freudian doxography. Derrida points out that part of the confusion in Freud's work derives from the acknowledgement that he is "unarmed concerning the question of knowing what pleasure-unpleasure *is*" (Derrida 1987, 279). According to Derrida, Freud privileges the economic point of view, thus establishing a first relation between *quantities* rather than between two *essences*. "The law is one of relation between the quantity of something whose essence is unknown to us...and a quantity of energy...whose presence in psychic life is presumed" (ibid., 279). In this sense, we may say that Khabzela did not create a new kind of positivity as much as he called into question the idea of positivity as essence. Khabzela taught us the uncanny lesson that the essence of the positive is unknown to us.

CONCLUDING REMARKS

I hope to have shown that kwaito is closely connected with HIV/AIDS in many, often only implicit, ways. These intricate lines of flight scatter images, sounds, and signifiers across the domain of lived experience in ways that are not fully controlled by individual subjects. The "connection" (such an impotent word) between kwaito and rape is both equivocal and indeterminate, and yet this does not mean that there is no connection at all. I have attempted to illustrate various types of supplementary and dialectical relationships, derivations, and correlations without settling too comfortably on some putative "conclusion."

Zola and Khabzela illuminate the ways in which individuals may impact entire communities. However, in neither case are we dealing with a heroic autonomous subject. Zola's AIDS activism is framed in terms of ethical responsibility: it is only by acknowledging and affirming his own subjective interpellation that Zola is able to "come into himself." Khabzela at times seems to embody and materialize the abstract concept of the "positive" (or the negative, depending on one's interpretation), and at other times wreaks havoc with the entire economy of the positive/negative. Both Zola and Khabzela play a double game of affirmation and rejection. Both Zola and Khabzela have offered imaginative—but perhaps somewhat troubling and uncomfortable—responses to the crisis of HIV/AIDS. Despite their similarities, however, there is one fundamental difference between the two stars: Zola is alive, and Khabzela is dead.

As a final gesture, I briefly turn to the boundary that separates those who are HIV-positive from those who are not (such as myself). I will spare the reader the details of my personal history as a white South African growing up during the last years of apartheid; I simply state here that I have never lost anyone close to me to AIDS. This is a very significant fact. Rather than discuss my personal history in detail, however, I would like to end this essay with a brief meditation on the "healthy" and the "unhealthy" more generally. In the *Genealogy of Morals*, Nietzsche writes: "[T]he sick should *not* make the healthy sick...this requires above all the healthy should be *segregated*, guarded even from the sight of the sick, that they may not confound themselves with the sick" (cited in Ronell 1994, 54). Allow me to quote Avital Ronell's commentary on Nietzsche's words at length:

> The healthy are so vulnerable, so susceptible to infection, that they must be placed in heavily immunized zones, in emergency wards for the healthy. They are so weak, or potentially so weak, these healthy ones, that they need to be protected from the sight of the sick...[T]he structure itself of Nietzschean health bars any one-to-one correspondence between a symptom of disease...and a sign of decadence or weakness: the strongest and most active are also the most vulnerable; they are immunodeficient. (Ronell 1994, 54)

It is by shying away from all that contaminates (illness, music) that we realize our ultimate weakness, our ultimate deficiencies.

30

Positive Disturbance

TAFASH, TWIG, HIV/AIDS, AND
HIP HOP IN UGANDA

Gregory Barz (Vanderbilt University/
University of the Free State)
Gerald C. Liu (Vanderbilt University)

INTRODUCTION

A CD compilation of local Ugandan rap recorded and produced by the authors in May 2008 shows how musical intervention and theological extension augment ethnomusicological research. Engaging lyrical and biographical analysis theologically, especially with respect to the disciplines of homiletics (preaching) and liturgics (worship), we consider two female MC participants, Tafash and Twig, as theologically minded agents who maneuver within our ethnomusicological intervention for social critique in unexpected ways. Balancing examination of the musical contributions from Tafash and Twig with additional survey and critique of scholarly literature related to the study of religion, music, and expressive culture, we weigh the specific and possible future contributions of theological analysis to medical ethnomusicology. In conclusion, we suggest future directions for ethnomusicological research with relation to the intricate contributions of fieldwork driven by musical intervention and theological investigation.

Do two female MCs in East Africa help us reconsider the public perception and consumption of HIV/AIDS relief in Uganda? If so, are their efforts religious, or even, theological?

We suggest that Tafash's rapping is proximate to theological proclamation, whereby she pronounces the evil of AIDS and the potential for its eventual demise through redemptive human choice. Tafash's musical message displays traces of her Rastafarian commitments and is embodied responsively by the surrogate motherhood of her fellow rapper, Twig. To oversimplify, Twig does what Tafash says in terms of new measures for opposing AIDS. Such aesthetic and ethical convictions have produced unusual and uncommon acts of courage to resist the deadly complacency and collateral damage associated with HIV/AIDS itself and campaign efforts for relief that, according to Tafash, do more harm than good. As Twig and Tafash cleverly counter the fatality of the disease, they engage in uncommon and unignorable cultural critique that both judges current campaigns for preventing the spread of HIV/AIDS and encourages more imaginative and female-specific forms of relief and female-centric restoration of persons and communities.

KAMPALA FLOW

In the Beginning...

During the summer of 2008, we collaborated with a variety of young East African rap artists from Kampala, the capital city of Uganda, to archive and discover how rappers like Twig and Tafash act as public witnesses who provide musical metrics for measuring the status of HIV/AIDS relief and infuse their music with religious conviction that results in extraordinary measures of healing and hope for their listeners and their own lives. When we approached rap artists in Kampala, we first explained that our interests were firstly and lastly educational. We wanted to document their rap biographies and record examples of their music. Many of them, When we approached rap artists in Kampala, we first explained that our interests were firstly and lastly educational. We wanted to document their rap biographies and record examples of their music. Many of them, however, saw our research interest and offer to record them as an opportunity to legitimate their music in ways that would guarantee public acceptance and popularity. Some, like Twig and Tafash, identified a primary difficulty with the local radio stations' unwillingness to allocate appropriate airtime to local rap and hip hop recordings. Curious about Twig and Tafash's characterization of the commercial plight of local rappers in Uganda, we sought the perspectives of Uganda music industry personnel. Radio executives such as Peter Kizito, Betina Tumhaire, Bryan Mackenzie, and David Wodmol explained that local radio resisted local Ugandan rap because rap music was associated with sexual and violent imagery frequently heard in the genre's lyrics from exporting markets like the United States. This reason seemed curious, however, because Kampala stations still played artists from the United States such as 50 Cent, T.I., and tracks like Usher's "Love in this Club," featuring Young Jeezy. Was there another dimension to the lack of appeal to radio listeners of local hip hop? Given the airplay of rap music from the United States, we also wondered if language might be an issue related to the acceptance of local Ugandan hip hop. Could popularity be gained by rapping as a socially conscious artist in Kampala? Could such popularity and rap method be sustained financially? Or, would a socially conscious approach to rapping require an artist to work in other genres of music, or other jobs altogether, or even other countries?

Facing the misperception of their music with regards to the international distribution of mainstream rap music from the United States, local producers such GK and Dawoo as well as longtime Ugandan rap pioneers like Bataka Squad also verified the sentiments of Twig, Tafash, and the industry personnel with whom we spoke. On more than one occasion we were told that local radio audiences wanted socially conscious music, not "thug rhymes" or club mixes.[1] Yet at the time of our writing, none of the recording studios had yet found it worth the financial risk to regard socially conscious music, perhaps because of some unstated mistrust of the Kampala radio stations. Nevertheless, some Kampala-based groups such as

Klear Cut and Bataka Squad saw potential in socially conscious rapping in the late 1990s and built solid followings as a result. Yet because of the public stereotype of rap as being violent and sexually illicit music, studio owners and operators such as GK and Dawoo make most of their income outside of hip hop. Supplementing, or at times even supporting their work with local rap artists, GK and Dawoo undertake what they see as more sustainable jobs such as advertising for local businesses and multinational corporations, or producing radio dramas with local NGOs. And it is difficult to say whether GK and Dawoo have been misguided in their decision making. Or more sinisterly, and to revisit the question of why producers have not invested heavily in socially conscious rap, perhaps this is because working in local radio advertising has proven more lucrative than socially conscious hip hop for Kampala airwaves. Whatever the case, on the artists' side, even with their local fame, the contemporary rap group Klear Cut banks on contributing to local radio advertisements and touring outside of Uganda. Especially with regards to their outside touring, they make the choice to "spit" their socially conscious rhymes in English, while remaining rooted in local culture by adopting regional instrumentation. Two-time Pearl of Africa Award winner Lyrical G, the only Ugandan hip hop artist to win the "African Grammy" in the category of Best Solo Hip Hop Artiste/Group twice, also spits exclusively in English.

Local rap artists in Uganda do indeed have their own local language rhyming style, referred to as "Lugaflow."[2] Pioneering groups mentioned above such as Bataka Squad and solo artists like Rocky Giant have popularized the style among rappers and gained some mainstream appeal in Uganda, including limited radio and video play. Artists that we recorded, such as GNL, Eazy Tecs, and Twig have made names for themselves as up-and-comers in the Lugaflow tradition. Some rappers such as Lumix and Rawfam even go further in the use of local language by rhyming in non-Bantu derived languages such as Acholi and Ateso, spoken mostly in the northern areas of the country.[3] Nevertheless, in the urban rap scene, pan-African and blended approaches to music-making are understood by many in the Ugandan popular music industry as alternative, and often necessary, options to navigate routes of support for their music-making. For example, an artist such as Derique BC includes in his English rapping Kiswahili hooks and choruses. Kiswahili is a language understood by many beyond the Ugandan borders in neighboring Kenya and Tanzania, but seldom embraced within the national borders of his homeland. Derique BC also collaborates with both English rapping and Lugaflow artists when possible. Yet there are also inverse examples, such as Tafash, who is Kenyan-born. She manages to carve a musical niche in Kampala with exclusive use of her native language—Kiswahili. Despite being a "foreigner" and despite local rap's lack of public popularity, Tafash works with Uganda's few professional rappers like Bataka Squad, Lyrical G, and GNL. She also draws significant attention from audiences at public performances in Kampala. Even so, she and other MCs continue to experiment with a range of languages and seek work outside Uganda, such as collaborating with Kenyan producers and recording in studios located in Nairobi. She also performs in Rwanda, Tanzania, and, less frequently, in the United Kingdom and the United States, in hopes of having her work heard by the largest possible audience.

The Collaborative Creation of Kampala Flow

Conflicted about how to situate our ethnomusicological investigations with artists' musical ambitions on the one hand, and what seemed like a multifaceted popular neglect based upon public association of local rap with the morally suspect content of mainstream international rap music on the other, we decided to take a risk and develop our compilation project as a direct ethnomusicological intervention. Would having studio time to create socially conscious tracks suitable for radio airplay in Uganda allow these rappers both to remedy their negative reputation and to increase their public reach?

Our invasive methodology was an attempt to raise popular support of Ugandan rap by providing studio time for artists and asking them to write from their "socially conscious notebooks" rather than consistently draw from their "club tracks."[4] Thus, we readily claim our role as both collaborators and producers of the recent *Kampala Flow* album that documents our efforts to highlight local rap artists and their ability to address local concerns. Yet it should also be clear that the request for "socially conscious" music was a *request*. We did not police the creative output of the contributors or enforce a "socially conscious" direction in their musical expression in any way. While the artists were asked to write "socially conscious" lyrics, this request referenced language from conversations with artists and music industry personnel when they characterized how Ugandan rap must present itself in order to gain widespread public support. In other words, the phrase "socially conscious" was already indigenous to the vernacular of local musicians and industry personnel in Kampala. Though all of the artists we recorded had already produced socially conscious rhymes, and though they had the awareness that socially conscious music was needed to bolster Ugandan rap, they still struggled to feel confident that a socially conscious style would benefit their musical ambitions. Recall that this is because there seemed to be a double-standard at work in the radio-play of rap in Kampala. Local artists were frequently refused airtime because their lyrics were deemed morally suspect. Yet local stations still occasionally played American music filled with explicit lyric content. Therefore, our presence as active and supportive *intervenors* may not have eliminated this contradictory tension in the Kampala rap scene and its relationship with local radio. Because we did provide a platform for the artists to record socially conscious music without any personal cost or personal financial investment, however, we helped the local MCs create music, with minimal financial risk to the artists, so that they could then plug to the radio stations as filling the criteria of being socially conscious.[5]

Even with our thematic request as part of the recording agreement with the artists, the rappers and studio colleagues were far from docile bodies. Not all of the tracks concerned HIV/AIDS, for example. Topics ranged from rape, to school fees, to HIV/AIDS, to gender issues, to spousal abuse, and to inheritance rights. Furthermore, the artists often engaged in lyrical *perruqué* (a trope for doing their own work in the guise of "working for us"), and we did not stop their spontaneous and free interpretation of our request for socially conscious music. Also, not all of the tracks on our forthcoming compilation were recorded with our thematic request for socially conscious music. Twig raps about love in "Man's Lady." Rawfam raps about street survival in "Igwaik akon kau kuju" ("Keep Your Head Up"). Tracks by Lyrical G and Xenson that concern civil war, child soldiers, prostitution, the corruption of Luzira prison, and pollution were solo works finished prior to our arrival in Uganda. Thus, tracks like these balance others that may be seen as constrained by recording instructions.

Though our approach may at first seem contrived, we see ourselves extending an already extant scope of ethnomusicological studies. Be they print studies or audio recordings, ethnomusicological studies have long introduced and supported (if not directly encouraged) change, even when they had no direct intention of doing so.[6] One need only reflect on the reception history of the recording and writings of John Lomax and Alan Lomax to identify such cultural production as direct and at times invasive interventions effecting change in cultural perceptions regarding American music.[7] Moreover, with the current move to greater advocacy in ethnomusicological research, we eagerly supported these particular artists, intending to eliminate economic concerns associated with making socially conscious music. We contractu-ally agreed with the artists not to profit from any sales of the recordings, confirming that any and all profits generated from the sale of the recording would be returned to them. We also wanted to lift pressure on the artists to conform to the desires of local radio stations. With the application of this experimental methodology we aimed to remove limitations on the artistic voice of the collective rap artists by helping the artists negotiate the expectations of the Ugandan radio public—a desire for socially conscious music.

Covering the expenses for beat production (a "beat" is the music accompaniment of a hip hop track, often made by another collaborator called a "beatmaker"),[8] studio time, pro-ducers' and engineers' fees, and the actual CD production allowed each rapper a full day (or in some cases longer) to produce a high-quality track focusing on the social issue of his or her choice. The tracks we recorded and produced in Kampala were released in the United States in the form of a commercial product that should have direct consequences for the popular music industry back in Uganda. The export of the CD back to Uganda will also make a public statement on the value of the rapper's chosen lyric content by the global rap community.[9] Will this intervention effect change? Will there be a greater acceptance of socially relevant rap "back home" in Uganda? Will rap artists be encouraged to use their craft to further reach out to the country's youth? It seems that change has already taken place since our initial 2008 recording sessions, and further analysis is needed to decipher the influence of our project. A 2009 concert, titled *Koi Koi* ("Riddles of Life") by GNL, an artist featured on *Kampala Flow*, became the first Ugandan rap show to gain sponsorship from a major corporation—MTN—a South Africa based telecommunications company, which is now the largest telecommunications provider in Uganda. Such sponsorship evidences increased private interest and arguably increased public support for local rap music. In performing tracks such as "Story ya Lukka," GNL openly raps about issues related to HIV/ AIDS in Uganda. "It seems though, that GNL can also hold his own, especially on Lukka. The slow, sad track, which is a social conscious offering about the devastation of HIV among the young of Uganda brings him down to a pace that he can work wonders with" (Tendo 2009). Has GNL turned activist? Also, at the 2008 Pearl of Africa Awards public audiences seem to have teetered between club and conscious taste. They voted for Navio, leading member of socially conscious group Klear Cut, as winner of the Best Hip Hop Artiste/ Group Award. GNL won Best Hip Hop Single. Yet the award went to his club track "Soda Jinjale" rather than a conscious release such as "Ekikufula Omusajja," a now popular tune in Kampala that concerns domestic violence. Returning to our project, did the local rap art-ists at the time of recording desire an opportunity to introduce a variety of cultural interven-tions? Yes. Did the ethnomusicologists also want to evaluate and analyze these interventions, and thus support and encourage the project? Certainly. Can the two groups—observer and observed—comfortably coexist? Absolutely.

Therefore, what may have seemed ethically questionable in regards to our field research—its quality of direct intervention and collaboration—actually follows and expands on trajectories in historical ethnomusicological research. What diverges and challenges eth-nomusicological thought is the inclusion of sustained theological attention to the "religious" dimension that was found to be integral to nearly all of the artists with which we worked.[10] The study of religious music or religion and music has long been a part of musicology's understanding of the Western art music canon. Ethnomusicology has roots in the theological encounter with music, perhaps best demonstrated in the 1779 writings about the complexities of Chinese music from Jesuit Jean Joseph Marie Amiot during his missionary stay in Beijing.[11] Recent scholarship such as Deborah Wong's *Sounding the Center: History and Aesthetics in Thai Buddhist Performance* (2001) and Kay Kaufman Shelemay's writings on the role of the Ethiopian *däbtära* also describe the religious history and understandings of musical cultures.[12] Yet writings such as these and others exploring religion and music in ethnomusicology have two key differences from the recommendations suggested by this essay.

A primary recommendation for theology is to serve as a viable hermeneutic for grasping how music functions in a given culture. Specifically, we suggest in this chapter that theology helps readers to see Tafash as a type of religious proclaimer, and Twig as one who responds to Tafash's proclamation, and also with a theologically based intention. The two key differences from these recommendations are as follows. First, previous ethnomusicological scholarship remains largely agnostic in regards to the types of religious claims made by the music and related musicians.[13] Granted, Shelemay has also recently collaborated with theologian Sarah Coakley in the volume, *Pain and Its Transformations: The Interface of Biology and Culture* (2008). As groundbreaking as this interdisciplinary collection of essays is, and though healing and theology are central themes, theological analysis does not always directly interface with ethnomusicology, and neither is this a primary purpose in the volume. Nevertheless, theological analysis still seems to function as a secondary or even sectarian discourse limited to a particular religious population, or a hermeneutic somewhere in between and dependent on medical knowledge and scientific verification.[14] Similarly limited is the second key difference. Prior studies, including the aforementioned, concern cultures and musics that are already circumscribed by religious context and already determined by explicitly religious content.[15] In contrast, what this chapter attempts—along with the already stated hopes of our intervention, collaboration, and documentation of Ugandan rappers and their music—is the recommendation for the possibility and value of theologically guided ethnomusicological interpretation.

What makes the following recommendation particularly interesting is that none of the artists chosen for the initial recording of the compilation were known to have religious commitments or theological claims.[16] Nor could their music be described as explicitly religious. Nonetheless, of the fourteen Ugandan rappers artists studied, only two did not associate religion with their music-making. Far from theology functioning as hermeneutical veneer that Liu has applied to his collaborative research with Barz, theological interpretation exposes how religion and its practice have been instrumental and often foundational to the music-making of the Ugandan rappers studied. Theological interpretation also helps to clarify the meaning that the artists attribute to their music, not only for themselves, but for us who hear it as well. The roles of religion and theology have not only shaped their current music-making process and its ethical tone, which is the central premise of this particular chapter. But in brief, religion and theology have also played a role in how the artists have (re)conceived of the historical continuity of Ugandan rap with relation to hip hop music in the United States and how they understand its continued reception by would be listeners.

Producer GK, in whose studio the majority of the compilation tracks were recorded, referenced the religious ritual known as *okuhingira,* where a suitor "raps" to the father of a potential bride in order to win her hand in marriage.[17] According to GK, this historic rhyming ceremony is a long-forgotten root of American rap musical traditions. Thus, in this way African rap predates what began in the Bronx. Diasporic artist Tshila echoes GK's recanonizing and reterritorializing of rap history when speaking of the deeper purposes of her own music. Tshila was born in Kampala, graduated from Valdosta State University in Georgia, and is now a fixture in Kampala's hip hop and traditional music-influenced R&B scene. Describing the "spirituality" behind her own music, she also syncretistically calls for a shared vision of comprehensive reconciliation and social cohesion among African and African American musicians. This vision may entail closer attention to less "trendy" but no less popular initiatives within African and African American mass culture, such as HIV/AIDS relief:

> *Tshila*—I want them [African Americans] to be more aware of the whole-someness of who we are as black people, the wholesomeness of our cultures, how music originated in Africa, and how we need to keep it, OK, lots of forms of music originated in Africa, like blues, you know, which later evolved into rock 'n' roll, which later evolved into jazz and other forms. And now it's modern music, you know and we listen to the radio, and gyrate, and shake to it, you know. But you know, looking back, I would feel, I personally would say to African Americans not to just keep, not to just keep being trend, trend makers, you know and just grab a trend, go go with it, abandon everything else, you know, and let other people take care of that. You know, they should, actually embrace everything that's a part of their history, including Africans as well. And you know, um, hopefully that way we can move together and create a force that's bigger and you know more powerful. (Interview with Liu, June 6, 2008)

So far, Tshila's artistic demand for more social consciousness within hip hop music-making has echoed no further into the United States than the sound files related to this chapter. Nevertheless, perhaps the "bigger force" desired in her exit interview had already begun to take shape during our collaborative compilation of Ugandan hip hop produced during the summer of 2008.

Through the analysis of Twig and Tafash that follows, and with particular attention to their contributions to HIV/AIDS relief in Kampala, we hope to describe how on the one hand, music like theirs both challenges and modifies directions for ethnomusicological research. On the other hand, and more dramatically, we hope to show musically and theologically how Tafash and Twig's proclamation and progressive living attests to a cohesive and redemptive African power that challenges and just might transform the scope of HIV/AIDS relief in Uganda.

TAFASH

Her Musical Center
May, 2008. Kampala Road (downtown Kampala).

The tin roof of Sabrina's Pub in downtown Kampala resonates like a snare drum from the rain. "Is the interview recording being drowned out?" I adjust the levels on the microphone. I manage to balance the audio just as Tafash reveals a religious ethic that fuels her music making. "Ummm...yah, it can, cuz like, you know, once you are a rasta, you are supposed to be with a clean heart and a clear conscience. Yah. So everything you want to do, you always keep it positive, you know. You wanna live good, you know. And you wanna live righteous, you know. Soooo, everything I try to do, I think about the people. And what I want them to hear. And how I want them. You know, it's like, I don't know how to explain this, but it's just righteousness, you know, yeah, righteousness, that's what I can say, yeah." (Gerald Liu, field-notes, 2008)

The religious conviction in her music is not something injected from outside. Rather it emerges with her identity as a Kenyan in Kampala intent on making music that demands attention. "You know what Tafash means in Swahili? Tafash means 'stubborn.' It's not really, you know, stubborn, like every time I get on the mic, OK that's my meaning of Tafash, ya. Every time I get on the mic I always cause that kind of disturbance. Everyone wanna know who I be and what I'm saying, you know? I just disrupt them, you know. Yeah, that's why I call myself Tafash, you know? Stubborn" (Barz and Liu interview with Tafash, 2008). Tafash's unusual mix of Rasta righteousness and self-assertion as a "foreign" woman claiming her space in an insiders' rap game would secure her a spot on our compilation of socially conscious Ugandan hip hop. We needed her stubbornness, her outsider's perspective, her conviction, and her "positive" approach to rhyme. What we did not expect however, was that in addition to her lyrical prowess, an equally powerful and paradoxical biography also saturated the track that Tafash would ultimately lay down in a Bukoto recording studio.

Her Life as a Female MC

June, 2008—I [Liu] meet Tafash in her "apartment," an 8 x 10 ft. concrete room that sits within a row of residences in a community compound. Her room is furnished with a bunk bed and a couple of wooden and wicker shelves that contain mostly shoes. Yet perched on one of these shelves is also a TV, DVD player, a stereo. Below this entertainment center is her "kitchen," which amounts to an electric carafe for boiling water, a handful of pots and pans, and plastic soft-drink bottles with various unidentifiable contents. There is no running water, and the shower is next door at her "cousin's." The toilets are latrines and outhouses shared by all residents.

She wears a white, woven skull cap whose border consists of gold, green, and red bands. Presumably, these colors refer to Rastafarianism: gold representing the economic wealth of the Rasta homeland Ethiopia, green the agricultural richness, and red an homage to the Rastafarian church triumphant and its martyrs. These colors are not simply located on Tafash's cap. The caramel colored dreadlocks that fall from the edges are also ornamented with matching gold, green, and red beads. Likewise, her wrists have gold, red, and green braided bracelets. Around her neck is a beaded necklace with an amulet that appears to be some miniature restatement of her look from the shoulders up. The talisman, or "talis-woman" as she calls it, is the profile of a dreadlocked female head whose neck is again wrapped in layers of gold, green, and red. In addition to these accessories, Tafash also wears a slightly oversized red *Akademiks* T-shirt that drapes over a baggy pair of grey tracksuit trousers. The cuff of each pant leg is pulled up above her calves. Her footwear at the moment is ankle socks and sandles.

She crosses her legs and asks if she can smoke a joint. "Sure," I [Liu] reply. Her countenance is nostalgic, optimistic, and sad all at the same time. Perhaps the adamancy of Tafash has something to do with an image that is meticulously crafted and yet resistant to casual interpretation (figure 30.1).

Tafash's real name is Zaitun Zahra. She is Kenyan and first moved to Kampala to attend Kampala International University (KU). Before moving to Uganda's capital city, she did secretarial work in Kenya. She began her studies at KU in Information Technology, but changed her focus to Mass Communications after experiencing financial difficulties following the death of her father. School fees were cheaper for Mass Communications. She eventually finished diplomas in Mass Communication and Voluntary Counseling and Testing, an HIV/AIDS-relief credential. Not using her degrees vocationally now, she divides her time between trying to escape from Kampala (most recently attempting to get a plane ticket and visa to do hotel work in Dubai) and attempting to embed herself as a fixture in the local hip hop scene. Tafash raps in her native language, Kiswahili.

Of her life prior to Uganda, Tafash explains that she grew up in an area that was "not really a hood" but geographically where there was a "ghetto up" and a "ghetto down" from her. Of her immediate family, she tells me that her dad died and her mother lives in Kenya. When

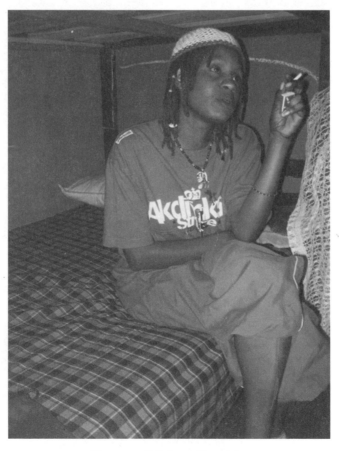

Figure 30.1 Tafash smoking a joint

I ask whether she has siblings, she replies, "uhhh, yeah." And then in the midst of vaguely mentioning some older and "much younger" brothers and "older step-sisters," she discloses that a sister died of an asthma attack while only in the Form 6 year of schooling.[18] Perhaps this is why she first sounded reluctant to answer my question. Tafash goes on to say that an older brother who had moved to North America also passed away of a "road accident" in Vancouver, Canada. When I try to acknowledge the tragic nature of her losses with a soft interjection of "That's hard," she immediately replies with detachment in her voice and a tear trickles down her face. "Yeah, but that's life, when you're hustling." For Tafash, it seems that "hustling" means balancing her musical dreams with practical aspirations, and hiding delicate memories like the ones she described to me. Hustling requires that Tafash numb her personal pain, and negotiate the fantasy of "making it" as a female MC with the reality of "looking for a job" so that she can live a better life than what she knows "here in Africa." Because "you can't just live by hip hop, hip hop only, here in Africa? Mm-mm. It's next to impossible. Maybe people who are lucky, you know? It happened to them."

Besides the Ugandan-born Twig, Tafash is the only other female rapper to appear on the recent *Kampala Flow* CD compilation.[19] As of 2008, Twig and Tafash were the only female MC's that we encountered in Kampala's still burgeoning local rap scene.

Prophet and Mother?

Tafash stuns her audiences. Everytime we [Barz and Liu] saw her perform at Sabrina's night club in Kampala, the audience seemed both shocked and riveted by the fury of her flow and stage presence. She lyrically blends contradiction and confidence as she problematizes and promotes measures to reverse the devastation of HIV/AIDS. In her carefully constructed rhymes she voices inscrutable challenges (such as a chorus that ends with "You do not know, Maybe drugs are a measure," follows) that border upon the prophetic. She blasts a rapid-fire knowledge of the way things really are with regards to HIV/AIDS relief in the everyday of Kampala, Uganda, at least according to other female MCs and herself.

"UKIMWI" ("AIDS"), LYRICS BY TAFASH

I am AIDS and AIDS is me	Ndiyo ukimwi na ikimwi ndiyo mimi
They call me danger 'cuz they were not ready for me	Wanamita hatari 'cuz hawakuwa tayari
I am coming worse than a car accident	Nakuja vibaya shinda accident ya gari
I am like a gamble	Nakucheza kaa kama kamari
I am spreading worse than news	Na spread kushinda habari
I cause a lot of worries	Naleta worries
When I arrive you cannot see me	Nikitokea huwezi ni ona
You get infected by me and you cannot heal	Nikikushika huwezi ni pona
Most people do not believe that I exist	Wengi hawaamini kuwa niko
I am hotter than fire	Mini moto shinda jiko
They take me as so simple	Wananitake so simple
They think I am like a pimple	Wanadhani mi ni pimple
They sing about me like some jingle	Wananiimba kaa kamaa jingle
I am illegal	Mini illegal
They have advertised me on billboards	Wameni advertise mpaka kwa bilboard

CHORUS: AIDS, I am a danger to your life / Ukimwi mini hatari kwa maisha yako

You didn't claim me as yours / Usiclaim vako

AIDS, I am a danger to your life / Ukimwi mini hatari kwa maisha yako

You didn't claim me as yours / Usiclaim vako

You do not know, maybe / [niko] Huweza jua labda niko

Drugs are a measure? / Dawa ni kupima

I like fools a lot / Napendaga sana wajinga

'Cuz they like doing it without protection / Wanpendaga kupanya bila kinga

Especially when they see you with a car / Kwanza nikiwa nadinga

I do not choose and I do not discriminate / Sichagui wala si bagui

I am a criminal / Mini mrui

I do not care if you are a kid or an elder / Sijali kaa we ne mtoto au mtu mzima

I do not care if you are rich or poor / Sijali kaa we ni tajiri au maskini

I do not care if you are light skinned or dark skinned / Sijali kaa we ni mweupe au mweusi

I just want to get into your body / Nataka tu kuingia kwa hiyo mwili

Into your brains / Nikuingie mpaka kwa akili

Then you die / Kisha udedi

I have killed so many / Nimeuwa wengi

I have infected so many and they do not know it / Bado niko ndani ya wengi

They are helping me spread / Wananisaidio kusamboza

'Cuz they are scared of exposing themselves / 'Cuz wanaogopa kujitangaza

CHORUS

I am a big problem to this world / Mini shida kubwa duniani

They are advertising me everywhere / Wananitangaza kila pahali

They are told to beware / Wanaabiwa wajitahadhari

Everyday in the news / Kila siku kwa habari

If you abstain, have safe sex, / Uki abstain, uki have safe sex, na ukitumia

and use sterilized objects / sterilized objects

You will have protected yourself / Utakuwa umejikinga

You will also be against me / Pia utakuwa umenipinga

Mothers are now boasting / Mothers wanaringa

That they can beat me / Ati waneza ni tunga

When they are pregnant / Wakiwa na mimba

They can have AIDS-free kids / Wazae watoto wako poa

Human beings can save themselves from me / Binadamu mnaeza jiokoa

You can eradicate me / Ukimwi mnaeza nitoa

These can truly happen / Mnaeza ni toboa

It is your choice / Chaguo ni lako

CHORUS[20]

Where did Tafash acquire such honest passion and profundity in her music-making? Are her lyrics deliberately esoteric or unconsciously polysemous? Do they exhibit a production, negotiation, or subversion of our request for socially conscious music? Or do they display deeper intentions and interplay, inclusive of but not contained by the parameters (or constraints) we set of her time in the studio? Was there a foreshadowing in her deep-seated reggae and Rasta beliefs and influences? As questions like these emerge from a rap like hers, what is clear is that there is no easy way to go about answering them. And her overall social critique provokes many more.

June, 2008—The compilation is finished. I (Liu) met Tafash for one last conversation. "Do you like Peter Tosh?" Tafash asked as she pointed to a TV placed on the bar of a local social club.[21] We sat only yards from local vendors in the busily trafficked main dirt road of the Namuwongo district of Kampala. The bar, a fly-infested area, provided the venue for meeting Tafash on her home turf. After some commentary on the Tosh concert video and how he kept it real, Tafash revealed a slice of her own reality. She had a son. Perhaps he had something to do with the lines about motherhood in "Ukimwi" and her other track, "Mama." "Would you like to meet him?" Tafash, mainly known as a Rastafarian rapper with a knack for elliptical rhymes about social change, was also a mother (Liu, fieldnotes, 2008).

Besides this surprise invitation to meet Sizzla, who is named after the Jamaican Rastafarian artist Sizzla Kalonji, Tafash doesn't say much more about her son (figure 30.2). I also refrain from inquiring further in order to respect her privacy. On the way to the home of the family friends that babysit Sizzla, who seemed around five or six years of age at the time, Tafash does mention that she rarely speaks with Sizzla's father, who still lives in Kampala. Perhaps this is why earlier in our exit interview, she sighed and explained how she considers "getting out of the [rap] game" on a daily basis. She dreams of moving to the United Kingdom. She also wonders if taking up hotel work in Dubai ("Cause like there are agencies that come to enroll people like every three months") might be another option to "live larger, buy houses...represent and maybe help my family."[22] In our last e-mail correspondence, Tafash told me that she is currently working on "four new joints" for an album titled "*Bindamu*" Kiswahili for "human being." She also hopes to shoot videos to accompany her new tracks, but struggles to finance such ambitions, as well as survive everyday life in "UG" [slang for "Uganda"].[23] At the message's end, she also lets me know that Sizzla has recently moved back to Kenya to live with Tafash's mother who makes a living selling African artifacts.

Her Rhymes About AIDS

A comprehensive analysis of Tafash's lyrics to "Ukimwi" ("AIDS") exceeds the scope of this chapter. Yet her lyrical content is not the express focus of our inquiries. Nevertheless, selections from each of her three verses demonstrate how on the one hand, Tafash aims to utterly disturb the complacency of her listeners with regards to HIV/AIDS, and on the other, to leave them with the possibility of eliminating the disease through the exercise of an unexplained, but nonetheless, saving communal agency. A dialectical back-and-forth where the negativity of AIDS is balanced by words of hope does not adequately describe the oscillation in her rhyming. Rather, what actually happens is a constant and sustained interplay where total destruction is imminent for neither human beings nor the disease, but it remains in the realm of possibility. Also, though Tafash judges the effectiveness of mass-campaign efforts for HIV/AIDS relief, it is not as if her call for responsible decision making is a social solution that cancels what has already

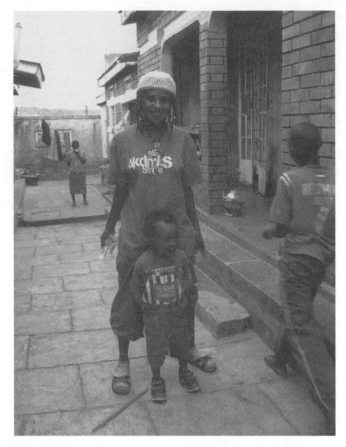

Figure 30.2 Tafash and her son Sizzla

been promoted by relief efforts. Indeed, it presumably includes much of what has been promoted with regards to HIV/AIDS relief in Uganda. "If you abstain, have safe sex, and use sterilized objects, You will have protected yourself, You will also be against me." Therefore, her particular call for decision making is a negotiation of messages for relief that have preceded her own. Yet striking is how Tafash builds on what she sees as ineffective efforts from the past in order to point toward an alternative and ambiguous horizon of healing characterized by motherhood and human choice. "Mothers are now boasting, That they can beat me [AIDS]...These [things] can truly happen. It is your choice." Whether people are saved or AIDS continues to rampage across Uganda is contingent upon a human decision-making process not fully described. Perhaps this is because such deciding is ultimately reliant upon something incomprehensible within humanity.[24]

The first selection from verse 1 critiques the ineffective cultural production and distribution of HIV/AIDS relief awareness in Uganda. "I am hotter than fire / They take me as so simple / They think I am like a pimple / They sing about me like some jingle / I am illegal / They have advertised me on billboards." For Tafash, mass cultural programs that seek to raise awareness have trivialized the disease and, ironically, contributed to its spread by overly simplistic advertising.[25] In the second selection located in verse 2, the relentless deadliness and sinister nature of AIDS saturates and trangresses Ugandan society indiscriminately. Generational, socioeconomic, and racial lines mean nothing to AIDS. "I do not care if you are a kid or an elder / I do not care if you are rich or poor / I do not care if you are light skinned or dark skinned / I just want to get into your body / Into your brains / Then you die." Not long after this blunt reminder of the core ambition of AIDS, Tafash returns in the third verse to the irony that campaigns aimed at mass prevention ironically contribute to the spread of HIV/AIDS. Paraphrasing the message of Tafash's track, she asserts that cultural complacency and heightened sexual curiosity has been fostered by mass appeals for safer sexual practices and larger consciousness regarding the threat of HIV/AIDS. Again, consider lines from her third verse: "I'm a big problem to this world / They are advertising me everywhere / They are told to beware, Everyday in the news / If you abstain, have safe sex, and use sterilized objects / You will have protected yourself / You will also be against me / Mothers are now boasting / That they can beat me / When they are pregnant." Nevertheless, Tafash does not end her track with cynicism. Rather, she extends an elusive reliance on a salvation discourse (soteriology)—"Human beings can save themselves from me"—offering hope for humans if they can exercise responsible decision making.

The self-saving agency that Tafash recommends is elusive because she never specifically describes exactly what her audience should do to eliminate AIDS. Her final challenge is also foregrounded by her redemptive challenge. Her positive disturbance—that listeners take it upon themselves to completely defeat the disease—is made more mysterious because the final repetition of the chorus is a final statement of threat, dispossession, and unintelligibility.

AIDS, I am a danger to your life	Ukimwi mini hatari kwa maisha yako
You didn't claim me as yours	Usiclaim vako
AIDS, I am a danger to your life	Ukimwi mini hatari kwa maisha yako
You didn't claim me as yours	Usiclaim vako
You do not know, maybe	[niko] Huweza jua labda niko
Drugs are a measure?	Dawa ni kupima

According to Tafash's rhyme, the self refuses to admit having AIDS. For some unstated reason, the possibility of drugs as a means of treatment is unintelligible. Or, ignorance prevents one from seeing drugs as viable treatment. The last verse locates eradication of the disease in agency. Yet the chorus attempts to fictionalize this agential hopefulness. It restates the way in which AIDS either escapes or proliferates as a result of a refusal to claim the disease. Thinking about pharmaceutical treatment becomes abstruse. How then does one respond to such cryptic advice from Tafash? And do Tafash's lyrics accurately diagnose what is occurring with regards to HIV/AIDS relief in East Africa? Or, do the lyrics of "Ukimwi" satirize the efforts to prevent and eradicate the disease in an uninformed way? Does the cultural ignorance she depicts in her lyrics function as unfounded generic irony or subversively sound speech to complacent ears? "I have killed so many / I have infected so many and they do not know it / They are helping me spread / 'Cuz they are scared of exposing themselves." Perhaps clear address to the constellation of questions occurs in the last lines of "Ukimwi," where Tafash's call for agency is preceded by the image of new birth. But clarity is not reached by what these lines say. Rather they must be seen with respect to how they are affirmed and unusually verified by the life of this chapter's second protagonist, Twig. Twig answers Tafash's call.

TWIG

Her Life as a Female MC: A Mother and an Affirmer of Tafash's Lyrics

Twig, whose birth name is Shannon Kayiga Nankeeze, was twenty-two years old at the time we recorded her in 2008. She typically raps in Luganda in the local Lugaflow style. A local female rapper in Uganda, she is the embodiment of Tafash's last stanza. She is a mother choosing survival, but her motherhood is defined by surrogacy. Twig has an adopted an AIDS orphan named Carol that she cares for full time.

> *Twig*—So this kid. She was so young. And she didn't know what really happened to her mother. Every time she would ask us, "Oh, but when is mom coming back?" And so I looked at her. That she was still a young kid. And she wanted help. Little help. They never had food to eat. They never had nothing. Like everyday the kid used to come to me crying. "Auntie, ok, give me 100. I go out at least I find something to eat. Daddy left me in the house. I have nothing. Brother walked away. He left me home so I'm there." So I decided to take care of this kid. (Interview with Liu, June 11, 2008)

The interview above ends a memory about how Twig adopted Carol. Carol's mother relocated near to where Twig lives in 2005. Carol's biological mother was suffering from AIDS at the time, but she didn't approach Twig at first due to that fact that Twig's mother was known to be a women's health care counselor. One day Carol's mother was found dead, and the father, known as a heavy drinker who was also HIV-positive, wouldn't take his antiretrovirals. Twig stepped in to take take care of the child and adopted her with the father's blessing. Carol had been with Twig for a year at the time of our recording, and the child was present in the recording studio whenever Twig performed (figure 30.3).

Twig is not "beating" AIDS by birthing an HIV/AIDS-free child. She "truly" lives into the last hopeful sentences of Tafash's conclusion by representing an unexpected permutation of what Tafash raps. Carol is not her biological daughter. Carol may also be infected. Thus, Carol is not an HIV/AIDS-free child born from a "boasting" mother to follow the illustration of Tafash's rhymes. Nevertheless, Twig's version of Tafash's maternal solution "eradicates" (even if temporarily) the devastation of AIDS by providing rescue for an HIV/AIDS orphan. We also suggest that Twig's decision to adopt Carol is an act of faith, that is more circuitously expressed in her music-making.

Her Musical Center
June, 2008. Cooper Road (Kampala).

> *Greg has departed. Feeling like we need one more female MC on the album, I have set up a meeting with Twig, who joined GNL ("Greatness with No Limits") last night on stage at Sabrina's. After asking her how she "got into the game," she explains that she first started rapping in church. Curious about the religious roots of her rhyming, I follow up with whether she considers herself a "person of faith." She responded, "I have to trust myself in the first place. And that means, if I trust myself, I trust God, everything I do, I mean I do it for myself and I do it for people. As well as, God is there. Everything of mine I need to be straight. Yeah, I need to be straight. So that's the reason why I put this faith in me. I don't*

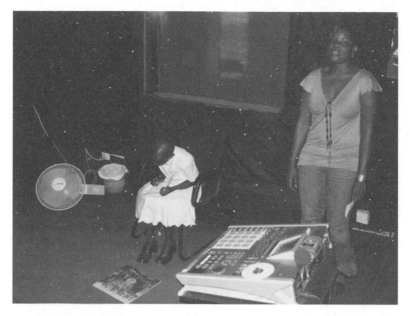

Figure 30.3 Twig and Carol in GK's Recording Studio

wanna lie, I don't wanna, do anything but. I just wanna be straight. Yeah.
Cause, I mean, if I didn't have God in me, I think I would have, I would've been
this crazy girl on the planet. Yeah, but just because I have someone who is guid-
ing me and listens to my heart, that's the reason why I have this, yeah." (Liu,
fieldnotes, 2008)

Like Tafash, Twig (who often refers to herself as "Twiggy") articulates a comprehensive
and complicated coinherence between her religious belief, her personal identity, and her
musical endeavors.[26] During the interview, when asked for further explanation, she states
that God does not affect her music-making. Then only seconds later, she reverses her position by portraying God as a writing muse, a "character" to which she appeals. Before any
line is written, she always asks God, "Is this right, do I have to do this?" Also like Tafash,
Twig approaches doing music as a self-assertive form of artistic expression as well as an
acknowledgment of religious underpinning. "I'm going to write about Twiggy. Why?
People will really want to know who Twiggy is. 'Cause some of them are not sure about
Twiggy. Yeah, so if I want to write about myself, I'm going to get like, 'Twiggy is so and
so.' I introduce myself. 'Twiggy started like this. Twiggy means this.' And, 'This is the
Twiggy!' And at the end of it, I say, yeah, 'if you want to know more about Twiggy, listen
to this.'"

ETHNOMUSICOLOGY AND THEOLOGY

Though it would not be difficult to characterize Twig's demand for attention from her listeners
as ego-driven and artistically self-absorbed, we wish to suggest that her attention to the self is
directly related to what she means by living with "God in me." In fact, Twig's self-understanding

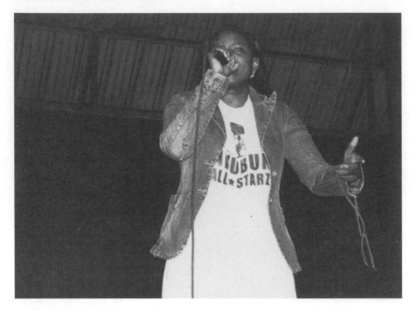

Figure 30.4 Twig spitting at Sabrina's Pub (downtown Kampala)

is inseparable from her belief in God. It is inseparable from how she understands her identity as an aspiring rap artist. It is inseparable from how she understands the activity of God in her life ("Is this right, do I have to do this?"). And for her listeners, it is requisite for grasping how she negotiates explanations of faith and belief that reverse, unravel, reassemble and generally proceed in unexpected directions. Therefore, Twig's belief in God not only links statements that at first appear to have no relation: it also helps Twig to model a theological epistemology pushing the limits of Western metaphysics. "[I]f I didn't have God in me, I think I would have, I would've been this crazy girl on the planet."[27] Twig's explanation challenges the boundaries of metaphysics because she does not pretend to know herself without God. Nor does her theological epistemology originate in her self understanding.[28] Rather God makes Twig knowing herself possible and coherent. Thus, Twig arrives at self-understanding by theological justification. Yet such interpretation of Twig's responses still may not necessarily be theological. Her logic of the self is plausible even from an agnostic view, if our analysis simply relies upon the defense, "Well this is what she said." What we more provacatively suggest is that Twig may be saying something about God, one that neither belongs to nor is contained by her, and one that is perceptible by others including her.

The above argument that Twig's belief in God is crucial for understanding her personhood and her music-making and significant for our consideration of God is why homiletics and liturgics can provide insightful contributions for ethnomusicology. For if Twig's music-making necessarily ties to her self-stated "trust [in] God," then Twig also functions "homiletically" as a religious "proclaimer" suggestive of how other persons might also associate and even attribute their self understanding to God. Homiletics concerns itself with the nature of proclaimed belief. As she states, Twig's being necessarily depends upon an indescribable "someone who is guiding me and listens to my heart" that also serves as inspiration for her creative work. Therefore liturgics, which concerns the work of the people (*leitourgia*) or how persons are wrought by God, becomes a viable field of orientation for understanding who Twig is and what her music means.

The theological scope of homiletics and liturgics likewise brings attention to the underlying Rastafarian purposes informing Tafash's music in general and how such purposes emerge in her HIV/AIDS rapping, which is the focus of this chapter. A hermeneutic with its basis in homiletics and liturgics also suggests how these purposes may bring us back to the confessional language and faithful life of someone like Twig, who symbolizes and embodies a second social, public, and ethical performance of Tafash's HIV/AIDS rhymes. Granted, her adoption of Carol is not a literal reaction to the rhymes of Tafash. On one hand, Twig's decision for surrogate motherhood coincidentally responds to what Tafash raps. On the other hand, however, the meaning of Tafash's lyrics becomes unexpectedly accessible in Twig's choice. We suggest that this meaning is not merely an unusual ethical expression that is helfpul for deciphering the ambiguity in Tafash's rhymes. Twig answers Tafash's call, but Tafash's rhymes do not begin at the site of the self, but with religious conviction that travels alongside her musical identity. Similarly for Twig, "God is there" and "in me." Therefore, the significance of the symbolic connection between them requires a theological mode of analysis. Yet before some concluding remarks regarding how theology helps bridge the music of Tafash to the life of Twig, and why we should be interested, some foregrounding of medical ethnomusicology is needed.

MEDICAL ETHNOMUSICOLOGY

The rapprochement of health-related issues, religion, and musical performance that exists within the culture of contemporary rap artists in Uganda relates directly to the concerns of the emergent academic field of medical ethnomusicology. A brief divergence into the historiography of medical ethnomusicology will serve to reveal the nuances and complexities in the lyrical work of Tafash and Twig. As will become clear, most scholars in the emergent field have laid a strong theoretical basis for positing the performance of religion, but we suggest that our work in Uganda would be more productively interpreted by applying a rationalized approach to the theology of healing proclaimed. The two inceptive full-length studies in medical ethnomusicology that deal with this issue include a dual emphasis on health and religious concerns. For example, Ben Koen's path-breaking book, *Beyond the Roof of the World: Music, Prayer, and Healing in the Pamir Mountains* (2009) and his dissertation on music of the Pamir Mountains in Tajikistan on which the book is based (2003), both position prayer within everyday contexts of individual and communal healing. Similarly, Barz problematizes one-dimensional understandings of religion as they pertain to medical and musical outreach efforts that address HIV/AIDS in Uganda in *Singing for Life: HIV/AIDS and Music in Uganda* (2006a). Neither of these ethnographies avoids the problematics of addressing religion within confusing and often conflicting cultural contexts. Yet both Barz and Koen tend to emphasize the physiological and communal in their investigations. Missing still are formal statements concerning how the revelatory may have been and may still be accesssible, not only for them as ethnomusicologists and for the musics and musicians they studied, but also for their readers and listeners. In *Singing for Life*, when asked about "the *future* of AIDS prevention, diagnosis, and care," healer Maboni Nabanji expresses the need "to learn each other's songs" with regards to the coalition work of "witch doctors, modern medical doctors, mosques, and churches."[29] Barz interpretively echoes Nabanji's words by pointing to a lack of ethnomusicological fieldwork that focuses on the relationship between music, faith, and expressive culture.[30] To what extent, then, does theology as an interpretive lens become a vital part of such focus and learning of other's songs? Koen speaks of the "culturally-transcendent" quality of Pamir devotional music, and even goes so far as to admit his increasing identification as an *âsheq* ("lover" of God); upon his return from fieldwork, moreover, he forms focus groups to test the healing qualities of Pamir music. Yet Koen's methods remain firmly rooted in the social sciences, with heavy reliance on statistical and cognitive data collection (Koen 2009, 154ff.). The epistemology we see functioning in the lyrics and lives of Tafash and Twig derives from an academic disposition similar to the empathy that Koen shares with his reader. In contrast to Koen, however, the words and actions of Tafash and Twig are shown to elude justification via quantification. They also communicate theologically with lived and spoken rationalities that are paradoxically incommensurable with how ethnomusicology may have previously studied religion, and therefore represent a critical opportunity to shift modes of analysis. Yet the current theological interpretation of their musical expression and lives has been widely prefigured by prior scholarship exploring the interplay between religion, health, and music.

Even in the critical historical texts that inform current efforts in medical ethnomusicology that preceded the two studies of Barz and Koen, there is a degree of reliance on positioning religion as central to the study of health and healing. In Marina Roseman's seminal text, *Healing Sounds from the Malaysian Rainforest* (1991), specific Temiar healing practices are positioned within an overarching cosmology. Roseman, perhaps more than any other scholar to date, attempts to fuse the study of music, healing, culture, and religion by focusing on the musical and medical ceremonies of the Temiar people as central to Temiar identity. Music and medicine draw on forms of local knowledge that are, according to Roseman, related to local Temiar gender issues, religious and spiritual concerns, kinship, and specific economic concerns. In the study of African religions as they pertain to healing, we are often confronted with the intricacies of African indigenous health care systems. The role of music within spirit possession ceremonies has proven to be most complicated. In his ethnography of Tumbuka healing practices in Malawi, *Dancing Prophets: Musical Experience in Tumbuka Healing* (1996), based on field research conducted in the northern area of the country, Steven Friedson provides answers from the philosophical method of phenomenology. Friedson is particularly interested in the forms and rituals that contribute to what he calls the Tumbuka people's construction of a "sacred clinical reality" (a concept drawn from Arthur Kleinman [1981]), in which music, divination practices, trance, spirit possessions, and medical treatment become intertwined within a single coextensive moment.

Contemporary ethnomusicological thought regarding music, medicine, and healing can be found in the recent collected volume of essays, *The Oxford Handbook of Medical Ethnomusicology* (Koen et al. 2008). A compendium of fundamental issues related to the study of medical ethnomusicology, *The Oxford Handbook*, while not intended to focus on religion, nevertheless provides scant attention to direct issues related to the expressive culture surrounding religious traditions.[31] A notable exception in the volume is Harold Koenig's study, "Religion, Spirituality, and Healing: Research, Dialogue, and Directions" (2008). In his study, Koenig outlines issues related to the historical resistance to religion and spirituality in science and biomedical research and practice (2008, 47), while also providing substantial research history pertaining to opportunities for future, collaborative work. Perhaps to a greater extent than any other author in *The Oxford Handbook*, Koenig values the agency of the health care practioner, the musician, and the ethnomusicologist in the study of music and religion as a collaborative art. Koenig's schema and suggested outline for research in medical ethnomusicology provide an invaluable resource for studies of religion and healing in East African popular musical traditions, which have yet to develop research protocol along these lines. In addition to the previously mentioned lack of theological proclivity in ethnousicological cultural analyses there is also an underdeveloped application of the basic tenets of medical ethnomusicology to studies involving popular music beyond basic songwriting and world music platforms for situating the therapeutic within musical healing.

East African MCs and HIV/AIDS

By pointing to a distinct lack of scholarship focusing on the critical reflection on HIV/AIDS or health care outreach efforts and African hip hop, we must also mention a paucity of academic studies involving the voices of East African rap artists. In *Global Noise: Rap and Hip Hop Outside the USA*, Tony Mitchell (2002, 50, 87) discusses hip hop in countries such as Japan and with peoples like the Maori, but discussion directly related to postcolonialism is limited to the European context. According to Mitchell, most scholarship of African rap has focused on South and West Africa, with groups such as Zimbabwe Legit, Positive Black Soul from Senegal, Jarring Effects from Morocco; there is little focus on female MCs (ibid., 8). Likewise, little interest or attention has been given to Uganda or more robust hip hop scenes such as those found in Tanzania and Kenya. While Halifu Osumare raises the issue of the African female voice in hip hop, little is documented in *The African Aesthetic in Global Hip-Hop: Power Moves*. Yet, Osumare quotes an interview with Afrik Image that begs for such scholarship: "'We have a rage inside of us. We want to succeed. If women can rap in the USA, [we say] why don't [we] try it in Ivory Coast?'" (2007, 29). Abdoulaye Niang (2006) confirms the position of African women in the margins of hip hop in West Africa. According to Niang, hip hop is still primarily a "masculine domain" in Senegal (2006, 166), with men and women fulfilling prescribed roles in the popular culture as either "b-boys" (bad boys) or as "fly-girls." It is interesting to note that Niang suggests that "'[m]ainstream' Senegalese society is calling more and more often on the rappers to raise public awareness of social problems such as HIV and AIDS" (ibid., 183). Thus, it appears that local cultures value the ability of rap to "speak" to the youth of contemporary Africa. Despite its promising subtitle's allusion to African rap, meanwhile, the focus of David Toop's *Rap Attack #3* is primarily on the history of African American rap and its influences around the world. That global women's voices hold little place in this writing of popular history was in part a primary motivation for writing the present chapter.

In East Africa, rap emerged as a primarily male-centric oratory art in the early 1990s, as confirmed by Haas and Gesthuizen's overview of early rap in Kiswahili—primarily in the country of Tanzania, but now performed throughout the region (2000). This conforms to Gregory Barz's own experiences with early rappers such as Saleh J. in Tanzania in the early 1990s. With the recent publication of Mwenda Ntarangwi's *East African Hip Hop* (2009), however, the depth of the expressive culture of youth in East Africa is well investigated. In his chapter, "Move Over, Boys, The Girls Are Here: Hip Hop and Gendered Identities" (2009), Ntarangwi introduces the key female performers who have enterred the heretofore male-dominated realm of hip hop in East Africa (limited, however, to examples in Kenya and Tanzania). In addition, Ntarangwi introduces several critical issues related to healthcare in his chapter, "Morality, Health, and the Politics of Sexuality in an Era of HIV/AIDS" (2009).

HOMILETICS AND LITURGICS

Returning to the theological analysis of the music and lives of Tafash and Twig, several arguments have shown why the use of homiletics and liturgics as a hermeneutic is not an attempt to adorn ethnomusicology with Sunday dress. The following statements further explore ways in which Tafash and Twig could be respectively seen as a religious proclaimer and an enactor of public liturgy, and how the theological roles attributed to them fit together.

What Tafash and Twig demonstrate are practices of radical hope in the face of cultural devastation.[32] Their hope is radical because they continue playing the "rap game" despite allergic reaction from the Ugandan public both to local hip hop and to their gender. Their hope is radical because when facing opportunities creative and personal, they refuse easy approaches to making an artistic statement about HIV/AIDS relief in Kampala. Nor do they circumvent possibilities within their own artistic lives for counteracting the carnage of AIDS. Not only illustrative of radical hope, the practices of Twig and Tafash function theologically because for Tafash, her esoteric rhymes operate out of a clear commitment to Rastafarianism. The ethical proclamation of her track has an underlying ethos that arguably makes her rhyming a religious proclamation as well. This is not because of the apocalyptic personification of AIDS in her lines. Rather, it is the parting call for choice that leads to eradication of AIDS and salvation of human beings: "you wanna live good, you know. And you wanna live righteous, you know. Soooo, everything I try to do, I think about the people. And what I want them to hear. And how I want them. You know, it's like, I don't know how to explain this, but it's just righteousness, you know, yeah, righteousness, that's what I can say, yeah." Like the trace of Rastafarian righteousness that can be perceived in Tafash's rhymes, Twig knows that "God is there." Attending to this divine presence even in the absence of Carol's biological parents, Twig enacts the concluding stanzas of Tafash's by choosing surrogate motherhood. This is not only an act of faith. It is a response to Tafash's words. Whereas a homiletic operative in Tafash's Rastafarian grounded rhymes has been suggested, Twig's choice of surrogate motherhood is also a proclamation in its own right. As Chauvet states, corporality can function as the liturgical speech of the body (Chauvet 1995). Therefore, Twig's embodied response of surrogate motherhood speaks back to Tafash's ultimatum with as much defiance toward the destruction of HIV/ADS, but also negotiated hope borne out of faith and attention to the reality of Carol and her. It is as if Twig's care of Carol says, "I have chosen to rescue this child even though the elimination of AIDS may not 'truly happen' for my daughter or Kampala."

CONCLUSION

Acting as agents of alterity who relentlessly negotiate, reinvent, and author their faith commitments within an uncompromising reality of HIV/AIDS, and a musical environment inhospitable to their hip hop and nearly intolerant of their pursuing rap music as females, these two women rappers in Uganda have made themselves pioneers in new endeavors for defeating the pandemic of HIV/AIDS in Africa.[33] Tafash lyrically indicts mass campaign efforts as propaganda that promote the spread of HIV/AIDS instead of societal commitment to prevention. She does not however, finish "Ukimwi" as a satirical tirade. Instead, following her hip hop aspiration for rhyming that *positively disturbs*, she ends the track with a proleptic proclamation that something as unimaginable as the elimination of AIDS can "truly happen" if humans undertake what seems to be an uncomplicated route of choosing to save themselves. By doing so, Tafash creates a personification of AIDS that excoriates current campaign efforts for relief and requires newly imagined mother-based human intervention as an alternative solution. In this way, Tafash takes our musical intervention to increase public attention to local Ugandan rap, and our request for socially conscious music, and makes them unmistakably her own. She intervenes within our intervention. She simultaneously attends to our research interests and subverts and supercedes them by rapping an unexpected social critique that functions as social and implicitly religious proclamation for her hearers not only to do something about AIDS, but also to make decisions toward living "righteously."[34]

Twig, an embodied affirmation and possible verification of Tafash's lyrics or proclamation, however, lives a nuanced version of "Ukimwi"'s final challenge. Of course, chronologically or even empirically, it is not as if Twig literally hears Tafash's track and then chooses to live accordingly. Rather, Twig represents an unanticipated and already extant form of the motherly redemption that becomes the culminating image in "Ukimwi." In her adoption and care of Carol, Twig diverges from Tafash's already obscure and open-ended vision of redemption.[35] She decides for motherhood that is simultaneously marginal, manifest, and different from the sense of motherhood implied by Tafash's mother boasting about having "AIDS-free kids." As Twig states: "And that means, if I trust myself, I trust God, everything I do, I mean I do it for myself and I do it for people." It seems to follow then that what Twig has done for Carol must be included in the "everything" what she does out of "trust" in God. Therefore, Twig exercises choice that responds to a call like Tafash's. Yet Twig demonstrates that such choice cannot happen without God. With God, however, Twig can and does rescue Carol from the destruction and ruins of HIV/AIDS toward the promise of life nurtured for a reimagined and hopefully better present and future. This divine enabling may not only activate saving acts within a life like Twig's, but perhaps have its place in others, including ours, as well.

Ethnomusicology in general—and medical ethnomusicology specifically—infrequently moves beyond the collection and representation of musical and cultural data in ways that are any more than cognitive, statistical, analytical, or observational. By listening to two female East African rappers in a theological register we begin to hear the subaltern voices of Uganda's rap community resonating with the performance of religious proclamation. In so doing there is a marked shift in these women's lyrics as they spit new ways of healing their communities. Enigmatically, they may also help us, including but not limited to the two authors of this chapter, reconceive of how rescue becomes possible in our own locales. It might seem a bit risky to focus on the marginalized treatment of lived religious experience in ethnomusicology, yet in so doing we approach the consumption of health care interventions among rap artists working in East Africa from a decidedly theological perspective that unveils an ability for the ethnomusicologist to experience an alterity of the very *positive disturbance* of that which Tafash and Twig proclaim and live.

31

"EDZI Ndi Dolo" ("AIDS is Mighty")

SINGING HIV/AIDS IN MALAWI, 1980–2008

John Chipembere Lwanda (Dudu Nsomba Publications)

INTRODUCTION AND THEORETICAL FRAMEWORK

Early cases of HIV/AIDS in Malawi, circa 1977, at first confused musicians just as they confused the general public and the government (Lwanda 2002, 151–52). After an initial silent phase, musicians began to create jingles, songs, and musical dramas that expressed emotions ranging from bewilderment, blame, and paranoia to a surge in religious activity. Many initial musical reactions were created by request for non-governmental organization-based (NGOs) or government-inspired HIV/AIDS campaigns. Only after experience and reflection did musicians eventually take ownership of their musical compositions, leading them to produce some of the often humorous proverb- and metaphor-rich, if at times controversial, music of the late 1990s and 2000s. In this chapter, I will discuss some of the songs documenting the arrival of HIV/AIDS in Malawi, describing the features of the disease, interpreting the associated awareness-raising and Voluntary Counseling and Treatment (VCT) campaigns, and reflecting on the epidemic's social, economic, political, and cultural effects.

I organize this chapter to address music and HIV/AIDS in five chronological periods: before HIV/AIDS had a local name; the initial period of "silence" from 1985 to 1990; the transitional period from one-party rule to multiparty between 1990 and 1994; the first multiparty years, 1995 to 1999; and 2000 and beyond. I will also discuss how several musicians addressed their own personal involvement with HIV/AIDS.

As in the rest of Africa (see Nketia 1982), music in Malawi is integrated with most activities of daily life; many health and medical issues, moreover, manifest themselves within the social public sphere (Lwanda 2003a, 113–26 and 2008, 71–101). This social arrangement makes popular music highly relevant to the HIV/AIDS discourses.

Musicians in Malawi have, from the beginning of the epidemic, largely adopted war-like metaphors or *kunja kuno kwaopsya* (adverse environment scenarios) when dealing with

HIV/AIDS. Pongweni argues that the "[s]ongs that won the liberation war" can be divided into a number of categories: those that raised consciousness and awareness; those containing an argument; those that "appealed to ancestral spirits"; "songs appealing for help from," and thanking, "progressive countries"; stocktaking songs; "songs appealing for unity"; "songs inspired by tribulation"; and "songs defying and deriding the colonial system" (1982, preface). Although we could easily add "songs appealing to morality and the need for self-preservation," and replace "colonial" with "governmental," Pongweni's classification, given its "war" background, could also roughly classify the HIV/AIDS songs in Malawi.

Malawi was, between 1964 and 1994, a one-party, male-dominated state led by Dr. Hastings Banda, whose political philosophy of "loyalty, unity, obedience, and discipline" (Africa Watch 1990) was tinged with Presbyterian public moral values (Forster 1994, 477–97). This constrained environment of limited public discussions of sexual issues set the background for the arrival of HIV/AIDS into Malawi (Lwanda 2003a, 113–26; Chimombo 2008, 213–23).

Dr. Banda loved, encouraged, and patronized traditional music. The women of his Malawi Congress Party sang *mbumba* praise music (appropriated traditional tunes and dances with political lyrics) at all of his public functions (Chimombo and Chimombo 1996, Muyebe and Muyebe 1999, Lwanda 2003b, 119–42). Some men felt emasculated by *mbumba* music (Mapanje's "The New Platform Dances" in 1981, 12), sowing the seeds of later gender tussles. At the time there was also a tradition of popular music despite the limited recording industry (Lwanda 1994, 210–11).[1]

When the National AIDS Committee was formed in 1989, IEC (information, education and communication) campaigns, partly influenced by the political environment of the time and partly by the lack of a cure, had led the general population to link action on HIV/AIDS with government power (Chimombo 2007, 12). Dr. Banda—the father, founder, and all-powerful *ngwazi*—was the one to whom Malawians sang "Zonse zimene za Kamuzu Banda" in which everything regarding "development" was ascribed to Dr. Banda (Malawi Broadcasting Company [MBC] recording):

Zonse zimene za Kamuzu Banda	Everything belongs to Kamuzu Banda
Nyumba zonsezi	All these houses
Za Kamuzu Banda!	Belong to Kamuzu Banda!
Anthu onsewa	All these people
—MBC recording (author archives)	

Inevitably, some humorists singing in private added more critical issues such as cholera, hunger, suffering, and other ills to this list. The government consequently responded by limiting access to those infected with HIV. When the dead bodies of early AIDS victims were transported to burial, they were typically escorted only by "doctors, government officials, even police and prisoners, with strict instructions for burial, without the ceremony of viewing the body...[and] only prisoners...allowed to bury the body" (Chimombo 2007, 12). Such secretive actions led people in Malawi to call the new disease *matenda a boma* (the government disease). Understandably, not even the bravest musician in the country was going to be the first to sing publicly about the new "government" disease.

But popular musicians had long sung about their culture, a culture that in fact was later blamed for escalating the HIV/AIDS epidemic. The Ndingo Brothers, for example, was a popular band in the 1970s that popularized aspects of Malawi's male-dominated society (Ndingo ca. 1975):

Anamwaliwa muwalange!	These girls need instructing!
Lero akula muwalange, muwalange!	They are mature now, instruct them!
—Ndingo Brothers (n.d.)	

We note that "only women" required instructions in sexual and marital issues. Traditional wedding songs also emphasized the dominance of males in marriage and society (see Kanjo and Gomile 1993):

Wamkulu ndani m'banja?	Who is the boss in the family?
Wa'mkulu ndani m'banja?	Who is the boss in the family?
Wa'mkulu ndi mwamuna!	The man is the boss!
—Kaliati and Ning'ang'a (n.d.)	

These attitudes were later reflected in songs that stigmatized females as spreaders of HIV. Examples included Albert Khoza's "*Akunenepa nako kachilombo*" ("She looks nice and plump despite the virus") and rapper Anne (sic) Matumbi's "*Mkazi wa Neighbour*" ("Neighbor's wife"), which described bored HIV-positive housewives seducing and infecting eligible bachelors living next door.

BEFORE THE NAME

Even before HIV/AIDS officially arrived in Malawi, musicians sang about "something" they had noted since the late 1970s. In the early 1980s, Jivacort Kathumba had given some indication in "*Mabvuto simaliro okha*" ("Death is not the only problem"). The title was an ironic comment on a subject regarded as politically sensitive; death indeed was the problem:

Mabvuto simaliro okha,	Death is not the only problem,
mabvuto!	problems!
Ukhale opanda chakudya, amenewo	Be without food; that is a
ndi mabvuto!	problem!
Ana ako adzidwala, amenewo	Your children are ill, that is a
ndi mabvuto!	problem!
—Kathumba (1995)	

In retrospect, it appears that musicians started singing about the epidemic even before it had a name. Robert Fumulani's early 1980s "*Kunja kuno imfa ikuthamanga*" ("Out here deaths are accelerating"), couched in a gospel idiom, predates the first official diagnosis of HIV/AIDS in 1985 (cf. Cheesbrough, 1986, 5–13) and presages the official IEC programs both in its vision and urgency:

Kunja kuno, kulibe chabwino.	In this world there is nothing good.
Tili m'masiku oopsya padziko lapansi	We live in dangerous times on earth
Imfa ikuthamanga, tsiku ndi tsiku	Deaths are escalating day by day
Modetsa nkhawa.	In such a frightening way.
Mulungu wanga ndiululileni	My God, please reveal to me
Chinsinsi cha imfa yanga, nditsikulo	The secret and day of my death
Inu pakudza, mudzandipeze ndili	So when you come I will be ready
wanu.	for you.
—Robert Fumulani (n.d.)	

Fumulani's phenomenological observations were echoed by Saleta Phiri in "Ife tinali ndi anza-thu ife" ("We had friends").

Ife tinali ndi anzathu ife, ife tinali ogwirizana.	We had friends, we were united.
Koma onse anapita pa ulendo wosabwelera.	But they all left us on a one way trip.
— Saleta Phiri (1997)	

And to confirm that people were dying, Alan Namoko, against the background of significant orphan abuse, asked Malawians to look after the many "*Ana Osiidwa*" ("The orphans"):

Msawatemere m'manja ana a masiye!	Do not be mean to the orphans!
Ana osiidwawa, opanda mai wawo	These orphans, without mothers
Zoona kwalera kwache mwatere?	Is this the way to raise them?
— Alan Namoko (1992)	

THE PERIOD OF SILENCE, 1985–1990

Because of Malawian President Dr. Hastings Banda's generally negative attitudes toward family planning and public discussions of sexual issues, there was no leadership from the Ministry of Health, the National AIDS Secretariat (formed in 1987), and from the National AIDS Committee (instituted in 1989). Both musicians and health promotion workers were afraid to act due to the possible consequences. Between 1985 and 1990 there was therefore an artistic "silence," challenged only by tentative foreign-led attempts to tiptoe around Dr. Banda's sensibilities. These NGO-led efforts soon began to make an impact, allowing music to be employed as a consciousness-raising tool.

Beginning in late 1985, the MBC began to feature "traditional" sounding anti-AIDS jingles and songs. Their theme, *Kwabwela Edzi* (*AIDS has come*), acknowledged AIDS as a new disease introduced into the country. An example is the Kaluluma Hospital Choir's *chimtali* rhythm-backed "*Edzi ndi matenda oopsya*" ("AIDS is a dangerous disease").

Tichite bwanji kuti tiipewe?	How can we prevent it?
Chiwerewere tingoleka	We should stop being promiscuous
Tisamale banja.	Let us look after our families.
—Kaluluma Choir (n.d.)	

Some musicians, such as the young Kasambwe Brothers Band, were inspired by these jingles. The Kasambwe even sang their song "AIDS is a killer" in English (1992).

I mean you boy
Check your step!
I mean you girl
Check your step!
AIDS is a killer,
AIDS is a fatal disease!

NGO tracts advocating HIV prevention tended to be "preachy," often leveraging "protective" Western family planning concepts of condom use over traditional ideas. The so-called "cultural imperialism" of Western NGOs has persisted, with many jingles and songs played on radio still carrying the banner, "brought to you by the European Union, USAID or DFID."

The period of silence was followed by an era of blame, usually toward the then-traditional targets: "homosexuals, hemophiliacs and Haitians." Some musicians reflected the "God's wrath" argument becoming prevalent; the Masaka Band, for example, sang "*Watenga AIDS iwe*" ("You have contracted AIDS"), adding "sinners and prostitutes" to the list of the condemned. Ultimately, however, few musicians took this perspective. In general this period was characterized by musicians singing to medical and NGO-based texts.

Instead, from behind this publicly silent screen emerged a disease that was, as seen by musicians, "ravaging" the area and threatening the "survival of the nation." This *tikutha* (we perish) theme was best encapsulated by the Malawi Police Orchestra. Their late 1988 hit "*Kunja kuno kwaopsya*" ("The world is now dangerous") also used a communal "at war" approach, that for decades afterward remained a common strategy for describing the disease:

Tonse tili pankhondo ndi Edzi eh!	We are all at war with AIDS
Zipolopolo zao ndi tizirombo eh!	Its weapons are the viruses!
Pothawira peni peni tilibe ife.	We really have nowhere to run to.
Zishango zathu zikhale makondomu eh!	Our shields are condoms eh!
Masiku ano kunjaku kwaopsya	Nowadays it is dangerous out there
Tizirombo tikukhala m'magazi.	These viruses are living in the blood.
Masiku onse tikulira maliro.	Every day we have a funeral.
Nkhondo yomwe ndikunena ndi matendawa.	The war we are talking about is this disease.
Madotolo akuti mankhwala kulibe kuchipatala.	Doctors say there is no medicine in hospitals.
Asing'anga akuti mitengo kulibe uko ku dondo!	Herbalists say there are no herbs for it in the forest!
Opezeka ndinthendayi tiwasunge bwino,	Let us take good care of those who are found to have this disease,
Pothawira peni peni ife tilibe eh!	We have really nowhere to run to!
—Malawi Police Orchestra (1988)	

Singing of overtly-themed AIDS songs by popular musicians could thus be said to have started circa 1988–1989, a full four years after HIV arrived in Malawi. The Malawi Police Orchestra led this shift both because it included experienced musicians and because the Police, like the Army, had been badly affected by HIV/AIDS (Lwanda 2002, 158).

THE TRANSITIONAL PHASE: AIDS AS CULTURE DESTROYER/BUILDER, 1990–1995

After the 1989 visit of Pope John Paul II to Malawi, the debate between "condomist" and "fidelitist" religious and nonreligious groups became heated. The visits by the Pope, Archbishop of

Canterbury Runcie, and Margaret Thatcher to Malawi bolstered many fundamentalist Christians. Some firmly believed that fidelity and abstinence were the only answers; others went as far as claiming that "HIV/AIDS was God's wrath" on sinning Malawians. To this end some Christian gospel groups used the musical couplet "*Edzi inabwelera anthu, osati nyama*" ("AIDS came for humans not animals") to illustrate the moral dimensions of the disease (see Mt. Sinai Choir 2001).

At first it was thought HIV/AIDS would destroy the fabric of Malawian cultural life. Initially, bosses denied many workers their cultural rights to attend the escalating numbers of funerals. In 2005, Nhlashi and Miye noted that bosses still thought workers lied when they asked to attend funerals "every week." Only when the disease had come to affect every level of society and every company did bosses understand the cultural need for workers to attend funerals.

But, paradoxically, as extended family systems are the basis of social cohesion, it was not long before the numerous funerals actually became the basis for an increased cultural vibrancy: since the memorials would include hymn singing, gospel all-nighters, traditional mourning music, and other activities related to disease and death. Saleta Phiri, an astute observer of social behavior, used satire to record the confluence of a mourning culture, the economy, and the nature of seduction in his song "*Ulemu/ndilekeni*" ("Respect/let me"). Funerals, in his portrayal, became hunting grounds for sugar daddies, widowers, and desperate widows:

Amai ena akavala nsalu yakuda	Some women when mourning in black
Achita kuyenda nyamu nyamu *Gwede gwede*...	Walk provocatively, shaking hips...
Naonso amuna ena akaona azimai *pamaliro*	When some men see widows at funerals
Achita kuti basi mai inu ndi ine *khete khete!*	They swear: you are mine now!
—Saleta Phiri (2001)	

In rural areas, traditional musicians were less constrained by urban political censorship, and more influenced by radio advertisements, NGOs, and health extension workers. Consequently, artists began to incorporate HIV awareness lyrics into traditional dances. An *Ingoma* group from Ncheu provides an example:

Kulibe nthenda ina makosana	There is no other disease folks
Yoposa Edzi!	Worse than AIDS!
Chigololo n'chibwana!	Adultery is playing with fire!
—Ncheu Ingoma Group (1994)	

Cleverly, the group had created this song by adapting one of the praise songs for Dr. Banda: "*Palibe fumu ina*" ("There is no other chief").

At this time a number of musicians were asked to compose HIV/AIDS awareness songs, either as a public service or for a competition. Saleta Phiri's composition "*Iri mu ufa*" ("It is in the flour") suggested that HIV was an elemental issue, as elemental as sex.[2]

Anzathu tafuna mumve	Friends we want you to listen
Tabwela ndi uthenga wabwino.	We bring a good message.
Chiwerewere anzathu lekani	Please stop being promiscuous
Kunja kuno kwaopsya.	The world is now dangerous.
Kuli matenda alibe mankhwala!	There is an incurable disease!
—Saleta Phiri (1990)	

When the Chishango condom was launched in 1994, meanwhile, Population Services International's (PSI) promotional jingle for the item reflected the form of the popular songs of the era:

Tinapangana, kunja kwabvuta	We agreed things are now dangerous
Nthenda zachuluka.	There are now too many diseases.
Tichitenji, tachulukana?	What shall we do, we are many?
Kupewa moyo ndi kwako mbale	Prevention is up to you
Chishango chilipo pewera!	Chishango (condoms) are there, stay safe!
—PSI advertisement (1995)	

The content of these advertisements in turn acted as templates on which musicians built their songs.

MULTIPARTY *ALANGIZI*, 1995–1999

The onset of multiparty rule liberated the arts from silence and censorship, unleashing the various perspectives and prejudices of the musicians. Musicians' various identities—gospel, secular, political, reggae, pop, and particularly rap or ragga—became more obvious. (During the one-party era, some musical identities such as rap and raga had not been permitted for political reasons.) Some musicians adopted traditional roles, such as *aphungu* (prophets or messengers) and *alangizi* (counselors). In traditional cultures *aphungu* and *alangizi* are given considerable latitude to critique chiefs and other powerful societal groups, though this latitude had disappeared during Dr. Banda's dictatorship. These developments paralleled the (re)cementing of strained extended family systems as a public culture of "attending funerals and compassion" began to emerge. Funerals of MPs and other elite citizens, many who died from HIV-related illnesses, transformed into events of "national theatre" with copious hymns and secular music: President Bakili Muluzi recognized the political significance of these moments, and gained a reputation as a "man of the people who attended funerals" (Lwanda 2005, 248–52).

Because of the censorship during Dr. Banda's rule, musicians developed ways of communicating to and with various sectors of society without getting into trouble. Popular music lyrics usually employed vernacular languages, but occasionally engaged in code-switching (cf. Kayambazinthu 1998, 19–43), with English generally reserved for harmless, ironic, or comedic phrases. The younger rap and ragga musicians, for example, generally mixed English with the vernacular to address their issues (see Gilman and Fenn 2006). Deep vernacular, proverbs, metaphors, colloquialisms, and other masking modes of social discourse, meanwhile, were often used by *alangizi* to address problematic subjects.

Songs from this period emphasized prevention, continuing the "no cure" and *tikutha* (we perish) refrains from earlier. The extent of the epidemic was observed by Billy Kaunda in his song "Coffin workshop." Carpenters were "making coffins, one after another" as the Tiyamike Band implored:

Inu anzanga mverani!	My friends, listen!
Kunja kuno kwaopsya!	It's frightening out here!
Ichi chakoma chakoma	Yielding to multiple temptations
fisi anagwa chagada.	Killed the hyena.
— Tiyamike Band (1995)	

Toward the end of the song the group alludes to the evils of sugar daddies:

Abambo yawa kuipa mtima	This man is heartless
Kuononga tiana taweni!	Spoils other people's kids!

The younger ragamuffin and rap singers, given the austerity of the Banda era, only significantly started addressing HIV/AIDS publicly after the onset of multiparty rule. Rap artist Albert Khoza revisited the issue of *Chidyaximan* (*chidyamakanda* or sugar daddy), but then became controversial with the release of *"Akunenepa ndi kachilombo"* ("She is getting fat despite the virus") which stigmatized asymptomatic HIV-positive women as spreaders of the disease.

This period also saw the emergence of some of the most reflective music. Set to a funereal *ingoma*, Dennis Phiri's magisterial *"Tikutha"* ("We are perishing") is one of the most nuanced Malawi HIV/AIDS awareness songs to date:

Ine chomwe ndaona:	What I have seen is this:
Satana wamanga masiku	Satan is now in charge
kulamulira aliyense	Controlling everyone
zibale ziti zipita?	Which relatives will go next?
Maliro ndi akale	Death has always been with us
koma lero zanyanya!	But now things are too much!
Tawafunseni agogowa	Ask grandmother
momwe zimakhalira kale.	How things were in the old days.
Magulu onse a wanthu	All groups of people
alowelera inu	Are engaged in this process
sitikuopa kuti kunjaku zinthu zabeba.	Not fearing that the world has gone bad.
Imvani anthu kusewera ndi moto	See people playing with fire
ungadziotche chabe.	You will merely burn yourself.
Chala mkamwa mwa njoka	Sticking a finger in a snake's mouth
ndikuziputa dala!	Is asking for it!

Refrain:

Tikutha! Tikutha anthu!	We are perishing, people we are perishing!
Taganizani inu ku mortuary	Imagine at the mortuary
kusowa koponda inu	You cannot find a space to step on
abale athu ngunda ngunda ngati	Our relatives lying scattered as if play
achitira dala.	acting.

Mabokosi kale lija amatiopsya zedi	Coffins used to scare us stiff in the old days
lero siawaagulitsidwa pali ponse wawa.	Now they are sold everywhere.

Phiri continues his song by claiming that sacrifices would have been made in the old days, adding:

Koma lero mizimu yatitembenukira.	But today the ancestral spirits have turned against us.

He attributes this turnabout to "too much sin," and graphically describes the nocturnal "wild side" of Malawi cities:

Tadzayeseni tsiku lina mudzayende ku Lilongwe	Try one day walking around Lilongwe
kuKabula kumahotela awa mudzawaona	and Blantyre hotels you will see them
anamwali anu ali mbwanda mbwanda kuonetsatu	your maidens spread-eagled indecently showing
kuti imfa alibe nayo mantha!	that they do not fear death!

Phiri then describes what happens when someone falls ill with HIV/AIDS:

Mukadwala adzimvetsa anzanu	But when you fall ill your friends suffer
amakayikira makolo akale, akazi anu	blaming your ancestors, your wife
kudandaula, kunamiza anzanu	you complain, deceiving your friends
anandilodza ine!	"I was bewitched!"
Mwaiwala nchito zanu zakumdima dzana	You forget your nocturnal activities of yesteryear.

He then notes how the victim spends all his savings on false cures and inevitably dies:

kuti mupeze moyo	So that you can extend your life
Lero siwo apuma,	Today he goes to his rest,
katundu watha kugulitsa kufuna moyo.	his inheritance exhausted in the quest for life.
Makolo kulira mkazi kulira	Parents weep, the wife weeps
ndi ana omwe kulira!	and even the children weep!
Nchito zonse panyumba pano zafa lero bambo.	All is dead in this household, father.

— Dennis Phiri (1999)

The song mixes Christian and traditional moral perspectives, attributing the graphic and epidemic rise in deaths to "playing with fire," an "abundance of sin," and "deliberate activities of the night in the full knowledge of the consequences." The deaths overwhelm available mortuaries, thus reducing the dignity of the dead. Phiri assumes that the pathways of infection are widely known, since he portrays the victims as "playing with fire." He also alludes to the economic desperation of the young women, which causes them to lose their fear of death. Interestingly, the song has a pro-feminist stance in that it does not give women a disproportionate amount of blame for the epidemic. Rather, he describes how men use denial, embedded in the discourse of witchcraft, to legitimate their squandering of family resources in the pre-antiretroviral (ARV) era, leaving the nuclear and extended family destitute. The song thus offers a particularly nuanced engagement with the various sociocultural, medical, gender, economic, and religious discourses of the period.

SINGING AIDS IN THE TWENTY-FIRST CENTURY: PREVENTION, VCT, ARVS, AND ANGER

At the turn of the millennium, one of the most popular songs on the radio was "*Mbuyo kucheta*" ("Out of sight") by Austin Skeremu. Its lyrics, addressing the paradox of the popularity of *ufiti* (witchcraft-based) discourse in relation to HIV/AIDS, deconstruct a popular excuse by youths:

> *Inu achinyamata*　　　　　　You the youth
> *kumbuyo kucheta!*　　　　　　Out of sight, out of mind!
> *Tikayendayenda tidzipita kumudzi.*　After some wandering, we should
> 　　　　　　　　　　　　　　visit home.
>
> *Tisamati tikapita moyenda*　　We should not say, once away
> 　　　　　　　　　　　　　　from home
> *kumudzi sindifunako*　　　　　I don't want to go home
> *adzangondilodza ine!*　　　　They may bewitch me there!
> *Anthufe tinalodzedwa kale*　　We humans are cursed already
> *imfa tingoyenda nayo...*　　　we walk with death all our lives...
> *Palibe chozemba ngati imfa*　Nothing is as cunning as death
> —Austin Skeremu (2000)

The following year, 2001, saw Peter Chidzanja rework an Anansi-type folk tale involving *Chechule* (Mr. Frog) into an effective HIV/AIDS awareness song. Ordinary people found resonance in this folktale because it situated a humorous message in the arena of social change rather than in the more direct personal messages from NGO jingles. After describing the nocturnal activities of young men in the townships of Lilongwe, including the drinking dens of Bwandiro suburb, the song (replete with double entendres) concludes:

> *Ndinapita ku Malawi*　　I went to Malawi
> *ndinapeza Chechule*　　and found Mr. Frog
> *Atavala condomu!*　　　Wearing a condom!
> —Peter Chidzanja (2001)

The message seemed clear enough: such was the magnitude of the HIV/AIDS epidemic that even Chechule (Mr. Frog) was now using condoms.

Popular music competitions, favoring local music, also began to generate significant numbers of musical compositions about HIV/AIDS. Ben Michael won several of these. In 2001, for example, he composed "*Tilire tilire*" ("Let's all cry"), a song that involved a call-and-response pattern:

> *Tilire tilire*, let's all cry!
> Not for the dead, but for ourselves!
> *Tilire tilire*, let's all cry!
> Not for the dead, their turn is gone!

Coss Chiwalo used a call-and-response chorus in his song "*Mudzingoti toto*" ("Just say no") as well, appealing to teenagers to avoid behavior likely to bring *Edzi* (AIDS):

Ananu mudziti	Kids, you should say
Akati lawa chamba	If they say smoke dope
Aah! Toto!	Oh! no!
Akati imwa mowa	If they say drink some beer
Aah! Toto!	Oh! no!
Chidyamakanda	Sugar Daddy
Aah! Toto!	Oh! no!
Coss Chiwalo (n.d.)	

After 2003, when antiretrovirals (ARVs) became available in government hospitals, the "'no cure' excuse" became less valid. Instead, the issue became one of persuading members of the public to accept Volunteer Counseling and Testing (VCT). Malume Bokosi reflected this state of affairs in "*Wakana kukayezetsa*" ("She's declined the test"):

Tinatengana ndi wachikondi wanga	My love and I agreed
kuti tikayezetse	to go for VCT
ndicholinga kuti tilowe m'banja	the better to enter marriage
opanda chikaiko.	with total trust.
Adzandityola bwanji	How will she affect me?
Sindidziwa.	I do not know.
Wanditengela zotani?	What has she brought me?
Sindidziwa.	I do not know.
Kuchipatala ndiko kuli mayankho!	The answer is at the hospital!

However, while at the hospital, Bokosi's intended does not return from "powdering her nose," and instead evades the prenuptial HIV test. He has no choice but to cancel the wedding:

Mwauze Makolo ake	Tell her parents
kuti chikwati ndachilephela.	I have failed to get married.
Fupa lokakamiza	Forcing a bone in
silimachedwa kuswa mphika!	Is the quickest way to break a pot!

He asks ruefully:

Wakana kukayezetsa, akuopa chiani?	She won't test; what is she scared of?

Then, like Dennis Phiri, Bokosi harkens back to the good old days of his parents' youth:

Munali odala inu mai ndi bambo,	You were lucky mum and dad,
agogo ndi anganga.	gran and granddad.
Chinyamata chanu mukusimba	Your youth as you tell it
chinali chokoma.	was sweet.
Polowa m'banja simumawerenga	You had few qualms before marriage
zambiri	
bola mkhalidwe, kugwirizana	just good behavior, love and
Chichewa.	understanding.
Koma zililero ngondo amawo	But today, please it is like war!
choonde!	

—Malume Bokosi (2006)

This theme of "testing before marriage or commitment" was also pursued by Mt. Sinai Choir, whose members addressed the phenomenology of HIV infection in "Tilalikire za Edzi" ("Let us preach about AIDS").

Nanga munthu ali ndi kachiromboka	Does the HIV-infected person
kodi amadziwika?	Look distinguishable to the
	naked eye?
Munthu ali ndi kachirombo sadziwika,	An infected person is not
	identifiable;
chimunthu chonenepa,	a chubby person,
wathupi losalala,	a beautiful looking person,
chikome kome chankuyu mkati muli	could be like a fig, pretty on the
nyerere.	outside, full of ants inside.
Azimai sinthani,	Women change your behavior,
azibambo kalamukani,	men wisen up,
dziko la pansi laipa.	the world is spoiled.
Mtendere supezeka	There is no peace
Tsiku ndi tsiku maliro!	Every day there are funerals!

—Mt. Sinai Choir (2007)

Mount Sinai Choir, located in the densely populated Ndirande Township, offered an example of a gospel choir that mixed church and secular traditions. Their music, while containing serious messages, was also infused with humor and drama and was popular because it was not overtly "preachy." They performed as often at secular occasions as in churches.

EXTENDED MUSICAL FORMS

Apart from commissioned works, few musical artists have gone so far as to create entire HIV/AIDS concept albums. Joe Gwaladi, for example, has incorporated HIV/AIDS into much of his work. His individual songs tend to ramble through a number of subjects, with HIV being a favorite of his. However none of his two major works could be considered HIV/AIDS concept albums.

Charles Nsaku's 2006 *Tiwana ku ndende* ("Little children in prison"), on the other hand, comes close, with seven out of ten tracks addressing HIV/AIDS problems. In *"Amasiye,"* a mother asks from the grave why her orphaned child is not benefiting from the inheritance he left her, but is instead being ill-treated. The chorus tells us the message has a wider target:

A President	Mr. President
kondani a masiye!	Love the orphans!
A minister	Cabinet Minister
mukondane ndi amasiye!	Love orphans!
Amabungwe	NGOs
Tikondereni anawo	Love the kids on our behalf
—Charles Nsaku (2006)	

"Akazi m'Field" describes a wife working on contract in Mbeya, Tanzania, while her husband remains in Malawi. There, she is seduced by a rich Nigerian. Nsaku warns the husband that the gifts she brings him, as she professes her love for him, have been bought by the Nigerian boyfriend and are a smokescreen to prevent him from being suspicious. He should wise up to the facts as he risks getting sexually transmitted diseases. *"Dyela"* ("Gifts," 2006) describes how sugar daddies and sugar mummies unashamedly seduce the young, while the young, seduced by money, forget the dangers involved:

Matenda lero ndi obadwa nawo	One can be born HIV-positive
Safuna saizi	But they do not care about age
Agogo kupanga chikwati ndi zidzukulu	Grandfathers marrying their own
zawo	grandchildren

In this case, Nsaku turns the tables on the standard expectations, and describes the child infecting an older person.

"Economy" describes the poverty that grips a Malawi affected by HIV. *"Tiwana ku ndende"* talks about children forced to share their mothers' prison sentences due to authorities not bothering to build mother and baby units in prisons, despite the millions given by donors. The child in the song, brought up in a "smelly environment" and fed on "saltless porridge," wishes he could sue the government. *"Zelo zelo"* ("Zero Zero") critiques an agro-economy that has peasant farmers breaking their backs only to end up returning with "zero" money after selling their produce.

In *"Zidzakutsalira"* ("You may regret it"), a parent beseeches his child to be wary of prostitutes, drug dealers, and others of ill repute who may leave him HIV-infected. Like some Malawi musicians, Nsaku mixes HIV/AIDS awareness with issues of delinquency, crime, and drugs.

Tazisiya iwe	Let it go
Zidzakutsalira!	You may regret it!
Tazitaya iwe,	Let it be,
mwana wanga zisakutsalira.	My child there will be consequences.
Anzako ndima carrier za edzi	Your friends are carriers anyway
samacheuka	
angasinthe mahule	promiscuous or not they have
	nothing to lose
maka zodwala ndi apongozi.	they are already ill.

Ngati mowa wa Ntojaniwo	Like stale *Ntojani*beer
ii ndithu wafika moipa	you have reached a dangerous level
ukundipotozera mwana wanga!	This is heartbreaking my child!
John unali wana wabwino	You used to be a nice lad
mahule unkawaopa,	afraid of prostitutes,
nanga tsopano wayamba chiani	so what is this now?
ungogona ndi nkhalamba zomwe.	you even sleep with older women.
Kodi kapena wapepereredwa?	Have you been cursed?
Akuti condomu sulabadonso	You don't even use condoms
bola mwendo ukawala bwino.	as long as she has a nice leg.
Paeyerepayere live wire	Beware live wire
podzi limbinsa aliyense adzafa!	you bravely shout: we all die!
Zoona aliyense adzafa	True everyone will die
koma Edzi imfa yachabe.	but an AIDS death is a horrible one.
Iwe chonde ipewe edzi mtembo	Please avoid AIDS so your remains
wako usadzanyozedwe	will not be disrespected
Zidzakutsalira!	You will reap what you sow!
Umphawi usadzatipezetse.	Poverty will befall us.
Zodwala ndi apongozi	Illness is to be avoided
samalani kutenga manyuwani.	be careful with new partners.
Mwanawanga upita	My son you will die early
udzafera za eni	You will die for other people's business
Zidzakutsalira!	You will be left holding the baby!
—Charles Nsaku (2007)	

Nsaku includes the issue of youth being seduced into delinquency and criminality in the subsequent verses.

In "Technology" Nsaku discusses how ARVs, steroids, and other drugs can affect the outward appearance of HIV-positive people, making them sexually attractive to HIV-negative people. It is clear from all these songs that Nsaku uses music as a tool for social critique as well as entertainment, complementing a broader musical oeuvre of his that regularly addresses class and inequality (Lwanda 2008, 97–135).

But it is Gwaladi who currently has the highest visibility of musicians singing about HIV/AIDS. Gwaladi's status as a singer who cares about HIV issues emerged in 2006, at a time when the rolling out of ARVs in government hospitals was being "escalated." Although the program treated at best a minority of eligible patients, Malawi authorities described the rollout as a "success" (see Avert 2008). As the authorities were congratulating themselves on running "one of the best organized African HIV programmes in Africa," Joe Gwaladi, seeing the misery of the majority around him, and articulating what many recognized, disagreed, ruthlessly critiquing both Western and traditional medicine in "*Edzi ndi dolo*" ("AIDS is mighty"). He started by stating his case directly:

Edzi ndi dolo!	AIDS is mighty!
Adotolo mukuchepera	Doctors you are inadequate
mukuchepera kaba!	you are inadequate to the task!
Asinganga mukuchepera!	Traditional healers you are failing!

Gwaladi goes on to give vivid clinical descriptions of an HIV/AIDS victim:

Mupite Kuchipatala	Visit a hospital
Munthu atakhala atachita kuphwela	A person so emaciated
Pagona iye	Where he/she sleeps
Ngati pagona mwana	You would think it was a child sleeping
Ma kg 80 atafika ma kg 18	From 80 kg down to 18 kg
Edzi ndi dolo	AIDS is mighty
Edzi ndi shasha	AIDS is something else

And in a sideways glance at the issue of class, he notes:

Bwana akusilira thupi lawamisala!	The big man now envying the vagabond's body!

He concludes:

Tengani ochenjera onse	Take all the clever people
Tengani madokotala onse	Take all doctors
Kuwaunjika pamodzi	Lump them together
Akuchepera akuchepera kaba	They are not enough to fight AIDS
Edzi ndi dolo!	AIDS is mighty!
—Joe Gwaladi (2006)	

But not all musicians were so critical of the health care and social services establishments. In "*Osaiwala*" ("Do not forget") Dennis Phiri reminded people of the fact that HIV/AIDS could be acquired via other means, and that some of those affected, including doctors, nurses, and charity workers, were infected during the course of their professional work. Paul Banda also reminded Malawians that "*Edzi ndi yatonse*" ("AIDS is for us all"), noting the ubiquity of AIDS in towns and villages, as well as its ravages, leaving "dry grandmothers breastfeeding orphans."

In the meantime, religious discourses about the causes, spread, and morality of HIV/AIDS had continued into the twenty-first century through both circular and progressive arguments. In "*Mkwapulo*" ("The lash"), the Chitsitsimutso Choir essentially continued the 1989–94 arguments of AIDS as a form of divine message:

Dziko la Malawi lachita misala!	Malawi has gone mad!
Ndikunena azibambo ndi azimai	I mean men and women
anyamata ndi asungwana	Girls and boys
Zimene akuchita anthu	What people are doing
Zikufanana ndi nyama zakuchile	Behaving like wild animals
Kapena ziweto m'mudzimu	Or domesticated animals
Miyoyo yawanthu yawonongeka	Peoples lives have been destroyed
Ine ndalila	I cry
Ndalila mtundu wa Malawi	I cry for Malawi
Malawiyo kalelo linali dziko laulemu	Malawi used to be a respectful nation
Loopa Yehova	God fearing
Komatu lero zasintha	Today things have changed

Malawi uja wapenya	Malawi has changed
China chirichonse kuno chasokonekera	For the worse
Makhalidwe achiMalawi asintha	Malawi culture has changed
Mayendedwe asintha	People's behavior has changed
Demokalase yalowa	Democracy has come in
Mwalowa chizungu	European culture has come in
Chaononga	Destroying ours
Lachita misala dziko	The country has gone mad
Koma Mulungu ananena mBaibulo	But God said in the Bible
Kunena zamasiku ano	Talking of these days
Masiku otsiriza ngati ano	These last days
Chuma chidzakoma ngati uchi	Riches will taste like honey

The song then cites *umbava* (crime), *chiwerewere* (promiscuity), *kuledzela mowa* (drunkenness), and drugs as some of the liberties and sins of the multiparty era. It is then suggested that, despite harsh summary punishments to criminals, crime proved as resilient as promiscuity in the democratic period. God therefore decided to send *Mkwapulo* (his wrath) in the form of HIV/AIDS to warn his people to stop being promiscuous and to punish the recalcitrant; it would be a lesson to the rest. But did it work? *Ai?* (No!)

The Chitsitsimutso Choir then claims that most diseases, including HIV/AIDS, are due to God's *mkwapulo* (wrath). Toward the end of the song some humor, sarcasm, and irony are introduced. "*Ndi Mkwapulo uwo! Ndi mkwapulo!*" (It's the punishment! Everywhere!) The group's well-executed, but historically inaccurate song, criticizes the public deterioration in security and morality.

Hax Momba's "*Samala*" ("Take care") blamed multiparty culture and condom makers for increased promiscuity:

Kodi edzi ingathe bwanji	How can AIDS be overcome
ngati anthu akuyenda maliseche?	if people walk naked?
Mpikisano wanji wochita uli maliseche	What kind of [beauty] contest is held naked
kuchititsa manyazi yemwe anakulenga?	shaming your creator?
Nanunso opanga makondomu	And you condom manufacturers
ona mukulimbikitsa chigololo;	see how you promote promiscuity;
musawauze zamakondomu ai,	don't tell them about condoms,
musawaonetse anawa	don't show these children
zinthu zolaula...	things we consider taboo...
Aphunzitseni kuwerenga Bukhu laMulungu	Teach them to read God's Book
—Hax Momba (n.d.)	

The social effects of HIV/AIDS, including increased mortality, orphans, and worsening poverty, led to a re-emergence of traditional *umunthu* (human) cultural values, strengthening extended families in the face of illness and death. However, Malawi, like everywhere, has its share of selfish individuals. In the duo Edgar & Davis's eyes, people who live selfish lives in the city refuse to help their rural folk while working; but as soon as they hit hard times they want to return home "to be looked after by the family":

Musamakonde kuti mukadwala	When ill you are inclined to say
Ine ndikunkha kumudzi	I am going home
Mwaona kuti chuma chabvuta	When your wealth is gone you say
Abale anga akandithandiza	My village folks will look after me
Mwaona kuti muthupi mwabvunda	When your body is rotting you think
Abale anga akandisamala	My village folks will look after me
Mwaiwala kuti kumudzi mabvutonso aliko	Forgetting that there are problems there too
Musamati bola ine ndikafele kwathu	Don't say better to die at home
Musamabwele kumudzi	Don't come home
Kumudzi sikofela	Home is not where you come to die
Musadzabwelelenso!	Don't ever return!

Then the song reminds them of their selfishness in good times:

Mulindimtima wachabe	You are bad
Wokumbukira abale mukabvutika!	Only remembering your family when in trouble!

—Edgar & Davis (2007)

The reason for the subject of the song being unwanted is given: he had lived a selfish life of relative plenty over the years, ignoring letters from home for assistance.

Toward the end of the period under study musicians are still observing and describing the epidemic with degrees of humor, irony, sympathy, sadness, and anger. In *"Mwanadala"* ("pedophile" or "cradle-snatcher") Joe Gwaladi complains that his generation is unlikely to survive "to a ripe age" due to sugar daddies and sugar mummies who employ various strategies to look young in order to seduce youths. Women "shove their breasts into" bras to get younger-looking busts, and men shave their "graying locks and beards."

But one of the major issues of the HIV/AIDS epidemic still looms large: orphans. Musicians tend to regard those who run orphanages with suspicion. In *"Sinkhalidwe"* ("That is not good behavior") Patrick Jumbe rails against those who abuse orphans and donor funds. Jumbe and other musicians (including Nsaku) target their ire directly at the non-governmental organizations (NGOs) formed largely to obtain donor money for the benefit of the NGO owners rather than the children they claim to look after. Criticism is typically directed at the large, four-wheel drive opulent lifestyles enjoyed by these NGO owners, including sending their children abroad for education, in contrast to the basic orphanages they run.

MUSICIANS AS INFORMANTS AND CRITICS

A wider examination of some of the Malawi musicians' lyrics and behavior shows that they were, as a group, ambivalent toward discussions of sex and still more ambivalent about people contracting and living with AIDS. Largely a male group, musicians frequently reflect some of the misogynistic views found in a male-dominated country such as Malawi. Lyrics also show that musicians as a group had erroneous perceptions about HIV/AIDS (cf. Lwanda 2003).

The contradictory messages in HIV/AIDS musical discourse are exemplified in Ben Michael's *"Zina kambu zina leku"*:

Wona mwana wa zaka twenty!	Look at a girl of twenty!
Body structure!	Body structure!
Wona chest oh! Kumbuyo!	Look at the bust, the ass!
Body movement!	Body movement!
Wona mwendo wona hip!	Look at the legs, hips!
Ngakhale abusa amayamika:	Even the priest/minister will shout:
Alleluia!	Alleluia!
—Ben Michael (2004)	

This thinly disguised "girl watching" discourse is in contrast to Michael's usual lyrics (2001):

Thawa iwe ndi moto uwu!	Just run away! This is fire!
Kuchotsa fumbi!	Widow cleansing!
Is dangerous!	Is dangerous!
Chokolo practice!	Widow inheritance!
Is dangerous!	Is dangerous!
Chibwenzi cha mseri!	Extramarital affairs!
Is dangerous!	Is dangerous!

One thing popular musicians do not equivocate about is their criticism, whether of politicians or doctors. Since 1999, criticism has usually been quite direct. Alex Mataya Mphepo, for one, had harsh words for the "ignorant" political leadership of Malawi, which he blamed for Malawi's troubles in "*Tiona Mbwadza*":

Mtundu wa Malawi pampanipani!	Malawi is in hot water!
Tiona mbwadza!	We will experience bad times!
—Alex Mataya Mphepo (2007)	

In "*Mudzichita chisoni inu*" ("Have some sympathy"), Blessings Chimangeni is vicious in his criticism of the attitudes of young doctors and nurses toward HIV/AIDS patients:

Kwa olemera amphwawi odwala	Towards the rich and poor patients
Mudzichita chisoni inu.	You should be sympathetic.
Tikuthokoza madokotala	We thank you doctors
Inu nchito mumaigwira	You work hard
Koma chimodzi ndikuti ndikambe	Let me say one thing though
Sikuti mukavala dzina la udokotala	When you get your degree
Wachiwembu mukhale ndinu	Do not become the patient's enemy
Makamaka anyuwaniwa	The new doctors are particularly
Anyanya chipongwe awa	Prone to be abusive
Akamuona mbaleyo zabvuta	When they see your relative is critical
Angoyenda	They say, "let him go
Chithandizo kulibe kuno!	There is no medicine here"!

But could this criticism be that of a musician actually speaking up for doctors working with limited resources? He concludes:

Ndimayesa kunama	I thought it was a lie
Anzanga anandiuza	When friends told me
Aliyense kuchipatala	Everyone only goes to hospital
Angopitila bedi	Just for the bed
Chithandizo kulibe!	There is no treatment!

—Blessings Chimangeni (2008)

MUSICIANS' SILENCE ON HIV AMONG THEMSELVES

No major Malawian musicians have ever declared that they were HIV-positive and then sung about it. The few who have declared illnesses have usually suffered from cancer, never HIV. Paul Chaphuka and Stonard Lungu, for example, both succumbed to skin cancer. Chaphuka sang about his skin cancer in his farewell cassette *Ndichiritseni* ("Cure me"). In *"Tsalani"* ("Bye bye") he asks friends and family to look after his children. In the song, his colleague Lucius Banda, Malawi's most popular musician, promises to look after the children, a promise he has fulfilled. Chaphuka's title track pleads for treatment:

Ndichiritseni	Heal me!
Mundichiritse tsopano	Heal me now
Ambuye thandizeni	Lord help me!

—Paul Chaphuka (1997)

It was Stonard Lungu who sang about the many fellow musicians departed in *"Ndiyimba ndi yani?"* ("Who will I sing with?")—a song in which the artist paid homage to departed seminal musicians of the 1950s and 1960s such as Dr. Daniel Kachamba, Samangaya, Malikula, Stompie Kamwendo, and Morson Phuka. Lungu does not provide the causes of death. Billy Kaunda similarly mourns lost artists, musicians, dramatists, and broadcasters in *"Kumidima"* ("In the dark"):

Kumidima komwe muliko	From the dark depths where you are
simufuna kutiyendera aah!	You do not want to visit us!
Kapena mwina tinayambana	Or maybe we quarreled?
Mwachita kuchoka chotere eeh?	You departed prematurely?

The last line gives a hint that the singer is aware that some of the musicians died prematurely and very possibly from HIV/AIDS. But even he, a friend of the deceased, dares not say so explicitly. While these artists have effectively raised social consciousness concerning HIV/AIDS, no single major musician has yet gone public with his own status.

DISCUSSION

HIV/AIDS songs have to be viewed within the context of Malawi's wider socioeconomic fabric. Though initially seen as a threat to the extended family system, HIV/AIDS has paradoxically largely acted as cultural cement.[3] Funerals, social settings, and networks that had been threatened by the HIV pandemic in the 1980s and 1990s due to the sheer numbers of those who had died from AIDS have recently been refreshed, empowered by the realization that in the context of limited resources and facilities, it is important to mourn and bring about closure. Because it is cheap, communal, and healing, music has come to play a significant role, whether cosmetic or substantive, in these social contexts.

HIV/AIDS was initially seen as a "government disease," something that portended *kutha kwa mtundu* (the end of the nation). Its arrival induced a paranoia and paralysis among musicians that was largely created by the prevailing culture of censorship and autocracy. Early songs contained messages that assigned blame and saw HIV/AIDS as a brutal killer. Some musicians saw HIV/AIDS as contained in the basic fabric of sex—or as Saleta Phiri metaphorically put it, *Ili mu ufa* (It is in the maize flour [we eat])—and therefore unpreventable, essentially supporting the abstentionist religious view.

Songs slowly evolved and proliferated, incorporating messages of caution and prevention as well as comfort and confusion; the confusion arising from some musicians' "unscientific" prejudices. Underlying it all, a small but significant trend of blame has remained, emerging in some of the harder ragamuffin music recorded after 2004 around the "normalcy of appearance with ARVs." As most of the musicians are men, this stigmatization of women is obvious and, in the context of Malawi's male-dominated societies, presents some concern.

HIV/AIDS songs also reflect what some scholars see as "neocolonialism" or cultural imperialism, with foreign secular and religious NGOs leveraging various family planning and religious viewpoints on HIV/AIDS awareness initiatives. A number of musicians have benefited from working with various donor organizations. At the same time, these activities have become fodder for a potent form of social and sociopolitical critique. Saleta Phiri, for example, lamented the moral poverty of musicians forced to compose HIV songs in relation to politicians in "*Zinthu zasintha*" (Lwanda, 2008).

HIV/AIDS songs have also been widely used as prayers to offer hope and comfort to those affected, particularly within gospel settings.

Where musicians have been most effective, scientific aberrations and misconceptions notwithstanding, is where they have combined AIDS awareness messages with critiques of the medical service's inadequacy and the underlying sociopolitical economy, such as in Gwaladi's "*Edzi ndi dolo*" or Nsaku's "*Zidzakutsalira*." In these settings, musicians have been very effective in raising awareness about HIV/AIDS. But the jury is still out on the overall effectiveness of popular music in inspiring cultural change, given the ambivalence and ambiguity of some of the messages in the songs (see Lwanda 2003).

Beyond enacting political and social agendas, however, singing about AIDS has also become an important diversionary entertainment, offering solace via popular gospel that a country with massive sociomedical and socioeconomic such as Malawi needs. Along the way, singing about AIDS has also provided a considerable boost to the popular Malawi music industry, with many musicians benefiting from royalties (Kanjo and Lwanda 2009). These facets of cultural vibrancy have continued to develop in rich and complex ways in the face of adversity.

32

Representing HIV/AIDS in Africa

PLURALIST PHOTOGRAPHY AND LOCAL
EMPOWERMENT

Roland Bleiker (University of Queensland) and

Amy Kay (Centre for Development and Population Activities)

This essay explores the nature and political consequences of representing HIV/AIDS in Africa, where the disease has taken its greatest toll.[1] We examine how different methods of photography embody different ideologies through which we give meaning to political phenomena. We distinguish three photographic methods of representing HIV/AIDS: naturalist, humanist, and pluralist. Naturalist approaches portray photographs as neutral and value free. Humanist photography, by contrast, hinges on the assumption that images of suffering can invoke compassion in viewers, and that this compassion can become a catalyst for positive change. By examining a widely circulated iconic photograph of a Ugandan woman and her child affected by AIDS-related illnesses, we show that such representations can nevertheless feed into stereotypical portrayals of African people as nameless and passive victims, removed from the everyday realities of the Western world. We contrast these practices with pluralist photography. To do so we examine a project in Addis Ababa, which used a methodology that placed cameras into the hands of children affected by HIV/AIDS, giving them the opportunity to actively represent what it means to live with the disease. The result is a form of dialogue that opens up spaces for individuals and communities to work more effectively in overcoming problematic stigmas and finding ways of stemming the spread of the disease.

Over the last decades, HIV/AIDS has grown from a medical mystery to a truly global challenge. In 2000, the UN Security Council declared HIV/AIDS a security threat, stressing the increasingly serious implications of the pandemic's spread, especially in Africa. But despite extensive community efforts to address these implications, and despite significant resources being devoted to prevention and treatment, worldwide infection rates continue to increase.

Most experts see only very limited opportunities to reverse this alarming trend (UNAIDS 2003, 2004a, 2004b).

The difficulties of stemming the spread of HIV/AIDS are in part due to the fact that the disease is not only a medical problem but also a social, cultural, and political challenge. Perhaps more so than any other disease in history, HIV/AIDS has generated countless political debates, scientific publications, donor appeals, public protests, education campaigns, and artistic engagements (see Miller 1992; McNeill 1998; Elwood 1999, 3; Ogdon 2001; Crimp 2002). Paula Treichler (1999, 1) thus speaks of an "epidemic of signification," which is to say that the nature and political impact of HIV/AIDS is intrinsically linked to how the disease is represented, and how these representations influence key issues, such as the production of stigma and discrimination.

The purpose of this essay is to examine the nature and political consequences of representing HIV/AIDS. We do so by focusing on how different methods of photography embody different ways of understanding and dealing with HIV/AIDS in Africa, the continent where the disease has taken its greatest toll. Since the early 1980s, some 16.7 million Africans have died from AIDS-related illnesses. In South Africa alone there are 1,600 new infections everyday (Freedman and Poku 2005, 665–67). Africa is, of course, far too diverse a continent to be represented in homogeneous ways. That is, in fact, one of the stereotypical representations we critique in this essay. HIV infection rates for people between the ages of 15 and 49, for instance, range from 1 percent in Mauritania to almost 40 percent in Botswana and Swaziland. Major differences also exist with regard to key factors influencing HIV/ AIDS, such as gender disparity, poverty, mobility, and intravenous drug use. Sub-Saharan Africa is the most affected region, containing 25.8 of the estimated 40.3 million people living with HIV/AIDS worldwide in 2005 (UNAIDS 2005).

We focus on photographs in our essay because they play an important role in shaping private and public understandings of HIV/AIDS. The political dimensions of photographic representations become particularly acute when they enter the realm of mass media. Popular perceptions, policy frameworks, and development priorities are all influenced by the visions that mass media create with respect to a particular issue. Photographs are central to this process. The likelihood of a story making it to print, especially on the cover of a publication, increasingly depends on the quality of the pictures that accompany it. At a time when we are saturated with information stemming from multiple media sources, images are well suited to capture issues in succinct and mesmerizing ways. They serve as visual quotations (Sontag 2003, 22, 85; 2004, 22). Some of the most influential means of representing HIV/AIDS in Africa have thus been through photography. From iconic photographs in mass media to local artistic engagements, photographic portrayals of HIV/AIDS have created a range of powerful effects, from apathy and fear to empathy and engagement.

We distinguish among three photographic methods of representing HIV/AIDS: naturalist, humanist, and pluralist. Each embodies different forms of representation through which we give meaning to political phenomena. Exploring such sites of representation, we argue, reveals how different ideological assumptions generate different public understandings of— and thus reactions to—the HIV/AIDS pandemic.

Naturalist approaches portray photographs as neutral and value free, as reflecting an objective reality captured through the lens (see Hall 1997, 98). Photographs are seen as having a truth value, allowing the viewer realistic insight into the events and people they depict. In its pure form, such a position is, we believe, not tenable. Photographs cannot portray the world as it is. A photograph is no different from any other form of representation, even though the seemingly naturalistic reproduction of external realities may deceive us initially. A photograph is taken at a certain time of the day, with a certain focus, and from a certain angle. These choices make up the very essence of the photograph: its aesthetic quality. But they result from artistic and inevitably subjective decisions taken by the photographer—decisions that have nothing to do with the actual object that is photographed. As there is relatively widespread scholarly consensus about these limits to naturalist photography, we do not engage the respective practices—and their underlying assumptions—in detail. Instead, we focus our attention primarily on two alternatives to naturalism: humanism and pluralism.

Humanist photography is the first of two non-naturalist approaches we examine systematically. We do so by focusing on an iconic "AIDS photograph" taken by photojournalist Ed Hooper. It depicts a Ugandan mother and her baby, both in the last stages of fatal, AIDS-related illness. We examine the Hooper photograph as a particular type of image that symbolizes broader Western practices of representing HIV/AIDS in Africa. Taken in 1986, during the relatively early years of Western recognition of the HIV/AIDS epidemic as a major crisis, the Hooper photograph reveals how HIV/AIDS was first visualized in the press, and how such early visualizations of suffering and victimization have had implications that still shape the HIV/AIDS discourse today (Bhattacharya et al. 2005, 8). It also symbolizes how very specific, humanist forms of representations continue to influence our understanding of HIV/AIDS in Africa (for a recent example, see Annan et al. 2003). The political assumption behind such humanist approaches is that images of suffering can invoke compassion in viewers, and that this compassion can become a catalyst for positive change. Although accepting the basic premise underlying this position, we inquire further into the values involved in these practices and the form of change that issues forth from them. We show that humanist photographic engagements, well meant as they are, contain residues of colonial values. They are more likely to invoke pity, rather than compassion. They reflect how Western—and thus very often universalized—accounts of HIV/AIDS in Africa are based on very specific assumptions, even stigma, revolving around the portrayal of people affected by HIV/AIDS as passive victims, removed from the everyday realities of the Western world.

We then juxtapose humanist practices of photography prevalent in Western media sources with different, more local, and more diverse photographic engagements. We term them pluralist photography. They differ from both naturalist and humanist approaches. They share with the latter the belief that photographs can become important catalysts for social change, but actively oppose the humanist focus on iconic photographs and their implicit association with Western and often universalized positions. Pluralist photography, by contrast, seeks to validate local photographic practices in an attempt to create multiple sites for representing and understanding the psychological, social, and political issues at stake. To illustrate this form of engagement, we focus on the recent work of photographer Eric Gottesman and the Addis Ababa community of the Kebele 15 neighborhood. Gottesman worked with local children affected by HIV/AIDS, teaching them how to use photography to represent for themselves what it means to live with HIV/AIDS in a community that has both high-infection rates and high levels of related stigma. We examine the potential—and limits—of such local photography to overcome the stereotypical image of the passive victim. While we advocate the use of pluralist photography, we fully recognize that this tradition is not void of bias either. It cannot give us authentic local knowledge. But by generating multiple and creative ways of representing HIV/AIDS, it helps viewers recognize that the process of representation is inherently incomplete, and thus inevitably political. Such engagements with representation can offer more effective ways of addressing the spread and sociopolitical effects of the disease. This is why, we argue, pluralist photography should be used more widely in attempts to understand and contain the spread of HIV/AIDS.

Before we begin our inquiry, a few words on methodology are in order. The photographs we have chosen for our case studies are obviously not meant to provide a comprehensive account of how the issue of HIV/AIDS in Africa is being represented. Doing so is not—and cannot be—the purpose of a short essay. Our main empirical focus rests with an iconographic photograph portraying HIV/AIDS in Uganda during the mid-1980s and a series of photographs taken more recently by Ethiopian children affected by AIDS. These photographs are taken two decades apart, at times when HIV/AIDS occupied a very different place in public discourse. They deal with two completely different parts of Africa. We have chosen the photographs in question because they symbolize, in an ideal way, specific kinds of photography. Studying them allows us to understand the sociopolitical dimensions entailed in different representations of HIV/AIDS, which is the main objective of our essay.

A similar disclaimer is in order with regard to the three categorizations we use: naturalist, humanist, and pluralist. These concepts are meant to differentiate between ideal types of photography. We are fully aware that in reality, a photograph and its public use may simultaneously contain elements of multiple approaches—say a combination of humanist and pluralist traits. But by focusing on ideal types of photographs—archetypes, so to speak—we are able to identify more precisely what is at stake in the process of representation. We use our own, relatively ad hoc terms, in part because we wanted to use everyday language, rather than jargon, in part because there are comparatively few relevant conceptual discussions, at least in the literature on international relations. Among the similar studies that do exist, François Debrix and Cynthia Weber distinguish between practices of representation, transformation, and pluralization (Debrix 2003, xxi-xxii). While our approach is influenced by their typology we nevertheless retain our own, slightly different concepts. We do so because Debrix and Weber focus on how an image is being mediated in the process of creating social meaning while our own task is mostly limited to understanding practices of representation themselves.

BEYOND NATURALISM: REPRESENTATION AND WESTERN MEDIA CONSTRUCTIONS OF STEREOTYPES

Photographs deceive. They seem to give us a glimpse of the real. They provide us with the seductive belief that what we see in a photograph is an authentic representation of the world: a slice of life that reveals exactly what was happening at a particular moment. This is the case because a photograph is, as Roland Barthes (1977, 17) stresses, "a message without a code." As opposed to a linguistic representation, or a painting, a photograph is "a perfect analogon." Indeed, its very nature, as Barthes continues, is defined by this analogical perfection. In the realm of documentary photography, for instance, it was for long commonly assumed that a photographer, observing the world from a distance, is an "objective witness" to political phenomena, providing authentic representations of, say, war or poverty (see Strauss 2003, 45). Theoretically, such naturalistic positions hinge on the belief that a photograph can represent its object in a neutral and value-free way, transferring meaning from one site to another without affecting the object's nature and signification in the process. Debrix (2003, xxiv, xxvii-xxx) stresses that this belief is part of a long Western search for transcendental knowledge, be it of a spiritual or secular nature.

While most scholars who work on photography acknowledge that photographs mimic vision in one way or another, few if any claim that such representations, even if they are pictorial simulacra, are authentic representations of the world as it is (see Friday 2000, 356–75). We agree. But rather than critiquing naturalist understandings of photography in detail we find it more productive to explore how alternative approaches recognize that photographs are practices of representations and thus of an inherently political nature. Two aspects make such alternatives to naturalism convincing.

First, and as already mentioned, a photographic representation reflects certain aesthetic choices. It cannot be neutral because it always is an image chosen and composed by a particular person. It is taken from a particular angle, and then produced and reproduced in a certain manner, thereby excluding a range of alternative ways of capturing the object in question (see, for instance, Barthes 1977, 19; Sontag 2003, 46).

Second, and more importantly, a photograph cannot speak for itself. It needs to be viewed and interpreted. This is why Barthes (1977, 17–19) stresses that there are always two aspects to a photograph. There is the "denoted message," which is the above-mentioned analogically perfect representation of a visual image. But there is also a "connoted message," which includes how a photograph is read and interpreted, how it fits into existing practices of knowledge and communication. Some refer to this process more specifically as "secondary image construction," which takes place when photographs are "selected out from their original ordering and narrative context, to be placed alongside textual information and reports in a publication" (Hall 1997, 86). It is not our intention here to engage the complex and rather diverse literature on photography, visual culture, and media representation. Doing so would go far beyond the scope of this essay. But we would like to point out briefly that there is widespread scholarly agreement that a connoted message cannot take the form of an unmediated representation of reality. John Berger (1980, 55), for instance, points out that photographs "only preserve instant appearances." When we look at a photograph we never just look at a photograph alone. We actually look at a complex relationship between a photograph and ourselves (Berger 1977, 9). Our viewing experience is thus intertwined not only with previous experiences, such as our memory of other photographs we have seen in the past, but also with the values and visual traditions that are accepted as common sense by established societal norms. Guy Debord (1992, 4), likewise, stresses how everything directly lived becomes distanced through representation. It becomes part of a "spectacle," which he defines as a "social relationship between people that is mediated by images." For David Levi Strauss (2003, 45), the important aspect of this process is that there are always relations of power at stake, that there is always an attempt to tell a story, and that this story is always told from a particular, politically charged angle.

What makes photographs unusually powerful—and at times problematic—is that their analogically perfect representation of a visual image masks the political values that such representations embody. The assumption that photographs are neutral, value free, and evidential is reinforced because photography captures faces and events in memorable ways. For instance, if one looks at an image of a person affected by AIDS-related illnesses, one could easily believe that one actually sees that person as he or she was at that moment. Michael Shapiro (1988, 124, 134) writes of a "grammar of face-to-face encounters." And he stresses that the analogical nature of this encounter makes photographic representations particularly vulnerable to being appropriated by discourses professing authentic knowledge and truth. We may succumb to such a "seductiveness of the real" to the point that we forget, as photojournalist David Pearlmutter (1998, 28) warns us that "the lens is focused by a hand directed by a human eye." Add to this that the public rarely sees the news media as purveyors of commercially profitable stories and images. Instead, the news is perceived as a reflection of the actual, as a neutral mediator between a subject, and, in the case of most international news, an object usually located in another part of the world.

The fusion of information and entertainment, and the commercial need for recognizable headlines and simple stories, inevitably favors stereotypical representations over more complex ways of representing sociopolitical issues, such as HIV/ AIDS. Barthes (1977, 22) even goes as far as arguing that a photograph only achieves meaning "because of the existence of a store of stereotyped attitudes which form ready-made elements of signification." This tendency is exacerbated when a news item refers to events in the developing world. In such cases, Western media sources tend to fall back on the scripts of global news agencies circulated in wire services. Once the parameters of a news story have been set, coverage can lapse into a standard formula. Photography may thus give a pandemic such as HIV/AIDS the meaning of familiar crisis by cueing an audience to formulaic events via particular images. Such practices can, for instance, revolve around a micrograph picture of the virus or an image of a person dying of AIDS-related illnesses. They reinforce static pictures of HIV/AIDS and make it difficult to generate change (Watney 1990). Photographs can thus strengthen the perception that the disease is not part of daily life, but something less real and more remote, something that may resemble what Edith Wyschogrod (1973) once called a "death event" (Wyschogrod 1973).

HIV/AIDS AND COLONIAL PERCEPTIONS OF AFRICA

Portrayals of Africa epitomize how Western media sources produce and reproduce stereotypes. Since the early years of the HIV/AIDS epidemic, Western science and modern media have constructed a concept of "African HIV/AIDS" that is closely linked to the colonial heritage and its mystifications of Africa (see Watts and Boal 1995, 105). Part of this Eurocentric perception is the tendency to view Africa as a homogenous continent seen through a "prism of misery" (Kean 1998, 2). The Kenyan author and playwright Binyavanga Wainaina (2006) writes of the Western tendency to write as if Africa were one country, a place that "is hot and dusty with rolling grasslands and huge herds of animals and tall, thin people who are starving." Methods of photography that use standardized representational practices reinforce such colonial stereotypes, creating what David Campbell, in a series of innovative and convincing essays, calls an "iconography of anonymous victimhood" (see Campbell 2003a, 69, 70–71, 84; 2003b, 67; 2004, 62, 69).

The result is a fatalistic apathy in the Western viewer, leading to the impression that each crisis is simply part of a larger pattern of misery and gloom that is so deeply entrenched that it cannot possibly be reversed. Cindy Patton (1990, 83) points out how images of Africans suffering and dying from AIDS-related illnesses perfectly fit into such stereotypical images of "a wasting continent peopled by victimbodies of illness, poverty, famine." Patton stresses how this preconceived image neglects to recognize the many instances where development has actually taken place: moments, for instance, when local communities managed to thrive, when personal and societal achievements prevailed over doom and gloom.

Practices of representation are among the most influential elements in encounters between the North and the South (see Doty 1996, 2). This is particularly the case with Western representations of Africa, which correspond to what Edward Said (1979, 2–3) termed orientalism: a style of thought—and a corresponding mode of governance—that is based not on geographical, political, or cultural facts, but on a series of stereotypical assumptions about the values and behavior of people who inhabit far off and "exotic" places. Central here is a stark division between the orient and the occident. This division is characterized by the juxtaposition of fundamental opposites, which are presented as essential cultural traits. The West is characterized by values such as reason, progress, activity, optimism, and order, while Africa is associated with emotion, stagnation, passivity, pessimism, and chaos (see Mitchell 1998, 293; Bancroft 2001, 96). The practices of authority and domination that issue from such representations have insinuated themselves into all domains of life, from philosophy, science, history, and tourism to governmental regulations, economic structures, artistic traditions, and scientific methods. Early practices of photography are as much part of these colonial power relations (see Higgins 2001, 22–36) as are contemporary perceptions of HIV/AIDS.

Representations of HIV/AIDS do, indeed, fit into established patterns of orientalism. Consider, for instance, how some of the first media accounts of HIV/AIDS revolved around theories that traced the origin of the disease in Africa. One particular theory was based on the assumption that the HIV virus had actually been present in Africans for years but simply remained undiagnosed. That is, until they "passed it out to the world as civilization reached them" (Hilts 1988, 2). Another theory stipulated that HIV evolved from a parent virus discovered in wild African green monkeys. The disease was then said to have crossed species barriers and found a human host in Africans, who later passed it on to the rest of the unknowing world. Although debated by the medical community (see McNeill 1998, 11–17; Smith 1998, 330–333; Bancroft 2001, 92–94), theories based on the origins of HIV/ AIDS can often lead to a problematic practices of blaming others and generating racist stereotypes (Sabatier 1988). In this particular case, HIV/AIDS is represented as emerging in faraway places, from bodies of "others" that then "contaminate" the rest of the world. The result is an emphasis on questions of origins, rather than an engagement with the underlying causes of infection. It would be far more productive to emphasize how certain behaviors and practices put all people at increased risk for HIV infection. Equally important are efforts to understand factors that contribute to a person's vulnerability, such as power relations and societal norms that limit women's choices to protect themselves against infection (see Sarin 2002; Desantis 2003; Roudi-Fahimi 2003; UNDP 2007).

Stereotypical portrayals of Africa are epitomized by assumptions surrounding the sexual transmission of HIV. Rather than relying on scientific data or pragmatic policy deliberations, Western perceptions of HIV/AIDS in Africa have been dominated by moral judgments and prejudices (see Sabatier 1988, 1). This is, as Susan Sontag (1988, 27) stresses, not necessarily new or surprising. She points out that many diseases that are said to be linked to sexual fault (such as syphilis) tend to "inspire fears of easy contagion and bizarre fantasies of transmission by nonvenereal means in public places." But such tendencies have been particularly pronounced with regard to representations of HIV/AIDS in Africa. Sexual practices have been moralized and demonized by Western doctors and other experts. As with previous epidemics, such as cholera, the disease is being interpreted "as a sign of moral laxity or political decline" (Sontag 1988, 142). Representative of this practice is an American doctor, who stressed in a press interview that "there is a profound promiscuity in Uganda, and a virus which takes advantage of it" (cited in Hooper 1990, 28). The ensuing HIV/AIDS discourse mingles medical and moral assumptions, making it difficult to prevent the production and diffusion of stigmatizing ideas (Patton 1990, 105). The result is a public discourse based on an entrenched suspicion about the disease and, more important, about the people who live with it.

Prevalent journalistic styles of reporting further reinforce stereotypical images of HIV/AIDS in Africa. This is particularly the case of so-called "parachute reporters," who are flown in to a crisis zone for a short time and then report back to the "rest of the world." One of many examples: in the years immediately following recognition of the epidemic in Uganda, President

Museveni announced an "open door policy," designed to draw the world's attention to the impact of the epidemic in Africa (Sabatier 1988, 91). In the wake of this policy announcement, Western journalists entered the country, flooding hospitals in an attempt to visualize the pandemic though images of African AIDS victims. But such parachute reporters often lack knowledge of the political and cultural context that surround the issues they seek to cover. They are given only limited time and resources to do their work. The ensuing coverage almost inevitably leads to a reinforcement of existing stereotypes.

The reaction of some local African governments to the crisis often exacerbated the effect of the stereotypical images that prevail in the Western public discourse. Particularly fateful, Treichler (1999, 109) believes, is the combination of "doomsday predictions" by Western media sources and categorical denials by governments in developing countries. The latter not only increases fear, stigmatization, and the spread of the disease, but paradoxically reinforces stereotypes. When Western reporters seek to deal with HIV/AIDS in Africa, their representations often clash with the institutionalization of silence imposed by local public policies. Ministries in some African countries have often banned researchers and physicians from talking to the press. Various arguments are presented for such silencing, including fears that representations of HIV/AIDS could damage thriving industries, such as tourism, on which many African countries depend (Sabatier 1988, 96; Fleury 2004, 1). The result is an entrenchment of the problematic practices described earlier: foreign reporters rely more heavily on available foreign sources, thus reinforcing preexisting narratives of Africa and silencing the far more complex and intertwined local stories that characterize the epidemic's spread and sociopolitical consequences. The so-produced dehumanizing images of Africa are not just reflective of media representations, but permeate most Western engagements with the continent. Raymond Apthorpe (2001, 112), drawing on decades of experience with humanitarian work, emphasizes the deeply entrenched tendency of Western development workers and aid agencies to rely on stereotypical, reproducible, recognizable, and self-affirming views of Africa, thus reproducing a virtual reality that contains only "token roots in the actual, domestic reality of the land beneath."

The fact that HIV/AIDS is increasingly seen as a security issue may further add to these stereotypical attitudes. While many commentators welcome new ways of conceptualizing global health issues (see Singer 2002, 145–8), others are growing concerned that framing HIV/AIDS through the language and practices of security may further extend monitoring and surveillance traditions that go back to eighteenth-century Europe. This is why Stefan Elbe (2005, 403–19) fears that unless the securitization of HIV/AIDS is approached with great caution, the ensuing modes of governance could easily generate new forms of orientalism and racism. Extending the logic of security to health could, for instance, legitimize numerous, rather problematic practices designed to control, and contain parts of the population deemed "unhealthy" and seen as a risk to the vital and thriving core of global society.

CONFRONTING SUFFERING: HUMANIST REPRESENTATIONS OF HIV/AIDS

So far, we have portrayed a fairly grim picture, one that highlights how Western stereotypes about Africa render the problem of HIV/AIDS more difficult than it already is. Photography plays an integral part in these neocolonial practices of domination. But this is not the end of the story. Photography can also play an important role in overcoming stereotypes, creating alternative images of HIV/ AIDS, and thus new ways of understanding, discussing, and addressing the spread and impact of the disease. We begin our inquiry into these alternatives by focusing on humanist photography.

Humanist photography has a mission: it aims to use photography in the service of a human cause. Such photographic engagements emerged as a direct reaction against early naturalist tendencies to consider photographs as pieces of evidence, as authentic records that reflected a true image of the world. Humanist approaches, by contrast, stress that documentary photography can provide access to both facts and feelings. Lewis Hine (quoted in Beloff 1983, 171), one of the early proponents of this position, stressed that he "wanted to show things that had to be corrected." Photography can thus be used as a specific political tool, as a way of rallying public opinion in favor of a particular issue. We term this approach humanist because it contains key traits associated with humanism as it is broadly understood: a modern attempt to "replace God with man," that is, to reject the notion of a divine will in favor of a world where people take charge (Caroll 1993, 2). But humanism also created a specific understanding of agency and order, one that revolves around the search for certitude, one that sees humanity in absolute and often universal terms (see Doty 1996, 24, 125; Edkins 2005, 379).

Humanist photography is able to live up to many of humanism's key goals, most notably to the idea that human beings are able to shape their social and political environment. Few commentators would question that the reaction of the Western world to human suffering in other countries is linked to the influence of key photographs on the formation of public opinion. Pictures of impoverished children, of villages devastated by natural disaster, or of people dying of AIDS-related illnesses are often circulated with the hope that an outpouring of humanitarian support will help those who are in need (Schwartz and Murray 1996, 1; Sankore 2005). Humanist photography has become an important aspect of what Michael Ignatieff (1998, 10) calls the new "internationalization of conscience."

While the impact of photographs on public discourses is beyond doubt, the exact nature of this influence is far more difficult to assess. We now address this challenge by examining a widely circulated iconic HIV/AIDS photograph, taken in 1986 by Ed Hooper. Reprinted as figure 32.1, this picture epitomizes the key ideas behind humanist photography. It depicts a Ugandan woman named Florence and her child, Ssengabi, sitting outside their home in Gwanda, Uganda.

Both Florence and Ssengabi were visibly ill. Taken during the early period of Western public awareness about HIV/AIDS, the Hooper photograph provided a "face" that could symbolize the AIDS crisis in Africa. It was published widely in the international media, including *Newsweek* and the *Washington Post*. Florence died four weeks after the photograph was taken. Her baby Ssengabi died four months later. The photograph is very confronting in its direct visualization of illness, suffering, and death. It is part of a long tradition, deeply rooted in Christian art, of depicting the human body in pain. Some label this practice "demonic curiosity" (Friday 2000, 363). Some even compare it with pornography, for images of suffering and death expose in public a person's most intimate and vulnerable features (Dean 2003, 91–93; see also Scarry 1985; Sontag 2003, 41–42).

One of the most obvious problems associated with the Hooper photograph is the unequal power relationship between the photographer and his object. Any Western photographer, no matter how well meant and sensitive his or her artistic and political engagement is, operates at a certain distance from poverty, conflict, and disaster. And there is, of course, an even greater distance between the viewers of the photographs and the content they convey. Making public a person's private suffering may well draw attention to the issue of HIV/AIDS, but perhaps only by compromising the dignity of those being photographed. Hooper's

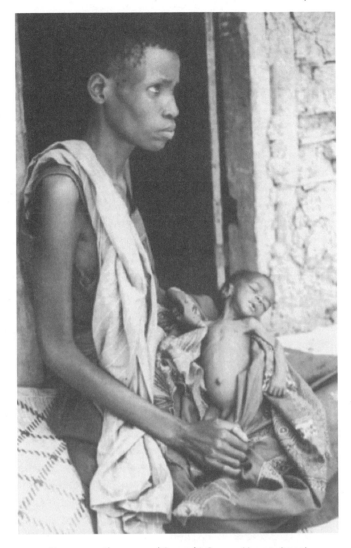

Figure 32.1 Florence and Ssengabi. Source: Hooper (1990)

subsequent reflections reveal that he was aware of this dilemma, oscillating between his humanist desire to draw attention to the AIDS crisis and an acute awareness of the privileged position he occupied as a Western photographer:

> I feel that we were right, that day in Kyebe, to use film and tape to record the brutal realities of Slim [HIV/AIDS]; for Florence had agreed, and in the end permission was surely hers to grant or withhold. Nevertheless, I also know that I participated in something of a media rape. For the next 15 minutes, barely containing...excitement...I photographed the mother and child from every angle, with every lens. Cameras clicked and whirred, pausing only for the changing of films...Some minutes later, we took our leave of Florence and her family...and I gave some money...On one level it was a simple gesture of assistance to people whom we had met...who were in a hopeless

situation. On another... it was payment for taking the photographs... payment to help ease our consciences. (Hooper 1990, 48–49)

Hooper's moral agonizing touches on a range of political and ethical dilemmas. But above all, it underlines one key point: the privileged position of the photographer and the consequences that issue from this position. The photographer controls the action, from staging and framing the photograph to deciding about the appropriate compensation for the so-captured object. Hooper depicts HIV/AIDS not unlike Baudelaire's famous flâneur observed the contradictions and undersides of urban life in the late nineteenth century. Peeking out of his secure bourgeois existence, the flâneur voyeuristically strolls through the city's darker parts, thereby discovering its neglected and suffering population (see Sontag 1977, 55–56; Debrix 2003, xxxii-xxxvi). And just as the disturbed flâneur uses his gaze in the hope that it might engender social change, Hooper's photograph too was taken and reproduced largely in the context of a humanist engagement for positive change. But this does not deflect from the fact that the ensuing practices of representation are unequal, perhaps even exploitative. This is the case because the photographer, and the Western press in general, have the privilege to frame, and thus politicize, another person's suffering.

Two main interrelated critiques have been raised against such forms of humanist photography: that it aestheticizes suffering and that it leads to compassion fatigue. The former critique is epitomized through a prominent essay by Ingrid Sischy (1991, 92) about Sabastião Salgado's beautiful and politically engaging photographs. She found them problematic insofar as they "anesthetize" the viewer. "The beautification of tragedy," she stresses "results in pictures that ultimately reinforce our passivity toward the experiences they reveal." This passivity, some commentators assert, is reinforced by the very confronting nature of photographs like those by Hooper. Shock can only work for a limited period of time before its mesmerizing capacity loses sway. Even the most horrific image becomes banal when it is repeated ad infinitum. It may end up normalizing suffering, and thus rending the viewer numb and indifferent (Sontag 1977, 19–20; Dean 2003, 88). The result, some stress, is what Susan Moeller (1999) termed "compassion fatigue" or, as it might be called in the case of our specific topic, "AIDS fatigue."

We believe that both critiques are not warranted, at least not in an unqualified manner. But as the issues at stake are rather complex, and as they touch only marginally upon our main objective, we only draw brief attention here to some of the scholars who have provided counterarguments. David Campbell (2004, 62), for instance, stresses that the compassion fatigue position cannot be sustained in an unqualified manner, not least because there is widespread evidence that the public often reacts generously when charity organizations appeal for help (see also Cohen and Seu 2002, 200). At a theoretical level, debates about the effects of aestheticized suffering go back at least to Walter Benjamin's (1977, 168) concern that all attempts to "render politics esthetic" end up in war, or Theodor Adorno's (1955, 31) controversial remarks that it is impossible to write poetry after Auschwitz, that even the attempt to do so would be barbaric. But these remarks emerged in a very specific political context, that of fascist Germany. As general statements, they are, we believe, neither tenable nor, for that matter, compatible with Benjamin and Adorno's overall scholarly positions. Various authors, such as David Levi Strauss (2003, 9), have thus questioned the idea that an estheticized image is somehow politically less relevant or that beauty cannot be a call to action. Rather than dismissing aesthetics as politically problematic per se, one should try to understand the nature and political consequences that are entailed in particular types of aesthetic representations. Doing so is our task here, and we engage it now through a closer reading of the Hooper photograph.

THE POLITICAL CONSEQUENCES OF DECONTEXTUALIZING SUFFERING

The Hooper photograph gives us a very particular image of suffering. It depicts a dying mother and child, sitting alone in an open doorway somewhere in Africa. No other people are visible, nor are there any features that can be recognized as part of a particular society or culture. Hooper displays Florence and Ssengabi passively, as if they were unable to do anything but wait for death. They are seen in one function only, as sufferers. Indeed, Florence and Ssengabi are entirely defined by their suffering. But this was, of course, not their only identity, even though they were facing imminent death. One could have just as well presented them in different ways, as being integrated in their surroundings, or as pursuing an activity. But the Hooper photograph is an attempt to capture the universal nature of death, stripped free of culture and context. As a result, it shows an image of passive victims, void of agency, history, belonging, or social attachment.

The decontextualized and universalized nature of Hooper's humanist photograph becomes, not surprisingly, further reinforced by its subsequent usage in Western media sources. The photograph was published in leading Western media outlets, including *Newsweek* and the *Washington Post* Journal of Health. The former used the picture with a generic caption that read: "Two Victims: Ugandan Barmaid and Son" (Nordland et al. 1986, 44). The names of the victims are already lost, having been replaced with more generic terms of "victim" and "Ugandan." Florence is, furthermore, framed pejoratively as an anonymous barmaid. The *Washington Post* story does mention the names and ages of Florence and Ssengabi. It does so in the caption accompanying the photograph. Given its shocking nature, the photograph stays in the reader's mind, but the corresponding article never mentions Florence and Ssengabi again. We never hear what Florence has to say about her situation. We only see a snapshot of her suffering and that of her baby, and even this picture is framed by someone, as Hooper (1990, 47–50) himself acknowledges, who barely knows her and her family. Further, the *Washington Post* story appeared two years after the *Newsweek* story but used the same photograph, rendering its use even more generic and universal.

As reproduced in the Western press, the Hooper photograph was meant to shock readers and draw their attention to the urgency of an issue. It was meant to "hook" them, not only to shocking AIDS images but also to a particular consumer product: a newspaper or magazine that operates according to profit-seeking principles of market economics. That in itself would not necessarily hinder representational sensitivity, but due to the lack of context provided by *Newsweek* and other media sources, the Hooper photograph soon turned into a symbol, an archetype used years after it was first taken. And from there, it is only a short step to stereotypes.

This is, we believe, the most characteristic and also the most problematic aspect of Hooper's humanist photograph: its attempt to capture a generic image of AIDS, a universalized and decontextualized notion of human suffering. We are left with an increasingly fixed image, frozen in time and place, inevitably feeding into stereotypical images of Africa we have already identified in detail earlier in the essay: a dark and homogenous continent, populated by passive victims stripped of either voice or agency. Although the Hooper photograph is meant precisely to escape from this doomsday scenario, its generic nature paradoxically feeds into the same problematic tradition. It also evokes a long photographic tradition, epitomized by *National Geographic*, which has represented Africa through typical orientalist images of "dark-skinned, bare-breasted women, in their customary dress, looking at the camera without awareness of their impending status as spectacles of adolescent Western eyes" (Grundberg 1990, 173).

Although corresponding reporting practices have become more sensitive, many of its key features remain intact, as demonstrated by issues of *National Geographic* on "Living with AIDS" (September 2005) and *Time* on "Global Health" (November 2005). Even the shocking nature of an AIDS photograph is not enough to break through such stereotypes. Sontag (2004, 23) even believes that the opposite may be the case, for "the image as shock and the image as cliché are two aspects of the same presence."

Several consequences emerge from the decontextualized nature of humanist photography. The basic idea behind this approach, as already stressed, is to generate compassion in viewers, which, in turn, ought to engender social change. But the universal nature of humanist photography is unlikely to generate compassion, at least if we define compassion as Hanna Arendt (1990) does: as sentiments that are directed toward particular individuals. Humanist photography is more likely to inspire what Arendt calls pity, a more abstract and generalized form of politics.

In a compelling application of Arendt's typology, Luc Boltanski (1999, 4) stresses how a politics of pity views the unfortunate collectively, even though it relies on singling out particular misfortunes to inspire pity in the first place. It is evident that the ensuing dynamics entail a fundamental dilemma, one that perhaps cannot be solved. A generalized portrayal of HIV/AIDS as a political problem is unlikely to inspire pity. Statistical data, for instance, cannot do this, no matter how much evidence it provides of the devastating impact of the disease. To arouse pity, Boltanski (1999, 11) stresses, "suffering and wretched bodies must be conveyed in such a way as to affect the sensibility of those more fortunate." That is the function of the Hooper photograph. But problems arise as soon as this image is used to establish and defend a more generic political stance. This is the case, for instance, when the Hooper photograph is being used to draw public awareness in the West about the general problem of HIV/AIDS in Africa. The image of suffering then inevitably becomes detached from both the sufferer and local circumstances.

Manifestations of pity often mask unequal power relations. It was precisely in the seemingly selfless Christian practices of pity that Nietzsche (1991, 947) detected a will to power, a thirst for triumph, a desire to subjugate. Pity then becomes linked to several features that fundamentally contradict the original humanist desire for social change. Images of suffering in Africa subconsciously contain a range of moral judgments and sentiments, including resentment and fear (see Sontag 2003, 75). They may also remind Western audiences of what they are free from. Paradoxically, the very disturbing nature of the Hooper photograph thus provides a certain feeling of safety and security to some of those viewing it. Death in a distant and dangerous elsewhere can then become a way of affirming life in the safe here and now, giving people a sense of belonging to a particular group that is distinct from others (Biehl 2001, 139; Radley 2002, 2; see also Nussbaum 2001, 297–454 for a more general discussion of pity and its distinctiveness from compassion, sympathy, and empathy).

LOCAL REPRESENTATION THROUGH PLURALIST PHOTOGRAPHY

Despite the humanist aspiration to change the world for the better, we are, then, back to a more pessimistic interpretation of photography and its ability to engage political dilemmas. Or are we? Not necessarily, for photography has the potential to break through stereotypes. It may even be able to engender compassion, rather than mere pity.

To scrutinize this potential, we now examine what we call pluralist photography. Just as humanist approaches do, pluralist ones oppose the naturalist belief that photographs are authentic and value-free representations of the world. Photography is seen in the context of sociopolitical practices. And it is endowed with the explicit mission to shape these practices actively. But as opposed to humanist photography, pluralist approaches do not aim to capture a generic and universal notion of suffering. Photography is, instead, seen as a method to validate multiple local knowledge and practices, thereby disrupting existing hierarchies and power relationships—as for instance the ability of Western photographers and media representations to frame the suffering of others. The basic idea behind this approach is to provide people affected by HIV/AIDS with the power to decide for themselves what kind of information and representation is most appropriate to capture the social, political, ethical, and psychological challenges they face. The ideal result of this practice is a form of dialogue that opens up spaces for communities to work through the problems that confront them. Photography would then facilitate what Debrix and Weber (Debrix 2003, ix) called a ritual of pluralization: a practice of mediation whereby the represented person takes an active role in the process of inscribing social meaning, but does so without attaching to it an exclusive claim that silences other positions and experiences. Our engagement with such pluralist photographic practices is strongly shaped by and indebted to the work of William Connolly (1995, 2005), even though we refrain from drawing specific linkages to his conceptual elaborations on pluralism.

We examine the potential and limits of pluralist photography by focusing on a project initiated by documentary photographer Eric Gottesman. Between November 2003 and March 2004, Gottesman (2003) worked on a photography project in Ethiopia, collaborating with HIV/AIDS-affected children in a particular neighborhood of Addis Ababa, in Kebele 15. Participation in the project, which has continued since then in different forms, was voluntary. It was coordinated through a local NGO, Hope for Children. It took place in a country with the second-highest population of HIV/AIDS orphans in the world. Some 720,000 children have been orphaned as a result of HIV/AIDS-related deaths or stigma. About 200,000 of them live with HIV/AIDS, many of them in the streets of Addis Ababa (USAID 2003, 19–23; UNICEF 2004, 26).

The objective of the Addis Ababa project was, in part, to place cameras in the hands of children affected by HIV/AIDS, giving them a tool to represent what it means to live with the disease in a community where HIV infection rates and HIV/ AIDS-related stigma are high. This practice includes providing a medium and space to share stories and visions, rather than giving this authority away to a professional photographer whose products are then reproduced to fit media priorities and preexisting narratives of Africa. Gottesman's project is based on a method pioneered by photographer Wendy Ewald, who worked with children in different contexts, from inner cities in the United States to small towns in Columbia and rural areas in India and Mexico. Ewald's understanding of photography evolved as she worked with students in different places. It began with the idea of sharing the camera with children but then moved into situations where children took charge and created images themselves (Ewald 1998, 1–3). These approaches are part of a larger set of development communication methods designed to promote multidimensional and dialogic ways of representing and engaging communities. They are meant to replace centralized, professionalized, and consumer-oriented communication practices, which tend to silence many people, particularly those who live at the margins of society. Pluralist photography is part of an alternative, more democratizing means of representation that seeks to create space for diverse and localized ways of communicating meaning (see Servaes 1986, 211–215).

Children involved in the Addis Ababa program were taught how to use the cameras themselves. On some occasions digital cameras were used, but in most cases the technology was as simple as possible, consisting of Polaroid Propack cameras that automatically produced a black and white photograph with negatives attached. Some of the so-taken photographs deteriorated relatively quickly, as is evident with some of the pictures represented here. But the method also has several advantages, including providing the young photographers with control over what was destroyed or kept for further use.

Pluralist local photography begins before any photograph is actually taken. It seeks to facilitate understanding of photographic representations and the type of values and power relations embedded in them. The children who participated in the project met each week with Gottesman, either on a one-to-one basis, or in a group. They were encouraged to develop their own methods of photography, so that they could tell their unique stories from their unique angle. Crucial to this process were preliminary discussions about the methods that would be used to represent their lives and those they loved and also lost. This included using photography to document not only the present but also the past. In one class, students were asked to reconstruct the history of their own parents who had died of AIDS—parents who often died before the children could get to know them. Thus, this process required using methods of photography to merge fact, fiction, and feeling into a composition that recovered and represented what had been lost in a parent's untimely death. Gottesman stresses that everyone involved was aware that they took decisions, and that these decisions affected the ways in which photographs represented them and their surroundings. This form of collaboration, he believes, is rather different from traditional photographic portrayals of developing countries as seen in *National Geographic* and other magazines. Both Gottesman and Ewald learned from their work that photographs taken by children are often more complex than the reality that professional representations usually assign to their experiences.

We now focus on the work of Tenanesh Kifyalew, a twelve-year-old girl who was living with HIV/AIDS and participated in the Addis Ababa project. Tenanesh means "she is health" in Amharic. She was named by her grandmother who, after her daughter had died of AIDS, refused to believe the doctor when he diagnosed her granddaughter with HIV. Tenanesh agreed to work with Gottesman while living with AIDS-related illnesses that often drained her energy. Like Florence and Ssengabi, Tenanesh died shortly after the photographs by and of her were created.

Tenanesh took over one hundred photographs, mostly in her home, where she spent much of her time confined by her illness. She either took the photographs herself or asked others to take photographs of her in particular situations. The impressions that these photographs convey are very different from the ones evoked by Hooper's picture of Florence and Ssengabi. Tenanesh's self-portrayal of what it means to live with HIV/AIDS is not nearly as dramatic, not nearly as shocking as Hooper's representation. When analyzing Tenanesh's photographs we found two types of pictures, each of them differing markedly from humanist photography. In the first type Tenanesh represented her illness; in the second she portrayed her daily life. Images of the first type are represented by figures 32.2 and 32.3.

We consciously resist the temptation to overinterpret Tenanesh's photographs. We do so in order to offer a form of commentary that illuminates the issues at stake but then refers authority back to the photographs themselves (see Heidegger 1981, 194). It would have been tempting indeed to speculate what the rubber-gloved hands exactly signify, or how the quasi-cling-wrapped doll may express a sense of suffocation or fear of the outside world. But the death of the photographer—in this case unfortunately not only metaphorical but also real—is as paramount a phenomenon as the much-discussed death of the author. We cannot know what Tenanesh intended to represent when she took the photographs, nor does it matter. She does not retain any control over how viewers subsequently see the photographs.

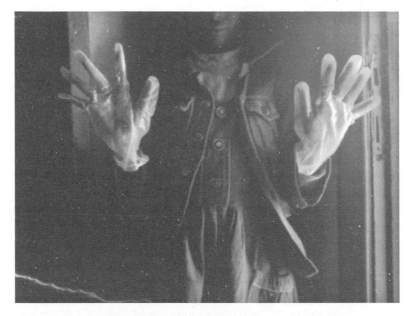

Figure 32.2 Tenanesh Kifyalew, "Untitled"

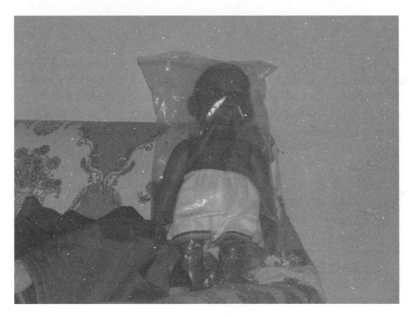

Figure 32.3 Tenanesh Kifyalew, "Untitled"

In order to leave the process of interpretation open to the reader and viewer, we only highlight how Tenanesh captures the nature of living with HIV/AIDS through a conscious process of abstraction. But the nature of Tenanesh's abstraction is fundamentally different from that of Hooper's. The humanist photographs of the latter contained elements of naturalism insofar as they sought to depict an authentic external reality: the "real" face HIV/AIDS as epitomized by a representative single person living with HIV/AIDS. A very particular image is frozen to then produce generalities from it. The process of representation and abstraction is masked by the shocking "reality" of the image. Tenanesh's portrayal of suffering, by contrast, makes representation its central theme. She does not take a photograph that is supposed to resemble some authentic external image of suffering. Her photographs are much more meta-phorical. She addresses the psychological and emotional dimensions of living with HIV/AIDS. And she does so by explicitly recognizing that photographs can never give us an authentic rep-resentation of the realities in which she lives. We, as viewers of the photographs, are con-fronted with the process of representation as well: we are asked to imagine what it means for her to face HIV/AIDS. As a result, representation becomes a site of politics, open to interpre-tation and debate.

The second type of photograph that Tenanesh took is illustrated in figures 32.4, 32.5 and 32.6. Here, her pictures do not represent suffering. They place her existence in a larger personal and social context. As opposed to the Hooper photograph, these pictures do not por-tray a decontextualized world of darkness and gloom. Instead, Tenanesh captures the dailyness of her life, its ups and downs, her determination to lead a relatively normal childhood. Perhaps, she does so precisely because she was confined by her disease, unable to attend school, or go outside for long. We cannot know that from the photographs alone. But we see a certain defiance, a playful defiance, and a way of demonstrating that she has not lost her agency. Tenanesh is not a passive victim in the way Hooper portrays Florence and Ssengabi. She has control of the camera, and with it she shows that she has some control over her surroundings too. As opposed to Florence and Ssengabi, Tenanesh's identity is not reduced to that of a sufferer alone. She is also a child, a Christian, a member of a family, part of a social community. We are inevitably confronted with the life of a single person, rather than an abstract image of a disease.

If Tenanesh's photographs shock, then it is not because we are graphically confronted with the agony of dying from AIDS-related illnesses. The pictures surprise because they portray Tenanesh living a seemingly normal, even vibrant childhood in the face of death. In a sense, her photographs symbolize a shift away from portrayals of people "dying of AIDS," which were par-ticularly dominant in the early days of the pandemic (see Watney 1990, 173–192; Nixon and Nixon 1991) toward an attempt to show people "living with AIDS" (see Mendel 2006, 42–51). Figures 32.4 and 32.5, for instance, depict Tenanesh in her surroundings. In figure 32.6, she photographs some of her family members. These pictures do not fit into a preconceived image of what it means to be living with and dying of AIDS in Africa. Western viewers cannot easily create a safe distance from these pictures by reassuring themselves that the life portrayed in them takes place in some far off, dangerous continent. The daily objects Tenanesh chooses as symbols to represent her life are uniquely personal and universal at the same time. From the teddy bear and the television set to pictures of Jesus, they suggest her attachment to "favorite things." They also capture her faith in the divine. Although such images can evoke shared expe-riences around the world, they do so without generating a generic picture of "AIDS in Africa." Tenanesh's unique environment is presented as an essential element of who she is and what it means to be affected by HIV/AIDS. It is thus much less likely that such context-specific pic-tures can feed into a preexisting neocolonial image of Africa as the dark continent, caught in a web of gloom and doom, populated entirely by helpless victims.

PLURALIST PHOTOGRAPHY AND COMMUNITY DIALOGUE

The practices of displaying pluralist photography are as novel as their composition. Tenanesh's photographs were an integral element of her activism. She used her remaining life to become an outspoken advocate for a movement called People Living with HIV/AIDS (PLWHA). She

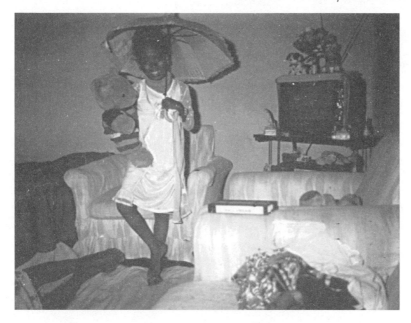

Figure 32.4 "My Favorite Things"

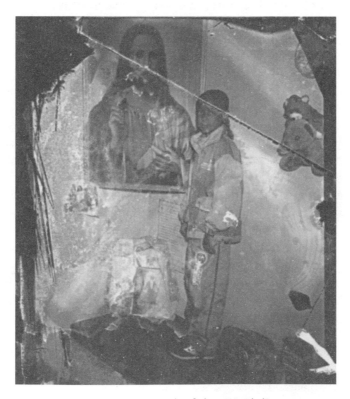

Figure 32.5 Tenanesh Kifyalew, "Untitled"

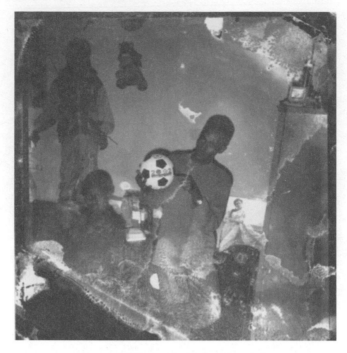

Figure 32.6 Tenanesh Kifyalew, "Untitled"

advocated the use of life-prolonging drugs, such as antiretrovirals, which were available only to a very small minority of people living with HIV in Ethiopia. Tenanesh spoke to thousands of people at public gatherings and eventually became an ambassador for UNESCO on behalf of HIV/AIDS-affected children. She wrote letters and postcards in which she made her claims public. They were addressed, among others, to Ethiopians abroad, students at Addis Ababa University, and the president of the United States. In these letters, she described what it meant to live with HIV/AIDS, telling, for instance, how she faced the social stigma that surrounded her. She also advanced specific political demands, such as access to free medical assistance for children affected by HIV/ AIDS.

Sixteen of Tenanesh's photographs, together with some of her letters and postcards, were included in an exhibition entitled "I was not a child when I was a child" (translated from Amharic). Tenanesh's original Polaroid photographs were scanned and then printed at a local advertising company that had a large-scale printer. During the month of March 2004, the exhibition, which also featured photographs by fourteen other children, traveled to twenty-one different kebeles in Kifle Ketema Subcity, as well as to City Hall in Addis Ababa (figure 32.7). Just as Tenanesh's photographs were created as a result of a dialogue, the exhibition too made dialogue one of its central themes. As members of a community, viewers were asked to add letters and pictures to Tenanesh's work, thus creating a verbal and visual dialogue that became an essential and constantly changing part of the exhibition. The idea that spectators are not just passive consumers but active contributors to the work of art is, of course, not new. It goes back at least to Marcel Duchamp and is practiced today by a range of prominent artists, such as Rirkrit Tiravanija (see Tomkins 2005, 82–95). By embracing such an approach, the Addis Ababa exhibition promoted new forms of discussion about what it means to live with HIV/ AIDS. It thus provided a creative and safe space for dialogue. The idea behind this dialogue was to break through some of the silences, taboos, and stigma that characterize HIV/AIDS in a city where almost everyone knows someone who lives with or has died of the illness. The objective was thus very practical: to influence the conditions under which people live with HIV/ AIDS and to find more appropriate ways of stemming the spread of the disease and related stigma. This is why, for instance, the Addis Ababa exhibition also provided information about local organizations that are engaged in dealing with the increase in HIV infections and the impact of HIV/AIDS.

The Addis Ababa exhibition told multiple stories about HIV/AIDS in the context of a unique local environment. By refusing to uphold one correct way of portraying the issues at stake, the exhibition drew attention to the political nature of representation. Such communication practices are, of course, rather different from those represented through the iconic images of humanist photography, where the flow of information is controlled, hierarchical, and works in only one direction.

While we believe that pluralist photography has the potential to challenge some of the taboos and stigmas that shroud HIV/AIDS, it is important not to idealize this form of representation. Two particular limitations stand out.

First: Just as any other photographic approach, the type of image that pluralist photography projects is neither authentic nor, for that matter, void of power relations. From Tenanesh's photographs alone, we do not know what her life is like, at least not entirely. We still have only snapshots of particular moments and situations.

Add to this that she was integrated in a photography project that was shaped by Western assumptions about representation. Gottesman provided not only the cameras needed for the project but also the know-how. He instructed the children involved in the project about the use of cameras and the different possibilities of capturing images with them. Although Gottesman was careful to teach the children how to make their own representational choices, his aesthetic influence cannot be extricated from the project. The same is the case with the subsequent exhibition, which was only possible as a result of Gottesman's know-how and funding from a variety of sources, including UNICEF and the Ethiopian HIV/ AIDS Prevention and Control Office. Funding does, of course, always come with constraints, either explicit or implicit ones. Gottesman retained some editing authority about the display at the exhibition, even though Tenanesh was actively involved in it from the beginning to the end. Power relations would have been present even had the project been organized without Western influence or participation. For better or for worse, taking and displaying photographs is a form of representation, and thus open to a range of political uses and abuses. The Addis Ababa exhibition, for instance, focused exclusively on the fate of Ethiopian children affected by HIV/AIDS. It did so, some would say, to the detriment of drawing attention to the affected adult population, thereby portraying a very particular, politically shaped image of the issues at stake. Many societal groups that are most vulnerable to HIV/AIDS, such as commercial sex workers, intravenous drug users, or men who have sex with men, remain marginalized and even criminalized.

Human relations cannot exist outside power. But the nature of pluralist photography minimizes the oppressive effects of these relations by consciously problematizing representation. The collaborative and dialogical nature of pluralist photography can provide ways through which multiple perspectives may be seen and validated. By undermining the authority of professional photographers and commercialized organizations to tell the truth about HIV/ AIDS, pluralist photography retains the ability to step out of preexisting narratives and to surprise the expectation of the viewer/reader.

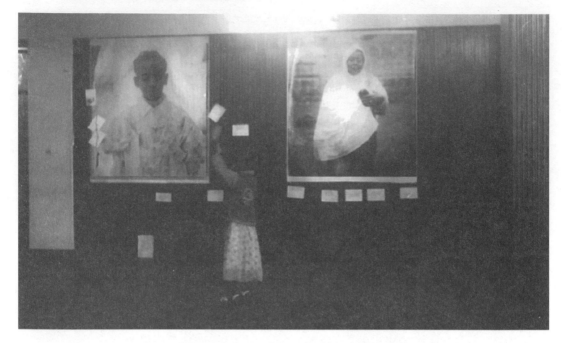

Figure 32.7 Tenanesh Preparing the Exhibition.

Second: The sociopolitical impact of pluralist photography can only be partial and gradual. As opposed to iconic humanist photographs, pluralist versions are less likely to be used by global media networks as symbols representing a particular issue. They cannot appeal to the same mass audience. But this does not mean that pluralist photography is void of social impact. The Addis Ababa exhibition may not on its own have transformed the situation in Ethiopia, where stigma, myths, misinformation and silence continue to surround HIV/AIDS and related issues of sexuality and health behavior. But the exhibition is part of a larger, ongoing effort to change the way people think about themselves and their surroundings. It reached some viewers who, in turn, may influence others through their experience. The exhibition was also part of an effort to convince the Ethiopian government of the need to make antiretrovirals available to the population. This has already started to happen, with the introduction of a first, although limited program aimed at supporting some 30,000 affected people (Thibodeaux 2005).

At times pluralist photographs may even have an impact beyond their local setting. The Addis Ababa project, for instance, reached an audience wider than the kebele, even though the mechanisms of diffusion were neither instant nor global. Ethiopian national television covered the exhibition in what were the country's first televised pictures of people living with HIV. In a society where one in six people is infected with HIV, this was an important and long-overdue step (see Hope for Children 2003, 2). The actual video images were provided by the children who participated in the exhibition. Versions of the exhibition also traveled to the United States and Australia. The exhibit changed as it traveled on, engaging new audiences and retaining its interactive and dialogical nature in an attempt to bring the children of Kebele 15 in contact with Western audiences. Even more opportunities would and will exist through the Internet, which is not only global, but pluralist itself. It may thus be particularly suited to diffuse pluralist photography.

CONCLUSION

In the twenty years since the recognition of HIV/AIDS as a pandemic, the disease has become a global challenge. This challenge is not only of a medical nature but also involves various political, social, and psychological factors. The lives of those who are infected or affected by HIV/AIDS have come to be decisively shaped by how we represent what it means to live with the disease. This is particularly the case in acutely affected African communities, where HIV/AIDS has taken its greatest toll. As in many parts of the world, people here live with a condition that is shrouded in silence, taboos, and stigma. The resulting practices of representation not only marginalize and oppress people affected, but also fuel the spread of the disease.

In this essay, we have examined how photographic representations either contribute to or break with stereotypical portrayals of HIV/AIDS. We began by discussing naturalist positions, which view photographs as authentic representations of external realities. Various problems emerge from such assumptions. When photographs are accepted as unquestioned factual representations, then our eyes become passive instruments rather than tools for broadening vision and understanding. We forget that the photograph was framed by a particular person who made a range of aesthetic and inherently subjective choices in this process. We have thus explored two approaches that use photography as an active catalyst for social change. Both acknowledge that photographs cannot portray the world as it is, that they always involve both facts and feelings. Humanist engagements seek to use iconic photographs as a way of visualizing the devastating aspects that can be a part of the reality of HIV/AIDS, hoping that the so-generated feeling of shock in Western viewers would serve as a catalyst for social and political change. Pluralist photography, by contrast, is more concerned with finding ways through which people can express the multiple and often local manifestations of what it means to live with HIV/AIDS. Such forms of representation can open up possibilities for a democratic and constructive public dialogue.

We examined humanist photography by interpreting one of the most influential iconic HIV/AIDS photographs; Ed Hooper's portrayal of a dying Ugandan woman and her child. The process here revolves around a Western photographer being in control of virtually all aesthetic and political choices involved in the process of representation. The object of the photograph, in this case Florence and her child, Ssengabi, are objects indeed. They are deprived of voice and agency—a loss that is further exacerbated by the manner in which iconic photographs are then used in global mass media. The result is a symbolic representation of HIV/AIDS, one that may shock Western viewers and evoke pity in them. But this shock comes at the expense of understanding the complexities of the local and personal situation. A symbolic representation of a person dying of AIDS-related illnesses can easily turn into an archetype, which feeds into deeply entrenched stereotypical images of Africa as a dark and homogenous continent, populated by nameless victims who are helplessly exposed to a never-ending series of crises. Suffering, then, becomes idealized and stigmatized at the same time, a combination that is particularly fateful with regard to a disease like HIV/AIDS, which is already surrounded by a range of prejudices and taboos. Gazing at the suffering of others in far off places may also become no more than a way of affirming the safety of the here and now, thus undermining the very humanist aspirations for social change that have inspired the respective photographic engagements in the first place.

There are alternatives to iconic humanist photography. These alternatives are of a more pluralist nature, consisting of attempts to open up spaces for people living with HIV/AIDS to decide for themselves how they would like to be represented, and how these representations should be used. Trying to understand the potential and limits of such approaches, we have examined Eric Gottesman's collaborative approach with HIV/AIDS-affected children in a community of Addis Ababa. Here, we see very different images of what it means to live with HIV/AIDS. We do not see victims stripped of voice and representational authority. Instead, each child finds her or his own way of representing life with a stigmatized disease. In the photographs we analyzed, for instance, we saw a twelve-year-old girl, Tenanesh, trying to capture her unique struggle and her normal daily routine of living with HIV/AIDS. The Addis Ababa project alone will not change the global image of HIV/AIDS, but it has empowered those who participated in it, giving them the opportunity to express their own visions of what HIV/AIDS means, using collaborative and dialogical means to do so. And, perhaps more importantly, it is part of a broader, long-term, and much-needed process of finding more diverse and appropriate ways of representing what it means to live with HIV/AIDS.

Pluralist approaches offer a viable alternative to naturalist and humanist photography. This is not to say that they are without problems. As any other form of photographic representation, pluralist approaches too are always open to political interpretation and appropriation, for better or worse. But because pluralist photography refuses to universalize suffering it is less likely to lead to stereotypical representations. Particularly when embedded in community projects that promote dialogue, pluralist photography—perhaps more so than any other photographic practice—has the potential to challenge some of the deeply entrenched and highly problematic taboos and stigmas that are associated with HIV/AIDS. Or so suggests the type of interpretative research and analysis we have conducted for this essay. Whether or not our results can be confirmed by empirical evidence remains to be seen. Doing so is no easy task, for, as Stanley Cohen and Bruna Seu (2002, 188) stress, "far more is known about the space between the pristine object—the tortured body, the massacred corpses, the homeless refugee—and its public representation than the space between the resultant image and its public perception." The exact impact of pluralist photography on sociopolitical practices remains to be investigated, and it can be done only through carefully designed case studies. But such studies are only possible once we have more systematic insight into the representative practices that characterize our knowledge of and political attitudes toward HIV/AIDS. Contributing to this process has been the main objective of our essay, and we hope that by doing so we have taken a modest step toward dismantling some of the stigma and discrimination that continues to shape the impact of HIV/AIDS.

33

Postlude
A Tam-Tam for Africa

IN MEMORIAM: MAMADOU KONTÉ (1945–2007)

Patricia Tang (Massachusetts Institute of Technology)

In recent decades, African musicians such as Manu Dibango, Salif Keita, Youssou N'Dour, Baaba Maal and Angelique Kidjo have all become household names in the world music scene. However, many listeners are unaware that the widespread exposure of these African artists was in large part made possible by an illiterate African laborer in France who, in the 1970s, began organizing aid concerts to improve the living conditions of immigrant workers. Through his creation of Africa Fête, this laborer-turned-businessman, Mamadou Konté (1945–2007), went on to become one of the most important and influential people in the African music industry. Founded by Mamadou Konté in 1978, Africa Fête is an organization dedicated to the promotion of African music and musicians. For over three decades, Africa Fête has managed numerous African artists, organized international tours and festivals, given exposure to new talent, and provided training in sound-engineering, production, and management. Currently based in Dakar, Senegal, Africa Fête has recorded numerous African musicians and distributed their songs through the creation of its own record label. It has also organized artistic residencies that foster collaborations between African artists and other artists around the globe. To date, the best-known African stars to grace world music stages have done so under the auspices of Africa Fête.

Although Mamadou Konté was a leader in the African music industry, he came to music production as a cultural activist, believing that music could and should be an important means for furthering economic development and social awareness among Africans both at home and in the diaspora. Throughout his life, Konté used music as a tool for raising money and awareness for important causes, from the plight of immigrant workers in France in the 1960s, to the fight against music piracy and, most recently, the HIV/AIDS epidemic at the turn of the twenty-first century.

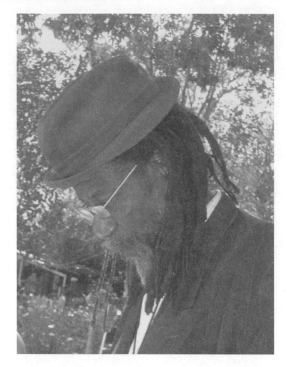

Figure 33.1 Mamadou Konté. Photograph by Patricia Tang

Since 2001, the Africa Fête festival has been held in Dakar every year in conjunction with World AIDS Day. Partnering with the condom manufacturer Protec, the annual festival showcases both new and seasoned talent in hugely successful mega-concerts, bringing HIV/AIDS-related issues to the attention of large numbers of youth who are in attendance.

One of the last projects spearheaded by Mamadou Konté before his death was the album entitled *Nous sommes les Tams-tams (We are the Drums)*. The album was produced by Africa Fête in collaboration with the "Africa 2015" initiative headed by the United Nations Development Program as well as the United Nations Office of Sports for Development and Peace, the United Nations Joint Program on HIV/AIDS, the United Nations Population Fund and the Millennium Campaign. The eleven songs on the album feature thirty-seven musicians singing in eighteen African languages as well as in French and English. The songs discuss the need to break the silence about AIDS, the importance of fighting discrimination and stigmatization of those with AIDS, and the importance of prevention against HIV infection. The title song, "*Nous sommes les Tam-tams,*" encourages Africans to take individual responsibility for halting the spread of HIV/AIDS so that the 2015 generation will not be affected by the disease. Africans are called on to act as the traditional tam-tam drums, passing on this important message to those who have not yet heard it. In this vein, the album and its message have been freely distributed to radio and TV stations in fifty-two countries throughout Africa.

Mamadou Konté believed first and foremost that music should play an active role in African economic development and social awareness. Although Mamadou Konté is no longer with us, Africa Fête continues his work through its commitment to humanitarian causes and the promotion of AIDS awareness in Africa.

ABOUT THE AUTHORS

E. Jackson Allison Jr. has been involved in public health education internationally since 1966 and holds fellowships in the American College of Preventive Medicine, the American Academy of Family Practice, the American College of Emergency Physicians, and the International Federation for Emergency Medicine. He has authored or co-authored more than 280 contributions to the medical literature. He is known for developing innovative approaches to health education involving nutrition and HIV/AIDS in Malawi and low-cost sanitation in Tanzania through the use of public health songs and jingles, which would also incorporate puppetry, dance, poetry, storytelling, videos, and drama. He is professor of emergency care at the College of Health & Human Sciences, Western Carolina University, and adjunct professor at the College of Health Professions, Upstate Medical University, Syracuse.

Ric Alviso is professor of music at California State University Northridge. He received his bachelor's degree in music composition from California State University, Long Beach, and his MA and PhD in ethnomusicology from UCLA. As an ethnomusicologist, he has conducted fieldwork in Senegal, Zimbabwe, and the southwest United States with a focus on applied ethnomusicology. He has written on a variety of subjects including applied ethnomusicology, music in prisons, Pentecostal music, and traditional and popular music in Africa. He is also on the music faculty at Santa Monica College.

Gregory Barz is associate professor of ethnomusicology in the Blair School of Music at Vanderbilt University, with appointments in Anthropology and the Divinity school. He is the producer of the 2007 Grammy-nominated album, *Singing for Life: Songs of Hope, Healing, and HIV/AIDS in Uganda* (Smithsonian Folkways) that draws on his field recordings in East Africa of the music of HIV-positive women's groups. His research in Uganda was supported by a senior research fellowship with the Fulbright African AIDS Research Program. His recent research involves documenting the role of music in contemporary reconciliation efforts in postgenocide Rwanda genocide and hip hop and medical ethnomusicology in South Africa. He is author or editor of nine books and CDs, including most recently *Singing for Life: Music and HIV/AIDS in Uganda* (Routledge, 2006) and the second edition of *Shadows in the Field: New Perspectives on Fieldwork in Ethnomusicology* (Oxford, 2008). He has also spent two years as a Franklin Fellow in global citizenship in Lugano, Switzerland, and is currently a Senior Research Professor at the University of the Free State (Bloemfontein, South Africa).

Roland Bleiker is professor of international relations at the University of Queensland. His previous books include *Popular Dissent, Human Agency and Global Politics* (Cambridge University Press, 2000), *Divided Korea: Toward a Culture of Reconciliation* (University of Minnesota Press, 2005) and *Aesthetics and World Politics* (Palgrave, 2009). His most recent co-edited volumes are *Security and the War on Terror* (Routledge, 2007) and *Mediating Across Difference: Pacific and Asian Approaches to Security and Conflict* (University of Hawaii Press, 2010). Bleiker is currently working on a project that examines how images shape responses to humanitarian crises. He has held visiting research and teaching affiliations at Harvard, Cambridge, Humboldt, Tampere, Yonsei, and Pusan National University as well as the Swiss Federal Institute of Technology and the Institute of Social Studies in The Hague.

ECKHARD BREITINGER received his education in English, History, and Archaeology in Tuebingen, Bangor North Wales and Geneva. He has taught at the University of the West Indies, Kingston, at Nkrumah University in Kumasi, Ghana. Since 1980 he has been based in Bayreuth University with regular appointments as a visiting scholar and examiner in Uganda, Kenya, Cameroon, and Malawi. He has published on English Romantic poetry, Gothic Novels, and American Radio Drama, but his main interest lies in postcolonial literatures from Africa and the Caribbean, with a special focus on theater and Theatre for Development. He has translated plays and poetry, written radio essays, and had his African theatre photographs exhibited at the Grahamstown National Arts Festival and various other international events. Recently he has engaged in comparative studies of Habsburgian postcolonial literature and Anglopohone postcolonial cultures. He retired in 2005 and has since held visiting posts in Cracow/Poland (Jagellonian University) and Maputo (Eduardo Mondlane) in Mozambique.

LAWRENCE H. BROWN, III has more than twenty years of emergency services experience. For the past twelve years he has worked primarily in research and academic settings. He is a member of the Board of Advisors for the Prehospital Care Research Forum, served as a co-investigator for the National EMS Research Agenda project, and is the lead author for the text, *An Introduction to EMS Research*. In 2006, Brown moved to Queensland, Australia, to study at the Anton Breinl Centre for Public Health and Tropical Medicine at James Cook University, earning a Master of Public Health and Tropical Medicine degree. Since then, he has worked to strengthen the links between research, emergency services, and public health, specifically in resource-poor settings. Brown currently serves as senior principal research officer for the Anton Breinl Centre.

JEFFREY CALLEN is an ethnomusicologist, writer and arts consultant, based in San Francisco. The bracketing of reactions, the deep hanging out and the willingness to be surprised, which are the *sine qua non* of the ethnographic method, are integral to his work. As a consultant, he assists artists, arts-related businesses, organizations and funders with writing, research, strategic planning, and project management. A former Fulbright scholar, his writing on popular music regularly appears in scholarly publications and popular outlets, such as *PopMatters, The Wall Street Journal, SF Weekly, East Bay Express, The Beat,* and *Afropop Worldwide*. He is currently writing a book on alternative music in Morocco and can be contacted through his professional blog, Deciphering Culture.

JUDAH M. COHEN is the Lou and Sybil Mervis Professor of Jewish Culture and associate professor of Folklore and Ethnomusicology at Indiana University. He is the author, with Gregory Barz, of the "Music and HIV/AIDS" chapter in the *Garland Handbook of African Music*, 2nd edition. In addition, he has published extensively on the history, identity, and music of Jews in the Americas, including the books *Through the Sands of Time: A History of the Jewish Community of St. Thomas, US Virgin Islands* (2004), *The Making of a Reform Jewish Cantor: Musical Authority, Cultural Investment* (2009), and *Sounding Jewish Tradition: The Music of Central Synagogue* (2011).

ABIMBOLA COLE is a PhD candidate in the Department of Ethnomusicology at the University of California, Los Angeles (UCLA). She is a former Fulbright scholar that has conducted research in Botswana and South Africa on the musical arts, popular music, and youth culture. Her involvement in HIV/AIDS initiatives has included various projects with the Botswana Business Coalition on HIV/AIDS (BBCA), Grassroot Soccer, the Youth Health Organization (YOHO), the Botswana Network on Ethics, Law, and HIV/AIDS (BONELA), and Schorer. She is currently completing her dissertation on the South African hip hop collective Cashless Society.

JONAH ELLER-ISAACS founded the Music is Life Project in 2003 to investigate musical responses to the African HIV/AIDS pandemic. On completing his research, he traveled around the United

States, educating a wide range of audiences on the transformative power of music in fighting the spread of the pandemic. Minnesota Public Radio aired his documentary *Singing in the Shadow of AIDS* in 2005, and a condensed version was nationally broadcast in 2006 for Public Radio International's syndicated news show *The World*. He currently works as a freelance writer and graphic designer in Brooklyn, NY where he lives with his wife Kathryn Wilening, a modern dance choreographer. He also keeps a blog at groinstrong.com and continues to explore the healing power of music after his 2008 diagnosis of late stage melanoma.

REBEKAH EMANUEL works at McKinsey & Company. A George Mitchell Scholar in Human Rights Law, she has worked in Uganda with Hospice Africa Uganda, focusing on the needs of cancer and AIDS patients and their families. A former Fox Fellow, she published "Informal Caregivers at Risk: Options for Preventive Interventions" in the *Journal of Palliative Medicine* (2008), based on her research in Uganda through the Jerome Medalie Endowment. Her interest in the social impact of illness and mourning has also encompassed research in India and Israel. In addition, she has served the Ugandan Parliament, conducting consultative meetings with women from northern Uganda as part of the Juba peace process.

MICHAEL GODBY is professor of History of Art at the University of Cape Town. He has lectured and published on a wide range of topics, including Early Renaissance Italian art, eighteenth-century English art (especially the work of William Hogarth), nineteenth-century South African art, contemporary South African art, and the history of photography in South Africa.

REBECCA HODES is the Deputy Director of the AIDS and Society Research Unit, Centre for Social Science Research, University of Cape Town. Her current research focuses on access to medicines and reproductive healthcare, new challenges and opportunities for HIV-positive prospective adoptive parents, and HIV in the media. Hodes completed her D.Phil at Oxford University in 2008, and a book adapted from her thesis about the history of HIV on South African television (working title, "Broadcasting the Pandemic") is under review for publication. Her most recent publications include "Televising Treatment: The Political Struggle for Antiretrovirals on South African Television," in *Social History of Medicine* 23, #3 (2010) and "Structure and Agency in the Politics of a Women's Rights Coalition in South Africa: The Making of the South African Sexual Offences Act," published in 2007 by the World Bank's Developmental Leadership Program.

DEBORAH JAMES is professor of anthropology at the London School of Economics. Her research interests, focused on South Africa, include migration, ethnomusicology, ethnicity, property relations and the politics of land reform. She is author of *Songs of the Women Migrants: Performance and Identity in South Africa* (1999) and of *Gaining Ground? "Rights" and "Property" in South African Land Reform* (2007), and co-editor of several volumes including *The Rights And Wrongs Of Land Restitution: "Restoring What Was Ours"* (2009) and *Culture Wars: Context, Models, and Anthropologists' Accounts* (2010).

AMY KAY is senior technical advisor for the Centre for Development and Population Activities (CEDPA). She is currently the Orphans and Vulnerable Children (OVC) technical team leader for the USAID Health Policy Initiative (HPI) Task Order One, a project that focuses on international public health and development; and she coordinates a portfolio of OVC activities in East and Southern Africa. Previously, Amy was the regional program officer for the UN Development Programme's HIV/AIDS Regional Program in the Arab States. She was also an HIV specialist for UN Development Programme and the UN Disarmament, Demobilization, and Reintegration programs in Sudan. She is currently a Board of Trustees member for Hope for Children, an NGO based in Addis Ababa serving OVC.

JENNIFER W. KYKER is assistant professor of ethnomusicology at the Eastman School of Music and the University of Rochester. She received her PhD from the University of Pennsylvania, where her dissertation explored music, morality, and politics in postcolonial Zimbabwe, through the songs of guitarist and vocalist Oliver Mtukudzi. Among her past and current research interests are music at the post-funerary rite of *kuroya guva*, the role of women *mbira* musicians, and issues of musical migration and circulation, including Zimbabwean and Brazilian musical diasporas. She has received both Fulbright and Fulbright-Hays doctoral fellowships in support of her research, and was honored as a Dean's Scholar at the University of Pennsylvania. In addition to her work in ethnomusicology, Jennifer is the founder and director of the nonprofit organization Tariro, which works to educate and empower teenaged girls in Zimbabwean communities affected by HIV/AIDS (www.tariro.org).

GERALD C. LIU is a Theology and Practice PhD candidate in the area of Homiletics and Liturgics at Vanderbilt University. He has a BA in Music from Washington University in St. Louis, MO and a Master of Divinity from Candler School of Theology. He also studied as a theological fellow at Georg-August Universität in Göttingen. He is an ordained United Methodist Elder, and, before beginning his doctoral studies at Vanderbilt, served British Methodist churches in the Nottingham Trent Valley Methodist Circuit of Nottingham, England. He is completing a dissertation that explores the possibility of perceiving God in music.

JOHN CHIPEMBERE LWANDA is a physician, social researcher, political historian, musicologist, former senior lecturer, and writer. His PhD was on the dynamics of culture, politics, and medicine with reference to the HIV/AIDS epidemic in Malawi. His seven books include *The Rhino's Lament*; *Music, Culture and Orature: Reading the Malawi Public Sphere, 1949–2006*; *Politics, Culture and Medicine in Malawi*; *Promises, Power Politics and Poverty: Democratic Transition in Malawi, 1961-1999*; *Black Thoughts from the Diaspora*; and the revised *Kamuzu Banda of Malawi*. He runs a small book publishing company and a music publishing company in Glasgow, Scotland that features Malawian musicians.

MJOMBA MAJALIA is a part-time lecturer in Jomo Kenyatta University of Agriculture and Technology in Kenya. He is also a visiting professor in St. Augustine University of Tanzania (SAUT). Mjomba's dissertation was on the use of local cultural performances in Kenya in HIV/AIDS intervention among Kenyan Youth. This work arose from his many years of experience as a teacher working with Kenyan youth in various high schools. Mjomba has written a number of articles in the area of HIV/AIDS interventions among the youth in Kenya. In addition, he consults and trains various organizations and institutions in areas of health communication, development communication, interpersonal communication, intercultural communication, and public speaking.

FRASER MCNEILL is a senior lecturer in the Department of Anthropology and Archaeology at the University of Pretoria. He has been conducting ethnographic research in the Venda region of South Africa for over 15 years, and is the lead guitarist in a popular Venda reggae band. His research interests include the role of music in HIV/AIDS education policies, the anthropology of knowledge, Tshivenda language, the politics of traditional leadership, female initiation, and poisonings. He is the author of *AIDS, Politics and Music in South Africa* (2011, Cambridge University Press), and *Magic* (with Isak Niehaus, AIDS Review 2009, Centre for the Study of AIDS, University of Pretoria).

Aldin Kaizilege Mutembei is a senior lecturer of literature and African philosophy and director of the Institute of Kiswahili Studies at the University of Dar es Salaam, Tanzania. He has researched on AIDS, literature, and communication since 1991 through the Sida-SAREC supported Kagera AIDS Research Project. From 2007 to 2009 he was a visiting scholar at Princeton University where he also taught courses on the Swahili Novel and AIDS and Literature. He has appeared in academic public talks as a main speaker at different universities including Tufts, Chicago, Georgetown, University of Florida and Goethe University. The author of four books, including the first Swahili historical novel on HIV/AIDS in Tanzania (which was translated into English as *The Dry Stump* in 2009), he has also published numerous articles in local and international journals. He conducts and sings with the University of Dar es Salaam chapel choir.

Leah Niederstadt is instructor of Museum Studies/Art History and curator of the Permanent Collection at Wheaton College in Norton, MA. Her research explores contemporary expressive culture and cultural heritage in Ethiopia, focusing on church-based and fine art painting traditions, circus performance, memorials, monuments, and museums, and the use of art and performance as a means of social education.

Austin Chinagorom Okigbo is currently on the faculty at Williams College, MA. He earned a doctorate in ethnomusicology from Indiana University; a master of music (M.M) in Sacred Music and Music Education from Westminster Choir College; and had previous training in philosophy and theology from the Pontifical Urban University, Rome. His research focuses on music in African, African-American, and African Diaspora religious experiences; Black World music and resistance movements; and music and the global politics of HIV/AIDS. His publications have appeared in the *Africa Today Journal* and *Du Bois Review* of the Cambridge Journals. He has conducted church, community, and college chorales in Nigeria, South Africa, and the United States, including the International Vocal Ensemble of the Jacobs School of Music at Indiana University.

Joseph Basil Okong'o is a lecturer in the Department of Literature, Theatre and Film, Moi University, Kenya. He teaches oral literature and African Theatre. He is currently completing his PhD in Embodiment in Luo Ohangla Music in the Department of Anthropology, Moi University. He has carried out research in the indigenous theatre of various communities in East Africa.

Daniel B. Reed is associate professor in the Department of Folklore and Ethnomusicology, and affiliated faculty in African Studies, at Indiana University. He is the author of *Dan Ge Performance: Masks and Music in Contemporary Cote d'Ivoire*, co-winner of the Amaury Talbot Prize from the Royal Anthropological Institute of London. He is also co-author, with Gloria Gibson, of the CD-ROM *Music and Culture of West Africa: The Straus Expedition*, and author of numerous articles and museum catalog entries on Ivorian music and masks. His current research projects include a study of Ivorian immigrant performers in the U.S. in the context of globalization, and a study of artistic responses to HIV/AIDS in Francophone Africa.

Gavin Steingo has published articles in *Popular Music and Society, Black Music Research Journal, African Music, African Identities,* and *Review of Disability Studies,* in addition to a number of book chapters on topics ranging from political economy and literature, to medical ethnomusicology and album cover aesthetics. Gavin recently edited a special issue of the journal *World of Music* on the topic of kwaito, a genre of South African electronic music that formed the basis of his dissertation. He is currently a Mellon Postdoctoral Fellow in the Department of Music at Columbia University and an Honorary Research Associate in the School of Social Sciences at Wits University.

ANGELA SCHARFENBERGER is a doctoral student in ethnomusicology with a minor in African Studies at Indiana University. She has presented two national conference papers on the topic "Musical Responses to AIDS in Ghana," based on fieldwork conducted in 2006. Her master's thesis examines the scholarship on women's participation in musical performance in West Africa. Her current PhD research engages Shona music and dance performance in transnational practice, with a focus on relationships between Zimbabwean and American practitioners. She is currently an adjunct instructor at Bellarmine University and IU Southeast, and performs and teaches African music.

PATRICIA TANG is associate professor in the Music and Theater Arts Section at the Massachusetts Institute of Technology. A specialist in Senegalese music, she is author of *Masters of the Sabar: Wolof Griot Percussionists of Senegal* (Temple University Press, 2007). She is the founder and co-director of Rambax, MIT's Senegalese drum ensemble and has performed extensively with Senegalese mbalax band Nder et le Setsima Group (violin) and with the Afro-mbalax band, Lamine Touré and Group Saloum (violin and keyboards). Her current book project looks at the humanitarian roots of the music management organization Africa Fête and its role in the globalization of Afropop music.

KATHLEEN VAN BUREN is lecturer in ethnomusicology in the Department of Music at the University of Sheffield, UK. She has presented at conferences worldwide on a variety of Africa-related topics, ranging from music and HIV/AIDS in Kenya to representing the Bible through African performing arts. Her work appears in journals such as *Ethnomusicology, Ethnomusicology Forum,* and *African Music,* as well as in the edited volumes *Interacting with Scriptures in Africa* (ACTON) and *African Folklore: An Encyclopedia* (Routledge). Her current research focuses on connections between music and health (e.g. for communication or therapy) in Sheffield. Van Buren received the MA and PhD from the Department of Ethnomusicology at the University of California, Los Angeles.

MELLITUS N. WANYAMA is a music educator, composer, arranger, choral trainer, dance choreographer and adjudicator of music and dance. He has taught music and dance at primary and secondary school levels in Kenya. Currently, he is a senior lecturer of music and dance in the Department of Literature, Theatre and Film Studies at Moi University, Eldoret, Kenya. In 2005, Wanyama completed his DMus degree in ethnomusicology at the University of Pretoria, South Africa. His doctoral thesis, *Form and Content of African Music: A Case Study of Bukusu Circumcision Music,* was published by VDM Verlag Dr. Muller in 2009.

ANNABELLE WIENAND is a Visual and Art History doctoral candidate affiliated to the AIDS and Society Research Unit at the University of Cape Town. Her dissertation focuses on the photographic representation of Africa, including HIV/AIDS. In the past her research interests have included visual and participatory approaches to HIV education in South Africa. Her masters thesis was short-listed for the African Thesis Award (Leiden, The Netherlands). After completing her masters degree, she was Outreach Project Manager at Community Media Trust and researched and wrote HIV education training materials before returning to academia.

SUSAN E. WILSON has been a teacher since 1970, a health educator since 1982, and a licensed marriage and family therapist (MFT) since 1998. She has served as Director of Learning

Disabilities and Preschool Deaf Programs, Department of Physical Medicine and Rehabilitation, University of Missouri School of Medicine; Health Education Coordinator of the Community Health Advocacy Program (CHAP), Brody School of Medicine, East Carolina University (ECU), Greenville, and Project Concern International; Health Education and Media Coordinator for the Center for Health Services Research and Development, Brody School of Medicine at ECU; Clinical Faculty in MFT, Division of Behavioral Medicine, Department of Family Medicine, Brody School of Medicine at ECU; Consultant for the Paramedic Intervention Program for Pregnant Teens, Department of Emergency Medicine, University of Pittsburgh Medical Center, Pittsburgh; therapist, Center for Counseling and Student Development, East Carolina University, Greenville; and therapist, Rape Crisis Center, Syracuse. Wilson has been in involved in two health education projects in Africa: health education and mass media aspects of low cost sanitation in the peri-urban areas of Dar es Salaam, Tanzania; and an AIDS awareness/education/ prevention project in Malawi.

JOHN ZARITSKY has won more than 40 awards for his documentary films. Some of his major honors include a 1982 Academy Award for his documentary "Just Another Missing Kid," a 1987 Cable Ace Award for "Rapists: Can They be Stopped," a Golden Gavel Award from the American Bar Association for "My Husband is Going to Kill Me," a Robert F. Kennedy Foundation Award for "Born in Africa," and an Alfred Dupont Award from Columbia University's School of Journalism in 1994 for "Romeo and Juliet in Sarajevo." He was an artist-in-residence at the Berkeley Graduate School of Journalism in 1995-1996, and taught documentary film at the University of British Columbia from 2002–2006.

REFERENCES

XVI International AIDS Conference. 2006. www.aids2006.org.

46664 Campaign Web site. 2007. www.46664.com.

Abah, Oga Steve with Faith, Mahmud and Nuhu. 2006. "Young People's Drama and Social Action in Northern Nigeria: A Case Study of the Zaria 'For Tomorrow...' Project." In *African Theatre Youth*, ed. M. Etherton, 42–60. Oxford: James Currey.

Abu-Lughod, Lila. 1986. *Veiled Sentiments: Honor and Poetry in Bedouin Society*. Berkeley: University of California Press.

———. 1993. "Islam and Public Culture: The Politics of Egyptian Television Serials." *Middle East Report*, 180 (Jan.–Feb.), 25–30.

———. 1997. "The Interpretation of Culture(s) After Television." *Representations* 59: 109–34.

———. 2005. *Dramas of Nationhood: The Politics of Television Serials in Egypt*. Chicago: University of Chicago.

Achieng, Judith. 2001. "Kenya: NGOs Seek to Import Generic Drugs from India." www.twnside.org.sg/title/generic.htm.

Acker, Kathy. 1997. "The Gift of Disease," *The Guardian*, January 18.

Adam, Gordon, and Nicola Harford. 1999. *Radio and HIV/AIDS: Making a Difference*. Geneva: Joint United Nations Programme on HIV/AIDS and Media Action International.

Adorno, Theodor W. 1955. *Prismen: Kulturkritik und Gesellschaft*. Frankfurt: Suhrkamp.

Africa Watch. 1990. *Where Silence Rules: The Suppression of Dissent In Malawi*. New York: Africa Watch.

African Comprehensive HIV/AIDS Partnership (ACHAP). 2006. *Setting the Stage for Scaling Up HIV Prevention—Discussion Paper*. Gaborone: ACHAP.

Agawu, Kofi. 2003. *Representing African Music: Postcolonial Notes, Queries, Positions*. New York: Routledge.

Airhihenbuwa, Collins, O. 1995. *Health and Culture: Beyond the Western Paradigm*. Thousand Oaks: SAGE Publications.

Allen, Lara. 2004. "Kwaito versus Crossed-Over: Music and Identity during South African Rainbow Years, 1994–1996." *Social Dynamics* 30 (2): 82–111.

Allison, E Jackson, Jr. 1977. "Mass Media Approaches to Nutrition Education in Developing Countries." In *Teaching Nutrition in Developing Countries or The Joys of Eating Dark Green Leaves*, ed. Kathryn W Shack, 97–104. Santa Barbara: Meals for Millions Foundation.

Altman, Dennis. 1986. *AIDS and the New Puritanism*. London: Pluto Press.

Alviso, J. Ricardo. 2003. "Applied Ethnomusicology and the Impulse to Make a Difference." *Folklore Forum* 34 (1/2): 89–96.

Amico, Stephen. 2001. "'I Want Muscles': House Music, Homosexuality and Masculine Signification." *Popular Music* 20 (3): 359–78.

Amu, Misonu. 2001. "Music and Health Messages." *Research Review* (Institute of African Studies) 17(1): 91–95.

Amuyunzu-Nyamongo, Mary, and Negussie Taffa. 2003. "The Triad of Poverty, Environment and Child Health in Nairobi Informal Settlements." www.aphrc.org/publication/wpapers.html.

Annan, Kofi, Nadine Gordimer, and Rory Kennedy. 2003. *Pandemic: Facing AIDS*. New York: Umbrage.

Appadurai, Arjun. 1996. *Modernity at Large: Culture Dimensions of Globalization*. Minneapolis: University of Minnesota Press.

———. 2000. "Grassroots Globalization and the Research Imagination." *Public Culture* 12(1): 1–19.

Apt, Nana Araba, and Ebenezer Q. Blavo. 1997. *Street Children and AIDS*. Legon: Social Administration, University of Ghana.

Apthorpe, Raymond. 2001. *Mission Possible: Six Years of WFP Emergency Food Aid in West Africa*. In *Evaluating International Humanitarian Action: Reflections from Practitioners*, eds. Adrian Wood, Raymond Apthorpe, and John Borton, 102–21. London: Zed Books.

Arbuckle, Katherine. 2004. "The Language of Pictures: Visual Literacy and Print Materials for Adult Basic Education and Training (ABET)." *Language Matters*. 35(2): 445–58.

Arendt, Hannah. 1990. *On Revolution*. Harmondsworth: Penguin Books.

ARHAP. 2006. "Appreciating Access: The Contribution of Religion to Universal Access in Africa." *Journal of Theology for Southern Africa* 12 (126): 120–26.

Aristotle. 2004. *Poetics*. Trans. S. H. Butcher. Kessinger Publishing. www.kessinger.net.

Aschwanden, Herbert. 1987 *Symbols of Death: An Analysis of the Consciousness of the Karanga*. Gweru: Mambo Press.

Ascroft, Joseph, and Sipho Masilela. 1989. "From Top-Down to Co-Equal Communication: Popular Participation in Development Decision-Making." Paper presented at the seminar Participation: A Key Concept in Communication and Change, University of Poona, India.

Ashforth, Adam. 2002. "An Epidemic of Witchcraft? The Implications of AIDS for the Post-Apartheid State." *African Studies* 61(1): 121–45.

———. 2005. *Witchcraft, Violence and Democracy in South Africa*. Chicago: University of Chicago Press.

Asiago, Sylvester M. 2004. "Let's Discuss AIDS." *Sunday Nation*, August 1, Buzz: We Got Mail, 2.

Askew, Kelly M. 2002. *Performing the Nation: Swahili Music and Cultural Politics in Tanzania*. Chicago: University of Chicago Press.

"A Strategy to Promote the Millennium Development Goals in Africa." www.ke.undp.org/Africa%202015.htm.

Austin, J. L., 1975. *How to Do Things with Words*, 2nd ed. Eds. J. O. Urmson and Marina Sbisa. Cambridge, MA: Harvard University Press.

AVERT. 2008. "HIV and AIDS in Malawi." www.avert.org/aids-malawi.htm.

The aWAKE Project: Uniting Against the African AIDS Crisis. 2002. Nashville: W Publishing Group.

Bähre, Erik. 2002. "Witchcraft and the Exchange of Sex, Blood, and Money among Africans in Cape Town, South Africa." *Journal of Religion in Africa* 32(3): 300–34.

Bakan, Michael B. 2008. "Preventive Care for the Dead: Music, Community, and the Protection of Souls in Balinese Cremation Ceremonies." In *The Oxford Handbook of Medical Ethnomusicology*, ed. Benjamin D. Koen, assoc. eds. Jacqueline Lloyd, Gregory Barz, and Karen Brummel-Smith, 246–64. New York: Oxford University Press.

Bamezai, Gita, and Archana Shukla. 1999. "The Impact of Enter-Educate Radio Broadcasts in Promoting AIDS Awareness Among the Youth: A Case Study of FM Radio's Broadcasts to Promote AIDS Awareness Among the Youth of New Delhi." In *Youth and the Global Media*, eds. Sue Ralph, Jo Langham Brown, Tim Lees, Marjorie Burton, and Edward Burton, 113–21. Luton: University of Luton Press.

Bancroft, Angus. 2001. "Globalisation and HIV/AIDS: Inequality and the Boundaries of a Symbolic Epidemic." *Health, Risk and Society* 3(1): 89–98.

Bandura, Albert. 1997. *Self-Efficacy: The Exercise of Control*. New York: W.H. Freeman and Company.

Banham, Martin, James Gibbs, and Femi Osofisan, eds. 1999. *African Theatre in Development*. Oxford: James Currey.

Barad, Dilip. 2008. "Aristotle's *Poetics*." WikiEducator. Wikieducator.org/Literary_Criticism

Barber, Karin. 1987. "Popular Arts in Africa." *African Studies Review* 3 (30): 1–78.

———. 1991. *I Could Speak Until Tomorrow: Oriki, Women and the Past in a Yuroba Town*. Edinburgh: Edinburgh University Press.

———. 1997. "Introduction." In *Readings in African Popular Culture*, ed. Karin Barber. Bloomington: Indiana University Press.

Barnett, Tony, Tsetsele Fantan, B. Mbakile, and Alan Whiteside. 2002. *The Private Sector Responds to the Epidemic—Debswana: A Global Benchmark (UNAIDS Case Study)*. Geneva: UNAIDS.

Barthes, Roland. 1977. "The Photographic Message." In *Image, Music, Text*, ed. Stephen Heath. London: Fontana Press.

Barz, Gregory. 2002. "No One Will Listen To Us Unless We Bring Our Drums! AIDS and Women's Music Performance in Uganda." In *The aWAKE Project: Uniting Against the African AIDS Crisis*, ed. Jenny Eaton and Kate Etue, 170–77. Nashville: W. Publishing.

———. 2003. *Performing Religion: Negotiating Past and Present in Kwaya Music of Tanzania, Church and Theology in Context*. Amsterdam: Rodopi.

———. 2004. *Music in East Africa: Experiencing Music, Expressing Culture*. New York: Oxford University Press.

———. 2006a. *Singing for Life: HIV/AIDS and Music in Uganda*. New York: Routledge.

———. 2006b. "'We are from Different Ethnic Groups, but We Live Here as One Family': The Musical Performance of Community in a Tanzanian *Kwaya*." In *Chorus and Community*, ed. Karen Ahlquist, 19–44. Urbana: University of Illinois Press.

Barz, Gregory and Judah Cohen. 2008. "Music and HIV/AIDS in Africa." In *The Garland Handbook of African Music, Second Edition*, ed. Ruth M. Stone, 148-159. New York: Routledge/ Taylor and Francis Group.

Barz, Gregory, and Timothy J. Cooley. 2008. "Introduction." In *Shadows in the Field: New Perspectives for Fieldwork in Ethnomusicology*, 2nd ed, 1-20. New York: Oxford University Press.

Baudrillard, Jean. 1987. *Forget Foucault*. New York: Semiotext(e).

Bauman, Richard. 2000. "Genre." *Journal of Linguistic Anthropology* 9 (1–2): 84–87.

Baylies, Carolyn. 2000. "Perspectives on Gender and AIDS in Africa." In *AIDS, Sexuality and Gender in Africa: Collective Strategies and Struggles in Tanzania and Zambia*, eds. Carolyn Baylies and Janet Bujra, 1–24. London: Routledge.

Bebey, Francis. 1975 [1969]. *African Music: A People's Art*. Brooklyn, NY: Lawrence Hills.

Beloff, Halla. 1983. "Social Interaction in Photographing." *Leonardo* 16 (3): 165–71.

Benjamin, Walter. 1977. *Das Kunstwerk im Zeitalter seiner technischen Reproduzierbarkeit*. In *Illuminationen: Ausgewählte Schriften*, ed. Siegfried Unseld. Frankfurt: Suhrkamp.

Bennett, Richard G., and Daniel W. Hale. 2009. *Building Healthy Communities Through Medical-Religious Partnerships*, 2nd ed. Baltimore: Johns Hopkins University Press.

Berger, Arthur Asa. 1990. *Scripts: Writing for Radio and Television*. Newbury Park: Sage.

Berger, Harris M. 2003. "Introduction: The Politics and Aesthetics of Language Choice and Dialect in Popular Music." In *Global Pop, Local Language*, eds. Harris M. Berger and Michael Thomas Carroll, ix–xxvi. Jackson: University Press of Mississippi.

Berger, John. 1977. *Ways of Seeing*. London: Penguin.

Berger, John, ed. 1980. *Uses of Photography*. In *About Looking*. New York: Vintage.

Berglund, Axel-Ivar. 1989. *Zulu Thought-Patterns and Symbolism*. Bloomington: Indiana University Press.

Berliner, Paul. 1993 [1981, 1978]. *The Soul of Mbira*. Chicago: University of Chicago Press.

Bhabha, Homi K. 1994. *The Location of Culture*. New York: Routledge.

Bhattacharya, Shivaji, Gulan Kripalani, Pramod Kumar, and Monica Sharma. 2005. *Arts and Media Transforming the Response to HIV/AIDS Strategy Note and Implementation Guide*. New York: UNDP.

Biblical Holistic HIV Care in Uganda: From Quality Safe Health Care to Caring for Communities. 2004. Discussion with Dr. Larry Pepper. www.ecuspace.net/contact.nsf/5e7350302ae3665 8c1256d0c004edeb3/779301F12245A988C1256EB4006784E4?OpenDocument.

Biehl, Joao. 2001. "Life in a Zone of Social Abandonment." *Social Text* 68 (19/3): 131–49.

Biressi, Anita, and Heather Nunn. 2005. *Reality TV: Realism and Revelation*. London: Wallflower Press.

Bishop, Sophie and Peter Bishop. 1998. "An Other Ethiopia." www.lefourneau.com/artistes/ circus/monde/presse/presse_tour_98.htm.

Blacking, John. 1962. "Musical Expeditions of the Venda." *African Music* 3: 54–72.

———. 1965. "The Role of Music in the Culture of the Venda of the Northern Transvaal." In *Studies in Ethnomusicology*, ed. M. Kolinski, vol. 2: 20–53. New York: Oak Publications.

———. 1967. *Venda Children's Songs: A Study in Ethnomusicological Analysis*. Johannesburg: Witwatersrand University Press.

———. 1969. "The Songs, Mimes, Dances and Symbolism of Venda Girls Initiation Schools, Part 1: Vhusha." *African Studies* 28(1): 3–35; (2): 69–107; (3): 149–79; (4): 120–44.

———. 1973. *How Musical is Man?* Seattle: University of Washington Press.

Blair, David. 2005. "White land grab has failed, Mugabe confesses." *The Telegraph*, March 3. www.telegraph.co.uk/news/worldnews/africaandindianocean/zimbabwe/1484864/White-land-grab-policy-has-failed-Mugabe-confesses.html

Blomfield, Adrian. 2001. "Activists Hail Kenya's First Generic AIDS Drugs." www.aegis.com/ news/re/2001/RE010634.html.

Boal, Augusto. 2000. *Theater of the Oppressed*. London: Pluto Press.

Bohlman, Philip V., Edith W. Blumhofer, and Maria M. Chow. 2006. *Music in American Religious Experience*. New York: Oxford University Press.

Boltanski, Luc. 1999. *Distant Suffering, Morality, Media and Politics*, trans. Graham Burchell. Cambridge: Cambridge University Press.

Bond, George and Joan Vincent. 1997a. "AIDS in Uganda: The First Decade." In *AIDS in Africa and the Caribbean*, ed. George Bond, John Kreniske, Ida Susser and Joan Vincent, 85–97. Boulder, CO: Westview Press.

———. 1997b. "Community Based Organizations in Uganda: A Youth Initiative." In *AIDS in Africa and the Caribbean*, ed. George Bond, John Kreniske, Ida Susser, and Joan Vincent, 99–113. Boulder, CO: Westview Press.

Bono. 2007. "Ich bin keine singende Mutter Teresa." 2007. Interview by Bartholomäus Grill and Ulrich Post, *Die Zeit*, 12 April: 65–66.

Boon, Richard and Jane Plastow, eds. 1998. *Theatre Matters: Performance and Culture on the World Stage*. Cambridge: Cambridge University Press.

———. 2004. *Theatre and Empowerment: Community Drama on the World Stage*. Cambridge: Cambridge University Press.

Bordowitz, Gregg. 2004. *The AIDS Crisis is Ridiculous and Other Writings: 1986–2003*. Cambridge, MA: MIT Press.

Bosch, Xavier. 2003. "Europe Refuses to Match US Cash for Ailing Global Fund." *Lancet* 362, no. 9380 (July): 299.

Botswana HIV and AIDS Second Medium Term Plan II 1997–2002. 1997. Ministry of Health. Gaborone: AIDS/STD Unit, Ministry of Health.

Botswana Millennium Development Goals Status Report 2004. Gaborone: Government of Botswana/United Nations.

Botswana National Broadcasting Policy (Draft for Public Consultation). 2003. Gaborone: Government Press, Department of Information and Broadcasting.

Bourgault, Louise M. 2003. *Playing for Life: Performance in Africa in the Age of AIDS*. Durham, NC: Carolina Academic Press.

Boutelle, Kerri N., Robert W. Jeffery, David M. Murray, and M. K. Schmitz. 2001. "Using Signs, Artwork, and Music to Promote Stair Use in a Public Building." *American Journal of Public Health* 91 (12): 2004–06.

Brice Heath, Shirley. 2000. "Seeing our Way into Learning." *Cambridge Journal of Education* 20 (1): 121–32.

Brunner, Elmar. 1998. "Circus Ethiopia: ein kleines afrikanisches Wunder. Eine sozialpädagogische Studie" (Circus Ethiopia: A Small African Marvel. A Socio-Pedagogical Study). BA Thesis, Department of Special Education, University of Cologne. Translated by Tobias Sperlich.

Bujra, Janet. 2000. "Target Practice: Gender and Generational Struggles in AIDS Prevention Work in Lushoto." In *AIDS, Sexuality and Gender in Africa: Collective Strategies and Struggles in Tanzania and Zambia*, ed. Carolyn Baylies and Janet Bujra, 114–32. New York: Routledge.

Burnim, Mellonee V. 2006. "Religious Music." In *African American Music: An Introduction*, ed. Mellonee V. Burnim and Portia K. Maultsby, 51–77. New York: Routledge.

Butler, Judith. 1993. *Bodies that Matter: On the Discursive Limits of "Sex."* New York: Routledge.

Cameron, Edwin. 2003. "AIDS Denial and Holocaust Denial–AIDS, Justice and the Courts in South Africa." *South African Law Journal* 120 (525): 525–39.

Campbell, Catherine. 2000a. "Selling Sex in the Time of AIDS: The Psycho-Social Context of Condom Use by Southern African Sex Workers." *Social Science and Medicine* 50: 479–94.

———. 2000b. "Social Capital and Health: Contextualising Health Promotion within Local Community Networks." In *Social Capital: Critical Perspectives*, ed. S. Baron, J. Field, and T. Schuller, 182–96. Oxford: Oxford University Press.

———. 2003. *"Letting Them Die": How HIV/AIDS Prevention Programmes Often Fail*. Johannesburg: James Currey.

Campbell, Catherine, and MacPhail, Catherine. 2002. "Peer Education, Gender and the Development of Critical Consciousness: Participatory HIV Prevention by South African Youth." *Social Science & Medicine* 55: 331–45.

Campbell, David. 2003a. "Salgado and the Sahel: Documentary Photography and the Imaging of Famine." In *Rituals of Mediation: International Politics and Social Meaning*, ed. François Debrix and Cynthia Weber. Minneapolis: University of Minnesota Press.

———. 2003b. "Cultural Governance and Pictorial Resistance: Reflections on the Imaging of War." *Review of International Studies* 29: 57–73.

———. 2004. "Horrific Blindness: Images of Death in Contemporary Media." *Journal of Cultural Research* 8 (1): 55–74.

"Can Musicians Save Africa?" 1994. BBC News, October 15. news.bbc.co.uk/2/hi/world/africa/3746666.stm[A]

"Care and Treatment Services at Sinikithemba." 2010. www.mccord.org.za/cgi-bin/giga.cgi?cat=1409&limit=10&page=0&sort=D&cause_id=1285&cmd=cause_dir_news

Carroll, John. 1993. *Humanism: The Wreck of Western Culture*. London: Fontana Press.

Carpenter, Diane J., Isaac A.K. Chirwa, E. Jackson Allison Jr., Kathleen A. Dunn, and Theodore Sneed. 1996. "Emergency Physician Involvement in Public Health: AIDS Education/Prevention Project in Malawi." *Annals of Emergency Medicine* 28 (5Abst): 563–64.

Carstens, Adelia, Alfons Maes, and Lilian Gangla-Birir. 2006. "Understanding Visuals in HIV/AIDS Education in South Africa: Differences Between Literate and Low-literate Audiences." *African Journal of AIDS Research* 5 (3): 221–32.

Center for Communication Programs. 2005a. "Wake Up Africa! Lève-toi, Afrique!" Baltimore: Johns Hopkins University Bloomberg School of Public Health, www.jhuccp.org/topics/enter_ed/eeprojects/02-11.shtml

Center for Communication Programs. 2005b. "Family Health and AIDS Project (Santé Familliale et Prévention du Sida): The Wake Up Campaign." Baltimore: Johns Hopkins University Bloomberg School of Public Health, Africa: Audio/Video, www.jhuccp.org/africa/av.shtml.

Chauvet, Louis-Marie. 1995. *Symbol and Sacrament*. Trans. Patrick Madigan and Madeleine Beaumont. Collegeville, MN: Pueblo Press.

Chavez, Vivian, Barbara Israel, Alex J. Allen, Maggie F. DeCarlo, Richard Lichtenstein, Amy Schulz, Irene S. Bayer, and Robert McGranaghan. 2004. "A Bridge Between Communities: Video-making Using Principles of Community-Based Participatory Research." *Health Promotion Practice* 5 (4): 395–403.

Cheesbrough, J.S. 1986. "Acquired Immunodeficiency Syndrome in Malawi." *Malawi Medical Journal* 3 (1): 5–13.

Chimombo, Steve. 2007. *Popular Responses to AIDS*. WASI 18 (1), December.

———. 2008. *AIDS Artists*.

Chimombo, Steve, and Moira Chimombo. 1996: *The Culture of Democracy, 1992–94*. Zomba: WASI.

Chisango, Tawanda. 2004. "Musicians Should Change Their HIV and AIDS Discourse." Kubatana.net, www.kubatana.net/html/archive/opin/040604tc.asp?sector=HIVAID

Chopyak, James D. 1987. "The Role of Music in Mass Media, Public Education and the Formation of Malaysian National Culture." *Ethnomusicology* 31 (3): 431–54.

Circus in Ethiopia. 2005. [Magazine] September.

Coakley, Sarah. 2007. "Palliative or Intensification? Pain and Christian Contemplation in the Spirituality of the Sixteenth-Century Carmelites." In *Pain and its Tranformations: The Interface of Biology and Culture*, ed. Coakley and Kay Kaufman Shelemay, 77–100. Cambridge: Harvard University Press.

Cobussen, Marcel. 2008. *Thresholds: Rethinking Spirituality Through Music*. Burlington: Ashgate.

Cochrane, James. 2006. "Of Bodies, Barriers, Boundaries and Bridges: Ecclesial Practice in the Face of HIV and AIDS." *Journal of Theology for Southern Africa* 126 (2): 7–26.

Cohen, Stanley, and Bruna Seu. 2002. "Knowing Enough Not to Feel Too Much: Emotional Thinking about Human Rights Appeals." In *Truth Claims: Representation and Human Rights*, ed. Mark Philip Bradley and Patrice Petro, 187–204. New Brunswick: Rutgers University Press.

Collins, John. 2002. "The Generational Factor in Ghanaian Music: Concert Parties, Highlife, Simpa, Kpanlogo, Gospel and Local Techno-Pop." In *Playing with Identities in Contemporary Music in Africa*, ed. Mai Palmberg and Annamette Kirkegaard, 60–74. Uppsala, Finland: Nordik Afrikainstitutet.

Comaroff, Jean, and John L. Comaroff. 1992. *Ethnography and the Historical Imagination*. Boulder: Westview Press.

———. 2000 "Millennial Capitalism: First Thoughts on a Second Coming." *Public Culture* 12 (2): 291–343.

———. 2004. "Notes on Afromodernity and the Neo World Order: An Afterword." In *Producing African Futures: Ritual and Reproduction in a Neoliberal Age*, ed. Brad Weiss. Leiden: Brill.

———. 2006. "Law and Disorder in the Postcolony: An Introduction," in *Law and Disorder in the Postcolony*, 1–56. Chicago: University of Chicago Press.

Communication Initiative Network. Accessed November 10, 2009. www.comminit.com

Comprehensive Health Sector Policy on Care and Treatment. 2001. Ministry of Health. Gaborone: Ministry of Health.

Connolly, William E. 1995. *The Ethos of Pluralization*. Minneapolis: University of Minnesota Press.

———. 2005. *Pluralism*. Durham: Duke University Press.

Cooper, Frederick. 2005. *Colonialism in Question: Theory, Knowledge, History*. Berkeley: University of California Press.

Coplan, David. 1994. *In the Time of Cannibals: The Word Music of South Africa's Basotho Migrants*. Chicago: University of Chicago Press.

———. 2005. "God Rock Africa: Thoughts on Politics in Popular Black Performance in South Africa." *African Studies* 64 (1): 9–27.

Cornwall, Andrea. 1996. "Participatory Research Methods: First Steps in a Participatory Process." In *Participatory Research in Health*. ed. K. Koning and M. Martin, 95–105. New Delhi: Vistaar Publications.

———. 2002. "Body Mapping: Bridging the Gap between Biomedical Messages, Popular Knowledge and Lived Experience." In *Realizing Rights: Transforming Approaches to Sexual and Reproductive Well-Being*, ed. Andrea Cornwall and Alice Welbourn. London: Zed Books.

Cornwall, Andrea, and Rachel Jewkes.1995. "What is Participatory Research?" *Social Science Medicine* 41 (12): 1667–74.

Correll, Joshua, Steven J. Spencer, and Mark P. Zanna. 2004. "An Affirmed Self and an Open Mind: Self-Affirmation and Sensitivity to Argument Strength." *Journal of Experimental Social Psychology* 40 (3) (May): 350–56.

Crimp, Douglas. 1988. *AIDS: Cultural Analysis, Cultural Activism*. Cambridge, MA: MIT Press.

———. 2002. *Melancholia and Moralism: Essays on HIV/AIDS and Queer Politics*. Cambridge, MA: MIT Press.

Crook, Timothy. 1999. *Radio Drama: Theory and Practice*. New York: Routledge.

Crowe, Sarah. 2006. "Hip-hop Star Zola Named UNICEF Goodwill Ambassador at African Development Forum." www.unicef.org/infobycountry/southafrica_36606.html.

Cueva, Melany, Regina Kuhnley, Anne Lanier, and Mark Dignan. 2005. "Using Theater to Promote Cancer Education in Alaska." *Journal of Cancer Education* 20 (1): 45–48.

Curwen, John. 1872. *The Standard Course of Lectures & Exercises in the Tonic Sol-Fa Method of Teaching Music*. London: Tonic Sol-Fa Agency.

D'Adesky, Anne-Christine. 2004. *Moving Mountains: The Race to Treat Global AIDS*. London: Verso.

Davis, Ronald M. 2003. "Kids Campaign Against Tobacco." *Tobacco Control* 12 (3): 243–44.

Davis, Susan R. 2003. "Climacteric Symptoms Among Indigenous Australian Women and a Model for the Use of Culturally Relevant Art in Health Promotion." *Menopause* 10 (4): 345–51.

De Bruyn, M. 1992. "Women and AIDS in Developing Countries." *Social Science and Medicine* 34 (3): 249–62.

de Certeau, Michel. 1998. "How is Christianity Thinkable Today." In *The Postmodern God: A Theological Reader*, ed. Graham Ward, 142–58. West Sussex: Blackwell.

de Fossard, Esta. 1996. *How to Write a Radio Serial Drama for Social Development: A Script Writer's Manual.* Baltimore: The Johns Hopkins University School of Public Health.

De Waal, Alex. 2007. *AIDS and Power: Why There is No Political Crisis—Yet.* New York: Zed Books.

Dean, Carolyn J. 2003. "Empathy, Pornography and Suffering." *Differences: A Journal of Feminist Cultural Studies* 14 (1): 88–124.

Debord, Guy. 1992. *La Société du Spectacle.* Paris: Gallimard.

Debrix, François. 2003. "Rituals of Mediation." In *Rituals of Mediation: International Politics and Social Meaning*, ed. François Debrix and Cynthia Weber. Minneapolis: University of Minnesota Press.

Della Porta, Donatella, and Mario Diani. 2006. *Social Movements*, 2nd ed. Malden, MA: Blackwell Publishing.

Deniaud, Francois. 1993a. "Musical and Clothing Invitations to Protection." *AIDS Health Promotion Exchange* 3: 12–14.

Deniaud, Francois. 1993b. "'Chaussez Capote': Des Chansons sur les Préservatifs Pour les Jeunes Africains." *Sociétés d'Afrique et SIDA: Comprendre et Agir* 1: 6.

Deniaud, Francois. N.d. "Presentation des Documents Audio-visuels sur la Prévention du SIDA." horizon.documentation.ird.fr/exl-doc/pleins_textes/dovers09-03/39152.pdf.

Derrida, Jacques. 1981. "Economimesis." *Diacritics* 11: 3–25.

———. 1987. *The Post Card: From Socrates to Freud and Beyond.* Trans. Alan Bass. Chicago: University of Chicago Press.

Desantis, Dominique. 2003. *HIV Prevention and Protection Efforts Are Failing Women and Girls.* UNAIDS: The Global Coalition on Women and AIDS.

DeShazer, Mary K. 1994. *The Poetics of Resistance: Women Writing in El Salvador, South Africa, and the United States.* Ann Arbor: University of Michigan Press.

Detterbeck, Markus. 2002. *South African Choral Music (Amakwaya): Song, Contest and the Formation of Identity.* PhD diss., University of KwaZulu-Natal.

District Response Initiative. 2003. "District Response Initiative on HIV/AIDS Action Research: Study Report-Mbarara District." www.aidsuganda.org/pdf/Mbarara_DRI_AR_Report.pdf.

Doctors Without Borders. 2007. "Treating HIV/AIDS in Malawi." doctorswithoutborders.org/publications/reports/2001/Malawi_12-2001.cfm

Donnelly, John. 2006. "HIV Hits Africa's Rich Hardest, Study Says: Analysis Disputes Long-held Beliefs." *The Boston Globe*, June 14.

Doty, Roxanne Lynn. 1996. *Imperial Encounters: The Politics of Representation in North-South Relations.* Minneapolis: University of Minnesota Press.

Dowling, Tessa. 2007. "HIV/AIDS and African Languages." www.africanvoices.co.za/research/aidsresearch.htm.

"'Dream Doctor' in Addis." 2007. *Capital* [Ethiopia], August 12.

Drewal, Margaret. 1991. "The State of Research on Performance in Africa." *African Studies Review* 34 (3): 1–64.

During, Jean. 2008. "Therapeutic Dimensions of Music in Islamic Culture." In *The Oxford Handbook of Medical Ethnomusicology*, ed. Benjamin D. Koen, assoc. eds. Jacqueline Lloyd, Gregory Barz, and Karen Brummel-Smith. New York: Oxford University Press, 361–392.

Ecks, Stefan. 2006. "Near-Liberalism: Global Corporate Citizenship and Pharmaceutical Marketing in India." Paper presented at London School of Economics Anthropology seminar.

"A Turning-point for AIDS?" 2000. *The Economist.* July 15: 77–79.

Edkins, Jenny. 2005. "Exposed Singularity." *Journal for Cultural Research* 9 (4): 359–86.

Ek, Anne. 2005. "Perilous Silence and Discriminatory Visibility: On Absent and Present Representations of HIV-positive Individuals in the South African Press, 1998–2003." In *No Name Fever: AIDS in the Age of Globalization*, ed. Maj-Lis Foller and Hakan Thorn. Lund: Studentlitteratur AB.

Elbe, Stefan. 2005. "AIDS, Security, Biopolitics." *International Relations* 19 (4): 403–19.

Elwood, William, ed. 1999. *Power in the Blood: A Handbook on AIDS, Politics, and Communication.* London: Lawrence Erlbaum Associates.

Epskamp, Kees. 2006. *Theatre for Development: An Introduction.* New York: Zed Books.

Epstein, Helen. 2007. *The Invisible Cure: Africa, the West, and the Fight Against AIDS.* New York: Farrar, Straus, and Giroux.

Epstein, Steven. 2005. "AIDS Activism and the State Policies in the United States." In *No Name Fever: AIDS in the Age of Globalization*, ed. Maj-Lis Foller and Hakan Thorn. Lund: Studentlitteratur AB.

Erlmann, Veit. 1991. *African Stars: Studies in Black South African Performance.* Chicago: University of Chicago Press.

———. 1996. *Nightsong.* Chicago: University of Chicago Press.

Etherton, Michael, ed. 2006. *African Theatre Youth.* Oxford: James Currey.

Euba, Akin. 1990. *Yoruba Drumming: The Dùndún Tradition.* Bayreuth, Germany: Eckhard Breitinger.

Evans, H. Martyn. 2007. "Medicine and Music: Three Relations Considered." *Journal of Medical Humanities* 28 (3): 135–48.

Evian, Clive. 1992. "Community Theater in AIDS Education in South Africa." *Progress Reports on Health & Development in Southern Africa* (Spring–Summer): 34–7.

Ewald, Wendy. 1998. "Innocent Eye, Conversation with Wendy Ewald." globetrotter.berkeley.edu/Ewald/ewald-con4.html.

Fadiman, Anne. 1997. *The Spirit Catches You and You Fall Down: A Hmong Child, Her American Doctors, and the Collision of Two Cultures.* New York: Farrar, Strauss, and Giroux.

Fanon, Frantz. 2004 [1963]. *The Wretched of the Earth.* Tr. Constance Farrington. New York: Grove Press.

Farber, Celia. 1998. "AIDS as Metaphor." *Impression* (November).

Farmer, Paul. 1988. "Bad Blood, Spoiled Milk: Bodily Fluids and Moral Barometers in Rural Haiti." *American Ethnologist* 15 (1): 62–83.

———. 1990. "Sending Sickness: Sorcery, Politics and Changing Concepts of AIDS in Rural Haiti." *Medical Anthropology Quarterly* 4 (1): 6–27.

———. 1994. "AIDS Talk and the Constitution of Cultural Models." *Social Science and Medicine* 38 (6): 801–09.

———. 2006 [1992] *AIDS and Accusations: Haiti and the Geography of Blame.* Berkeley: University of California Press.

Farmer, Paul, and Arthur Kleinman. 1989. "AIDS as Human Suffering." *Daedalus* 118 (2): 135–60.

Fassin, Didier. 2007. *When Bodies Remember: Experiences and Politics of AIDS in South Africa.* Berkeley: University of California Press.

Ferguson, James and Akhil Gupta. 2002. "Spatializing states: Toward an Ethnography of Neoliberal Governmentality." *American Ethnologist* 29 (4): 981–1002.

Fidzani, Boga. 2003. "HIV/AIDS Preventive Behavior in Botswana: Trends and Determinants at the Turn of the 21st Century." PhD diss., University of Southern California.

Figueroa, Maria Elena, D. Lawrence Kincaid, Manju Rani and Gary Lewis. 2002. "Communication for Social Change: An Integrated Model for Measuring the Process and its Outcomes." New York: The Rockefeller Foundation.

Fitzgerald, Timothy. 2000. *The Ideology of Religious Studies.* New York: Oxford University Press.

Fleury, Jean-Mark. 2004. "Development Journalism or Just Good Journalism." www.bbc.co.uk/worldservice/trust/2015/story/2004/06/040609_jean_marc_fleury.shtml.

Forster, P. G. 1994. "Culture, Nationalism, and the Invention of Tradition in Malawi." *The Journal of Modern African Studies*, 32 (3): 477–97.

Frank, Marion. 1995. *AIDS Education Through Theatre: Case Studies from Uganda.* Bayreuth: University of Bayreuth Press.

Freedman, Jane, and Nana Poku. 2005. "The Socioeconomic Context of Africa's Vulnerability to HIV/AIDS." *Review of International Studies* 31 (4): 665–86.

Freedman, Jo. 1973. The Origins of the Women's Liberation Movement. *The American Journal of Sociology.* 78 (4): 792–811.

Freire, Paulo. 1997 [1970]. *Pedagogy of the Oppressed.* New York: Continuum.

———. 1994. *Pedagogy of Hope.* New York: Continuum.

Friday, Jonathan. 2000. "Demonic Curiosity and the Aesthetics of Documentary Photography." *British Journal of Aesthetics* 40 (5): 356–75.

Friedman, G. 1992. "AIDS in South Africa: Puppet Power." *Links* 9 (1): 20–22.

Friedson, Steven M. 1996. *Dancing Prophets: Musical Experience in Tumbuka Healing.* Chicago: University of Chicago Press.

Galavotti C., M. Mooki, C. Collins Lovell, M. Kejelepula, K. Pappas-DeLuca, and P. Kilmarx. 2003. "M.A.R.C.H. and the Impact of *Makgabaneng* on the use of the *Ipoletse* HIV/AIDS Information Hotline." Presentation at the National HIV/AIDS Research and Other Related Infectious Disease Conference, December 8, Gaborone International Conference Center (GICC).

Galavotti, C., K. A. Pappas-DeLuca, and A. Lansky. 2001. "Modeling and Reinforcement to Combat HIV: The MARCH Approach to Behavior Change." *American Journal of Public Health* 91 (10): 1602–07.

Gausset, Quentin. 2001. "AIDS and Cultural Practices in Africa: The Case of the Tonga (Zambia)." *Social Science and Medicine* 52: 509–18.

Gell, Alfred. 1999. "Vogel's Net: Traps as Artworks and Artworks as Traps." In *The Art of Anthropology: Essays and Diagrams*, ed. Eric Hirsch and Alfred Gell. London: The Athlone Press.

Gere, David. 2004. *How to Make Dances in an Epidemic: Tracking Choreography in the Age of AIDS.* Madison: University of Wisconsin Press.

Gibson, Mawira. 2000. "The Role of Traditional Music and Dances in Primary Health Care Programme in Kenya Today." BEd thesis, Kenyatta University.

Gilbert, Shirli. 2007. "Singing Against Apartheid: ANC Cultural Groups and the International Anti-Apartheid Struggle." *Journal of Southern African Studies* 33 (2): 423–41.

Gillespie, Kelly. 2008. "Moralizing Security: 'Corrections' and the Post-Apartheid Prison." *Race/Ethnicity* 2 (1): 69–87.

Gilman, Lisa and John Fenn. 2006. "Dance, Gender, and Popular Music in Malawi: The Case of Rap and Ragga." *Popular Music* 25 (3): 369–81.

GNA (Ghana News Agency). 2004a. "Okuapeman wins Young and Wise singing competition," June 27. pda.modernghana.com/mobile/739/3/okuapeman-wins-young-and-wise-singing-competition.html.

———. 2004b. "Aggrey Memorial School Wins Debate Competition" June 15. www.modernghana .com/music/722/3/aggrey-memorial-school-wins-debate-competition.html

Goals Status Report. 2004. Gaborone: Government of Botswana/United Nations.

Godby, Michael. 1998. "Dismantling the Symbolic Structure of Afrikaner Nationalism: Gideon Mendel's Beloofde Land Photographs (1989)." *South African Historical Journal* 39: 111–28.

Good, Byron. 1994. *Medicine, Rationality and Experience: An Anthropological Perspective*. Cambridge: Cambridge University Press.

Gottesman, Eric. 2003. "Project Proposal, Hope for Children" (E-mail message).

Grey-Felder, Denise. 1997. "Communication and Social Change: Forging Strategies for the 21st Century." New York: Rockefeller Foundation.

Groombridge, Brian. 1972. *Television and the People: A Program for Democratic Participation*. Harmondsworth: Penguin.

Grundberg, Andy. 1990. *Crisis of the Real: Writings on Photography*. New York: Aperture.

Guay, L., Musoke, P., Fleming T., Bagenda, D., Allen, M., Nakabiito, C., Sherman, J., Bakaki, P., Ducar, C., Deseyve, M., Emel, L., Mirochnick, M., Fowler, M.G., Mofenson, L., Miotti, P., Dransfield, K., Bray, D., Mmiro, F. & J.B. Jackson. 1999. "Intrapartum and neonatal single-dose nevirapine compared with zidovudine for prevention of mother-to-child transmission of HIV-1 in Kampala, Uganda: HIVNET 012 randomised trial." *Lancet* 354: 795–802.

Guillemin, Marilys. 2004. "Understanding Illness: Using Drawings as a Research Method." *Qualitative Health Research* 14 (2): 272–89.

Gunderson, Frank. 2000. "Witchcraft, Witcraft and Musical Warfare: The Rise of the Bagiika-Bagaalu Music Competitions in Sukumaland, Tanzania." In *Mashindano: Competitive Music Performance in East Africa*, ed. Frank Gunderson and Gregory Barz. Dar es Salaam: Mkuki na Nyota Publishers.

Gunner, Liz. 2000a. "Wrestling with the Present, Beckoning the Past: Contemporary Zulu Radio Drama." *Journal of Southern African Studies* 26 (2): 223–37.

———. 2000b. "Zulu Radio Drama." In *Senses of Culture: South African Culture Studies*, ed. Sarah Nuttall and Cheryl-Ann Michael, 216–30. Cape Town: Oxford University Press.

———. 2005. "Zulu Choral Music—Performing Identities." Lecture in Music of Africa and the Middle East course, February 10, University of California, Los Angeles.

Haas, Peter Jan, and Thomas Gesthuizen. 2000. "*Ndani ya Bongo*: KiSwahili Rap Keeping it Real." In *Mashindano: Competitive Music Performance in East Africa*, ed. Frank Gunderson and Gregory Barz. Dar es Salaam: Mkuki na Nyota Publishers.

Hadland, Adrian, Michael Aldridge, and Joshua Ogada. 2006. *Revisioning Television: Policy, Strategy and Models for the Sustainable Development of Community Television in South Africa*. Cape Town: Human Sciences Research Council.

Hainsworth, Shawn. 2006. *Raising Their Voices: The Story of the Sinikithemba Choir* [Video Recording]. Philadelphia.

Hall, Stuart. 1997. *Representation: Cultural Representations and Signifying Practices*. London: SAGE Publications.

Hamm, Charles. 1991a. "'The Constant Companion of Man': Separate Development, Radio Bantu, and Music." *Popular Music* 10 (2): 147–73.

———. 1991b. "Music and Radio in the People's Republic of China." *Asian Music* 22 (2): 1–42.

Hamutyinei, M. A., and Albert B. Plangger. 1974. *Tsumo-Shumo : Shona Proverbial Lore and Wisdom*. Shona Heritage Series, Volume 2. Gweru: Mambo Press.

Hannan, M. 2000 [1981]. *Standard Shona Dictionary*. Harare: College Press.

Harris, Gregory E. 2006. "Practicing HIV/AIDS Community-Based Research." *AIDS Care* 18 (7): 731–38.

Harrison, Barbara. 2002. "Seeing Health and Illness Worlds—Using Visual Methodologies. A Methodological Review." *Sociology of Health and Illness* 24(6): 856–72.

Heald, Suzette. 2006. "Abstain or Die: The Development of HIV/AIDS Policy in Botswana." *Journal of Biosocial Science* 38: 29–41.

Heidegger, Martin. 1962. *Being and Time*. New York: Harper and Row.

———. 1981. *Erläuterungen zu Hölderlins Dichtung*. Frankfurt: Klostermann.

Heinonen, Paula M. 2000. "Anthropology of Street Children in Addis Ababa, Ethiopia." PhD diss., Durham University.

Henderson, Clara. 1995. "A Paradigm of Africanisation: Music of Mvano Women of the Church of Central Africa Presbyterian, Malawi." MA thesis, Indiana University.

Heywood, Mark. 2003. "Preventing Mother-to-Child HIV Transmission in South Africa: Background, Strategies and Outcomes of the Treatment Action Campaign Case Against the Minister of Health." *South African Journal on Human Rights* 19: 278–315.

Higgins, Nicholas. 2001. "Image and Identity: Mexican Indians and Photographic Art." *Social Alternatives* 20 (4):22–36.

Hilts, Philip J. 1988. "Out of Africa: Dispelling Myths about AIDS: Origins, Values, Politics." *Washington Post*, May 24.

Hladik, W., F. Kaharuza, R. Bunnell, J. Mermin, and J. Musinguzi. 2008. "The Estimated Burden of HIV/AIDS in Uganda, 2005-2010." *AIDS* 22 (4): 503–10.

Hodes, Rebecca. 2007. "HIV/AIDS in South African Documentary Film, c. 1990–2000," *Journal of Southern African Studies* 33 (1): 153–71.

Hodes, Rebecca & T. Naimak Holm. 2011. "Piloting ART in South Africa: The role of partnerships in the Western Cape's provincial roll-out", Centre for Social Research Working Paper, University of Cape Town, March. www.cssr.uct.ac.za/publications.

hooks, bell. 1994. *Teaching to Transgress: Education as the Practice of Freedom*. New York: Routledge.

Hooper, Edward. 1990. *Slim: A Reporter's Own Story of HIV/AIDS in East Africa*. London: The Bodley Head.

Hope for Children. 2003. *Annual Report 2003*. Addis Ababa: HFC.

Horrigan, Brian. 1993. "Notes on AIDS and Its Combatants: An Appreciation." In *Theorizing Documentary*, ed. Michael Renov. New York: Routledge.

Hospice Africa Uganda. 2003. *Tenth Annual Report: 1 April 2002 to 31 March 2003*. Kisubi, Uganda: Marianum Press.

Human Rights Watch. 2001. *In the Shadow of Death: HIV/AIDS and Children's Rights in Kenya*. Washington: Human Rights Watch.

Hunter, Mark. 2002. "The Materiality of Everyday Sex: Thinking Beyond Prostitution." *African Studies* 61 (1): 99–120.

Hussein, Ebrahim. 1969a. *Kinjektile*. Dar es Salaam: Oxford University Press.

———. 1969b. *Wakati Ukuta*. Dar es Salaam: EAPH.

———. 1983. "Hatua mbalimbali za kubuni na kutunga Tamthiliya kufuatana na misingi ya Ki-Aristotle." In *Makala za semina ya Kimataifa ya Waandishi wa Kiswahili: Fasihi III*. Dar es Salaam: TUKI.

Hyslop, Graham. 1957a. *Afadhali Mchawi*. Nairobi: Oxford University Press.

———. 1957b. *Mgeni Karibu*. Nairobi: Oxford University Press.

Ignatieff, Michael. 1998. *The Warrior's Honor: Ethnic War and the Modern Conscience*. London: Chatto & Windus.

Iliffe, John. 2006. *The African AIDS Epidemic: A History*. Athens, OH: Ohio University Press.

Impey, Angela. 2001. "Resurrecting the Flesh: Reflections of Women in Kwaito." *Agenda* 49: 44–50.

Ingstad, Benedicte. 1990. "The Cultural Construction of AIDS and Its Consequences for Prevention in Botswana." *Medical Anthropology Quarterly* 4 (1): 28–40.

Irobi, Esiaba. 2006. "African Youth, Performance & the HIV/AIDS Epidemic: Theatre of Necessity." In *African Theatre Youth*, ed. M. Etherton, 31–41. Oxford: James Currey.

James, Deborah. 1999. *Songs of the Women Migrants: Performance and Identity in South Africa*. Edinburgh: International African Institute, Edinburgh University Press.

———. 2002. "To Take the Information Down to the People: Life Skills and HIV/AIDS Peer Educators in the Durban Area." *African Studies*, 61 (1): 169–193.

———. 2006. "'Black Background': Life History and Migrant Women's Music in South Africa." In *The Musical Human: Rethinking John Blacking's Ethnomusicology in the Twenty-First Century*, ed. Suzel Reily. Aldershot: Ashgate.

———. 2007. *Gaining Ground? "Rights" and "Property" in South African Land Reform*. London: Routledge.

———. 2011. "The Return of the Broker: Concensus, Hierarchy and Choice in South African Land Reform." *Journal of the Royal Anthropological Institute* 17 (2): 318–38.

Jamil, Ishtiaq, and Roberts Muriisa. 2004. "Building Social Capital in Uganda: The Role of NGOs in Mitigating HIV/AIDS Challenges." Working Paper presented at conference of the International Society for Third Sector Research, July. Toronto.

Janis, Tim. 2002. *A Thousand Summers: Special AIDS in Africa Benefit Edition* (CD recording). Church World Service.

Jayaprakash, Yesudhassan Thomas. 2000. "Remote Audiences Beyond 2000: Radio, Everyday Life, and Development in South India." *International Journal of Cultural Studies* 3 (2): 227–39.

Johns Hopkins University Bloomberg School of Public Health. 2009. "Stop AIDS/ Love Life." October. www.jhuccp.org/africa/ghana/stopaids.

Johnson, Tuli. 2000. "Vision 2016 Update: The Present State of What Needs to be Done in the Next Five Years." In *Public Private Partnership in Development: Towards Vision 2016 Proceedings of the Sixth National Business Conference (2000)*, ed. A. Gergis, 36–42. Gaborone: Botswana Confederation of Commerce, Industry and Manpower (BOCCIM).

Jooma, Miriam. 2003. "South African Protest Songs Find Different Themes." *Reuters News Media* October 14. www.aegis/news/re/2003/RE031015.html.

Juhasz, Alexandra. 1995. *AIDS TV: Identity, Community, and Alternative Video*. Durham: Duke University Press.

Kahigi, K. Kulikoyera and Ahamad Ngemera. 1976. *Mwanzo wa Tufani*. Dar es Salaam: TPH.

Kaleeba, Noerine, and Sunanda Ray. 2002. *We Miss You All: Noerine Kaleeba: AIDS in the Family*, 2nd ed. Harare, Zimbabwe: SAfAIDS.

Kaliati, E., and K. Ning'ang'a. n.d. *Wamkulu ndani m'banja?* Blantyre: Studio K.

Kalipeni, E., J. Oppong, and A. Zerai. 2007. "HIV/AIDS, Gender, Agency and Empowerment Issues in Africa." *Social Science and Medicine* 64 (5): 1015–18.

Kamaldien, Yazeed. 2003. "Condom Wise," *Y Mag* Dec/Jan: 34–36.

Kanjo, C. and John Lwanda. 2009. "IT and Hits: Creating a Recording Industry from Scratch in Malawi," Unpublished paper.

Kanjo, G. and Gomile, F. 1993. "The Representation of Women in Malawian Mainstream Media." Research Publications Conference, August 25. Zomba.

Kant, Immanuel. 1987. *Critique of Judgment*. Trans. Werner S. Pluhar. Indianapolis: Hackett.

"Karibu Gadonet.com." 2007. www.gadonet.com.

Karkou, Vassiliki, and Judy Glasman. 2004. "Arts, Education and Society: The Role of the Arts in Promoting the Emotional Well being and Social Inclusion of Young People." *Support for Learning* 19 (2): 57–65.

Katalanos, Nikki. L. 1994. "When Yes Means No: Verbal and Nonverbal Communication of Southeast Asian Refugees in the New Mexico Health Care System." MA Thesis, University of Mexico.

Kaufert, Joseph M., and Robert W. Putsch. 1997. "Communication Through Interpreters in Health Care: Ethical Dilemmas Arising from Differences in Class, Culture, Language, and Power." *The Journal of Clinical Ethics* 8: 71–87.

Kayambazinthu, Edrinnie. 1998. "The Language Planning Situation in Malawi." *Journal of Multilingual and Multicultural Development* 19 (5/6): 369.439.

Kean, Fergal. 1998. "Another Picture of Starving Africa: It Could Have Been Taken in 1984, or 1998." *Guardian Media Supplement*, June 8.

Kebede, Ashenafi. 1982. *Roots of Black Music: The Vocal, Instrumental, and Dance Heritage of Africa and Black America*. Trenton: Africa World.

Kenya Music Festival Foundation Presents National Music Festival Programme. 1996. Nairobi: Ministry of Education.

Kenya Music Festival Foundation: Syllabus. 2004. Nairobi, Kenya: Ministry of Education, Science, and Technology.

———. 2005. Nairobi, Kenya: Ministry of Education, Science, and Technology.

———. 2006. Nairobi, Kenya: Ministry of Education, Science, and Technology.

Kenya Music Festival Programme. 2005. Nairobi, Kenya: Ministry of Education, Science, and Technology.

Kerr, David. 2002. "Theatre and Social Issues in Malawi: Performers, Audiences, Aesthetics." In *The Performance Arts of Africa: A Reader*, ed. F. Harding, 311–20. New York: Routledge.

Kerr, David, ed. 2008. *African Theatre: Southern Africa*. Trenton: Africa World Press.

Kezilahabi, Euphrase. 2005. "Signs of New Features in the Swahili Novel." *Research in African Literatures* 36 (1): 91–108.

Kiango, Saifu. 1973. "Maendeleo ya Fasihi ya Kiswahili upande wa michezo ya kuigiza," *Kiswahili* 43 (2): 88–97.

Kidula, Jean Ngoya. 1996. "Cultural Dynamism in Process: The Kenya Music Festival." *Ufahamu* 24 (2/3): 63–81.

"Kijani Kenya." 2009. www.kijanikenyatrust.org.

Kleinman, Arthur, 1981. *Patients and Healers in the Context of Culture: An Exploration of the Borderland Between Anthropology, Medicine, and Psychiatry*. Berkeley: University of California Press.

Koelble, Thomas A., and Ed Lipuma. 2005. "Traditional Leaders & Democracy: Cultural Politics in the Age of Globalisation." In *Limits to Liberation after Apartheid: Citizenship, Government & Culture*, ed. Steven L. Robins. Oxford: James Currey.

Koen, Benjamin D. 2003. "Devotional Music and Healing in Badakhshan, Tajikistan: Preventive and Curative Practices," PhD diss., Columbus: Ohio State University.

———. 2005. "Medical Ethnomusicology in the Pamir Mountains: Music and Prayer in Healing." *Ethnomusicology*, 49 (2): 287–311.

———. 2008. "Music-Prayer-Meditation Dynamics in Healing." In *The Oxford Handbook of Medical Ethnomusicology*, ed. Benjamin D. Koen, assoc. eds. Jacqueline Lloyd, Gregory Barz, and Karen Brummel-Smith, 93–120. New York: Oxford University Press.

———. 2009. *Beyond the Roof of the World: Music, Prayer, and Healing in the Pamir Mountains*. New York: Oxford University Press.

Koen, Benjamin D., ed., assoc. eds. Jacqueline Lloyd, Gregory Barz, and Karen Brummel-Smith. 2008. *The Oxford Handbook of Medical Ethnomusicology*. New York: Oxford University Press.

Koen, Benjamin, Gregory Barz, and Kenneth Brummel-Smith. 2008. "The Confluence of Consciousness in Music, Medicine and Culture," in *The Oxford Handbook of Medical Ethnomusicology*. ed. Benjamin D. Koen, assoc. eds. Jacqueline Lloyd, Gregory Barz, and Karen Brummel-Smith. New York: Oxford University Press.

Koenig, Harold G. 2008. "Religion, Spirituality, and Healing: Research, Dialogue, and Directions." In *The Oxford Handbook of Medical Ethnomusicology*, ed. Benjamin D. Koen, assoc. eds. Jacqueline Lloyd, Gregory Barz, and Karen Brummel-Smith, 46–71. New York: Oxford University Press.

Korfmacher, D. 2001. "Tuku Music: Reflections of Zimbabwean Society Through the Music of Oliver Mtukudzi." MA thesis, SOAS, University of London.

Kothari, M.P., and Kothari, V.K. 1997. "Cross-Cultural Health Challenges: An Insight into Small American Community Hospitals." *Journal of Hospital Marketing* 12: 23–32.

Kruger, Jaco. 1993. "A Cultural Analysis of Venda Guitar Songs." PhD diss., Rhodes University, South Africa.

———. 1999/2000. "'Of Wizards and Madmen': Venda *Zwilombe*, Part I." *South African Journal of Musicology*. 19/20: 15–29.

Kruger, Loren. 2004. "Theatre for Development and TV Nation: Notes on Educational Soap Opera in South Africa." In *African Drama and Performance*, ed. John Conteh-Morgan and Tejumola Olaniyan, 155–75. Bloomington: Indiana University Press.

Kuria, Henry. 1957. *Nakupenda Lakini*. Nairobi: Oxford University Press.

Kwami, Robert Mawuena, Eric Ayisi Akrofi, and Sean Adams. 2003. Integrating Musical Arts Cultures." In *Musical Arts in Africa: Theory, Practice, and Education*, ed. Anri Herbst, Meki Nzewi, and Kofi Agawu, 261–78. Pretoria: University of South Africa Press.

Kwaramba, Alice Dadirai. 1997. *Popular Music and Society: The Language of Chimurenga Music: The Case of Thomas Mapfumo in Zimbabwe*. Oslo: University of Oslo.

Kyker, Jennifer. 2009. "Carrying Spirit in Song: Music and the Making of Ancestors at Zezuru *Kurova Guva* Ceremonies." *African Music* 8 (3): 65–84.

LaChance, Marc and Sigfrid Soler. 1995. "Reach for the Stars." *The Magazine of the International Red Cross and Red Crescent Movement* 3: 22–23.

La Fontaine, Jean de. 1985. *Initiation*. London: Penguin.

Lambek. 2002. "Nuriaty, the Saint, and the Sultan: Virtuous Subject and Subjective Virtuoso of the Postmodern Colony." In *Postcolonial Subjectivities in Africa*, ed. Richard Werbner, 25–43. London: Zed Books.

Laplanche, Jean. 1976. *Life and Death in Psychoanalysis*. Trans. Jeffrey Mehlman. Baltimore: The Johns Hopkins University Press.

Latour, Bruno. 2000. "When Things Strike Back: A Possible Contribution of Science Studies." *British Journal of Sociology* 5 (1): 105–123.

Law, Sweety and Arvind Singhal. 1999. "Efficacy in Letter-Writing to an Entertainment-Education Radio Serial." *Gazette* 61: 355–72.

Lawless, Elaine. 1993. *Holy Women, Wholly Women: Sharing Ministries through Life Stories and Reciprocal Ethnography.* Philadelphia: University of Pennsylvania Press.

Lear, Jonathan. 2006. *Radical Hope: Ethics in the Face of Cultural Devastation.* Cambridge, MA: Harvard University Press.

Leclerc-Madlala, Suzanne. 2002. "On the Virgin Cleansing Myth: Gendered Bodies, AIDS and Ethnomedicine." *African Journal of AIDS Research* 1: 87–95.

Lee, Byoungkwan. 2004. "The Effectiveness of Entertainment-Education as Media Health Campaigns: The Effects of Entertainment Narrative and Identification on HIV/AIDS Preventive Behavior," PhD diss., Michigan State University.

Liddell, Christine, Louise Barrett and Moya Bydawell. 2005. "Indigenous Representations of Illness and AIDS in Sub-Saharan Africa." *Social Science & Medicine* 60 (4): 691–700.

Locke, Kevin, and Benjamin D. Koen. 2008. "The Lakota Hoop Dance as Medicine for Social Healing." In *The Oxford Handbook of Medical Ethnomusicology*, ed. Benjamin D. Koen, assoc. eds. Jacqueline Lloyd, Gregory Barz, and Karen Brummel-Smith, 482–99. New York: Oxford University Press.

Lomax, Alan. 1993. *The Land Where the Blues Began.* New York: Pantheon Books.

Long, Norman. 2001. *Development Sociology: Actor Perspectives.* London: Routledge.

Lugalla, Joe, Maria Emmelin, Aldin Mutembei, Mwitu Sima, Gideon Kwesigabo, Japhet Killewo, and Lars Dahlgren. 2004. "Social, Cultural and Sexual Behavioral Determinants of Observed Decline in HIV Infection Trends: Lessons from the Kagera Region, Tanzania." *Social Science & Medicine* 59 (1): 185–98.

Lusk, John. 2003. "Kwaito Right" *Roots Magazine* Jan.–Feb.: 42–45.

Lwanda, John. 1994. "Malawi." In *World Music: The Rough Guide*, 210–11. London: Penguin.

———. 2002. "Tikutha: The Political Culture of HIV/AIDS Epidemic in Malawi." In *A Democracy of Chameleons*, ed. Harri Englund. Uppsalla: Nordic Africa Institute.

———. 2003a. "The (In)visibility of HIV/AIDS in the Malawi Public Sphere." *African Journal of AIDS Research* 2 (2): 113–26.

———. 2003b. "Mother's Songs: Male Appropriation of Women's Music in Malawi and Southern Africa." *Journal of African Cultural Studies* 16 (2): 119–42.

———. 2005. *Politics, Culture and Medicine in Malawi: Historical Continuities and Ruptures with Special Reference to HIV/AIDS.* Zomba: Kachere.

———. 2008a. *Music, Culture and Orature: Reading the Malawi Public Sphere, 1949–2006.* Zomba: Kachere.

———. 2008b. "Poets, Culture and Orature: A Reappraisal of the Malawi Political Public Sphere, 1953–2006." *Journal of Contemporary African Studies* 26 (1): 71–101.

Lwihula, George. 1999. "Coping with AIDS Pandemic: The Experience of Peasant Communities of Kagera Region, Tanzania." In *Aids And African Smallholder Agriculture*, ed. G. Mutangadura, H. Jackson, and D. Mukurazita. Harare: Safaids.

MacDonald, C., and E. Schatz, 2006. "Coexisting Discourses: How Older Women in South Africa Make Sense of the HIV/AIDS Epidemic." IBS Working Paper.

Macharia, Wilson. 2004. "Why the Young Are in a Rebellious Mood." *Daily Nation*, August 16: 9.

Makgabaneng. 2003. *The Writing Process.* Gaborone: Makgabaneng Studios.

Makurdi, E. George. 2009. "Rapist Infects 3-Yr Old With HIV/AIDS." *The PM News*. thepmnews.com/2009/10/15/rapist-infects-3-yr-old-with-hivaids.

Manuel, Peter. 1988. *Popular Musics of the Non-Western World: An Introductory Survey*. New York: Oxford University Press.

Mapanje, Jack. 1981. *Of Chameleons and Gods*. London: Heinemann.

Marini, Stephen A. 2003. *Sacred Song in America: Religion, Music, and Public Culture, Public Expressions of Religion in America*. Urbana: University of Illinois Press.

Marion, Jean-Luc. 1991. *God Without Being: Hors-Texte*. Chicago: University of Chicago Press.

Marlin-Curiel, Stephanie. 2004. "Wielding the Cultural Weapon after Apartheid: Bongani Linda's Victory Sonqoba Theatre Company, South Africa." In *Theatre and Empowerment: Community Drama on the World Stage*, ed. R. Boon and J. Plastow, 94-124. Cambridge: Cambridge University Press.

Marks, Shula, and Neil Andersson. 1990. "The Epidemiology and Culture of Violence." In *Political Violence and the Struggle in South Africa*, ed. N. Chabani Manganyi and André du Toit, 29–69. New York: St. Martin's.

Mass, Lawrence D. 1994. *Confessions of a Jewish Wagnerite*. New York: Cassell.

Matumbi, Anne. 2007. *Chidzukulu*. MC Lilongwe: Nkhwazi Ngwazi.

Maughan-Brown, Brendan. 2010. "Stigma rises despite antiretroviral treatmean: a longitudinal analysis in South Africa." *Social Science & Medicine* 70 (3): 368–374.

Mayes, Stephen. 1993. "Photographing the Invisible—A Statement of Intent." In *Positive Lives: Responses to HIV—A Photodocumentary*, ed. Stephen Mayes and Lyndall Stein. London: Cassell.

Mbeki, Thabo. 2000a. "Remarks at the First Meeting of the Presidential Advisory Panel on AIDS," May 6. www.info.gov.za/speeches/2000/0005311255p1003.htm

———. 2000b. "Speech at the Opening Session of the Thirteenth International AIDS Conference," Durban, July 9. www.virusmyth.com/aids/news/durbspmbeki.htm

Mbembe, Achille. 2004. "The Aesthetics of Superfluity." *Public Culture* 16 (3): 373–405.

Mbowa, Rose, and Eckhard Breitinger. 1996. *Theatre for Development*. Bayreuth: Bayreuth African Studies.

McGann, Mary. 2004. *A Precious Fountain: Music in the Worship of an African American Catholic Community*. Collegeville, MN: Liturgical Press.

McGregor, Liz. 2005. *Khabzela: The Life and Times of a South African*. Johannesburg: Jacana.

McManus, Barbara. 1999. "Outline of Aristotle's Theory of Tragedy in the *Poetics*." www.cnr .edu/home/bmcmanus/poetics.html.

McNeill, Fraser G. 2007. "An Ethnographic Analysis of HIV/AIDS in Venda, South Africa: Peer Education, Politics and Music." PhD diss., University of London, School of Economics and Political Science.

———. 2008. "'We Sing About What We Cannot Talk About': Music as Anthropological Evidence in the Venda Region of South Africa." In *How Do We Know? Evidence, Ethnography and the Making of Anthropological Knowledge*, ed. L. Chua, C. High, T. Lau. Newcastle: Cambridge Scholars Press.

———. 2009. "'Condoms Cause AIDS': Poison, Prevention and Denial in Venda, South Africa." *African Affairs* 108 (432): 353–70.

———. 2011. *AIDS, Politics and Music in South Africa*. New York: Cambridge University Press.

McNeill, William. 1998. *Plagues and Peoples*. New York: Anchor Books.

Mead, Francis. 1998. *Finding the Right Frequency: UNICEF and Radio in the Twenty-First Century*. New York: UNICEF.

Meadows, Peter. 2003. "A Letter to the U.K. Church." In *The Hope Factor: Engaging the Church in the HIV/AIDS Crisis*, ed. Tetsunao Yamamori, David Dageforde, Tina Bruner, 147–56. Waynesboro, GA: Authentic Media.

Médecins Sans Frontières. 2003. "Antiretroviral therapy in primary health care: the experience of the Khayelitsha programme in South Africa." Geneva: World Health Organization.

Melkote, Srinivas. 1991. *Communication for Development in the Third World: Theory and Practice*. New Delhi: SAGE Publications.

Mendel, Gideon. 1998. *A Broken Landscape: HIV and AIDS in Africa*. London: Reportage.

———. 2001a. *A Broken Landscape: HIV & AIDS in Africa*. London: Network Photographers.

———. 2001b. Unpublished proposal to the South African National Gallery.

———. 2006. "Looking AIDS in the Face: An Activist Photographic Project from South Africa and Mozambique." *The Virginia Quarterly Review* 82 (1): 42–51.

Merinyo, Clement. 1988. *Kifo Cha AIDS na Hadithi Nyingine*. Dar es Salaam: Grand Arts Promotions.

Mezirow, Jack. 1991. *Transformative Dimensions of Adult Learning*. San Francisco: Jossey-Bass.

Mezirow, Jack and Associates. 2000. *Learning as Transformation: Critical Perspectives on a Theory in Progress*. San Francisco: Jossey-Bass.

Miller, James. 1992. *Fluid Exchanges: Artists and Critics in the HIV/AIDS Crisis*. Toronto: University of Toronto Press.

Minkler, Meredith, and Kathleen Cox. 1980. "Creating Critical Consciousness in Health: Application of Freire's Philosophy and Methods to the Health Care Setting." *International Journal of Health Services* 10 (2): 311–22.

Mitchell, Timothy. 1998. "Orientalism and the Exhibitionary Order." In *The Visual Culture Reader*, ed. Nicholas Mirzoeff. New York: Routledge.

Mitchell, Tony. 2002. *Global Noise: Rap and Hip Hop Outside the USA*. Middletown: Wesleyan University Press.

Mjomba, Leonard Majalia. 2002. "Reproductive Health and HIV/AIDS Prevention Campaign: Utilizing Creative Dramatized Traditional Dance and Music to Create Public Awareness about HIV/AIDS in Wongonyi Community." www.comminit.com/en/node/3895/38

———. 2005. "Empowering Kenyan Youth to Combat HIV/AIDS Using *Ngoma* Dialogue Circles: A Grounded Theory Approach." PhD diss., Ohio University.

Mlama, Penina. 1983. "Utunziwa Tamthiliya katika Mazingira ya Tanzania." In *Makala za semina ya Kimataifa ya Waandishi wa Kiswahili, Fasihi III*. Dar es Salaam: TUKI.

Moeller, Susan D. 1999. *Compassion Fatigue: How the Media Sell Disease, Famine, War and Death*. New York: Routledge.

Mogae, Festus. 2003. "Foreword." In *Botswana 2003 Second Generation HIV/AIDS Surveillance*, ed. Kereng Masupu, Khumo Seipne, Theirry Roels, Soyeon Kim, Mpho Mmelesi, and Sarah Gaolekwe. Gaborone: National AIDS Coordinating Agency (NACA).

Mokwena, Steve. 1992. "Living on the Wrong Side of the Law: Marginalisation, Youth and Violence." In *Black Youth in Crisis: Facing the Future*, ed. David Everatt and Elinor Sisulu, 30–51. Braamfontein: Ravan Press.

Moodley, D., J. Moodley, J. Coovadia, G. Gray, J. McIntyre, J. Hofmyer, C. Nikodem, D. Hall, M. Gigliotti, P. Rovinson, L. Boshoff and H. Sullivan. 2003. "A multicentre randomized controlled trial of nevirapine versus a combination of zidovudine and lamivudine to reduce intrapartum and early postpartum mother-to-child transmission of Human Immunodefiniciency Virus Type I." *Journal of Infectious Diseases* 187 (5): 725–735.

Mooki, Maungo, K. Pappas-DeLuca, P. Tembo, T. Koppenhaver, C. Galavotti, and P. Kilmarx. 2004. "Monitoring the Effects of an Issue Based Radio Serial Drama in Botswana: The Ups and Downs of *Makgabaneng*." Paper presented at the XV International AIDS Conference, July 11–16. Bangkok, Thailand.

Mosse, David, and David Lewis. 2006. "Theoretical Approaches to Brokerage and Translation in Development." In *Development Brokers and Translators: The Ethnography of Aid and Agencies*, ed. David Lewis and David Mosse. Bloomfield: Kumarian Press.

Mozes, Alan. 2002. "Tainted Blood Supply Spreads HIV/AIDS In Poor Nations." *Annals of Internal Medicine* 136: 312–19.

Mufamadi, S. 2004. Announcement of Commission of Traditional Leadership Disputes and Claims. South African Ministry of Provincial and Local Government. www.polity.org.za/pol/58365.

Muganda, Clay. 2004a. "Changing Tune in Line with the Times." *Saturday Nation*, May 22: 21.

———. 2004b. "Tipsy Students at Festival a Tip of the Iceberg." *Daily Nation*, August 18: 8.

Muhando, Penina. 1972. *Hatia*. Dar es Salaam: EAPH.

———. 1973. *Tambueni haki zetu*. Nairobi: EALB.

Mulokozi, M. Mugyabuso. 1979. *Mkwava wa Uhehe*. Dar es Salaam: DUP.

———. 1996. *Fasihi ya Kiswahili, OSW 105*. Dar es Salaam: Chuo Kikuu Huria.

"Music, Medicine, and Healing: Medical Ethnomusicology and Global Perspectives on Health and Healing" 2004. Conference website. www.med.fsu.edu/geriatrics/ethnomusicology/ethno_main.htm.

Mutembei, Aldin K. 2001. *Poetry and AIDS in Tanzania: Changing Metaphors and Metonymies in Haya Oral Traditions*. Leiden: CNWS Publications.

———. 2009. *UKIMWI katika Fasihi ya Kiswahili: Ushairi*. Dar es Salaam: TUKI.

Mutembei, Aldin K., Maria A. C. Emmelin, Joe L. P. Lugalla, and Lars G. Dahlgren. 2002. "Communicating About AIDS: Changes in Understanding and Coping With Help of Language in Urban Kagera, Tanzania." *Journal of Asian and African Studies* 37 (1): 1–16.

Muyebe, O. P., and S. J. Muyebe. 1999. *The Religious Factor Within the Body of Political Symbolism in Malawi, 1964–1994*. Parkland, Florida: Universal Publishers.

Mwaniki, Philip. 2004. "Now the UN Goes the Hip-Hop Way." *Saturday Nation*, September 11, Section 1: 20.

———. 2007. "Global Music Festival to Aid Local Projects." *Saturday Nation*, January 20: 29.

"Nairobi 2007: World Social Forum." 2007. wsf2007.org.

Namukisa, Noelina. 2002. "Meeting Point: Dignity, Value, and a Certain Degree of Humanity." In *The aWAKE Project: Uniting Against the African AIDS Crisis*, ed. Jenny Eaton and Kate Etue, 181–88. Nashville: W. Publishing.

Nariman, Heidi Noel. 1993. *Soap Operas for Social Change: Toward a Methodology for Entertainment-Education Television*. Westport: Praeger.

National AIDS Control Council. 2004. "Overcoming the HIV-Related Stigma." *Nation*, August 29: 32.

National AIDS Control Council and the National AIDS and STD Control Programme. 2009. "The Kenya 2007 HIV and AIDS Estimates and Interim Projected HIV Prevalence and Incidence Trends for 2008-2015." www.fpfk.or.ke/aids/images/Resources/Resources/Kenya%20National%20HIV%20Estimates%202007.pdf

National AIDS Coordinating Agency (NACA). 2003. *Botswana National Strategic Framework for HIV/AIDS 2003–2009*. Gaborone: NACA.

———. 2004. *Botswana AIDS Impact Survey II*. Gaborone: NACA.

———. 2005. *United Nations General Assembly Special Session on HIV/AIDS*. Gaborone: NACA.

———. 2006. *National Strategy for Behavior Change Interventions and Communications for HIV and AIDS*. Gaborone: NACA.

National AIDS Policy. 1993. Gaborone: Government of Botswana.

National Development Plan 9 2003-04-2008-09. 2003. Ministry of Finance and Development Planning. Gaborone: Government of Botswana.

National Immigration Project. 2004. "HIV/AIDS and Immigrants: A Manual for HIV/AIDS Service Providers." www.nationalimmigrationproject.org/HIV/2004HIVManual/2004hivmanual/page7.html.

National Policy on HIV Rapid Testing. 2005. Ministry of Health. Gaborone: Ministry of Health.

Nattrass, Nicoli. 2005. "Rolling Out Antiretroviral Treatment in South Africa: Economic and Ethical Challenges." In *Ethics and AIDS in Africa: The Challenge to our Thinking*, ed. Anton van Niekerk, and Loretta Kopelman. Cape Town: David Philip.

———. 2007. *Mortal Combat: AIDS Denialism and the Struggle for Antiretrovirals in South Africa*. Pietermaritzburg: University of KwaZulu-Natal Press.

———. 2008. "AIDS and the scientific governance of medicine in post-apartheid South Africa." *African Affairs* 107 (427): 157-176.

Nduati, Rose, and Wambui Kiai. 1997. *Communicating with Adolescents about AIDS: Experiences from Eastern and Southern Africa*. Ottawa: International Development Research Center.

Ndungane, Njongonkulu. 2003. *A World with a Human Face: A Voice from Africa*. Cape Town: David Philip.

Nettl, Bruno. 2005. *The Study of Ethnomusicology: Thirty-One Issues and Concepts*. Urbana: University of Illinois Press.

Neuwirth, Robert. 2005. *Shadow Cities: A Billion Squatters, a New Urban World*. New York: Routledge.

New HIV/AIDS Care Center. 2005. "New HIV/AIDS Care Center—Big Boost for the AIDS Support Organization (TASO) and Uganda Infrastructure." Pfizer Press Release, October 14.

Ngaira, Amos. 2004. "Abura Off to Dakar for AIDS Song Project." *Saturday Nation*, May 15: 21.

Ngugi, Gerishon. 1961. *Nimelogwa nisiwe na Mpenzi*. Nairobi: EALB

Nguyen, Vinh-Kim. 2005. "Antiretroviral Globalism, Biopolitics, and Therapeutic Citizenship." In *Global Assemblages, Technology, Politics and Ethics as Anthropological Problems*, ed. Aihwa Ong and Stephen Collier. Malden: Blackwell.

Niang, Abdoulaye. 2006. "Bboys: Hip-hop Culture in Dakar, Senegal." In *Global Youth? Hybrid Identities, Plural Worlds*, ed. Pam Nilan and Carles Feixa, 167–85. New York: Routledge.

Niederstadt, Leah. 2009. "Fighting HIV with Juggling Clubs: An Introduction to Ethiopia's Circus." *African Arts* 42 (1): 76–87.

Nietzsche, Friedrich. 1991. *Zur Genealogie der Moral*. Frankfurt: Insel Taschenbuch.

Nixon, Nicholas, and Bebe Nixon. 1991. *People with AIDS*. Boston: David R. Godine Publisher.

Nixon, Rob. 1994. *Homelands, Harlem, Hollywood: South African Culture and the World Beyond*. New York: Routledge.

Njagi, Anthony. 2004. "Original Tune Lights Up Stage." *Daily Nation*, August 11: 6.

Nketia, J. H. Kwabena. 1982 [1974]. *The Music of Africa*. London: Victor Gollancz.

———. 1995. *National Development and the Performing Arts of Africa*. Legon: International Centre for African Music and Dance.

————. 1998. "The Scholarly Study of African Music." In *The Garland Encyclopedia of World Music, Volume 1, Africa*, ed. Ruth M. Stone, 13–73. New York: Garland.

————. 2001. "The Arts in Contemporary Contexts: An Overview." Unpublished paper.

Noar, Seth M., Philip Palmgreen, Melissa Chabot, Nicole Dobransky, and Rick S. Zimmerman. 2009. "A 10-Year Systematic Review of HIV/AIDS Mass Communication Campaigns: Have We Made Progress?" *Journal of Health Communication* 14: 15–42.

Nordland, Rod, Ray Wilkinson, and Ruth Marshall. 1986. "Africa in the Plague Years." *Newsweek*, November 24.

Ntarangwi, Mwenda. 2009. *East African Hip Hop: Youth Culture and Globalization*. Urbana: University of Illinois Press.

Ntsimane, Radikobo. 2006. "To Disclose or Not to Disclose: an Appraisal of the Memory Box Project as a Safe Space for Disclosure of HIV Positive Status." *Journal of Theology for Southern Africa* 125 (1): 7–20.

Nussbaum, Martha. 2001. *Upheavals of Thought: The Intelligence of Emotions*. Cambridge: Cambridge University Press.

Nuttall, Sarah and Cheryl-Ann Michael, eds. 2000. *Senses of Culture: South African Cultural Studies*. Oxford: Oxford University Press.

Nyirongo, Edwin. 2005. "The Condom Controversy," *Weekend Nation*, 12–13 February: 23.

Nzewi, Meki. 2003. "Acquiring Knowledge of the Musical Arts in Traditional Society." In *Musical Arts in Africa: Theory Practice and Education*, ed. Anri Herbst, Meki Nzewi, and Kofi Agawu, 13–37. Pretoria: University of South Africa Press.

————. 2004. "The *Avu* of Alafrika: A Narrative on an Encounter with Musical Arts Knowledge." *Journal of the Musical Arts in Africa* 1: 55–83.

Odhiambo, Lewis. 2000. "Mass Media and the AIDS Pandemic in Kenya, 1997–98: A Moral Panic Perspective." In *Media and HIV/AIDS in East and Southern Africa: A Resource Book*, ed. S. T. Kwame Boafo and Carlos A. Arnaldo, 91–108. Paris: UNESCO.

Odhiambo, Christopher Joseph. 2008. *Theatre for Development in Kenya: In Search of an Effective Procedure and Methodology*. Bayreuth: Bayreuth African Studies Series 86.

Ogdon, Bethany. 2001. "Through the Image: Nicholas Nixon's 'People with HIV/AIDS.'" *Discourse* 23 (3): 75–105.

Ogot, Bethwell Allan. 2002 [1995]. "The Construction of a National Culture." In *The Challenges of History and Leadership in Africa: The Essays of Bethwell Allan Ogot*, ed. Toyin Falola and E. S. Atieno-Odhiambo, 155–81. Trenton, NJ: African World Press.

The Oikos Journey: A Theological Reflection on the Economic Crisis in South Africa. 2006. Durban: Diakonia Council of Churches.

Okigbo, Austin C. 2010. *Ingoma Yomzabalazo—Music of the Struggles: A South African Zulu Choral Music and the HIV/AIDS Struggle*. PhD diss., Indiana University.

Olsen, Dale A. 2008. "Shamanism, Music, and Healing in Two Contrasting South American Cultural Areas." In *The Oxford Handbook of Medical Ethnomusicology*, ed. Benjamin D. Koen, assoc. eds. Jacqueline Lloyd, Gregory Barz, and Karen Brummel-smith, 331–60. New York: Oxford University Press.

O'Manique, Colleen. 2004. *Neoliberalism and AIDS Crisis in Sub-Saharan Africa*. Basingstoke: Palgrave-MacMillan.

Onyango, Diana. 2001. "Communication for Prevention and Behavior Change." Unpublished paper, VIII Communication for Development Roundtable, Managua, Nicaragua, November 26–28.

Oomen, Barbara. 2005. *Chiefs in South Africa: Law, Power and Culture in the Post-Apartheid Era*. Oxford: James Curry.

Osumare, Halifu. 2007. *The Africanist Aesthetic in Global Hip-Hop: Power Moves*. New York: Palgrave Macmillan.

Otieno, Otieno. 2004. "Music Festival Turned into a Drama of Vice." *East African Standard*, August 10: 1, 3.

Owen, Theresa. 2006. "Zola for President." *Daily News*, October 6: 11.

PACSA. 2004. *Gender, Poverty and HIV/AIDS: What Ordinary People Living with HIV/AIDS Want Decision Makers to Know*, August, no. 52. Newsletter.

Papa, Michael J., Arvind Singhal, S. Law, S. Pant, S. Sood, Everett M. Rogers, and C. L. Schefner-Rogers. 2000. "Entertainment-Education and Social Change: An Analysis of Parasocial Interaction, Social Learning, Collective Efficacy, and Paradoxical Communication." *Journal of Communication* 50 (4): 31–55.

Pappas-DeLuca, K., J. M. Craft, C. Galavotti, L. Warner, M. Mooki, P. Hastings, T. Koppenhaver, T. H. Roels, and P. H. Kilmarx. 2008. "Entertainment-Education Radio Serial Drama and Outcomes Related to HIV Testing in Botswana." *AIDS Education and Prevention* 20 (6): 486–503.

Pappas-DeLuca, K., T. Koppenhaver, C. Galavotti, P. Tembo, and T. Roels. 2004. "Results from a Preliminary Evaluation of the *Makgabaneng* Radio Serial Drama in Botswana." Unpublished paper delivered at the 4th Annual Entertainment Education Conference. Western Cape, South Africa.

Parker, Beverly. 1997. "The Music Department, its Options, its Thinking in Terms of the Future." Interview with South African Broadcasting Corporation. Durban: SABC.

Parkin, David, Lionel Caplan, and Humphrey Fisher, eds. 1996. *The Politics of Cultural Performance*. Oxford: Berghahn Books.

Patton, Cindy. 1990. *Inventing HIV/AIDS*. New York: Routledge.

Pearlmutter, David. 1998. *Photojournalism and Foreign Policy: Icons of Outrage in International Crisis*. London: Praeger.

Peres, Camila A., Rodrigo A. Peres, Fernando da Silveira, Vera Paiva, Esther S. Hudes, and Norman Hearst. 2002. "Developing an AIDS Prevention Intervention for Incarcerated Male Adolescents in Brazil." *AIDS Education and Prevention* 14 (5 Suppl. B): 36–44.

Peterson, Bhekezizwe. 2003. "Kwaito, 'Dawgs', and the Antimonies of Hustling." *African Identities* 1 (2): 197–213.

Piot, Peter. 2005. "Foreword." In *The "Three Ones" in Action: Where We Are and Where We Go From Here*. Geneva: UNAIDS.

Planned Parenthood Association of Ghana. 2009. "Behaviour Change Communication," October. www.ppag-gh.org.

———. 2006. "IFPP Vision 2000 Strategic Plan," November. www.ppag-gh.org.

Plastow, Jane. 2004. "Dance and transformation: the Adugna Community Dance Theatre, Ethiopia." In *Theatre and Empowerment: Community Drama on the World Stage*, ed. R. Boon and J. Plastow, 125-154. Cambridge: Cambridge University Press.

Pongweni, J. C. 1982. *Songs that Won the Liberation War*. Harare: College Press.

Population Services International (PSI) Botswana. 2005. *Report of a Study to Plan, Monitor, and Evaluate PSI's Social Marketing Program on HIV/AIDS Prevention in Botswana*. Gaborone: PSI.

Presidential Task Group for a Long Term Vision for Botswana. 1996. *A Framework for a Long Term Vision for Botswana*. Gaborone: Government Printer.

Quist-Arcton, Ofeibea. 2001. "Senegal: 'This Is My Whole Life'—A Scientist's Dedication to Defeating AIDS." allafrica.com/stories/200107050030.html.

Radley, Alan. 2002. "Portrayals of Suffering: On Looking Away, Looking At, and the Comprehension of Illness Experience." *Body & Society* 8 (3): 1–23.

Rametsi, S., C. C. Lovell, A. Gasennelwe, E. Motse, and P. Kilmarx. 2003. "Getting Personal: Engaging a Mass Media Audience through Reinforcement Activities." Presentation at National HIV/AIDS Research and Other Related Infectious Disease Conference, December 8.

Rametsi, S., S. McClain, I. Bhowa, M. Masawi, and G. Osewe. 2004. "Community Reinforcement of an Entertainment Education Intervention: Botswana and Zimbabwe." www.ee4.org/Presentations/EE4_Rametsi.pdf.

Reed, Daniel B. in press. "Promises of the Chameleon: Reggae Artist Tiken Jah Fakoly's Intertextual Contestation of Power in Côte d'Ivoire." In *Hip Hop Africa and Other Stories of New African Music in a Globalized World*, ed. Eric Charry. Bloomington: Indiana University Press.

Reid, Graeme, and Liz Walker. 2003. "Secrecy, Stigma and HIV/AIDS: An Introduction." *African Journal for AIDS Research* 2 (2): 85–88.

Rhanem, Karima. 2005. "World AIDS Day: Over 17,000 HIV positive, 1839 full-blown AIDS cases in Morocco." friendsofmorocco.org/2005News/Dec05/1203News.htm.

Robins, Steven. 2006. "From 'Rights' to 'Ritual': AIDS Activism in South Africa." *American Anthropologist* 108 (2): 312–23.

Rogers, E. M., P. W. Vaughan, M. A. Ramadhan, R. M. Swalehe, N. Rao, P. Svenkerud, and S. Sood. 1999. "Effects of an Entertainment-Education Radio Soap Opera on Family Planning Behavior in Tanzania." *Studies in Family Planning* 30 (3): 193–211.

Román, David. 1998. *Acts of Intervention: Performance, Gay Culture, and AIDS*. Bloomington: Indiana University Press.

Rommen, Timothy. 2007. *"Mek Some Noise": Gospel Music and the Ethics of Style in Trinidad*. Berkeley: University of California Press.

Ronell, Avital. 1994. "Queens of the Night." In *Finitude's Score: Essays for the end of the Millennium*, 41–62. Lincoln: University of Nebraska Press.

Rørtveit, Bodil Lunde. 2003. "Tradisjonell musikk i Uganda 2002: Korleis tradisjonell musikk kjem til uttrykk gjennom tre ulike kontekstar i hovudstaden Kampala" ["Traditional music in Uganda 2002: How traditional music is expressed through three different contexts around the capital city Kampala"]. MA thesis, Institutt for Musikk, NTNU, Norway.

Roseman, Marina. 1991. *Healing Sounds from the Malaysian Rainforest: Temiar Music and Medicine*. Berkeley: University of California Press.

———. 2008. "A Fourfold Framework for Cross-Cultural, Integrative Research on Music and Medicine." In *The Oxford Handbook of Medical Ethnomusicology*, ed. Benjamin D. Koen, assoc. eds. Jacqueline Lloyd, Gregory Barz, and Karen Brummel-Smith, 18–45. New York: Oxford University Press.

Rosenberg, Charles. 1992. "Framing Disease: Illness, Society, and History." In *Framing Disease: Studies in Cultural History*, ed. Charles Rosenberg and Janet Golden. Piscataway, NJ: Rutgers University Press.

Rosenthal, Alan. 1980. *The Documentary Conscience: A Casebook in Film Making*. Berkeley: University of California Press.

Rosler, Martha. 1990. "In, Around, and Afterthoughts: On Documentary Photography." In *The Contest of Meaning: Critical Histories of Photography*, ed. R. Bolton. Cambridge, MA: MIT Press.

Rossi, Peter. H., Mark W. Lipsey, and Howard E. Freeman. 2004. *Evaluation: A Systematic Approach*, 7th ed. Thousand Oaks, CA: Sage Publications.

Roudi-Fahimi, Farzaneh. 2003. "Women's Reproductive Health in the Middle East and North Africa." *Population Reference Bureau, MENA Policy Brief*. Washington: PRB.

Ryerson, William N. 2004. "The Effectiveness of Entertainment Mass Media in Changing Behavior." www.populationmedia.org/programs/effectiv.html.

Sabatier, Renee. 1988. *Blaming Others: Prejudice, Race and Worldwide HIV/AIDS*. Philadelphia: New Society Publishers.

Said, Edward. 1979. *Orientalism*. New York: Vintage Books.

Samper, David A. 2002. "Talking Sheng: The Role of a Hybrid Language in the Construction of Identity and Youth Culture in Nairobi, Kenya." PhD diss., University of Pennsylvania.

Sankore, Rotimi. 2005. "Behind the Image: Poverty and Development Pornography." *Pambazuka News: Weekly Forum for Social Justice in Africa* 203, April 21.

Sarin, Radhika. 2002. "The Feminization of AIDS." In *Worldwatch Paper 161*, ed. Danielle Nierenberg. Washington: Worldwatch Institute.

Satyo, Sizwe. 2001. "Kwaito-Speak: A Language Variety Created by the Youth for the Youth." In *Freedom and Discipline: Essays on Applied Linguistics from Southern Africa*, ed. Elaine Ridge, Sinfree Makoni, and Stanley G.m. Ridge, 139–48. New Dehli: Bahri Publications.

Satyo, Sizwe. 2008. "A Linguistic Study of Kwaito." *The World of Music* 50 (2): 91–102.

Scalway, T. 2001. "Young Men and HIV: Culture, Poverty and Sexual Risk." The Panos Institute. www.panos.org.uk.

Scarry, Elaine. 1985. *The Body in Pain: The Making and Unmaking of the World*. New York: Oxford University Press.

Schoop, Kini. 2003. "UNICEF Lauds White House Leadership on AIDS Bill." www.unicef.org/media/media_7913.html

Schwartz, Joel and David Murray. 1996. "AIDS and the Media." *Public Interest* 125:57–71.

Seeger, Anthony. 1979. "What Can We Learn When They Sing? Vocal Genres of the Suya Indians of Central Brazil." *Ethnomusicology* 23 (3): 373–94.

———. 2008. "Theories Forged in the Crucible of Action: The Joys, Dangers, and Potentials of Advocacy and Fieldwork." In *Shadows in the Field: New Perspectives for Fieldwork in Ethnomusicology*, 2nd edition, ed. Gregory Barz and Timothy Cooley, 271–88. New York: Oxford University Press.

Seekings, Jeremy and Nattrass, Nicoli. 2005. *Class, Race and Inequality in South Africa*. New Haven: Yale University Press.

Seguin, A. and C. Rancourt. 1996. "The Theatre: An Effective Tool for Health Promotion." *World Health Forum* 17 (1): 64–9.

Semzaba, Edwin. 1980. *Tendehogo*. Dar es Salaam: TPH.

Senghor, Léopold Sédar. 1995 [1966]. "Negritude: A Humanism of the Twentieth Century." In *I Am Because We Are: Readings in Black Philosophy*, ed. Fred Lee Hord and Jonathon Scott Lee, 45–54. Amherst: University of Massachusetts Press.

Senkoro, E.M.K. Fikeni. 2006. "Fasihi ya Kiswahili ya Majaribio: Makutano Baina ya Fasihi Simulizi na Fasihi Andishi." In *Kioo cha Lugha* 4: 22–38.

Servaes, Jan. 1986. "Development Theory and Communication Policy: Power to the People!" *European Journal of Communication* 1 (2): 203–29.

———. 1996. "Introduction: Participatory Communication and Research in Development Settings." In *Participatory Communication for Social Change*, ed. J. Servaes, T. Jacobson, and S. White. New Delhi. Sage Publication.

———. 1999. *Communication for Development: One World, Multiple Cultures*. Cresskill, NJ: Hampton Press Inc.

Servant, Jean-Christophe. 2002. "Kwaito, Dagga, 'Edutainment,' and the Generation Gap in South Africa." *World Press Review Online*, June 11.

Setel, Philip W. 1999. *A Plague of Paradoxes: AIDS, Culture, and Demography in Northern Tanzania.* Chicago: University of Chicago Press.

Shapiro, Michael J. 1988. *The Politics of Representation: Writing Practices in Biography, Photography and Policy Analysis.* Madison: University of Wisconsin Press.

Sharan, Mona, and Thomas Valente. 2002. "Spousal Communication and Family Planning Adoption: Effects of a Radio Serial Drama in Nepal." *International Family Planning Perspectives* 28 (1): 16–25.

Shelemay, Kay Kaufman and Peter Jeffrey, eds. 1993/1994/1997. *Ethiopian Christian Liturgical Chant,* three vols., Madison, A-R Editions.

Shelemay, Kay Kaufman. 1991. *A Song of Longing: An Ethiopian Journey.* Urbana: University of Illinois Press.

———. 1992. "The Musician and Transmission of Religious Tradition: The Multiple Roles of the Ethiopian Dabtara." *Journal of Religion in Africa* 22 (3): 242–60.

Sherman, David K., and Geoffrey L. Cohen. 2006. "The Psychology of Self-defense: Self-Affirmation Theory." *Advances in Experimental Social Psychology* 38: 183–242.

Shisana, Olive, Thomas Rehl, Leickness C. Simbayi, Khanyisa Zuma, Sean Jooste, Victoria Pillay-van-Wyk, Ntombizodwa Mbelle, Johan Van Zyl, Warren Parker, Nompumelelo. P. Zungu, Sinawe Pezi, and SABSSM III Implementation Team. 2009. "South African National HIV Prevalence, Incidence, Behaviour and Communication Survey 2008: A Turning Tide Among Teenagers?" Cape Town: HSRC Press.

Shortell, Stephen M., and John Swartzberg. 2008. "The Physician as Public Health Professional in the 21st Century." *Journal of the American Medical Association* 300 (24): 2916–18.

Shorter, Aylward, and Edwin Onyancha. 1998. *The Church and AIDS in Africa: A Case Study: Nairobi City.* Nairobi: Paulines Publications Africa.

Sibanda, Silindiwe. 2004. "'You Don't Get to Sing a Song When You Have Nothing to Say': Oliver Mtukudzi's Music as a Vehicle for Socio-Political Commentary." *Social Dynamics* 30 (2): 36–63.

Singer, Peter. 2002. "AIDS and International Security." *Survival* 44 (1): 145–58.

Singhal, Arvind. 1990. "Entertainment-Education Strategies for Development." PhD diss., University of Southern California.

Singhal, Arvind, and Everett M. Rogers. 1999. *Entertainment-Education: A Communication Strategy for Social Change.* Mahwah, NJ: Lawrence Erlbaum Associates.

———. 2002. "A Theoretical Agenda for Entertainment-Education." *Communication Theory* 12 (2): 117–35.

———. 2003. *Combating AIDS: Communication Strategies in Action.* New Delhi: Thousand Oaks; London: Sage.

Singhal, Arvind, Shereen Usdin, Esca Scheepers, Sue Goldstein, and Garth Japhet. 2002. "Harnessing the Entertainment-Education Strategy in Africa: The Soul City Intervention in South Africa." In *Development and Communication in Africa,* ed. Charles Okigbo. Lanham, MD: Rowman and Littlefield Publishers.

"Sinikithemba: Our Story of Hope." 2009. *HIV Care Services at McCord Hospital.* www.mccord.org.za

Sischy, Ingrid. 1991. "Good Intentions." *New Yorker,* September 9.

Sitze, Adam. 2004. "Denialism." *South Atlantic Quarterly* 103 (3): 769–811.

Smith, J. Z. 1982. *Imagining Religion: From Babylon to Jonestown.* Chicago: University of Chicago Press.

Smith, Raymond A. 1998. *Encyclopedia of AIDS: A Social, Political, Cultural, and Scientific Record of the HIV Epidemic.* New York: Penguin.

Smith, René. 2003. "*Yizo Yizo* and Essentialism: Representations of Women and Gender-Based Violence in a Drama Series Based on Reality." In *Shifting Selves: Post-Apartheid Essays on Mass Media, Culture and Identity*, ed. Herman Wasserman and Sean Jacobs, 249–65. Cape Town: Kwela Books.

Sontag, Susan. 1977. *On Photography*. New York: Picador.

———. 1988. *AIDS and its Metaphors*. New York: Farrar, Straus and Giroux.

———. 2001. "AIDS and its Metaphors." In *Illness as Metaphor and AIDS and its Metaphors*, 89–183. New York: Picador.

———. 2001. *Illness as Metaphor* and *AIDS and Its Metaphors*. New York: Picador.

———. 2003. *Regarding the Pain of Others*. New York: Farrar, Strauss and Giroux.

———. 2004. "Regarding the Torture of Others." *The New York Times*, May 23. www.nytimes.com.

Sood, Suruchi, M. S. Gupta, P. R. Mishra, and C. Jacoby. 2004. "'Come Gather Around Together': An Examination of Radio Listening Groups in Fulbari, Nepal." *Gazette* 66 (1): 63–86.

Sood, Suruchi. 1999. "Audience Involvement with 'Tinka Tinka Sukh': An Entertainment Education Radio Soap Opera in India: An Analysis of Media Effects." PhD diss., University of New Mexico.

———. 2002. "Audience Involvement and Entertainment-Education." *Communication Theory* 12 (2): 153–72.

Southall, R. 2007. "The ANC State, More Dysfunctional than Developmental?" In *State of the Nation: South Africa 2007*, ed. S. Buhlungu, J. Daniel, R. Southall, J. Lutchman. Cape Town: HSRC Press.

Sprenkle, Sue. 2007. "Words of Hope Ministry Changes Outlook for People with AIDS." *The Baptist Standard*. www.baptiststandard.com/postnuke/index.php?module=htmlpages&func=display&pid=7113

Stadler, J. J. 2003. "The Young, the Rich and the Beautiful: Secrecy, Suspicion and Discourses of AIDS in the South African Lowveld." *African Journal of AIDS Research* 2 (2): 127–39.

Statistics South Africa. 2003. *Census 2001: Census in Brief*. Pretoria. www.statssa.gov.za/census01/html/CInBrief/CIB2001.pdf on 2/2/2007.

Stayt, Hugh. 1931. *The Bavenda*. Oxford: Oxford University Press for the International Institute of African Languages and Cultures.

Steinberg, Jonny. 2008. *Sizwe's Test: A Young Man's Journey through Africa's AIDS Epidemic* London: Simon and Schuster.

Steingo, Gavin. 2005. "South African Music After Apartheid: *Kwaito*, the 'Party Politic,' and the Appropriation of Gold as a Sign of Success." *Popular Music and Society* 28 (3): 333–57.

———. 2007. "The Politicization of Kwaito: From the Party Politic to Party Politics." *Black Music Research Journal* 28 (2): 75–102.

Stephens, Simon. 2000. "Kwaito." In *Senses of Culture: South African Culture Studies*, ed. Sarah Nuttall and Cheryl-ann Michael, 256–273. Cape Town: Oxford University Press.

Stephenson, H.C. and Davis, G. 1994. "Impact of Culturally Sensitive Aids Video Education on The Aids Risk Knowledge of African American Adolescents." *AIDS Education Preview* 6: 40–52.

Stone, Ruth M. 2000. "African Music in a Constellation of Arts." In *The Garland Handbook of African Music*, ed. Ruth M. Stone, 7–12. New York: Garland.

———. 2005. *Music in West Africa: Experiencing Music, Expressing Culture*. New York: Oxford University Press.

———. 2008. "African Music in a Constellation of the Arts." In *The Garland Handbook of African Music*, 2nd ed., ed. Ruth Stone, 7–12. New York: Routledge.

Strauss, David Levi. 2003. *Between the Eyes: Essays on Photography and Politics.* New York: Aperture.

Sugarman, Jane. 1997. *Engendering Song: Singing and Subjectivity at Prespa Albanian Weddings.* Chicago: University of Chicago Press.

Summerton, J. V. 2006. "Western Health Practitioners' View about African Traditional Health Practitioners' Treatment and Care of People Living with HIV/AIDS." *Curationis* 29 (3): 15–23.

Sunday Nation. 2004. "Ngodhe Steals the Show as Primary Schools Class Ends." August 8: 40.

Sypher, Beverley, M. McKinley, S. Ventsam, and E. E. Valdeavellano. 2002. "Fostering Reproductive Health through Entertainment Education in the Peruvian Amazon: The Construction of *Bienvenida Salud!*" *Communication Theory* 12 (2): 192–205.

Tandon, R. 1981. "Participatory Evaluation and Research: Main Concepts and Issues." In *Participatory Research and Evaluation: Experiments in Research as a Process of Liberation*, ed. W. Fernandes and R. Tandon. New Delhi: Society for Participatory Research in Asia.

Tanzania Commission for AIDS (TACAIDS). 2006. *UNGASS Indicators Country Report Template: Tanzania TACAIDS. Reporting Period 2003–2005.*

TASO Uganda Limited. 2002. *2001 Annual Report.* Kampala: TASO Uganda Ltd.

———. 2005. *2004 Annual Report.* Kampala: TASO Uganda Ltd.

———. 2006. *2005 Annual Report.* Kampala: TASO Uganda Ltd.

Taylor, Darren. 2005. "KENYA: From Bangkok, They Brought Hope for Millions Living with AIDS." www.aegis.org/news/ips/2005/IP050416.html.

Tembo, Prisca, Christine Galavotti, Todd Koppenhaver, Katina Pappas-DeLuca, and Peter Kilmarx. 2003. "'Dear *Makgabaneng*': An Analysis of Letters Received in Response to an HIV/AIDS Behavior Change Radio Drama." Unpublished presentation given at the National HIV/AIDS Research and Other Related Infectious Disease Conference, December 8.

Tendo, Steven. 2009. "GNL vs. Rocky Giant." *Daily Monitor*, May 22.

Thapisa, A. P. N. 2003. "The Use of Print and Electronic Media in Botswana." *Journal of Librarianship and Information Science* 35: 153–64.

Thapisa, A. P. N., and E. R. Megwa. 2002. *Report on the National Survey on Print and Electronic Media in Botswana TB 2/5/19/2001–2002.* Gaborone: Department of Information and Broadcasting.

Thibodeaux, Raymond. 2005. "Women, Children Hardest Hit by Ethiopia's Deepening AIDS Crisis." *Voice of America* February 11. www.aegis.com/news/voa/2005.

Thiong'o, Ngugi wa. 1986. *Decolonizing the Mind: The Politics of Language in African Literature.* Nairobi: Heinemann Kenya.

———.1999. "Forward." In *Community in Motion: Theatre for Development in Africa*, by L. Dale Byam, xiii-xv. Westport: Bergin & Garvey.

Thomas, Barbara, Renee S. Marshall, Susan B. Gold-Smith, and Anne Forrest. 2004. "Visual Art and Breast Health Promotion: Artists' Perspectives." *Canadian Oncology Nursing Journal* 14 (4): 233–43.

Thomas, Craig W., Bryce D. Smith, Linda Wright-DeAguero. 2006. "The Program Evaluation and Monitoring System: A Key Source of Data for Monitoring Evidence-Based HIV Prevention Program Process and Outcomes." *AIDS Education & Prevention* 18 (4 Suppl): 74–80.

Tomkins, Calvin. 2005. "Shall We Dance? The Spectator as Artist." *New Yorker*, October 17, 81/32: 82–95.

Toop, David. 2000 [1984]. *Rap Attack #3: African Rap to Global Hip Hop*, expanded third edition. London: Serpent's Tail.

Topan, Farouk. 1973. *Aliyeonja Pepo*. Dar es Salaam: TPH.

Touahri, Sarah. 2008. "Moroccan Artists Sign Artists' AIDS Pact." Magharebia.com, December 3. www.magharebia.com/cocoon/awi/xhtml1/en_GB/features/awi/features/2008/12/03/feature-01.

Towards an AIDS-Free Generation. 2001. Gaborone: Ministry of Education, Government of Botswana and UNDP.

Tracey, Hugh. 1963. "Behind the Lyrics." *African Music: Journal of the African Music Society* 3(2): 17–22.

Treichler, Paula A. 1999. *How to Have Theory in an Epidemic: Cultural Chronicles of AIDS*. Durham: Duke University Press.

Trengrove-Jones, Tim. 2002. "Simple Aids Vision Belongs in Museum," *Sunday Independent*, June 16.

Tshamano, Ndwamato Walter. 1993. "Radio Drama: A Critical Study of Some Radio Venda Broadcasts." MA thesis, University of Limpopo (University of the North).

Turino, Thomas. 2000. *Nationalists, Cosmopolitans, and Popular Music in Zimbabwe*. Chicago: University of Chicago Press.

Turner, Victor. 1987. *The Anthropology of Performance*. New York: PAJ Publication.

UNAIDS. 2001. "HIV and Young People." Joint United Nations Programme on HIV/AIDS Publications. Available online www.unaids.org/en/default

———. 2003. *AIDS Epidemic Update*, December 2003. Geneva: UNAIDS/WHO

———. 2004a. *AIDS Epidemic Update*, December 2004. Geneva: UNAIDS/WHO.

———. 2004b. *2004 Report on the Global AIDS Epidemic*. Geneva: UNAIDS.

———. 2005. *AIDS Epidemic Update, December 2005*. Geneva: UNAIDS/WHO.

———. 2006. "Ghana." www.unaids.org/en/Regions_Countries/Countries/ghana.asp.

———. 2007a. "Kenya." www.unaids.org/en/Regions_Countries/Countries/kenya.asp.

———. 2007b. "Sub-Saharan Africa." www.unaids.org/en/Regions_Countries/Regions/SubSaharanAfrica.asp.

———. 2008. *2008 Report on the Global AIDS Epidemic*. Geneva: UNAIDS.

———. 2009. "Ghana." www.unaids.org/en/Regions_Countries/Countries/ghana.asp.

UNAIDS/WHO Working Group on Global HIV/AIDS and STI Surveillance. 2008. "Epidemiological Fact Sheet on HIV and AIDS: Core Data on Epidemiology and Response: Kenya." apps.who.int/globalatlas/predefinedReports/EFS2008/full/EFS2008_KE.pdf.

UNASO Newsletter. 2003. "Mudinet." Uganda Network of AIDS Service Organisations, 8 (2).

UNDP. 2007. *Women's Rights Initiative*. www.harpas.org.

UNFPA. 2003. "Chapt. 9: Culture Matters—Malawi: Patnerschaften mit Kulturellen und Religiösen Einrichtungen im Kampf gegen HIV/AIDS." In *State of the World Population*, 81–89. New York: United Nations Fund for Population Activities,

UNICEF Response to AIDS in Uganda. 1991. *Expanded Communications Programme 1991–1995: Draft Plan of Operations*, August 29.

UNICEF. 2004. *Children on the Brink 2004*. www.unicef.org.

———. 2010a. *Zimbabwe PMTCT Factsheet*. www.unicef.org/aids/files/Zimbabwe_PMTCT Factsheet_2010.pdf

———. 2010b. *Humanitarian Action Report 2010—Zimbabwe*. www.unicef.org/har2010/index_zimbabwe.php

United Nations. 2005. *Report of the Fact-Finding Mission to Zimbabwe to assess the Scope and Impact of Operation Murambatsvina*. www.un.org/News/dh/infocus/zimbabwe/zimbabwe_rpt.pdf.

USAID. 2003. *USAID Project Profiles: Children Affected by HIV/AIDS*, 3rd ed. Washington: USAID.

————. 2009. *Integrating Multiple Gender Strategies to Improve HIV and AIDS Interventions: A Compendium of Programs in Africa*. pdf.usaid.gov/pdf_docs/PNADQ625.pdf

Valente, T. W., Y. M. Kim, C. Lettenmaier, W. Glass, and Y. Dibba. 1994. "Radio Promotion of Family Planning in the Gambia." *International Family Planning Perspectives* 26 (4): 148–57.

Vambe, Maurice T. 2004. "Versions and Sub-Versions: Trends in Chimurenga Musical Discourses of Post Independence in Zimbabwe." *African Study Monographs* 25 (4): 167–93.

Vambe, Maurice T. and Aquilina Mawadza. 2001. "Images of Black Women in Popular Songs and Some Poems on AIDS in Post-Independence Zimbabwe." In *Orality and Cultural Identities in Zimbabwe*, Ed. M. T. Vambe, 57–72. Harare: Mambo Press.

Van Buren, Kathleen. 2006. "Stealing Elephants, Creating Futures: Exploring Uses of Music and other Arts for Community Education in Nairobi, Kenya." PhD diss., University of California, Los Angeles.

————. 2007. "Partnering for Social Change: Exploring Relationships between Musicians and Organizations in Nairobi, Kenya." *Ethnomusicology Forum* 16 (2): 303–26.

————. 2009. "Locating Hope in Performance: Lessons from Edward Kabuye." *African Music* 8 (3): 144-161.

Van der Vliet, Virginia. 2001. "AIDS: Losing 'The New Struggle'?" *Daedalus* 130 (1): 151–84.

van Niekerk, Anton. 2005. "Mother-to-Child Transmission of HIV/AIDS in Africa: Ethical Problems and Perspectives." In *Ethics & AIDS in Africa: The Challenge to Our Thinking*, ed. Anton van Niekerk and Loretta M. Kopelman. Cape Town: David Philip.

Van Warmelo, N. J. 1989. *Venda Dictionary-Tshivenda English*. Pretoria: J. L. van Schaik.

Vaughan, P. W., A. Regis, and E. St. Catherine. 2000. "Effect of an Entertainment-Education Radio Soap Opera of Family Planning and HIV Prevention in St. Lucia." *International Family Planning Perspectives* 26 (4): 148–57.

Wainaina, Binjavanga. 2006. "How to Write about Africa." *Granta* 92. www.granta.com/extracts/2615.

Walser, Robert. 1995. "Rhyme, Rhythm and Rhetoric in the Music of Public Enemy." *Ethnomusicology* 39 (2): 193–217.

Wamitila, Kyallo Wadi. 2002. *Uhakiki wa Fasihi: Misingi na Vipengele vyake*. Nairobi: Phoenix Publishers Ltd.

Wanyama, M. N. 2007. "Policy and Implementation: A Case of Music Copyright Laws in Kenya." *Muzíkí* 4 (1): 27–41.

————. 2009. *Form and Content of African Music: A Case Study of Bukusu Circumcision Music*. Saarbruecken: VDM Verlag Dr. Müller.

Watney, Simon. 1987. *Policing Desire: Pornography, AIDS and the Media*. London: Methuen.

————. 1990. "Photography and HIV/AIDS." In *The Critical Image: Essays on Contemporary Photography*, ed. Carol Squiers. Seattle: Bay Press.

Watts, Michael and Iain Boal. 1995. "Working-Class Heroes: E.P. Thompson and Sebastiao Salgado." *Transition* 68: 90–115.

Weinberg, Paul. 1991. "Documentary Photography: Past, Present and Future," *Staffrider* 9 (4): 95–97.

White, Mike. 2006. "Establishing Common Ground in Community-Based Arts in Health." *Journal of the Royal Society of Health* 126 (3): 128–33.

"WHO African Region: Ethiopia." [2009.] www.who.int/countries/eth/areas/hiv/en/index.html.

REFERENCES

Wiehagen, Theresa, Nicole M. Caito, Vetta S. Thompson, Christopher M. Casey, Nancy L. Weaver, Keri Jupka, and Matthew W. Kreuter. 2007. "Applying Projective Techniques to Formative Research in Health Communication Development." *Health Promotion Practice* 8 (2): 164–72.

Wilson, Susan E., and E. Jackson Allison Jr. 1986. "Training Trainers in Developing Countries: Health Education and Mass Media Aspects of Low Cost Sanitation." *Journal of Environmental Health* 48 (3): 311–14.

Wojcicki, J. M. 2002. "'She Drank His Money': Survival Sex and the Problem of Violence in Taverns in Gauteng Province, South Africa." *Medical Anthropology Quarterly* 16 (3): 267–93.

Wolf, Angelika. 2006. *"Das was kommt schlägt nicht die Trommel:* Botschaften von Aids-Aufklärungsplakaten der postkolonialen Wendezeit in Malawi." In *Kommunikation über HIV/AIDS—Interdisziplinäre Beiträge zur Prävention im subsaharischen Afrika,* ed. Martina Drescher and Sabine Klaeger, 117–54. Berlin: Lit Verlag.

Wong, Deborah. 2001. *Sounding the Center: History and Aesthetics in Thai Buddhist Performance.* Chicago: University of Chicago Press.

Wong, Lana, ed. 1999. *Shootback: Photos by Kids from the Nairobi Slums.* London: Booth-Clibborn Editions.

Wood, Kate. 2005. "Contextualizing Group Rape in Post-Apartheid South Africa." *Culture, Health, and Sexuality* 7 (4): 303–17.

Work, John W., Lewis Wade Jones, Samuel C. Adams, Robert Gordon, and Bruce Nemerov. 2005. *Lost Delta Found: Rediscovering the Fisk University-Library of Congress Coahoma County Study, 1941–1942.* Nashville: Vanderbilt University Press.

World Bank Country. 2001. "Tanzania at the Turn of the Century: From Reforms to Sustained Growth and Poverty Reduction," study no. 2213.

Wyschogrod, Edith. 1973. *The Phenomenon of Death: Faces of Mortality.* New York: Harper & Row.

Yahaya, Mohammed Kuta. 2000. *Indigenous Music for Entertainment-Education: Lessons from AIDS.* Ibadan, Nigeria: Stirling-Horden.

Yankah, Kwesi. 2004. "Narrative in Times of Crisis: AIDS Stories in Ghana." *Journal of Folklore Research* 41 (2): 181–98.

Yoder, Stanley, Robert Hornick, and Ben Chirwa. 1996. "Evaluating the Program Effects of a Radio Drama about AIDS in Zambia." *Studies in Family Planning* 27 (4): 188–203.

Zaffiro, James. 1991. *From Police Network to Station of the Nation: A Political History of Broadcasting in Botswana 1927–1991.* Gaborone: The Botswana Society.

Zometa, Carlos S., Robert Dedrick, Michael D. Knox, Wayne Westoff, Rodrigo S. Siri, Ann Debaldo. 2007. "Translation, Cross-Cultural Adaptation and Validation of an HIV/AIDS Knowledge and Attitudinal Instrument." *AIDS Education & Prevention* 19 (3): 231–44.

Zvomunya, Percy. 2000. "The Female World and Female Authority in Tuku's Music." *Moto,* October: 21, 23.

DISCOGRAPHY

Aboutou Roots. 1995. "Jolie Femme Protège-toi." On *Protège-toi!, Volume 1.* Abidjan: EMI-JAT Music.

Banda, Paul. 2005. *Edzi ndi ya tonse.* On *Mwaonjeza.* Balaka: IY.

Barz, Gregory F. 2007. *Singing for Life: Songs of Hope, Healing, and HIV/AIDS in Uganda.* Washington, DC: Smithsonian Folkways.

Barz, Gregory F., and Gerald C. Liu. 2010. *Kampala Flow East African Hip Hop from Uganda.* Nashville, TN: Lime Pulp Records.

Bokosi, Malume. 2007. "Wakana kukayezetsa" On *Kukamwa kwangotiuma.* Blantyre: OG.

Border Klan. 2004. "Balaa." Unreleased single provided courtesy of Border Klan.

Chaphuka, Paul. 1997. *Ndichirtseni.* Balaka: IY.

Chidzanja, Peter. 2001. *Chechule.* MC Blantyre: Oreta.

Chimangeni, Blessings. 2008. "Mudzichita chisoni." On *Mphika wa nyemba.* Lilongwe: State records.

Chiwalo, Cosmas. N.d. "Mudziti toto." On *Mudzithandizana.* Balaka: IY Studio.

Dyoko, Beauler and Cosmas Magaya. 2000. *Afamba Apota.* Dandemutande.

Dzapasi Mbira Group. 2003. *Dzapasi Mbira Group: Nyamaropa Tuning.* www.mbira.org.

Edgar & Davis. 2007. *Musamabwelela kumudzi.* Blantyre: GME.

Fumulani, Robert. n.d. *Kunja kuno imfa ikuthamanga.* MBC Recording.

Gwaladi, Joe. 2006. "Edzi ndi dodo." On *Zakanika.* Blantyre: OG.

———. 2006. "Mwana dala." On *Tidzatuluka m'munda.* Blantyre: Defao.

Jumbe, Patrick. 2006. *Sinkhalidwe.* Blantyre: Ching'amba Records.

Kasambwe Brothers Band. 1992. "AIDS is a Killer, Check your Step." *Moyo wanga.* Glasgow: Pamtondo.

Katawa singers. 1995. "Kunja kwaipa." On *Tiimbire yesu.* Mzuzu: Spiritual Songs 6.

Kaunda, Billy. 1999. "Kumidima." On *Alibe Mau.* MC Balaka: Sounds of Malawi.

Khoza, Albert. 1998. "Chidyaximan." On *Bola kunthanzi.* MC Blantyre: Studio K.

Lungu, Stonard. 1997. "Ndiyimba ndi yani." On *Mukanene.* Blantyre: Deja Brew.

Malawi Police Orchestra. 1998. *Kunja kuno kwaopsya.* MBC Recording.

Maliro, Mlaka. 1997. "Toto." On *Maloto.* Balaka: IY studios.

Mapfumo, Thomas. 1994. *Hondo.* ZIMBOB Records.

Masaka Band. n.d. *Watenga AIDS iwe.* MBC recording.

"Masego and Cecilia Disclosure." 2004. *Makgabaneng* (English Version). *Makgabaneng* Studios. Prod. Idol Productions & Lewis, Jack.

Matshikiza, John. 2000. *South African Freedom Songs: A Documentary* [CD 1 of 2]. Cape Town: Making Music Productions.

Mhepo. 2001. *Mapapiro.* cdbaby.com/cd/mhepo.

———. 2003. *Thawa moto.* Blantyre: GME.

Micheal, Ben. 2001. "Ndimvereniko." On *Moyo wantauni* Blantyre: Mankhamba.

Momba Hax. n.d. *Samala.* On *Lilongwe Giants,* vol. 1.

Mount Sinai Choir. 2001. *Mau.* Glasgow: Pamtondo.

———. 2007. "Kukambirana za Edzi." On *Tiyeni Kumwamba.* Blantyre: Mt Sinai.

Mphepo, Alex Mataya. 2006. *Tiona mbwadza.* Blantyre: Mphepo.

———. 2006. "Ukwera zobanduka." On *Tiona Mbwadza.* Blantyre: Mphepo.

Mtukudzi, Oliver. 1999. *Tuku Music.* Putamayo World Music.

Namoko, Alan. 1992. "Ana osiidwa." On *Ana osiidwa.* Glasgow: Pamtondo.

Ncheu Ingoma Group. 1996. *Kulibe nthenda ina.* MBC Recording.

Ndingo Brothers' Band. n.d. *Anamwaliwa muwalange.* MBC recording.

Nowlin, Bill. 1996. *Radio Freedom: Voice of the African National Congress and the People's Army Umkhonto We Sizwe.* Burlington, MA: Rounder Records.

Phiri, Dennis. 1998. "Tikutha." On *Ulangizi.* Balaka: Sounds of Malawi, IY 1098043.

———. 2006. "Osaiwala." On MC Mwandidolola. Lilongwe: MC Studios.

Phiri, Saleta. 1989. *Iri mu ufa.* Blantyre: Saleta Phiri.

REFERENCES

————. 1995. "Zinthu zasintha." On *Ndirande Blues*. Glasgow: Pamtondo.

————. 1997. "Tinali ndi anzathu ife." On *The Last Pound*. Glasgow: Pamtondo.

SFPS and ACS. 1997. *Afrique Lève-toi*. Washington, D.C.: USAID.

Skeremu Austin, and Banda Manyowa. 2000. *Mbuyo kucheta*. Blantyre: Studio K.

The Soul of Mbira: Traditions of the Shona People of Zimbabwe. 1973. Various Artists, rec. Paul Berliner. New York: Nonesuch Records.

Tiyamike Band. 1995. "Edzi." On *Mudawona kuwala* Balaka: IY.

Young Messenger. 2004. "Get Ready for a Message." Field recording by Kathleen Noss Van Buren. Nairobi, Kenya: September 11.

FILMOGRAPHY

Afrique Lève-toi (Wake Up Africa): Les Artistes s'Engagent. 1998. SFPS (Santé Familiale et Prévention du Sida) and ACS (Artistes Associé Contre le SIDA). Washington, D.C.: USAID.

Born in Africa. 1990. dir. John Zaritsky. *Frontline* ep. 809. Frontline/WGBH in association with the Canadian Broadcasting Corporation.

Sharp Sharp: The Kwaito Story. 2003. dir. Aryan Kaganof. South Africa-Netherlands. Featuring Zola, TKZee, Oskido, Mzambiya, Don Laka, and Mandoza.

Siyayinqoba!/Beat It! [DVD]. Cape Town: Community Health Media Trust.

The Talking Drums Of Africa [musical Group]. 1998. Video recording of National Youth World AIDS Day Drama Festival performance provided courtesy of Edward Kabuye.

Why Must I Die? 2005. dir. Pierre Peyrot and Vincent Moloi, prod. Patrice Barrat. Cape Town: Mondopop Mediavision.

NOTES

CHAPTER 1

1. Sections of this introduction, in an earlier and substantially different form, appeared in Barz and Cohen 2008.
2. On October 30, 2009, Barack Obama lifted the United States' twenty-two-year-old ban on HIV-positive people visiting or immigrating into the country.
3. IDAAC (Integrated Development and AIDS Concern).
4. See www.aids2006.org, www.aids2008.org, www.aids2010.org, www.aids2012.org.

CHAPTER 3

1. Frontline episode #809, originally aired April 3, 1990. This transcription comes from the 90-minute version of the broadcast; a 60-minute version, broadcast at a later date, exists as well.

   Permission to publish this transcript courtesy of WGBH Boston. *Born in Africa* is a K. A.. Production for FRONTLINE/WGBH in association with the Canadian Broadcasting Corporation, © 1990 WGBH Educational Foundation.

   Many thanks to John Zaritsky, Gerald Bareebe, Stephen Ssendi, Anna Batcheller, and Lynn Mason for their assistance.
2. The first broadcast of *Born in Africa* was hosted and narrated by Peter Jennings (who also spoke what became the episode's starting titles). Subsequent airings of the episode replaced Jennings' narration with a nearly identical narration by actor Will Lyman (who became "the voice of Frontline" in 1984 and has served as the main narrator of the series ever since). This transcript comes from a video copy of the film, with Lyman's narration.
3. The name of this organization is actually the National Council of Women.
4. *Mafuta mingi* refers to Uganda's well-connected urban upper-middle class. Some political scientists note that this class arose in the 1970s, when Idi Amin's regime turned over land and business confiscated from expelled Asians to political associates, thus giving Lutaaya's reference here significant historical resonance.
5. According to King's College's Web site (http://www.kcbudo.sc.ug), the school was founded in 1906.
6. Considering that the capacity of Nakivubo stadium is between 12,000 and 18,000, it is likely that the actual attendance figure for Lutaaya's concert was considerably less.

CHAPTER 6

1. The other two countries that have experienced declines in HIV prevalence are Uganda and Zimbabwe. See UNAIDS 2007b.
2. Portions of this chapter have previously appeared in Van Buren 2006. See also Van Buren 2007 and 2009, which offer further information on some of the groups and issues mentioned here. Two comments should be made on spelling and translations. First, names of musicians are frequently spelled multiple ways in the Kenyan media and by the

individuals themselves (for example, the hip hop group Border Klan also spells its name Border Clan). Second, thanks are extended to the musicians discussed in this chapter as well as to Philip Noss and Chacha Leonard Mwita for assistance with printed song texts and translations.

3. Within Kenya, for instance, Nyumbani Children's Home was instrumental in lobbying the government to enable Kenyans to access generic drugs (Achieng 2001, Blomfield 2001).

4. As described by Peter Piot (2005, 7), former executive director of the Joint United Nations Programme on HIV/AIDS, the "Three Ones" approach is based on the following principles for action: "one agreed AIDS action framework that provides the basis for coordinating the work of all partners"; "one national AIDS coordinating authority, with a broad-based multisectoral mandate"; and "one agreed country-level monitoring and evaluation system."

5. A 2008 report by the UNAIDS/WHO Working Group on Global HIV/AIDS and STI Surveillance suggests that rates among young women may be at least three times higher than rates among young men. Rates among other parts of the population are also alarming; for example, rates among pregnant women in some rural areas are estimated to be as high as 26 percent (UNAIDS/WHO Working Group on Global HIV/AIDS and STI Surveillance 2008).

6. I have not been able to find details on the size and location of the test group for this National AIDS Control Council study.

7. Robert Neuwirth (2005, 22) critiques use of the term "slum," which he suggests carries connotations of despair, criminality, and disorganization, and which he argues masks the innovation and strength often visible in such spaces. I concur, and join other scholars (Neuwirth 2005, 17, Amuyunzu-Nyamongo and Taffa 2003) in combining the terms informal/low income and community/settlement (i.e., low-income community or low-income settlement) rather than using the term "slum."

8. Also see www.gadonet.com.

9. Differences between rural and urban programming can include, for instance, increased used of vernacular languages and traditional music in rural areas. For examples of work on arts and HIV/AIDS outside Nairobi, see Gibson (2000), who also addresses historical connections between music and healing; and Mjomba (2002 and 2005). Barz (2006) makes brief reference to Kenya.

10. *Benga* is a popular music style originally associated with the Luo of western Kenya.

11. "Artiste" is a common spelling of the word "artist" in Kenyan media.

12. "Balaa" is an unreleased 2004 single provided by Border Klan.

13. This English translation is by Border Klan. The musicians note that "mabeste" can also refer to a friend.

14. For more on the history of the Kenya Music Festival, see Ogot 2002 and Kidula 1996.

15. Other Kenya Music Festival themes have included immunization, prevention of drug and other substance abuse, child labor, and corruption.

16. Non-formal schools differ from formal schools in that they are not funded by the government and sometimes offer more flexible arrangements to students (for instance, on uniforms, school books, and attendance), yet they often still follow the formal curriculum.

17. The term "youth" is used broadly. Projects such as the one in Kawangware may involve young people (such as Martin) in their early and mid-20s.

18. As reflected in this chapter, and as asserted by many musicians and scholars, music is often combined with other arts (dance, drama, puppetry, acrobatics, etc.) in performances in Nairobi and other parts of Africa.

19. In his book on Yoruba drumming, for instance, Akin Euba (1990, 62) notes that music functions as "one of the principal media of general education." Francis Bebey (1975, 32), in turn, has asserted that the basic role of musicians is to "guide and coordinate" members of African communities. Hugh Tracey (1963), J. H. Kwabena Nketia (1982[1974]), and Ashenafi Kebede (1982), among others, have described the use of African songs to remind communities of the past, to teach about communal practices and values, and to communicate issues of concern.

20. For instance, when entertainment-education methods cannot directly teach literacy, they can stimulate audiences to seek literacy courses (Singhal and Rogers 1999, 13). On the effectiveness of programs, see also Yahaya (2000) and Ryerson (2004). For more on HIV/AIDS programs, see Singhal and Rogers (2003).

21. While more funding may be available for AIDS-related programs than for programs addressing other social issues, funding may still be restricted (i.e., it may be minimal, not covering rehearsal costs or material resources such as costumes needed for performances, and it may be available for single performances, but not for lengthier programs).

22. Such sentiments about government-run HIV/AIDS programs are also discussed by Shorter and Onyancha (1998).

CHAPTER 8

1. This chapter primarily reflects the commentary and ongoing involvement of the lead author (Allison) in AIDS awareness, education and prevention internationally, especially in Malawi, Southeastern Africa. Brown and Wilson were indispensable in researching, writing, and editing the manuscript.

2. Also known as grab or opportunity sampling, a convenience sample is a type of non-probability sampling in which individuals are selected at the convenience of the researcher. Findings from a convenience sample are considered less definitive. Results can be qualified by extrapolating them only to a much more targeted and narrowly defined population.

CHAPTER 9

1. Given the nature of their work as community health workers and treatment activists, I presumed that most participants would be familiar with the content of the workshop. This presumption was confirmed by data collected in a questionnaire that showed TAC and HOPE Cape Town participants had on average high levels of knowledge about HIV/AIDS and ART.

2. The Visual Body Map was developed by Colin Almeleh and Fiona Mendelson at the AIDS and Society Research Unit in the Centre for Social Science Research, University of Cape Town.

3. The failure of some exercises resulted in changing the sequence of exercises, while new exercises such as the disclosure of HIV-positive status and ways to support ART patients with treatment adherence were added.

4. The puzzle exercise proved to be the simplest and most accessible way of explaining the cellular structure of the human body. In the pilot workshop, two other exercises were tested and failed. In one I used a slice of onion and food dye to highlight the cellular composition of the onion. And in the other I tried the analogy of a house with bricks.

5. Note that some ART clinics, such as the Médecins Sans Frontières ART programme, require ART patients to have disclosed their status to at least one family member or to a friend who can assist them with their treatment.

6.   All participant names are pseudonyms but refer to specific individuals who took part in the project.

7.   Colleagues have suggested that drawing as a medium, as opposed to singing or drama, is not common in Southern African culture and could be seen as essentially "Western." I would suggest that regardless of cultural background, people are open to visual approaches to learning if it is participatory and fun and not framed as "art."

CHAPTER 10

1.   Matatus, public transport vehicles in Kenya, occupy a unique cultural space. It is believed that many of the drivers and conductors involved in this industry offer free rides to school girls in exchange for sexual favors.

CHAPTER 12

1.   I am indebted to Pia Thielmann, then of Chancellor College in Zomba, who provided the local press documentation, and to David Kerr for translations from Chichewa. Photographs by Eckhard Breitinger.

CHAPTER 13

1.   Radio serial dramas are not the sole form of HIV/AIDS communication; television serials are also a factor. One of the earliest comprehensive analyses of television serials was Heidi Noel Nariman's book *Soap Operas for Social Change: Toward a Methodology for Entertainment-Education Television* (1993). Alternative readings of television serials can be found in René Smith's article "*Yizo Yizo* and Essentialism: Representations of Women and Gender-Based Violence in a Drama Series Based on Reality" (2003), and Loren Kruger's article "Theatre for Development and TV Nation: Notes on Educational Soap Opera in South Africa" (2004).

2.   More information about HIV/AIDS serial dramas in southern African settings appears in "Community Reinforcement of an Entertainment Education Intervention: Botswana and Zimbabwe," a presentation delivered by Siphiwe Rametsi et al. (2004) and "Evaluating the Program Effects of a Radio Drama about AIDS in Zambia" (1996) by Stanley P. Yoder et al.

3.   The United States Department of Health and Human Services also participates in *Makgabaneng* activities.

4.   According to data on information and broadcasting provided in *Botswana's National Development Plan 9 2003-04-2008-09*, close to 80 percent of Batswana can access quality Medium and FM bands on their radios (Ministry of Finance and Development Planning 2003, 361–62). Additionally, statistics compiled from a 2003 national broadcasting survey revealed that 72.3 percent of Botswana's population listens to radio on a daily basis, confirming the significance of radio among the public.

5.   These studies were undertaken by staff at the Botswana-United States Partnership (BOTUSA), Centers for Disease Control (CDC), and the U.S. Department of Health and Human Services.

6.   David Gere looks at the significance of the musical arts in HIV/AIDS education in *How to Make Dances in an Epidemic: Tracking Choreography in the Age of AIDS* (2004).

7.   For more information on media in everyday life see "Wrestling with the Present, Beckoning the Past: Contemporary Zulu Radio Drama" (2000a) and "Zulu Radio Drama" (2000b) by

Liz Gunner; "Remote Audiences Beyond 2000: Radio, Everyday Life, and Development in South India" by Yesudhassan Thomas Jayprakash (2000); and *Dramas of Nationhood: The Politics of Television in Egypt* by Lila Abu-Lughod (2005).

8. Nzewi asserts that the musical arts also assist in physical fitness, stress management, self-discovery; social bonding, virtues, ethics, social mores, spiritual disposition, humane living, recreation, history; solidarity, mass communication, honor, reward, creativity, spontaneity, validation of public causes and events and peace (Nzewi 2003, 15–19).

9. James Zaffiro is one of the scholars who provided a full investigation of radio in Botswana. Although brief, his 1991 study *From Police Network to Station of the Nation: A Political History of Broadcasting in Botswana 1927-1991*, provides a comprehensive history of radio in the country.

10. Leading scholars have accentuated the need for building national awareness and consciousness through the arts. Material on the arts and nationalism can be found in Franz Fanon's "On National Consciousness" in *Wretched of the Earth* (1963), Léopold Sédar Senghor's "Negritude: A Humanism of the Twentieth Century" (1966), and J. H. Kwabena Nketia's "The Scholarly Study of African Music" (1998).

11. Once RB2 was established, the name of its parent station, Radio Botswana 1 (RB1), was changed to distinguish between the two. RB2 earned a reputation for being a contemporary radio station directed toward younger audiences.

12. Thomas Turino delves deeper into the relevance of the musical arts in promoting nationalism in *Nationalists, Cosmopolitans, and Popular Music in Zimbabwe* (2000).

13. Musicologist Charles Hamm provides further insights on the function of government radio and its promotion of national ideals in his articles "'The Constant Companion of Man': Separate Development, Radio Bantu, and Music" (1991a) and "Music and Radio in the People's Republic of China" (1991b).

14. In ensuing years, entertainment education became known as "the intentional placement of educational content in entertainment messages" (Singhal and Rogers 2002, 117). However one of the most comprehensive definitions of entertainment-education positioned it as "the process of purposely designing and implementing a media message to both entertain and educate, in order to increase audience members' knowledge about an educational issue, create favorable attitudes, shift social norms, and change overt behavior" (Singhal et al. 2002, 4).

15. According to youth communications scholars Gita Bamezai and Archana Shukla, radio serial drama is one of the preferred tools in HIV/AIDS entertainment-education strategies because it "provides quick, direct contact with large populations, and can encourage dialogue and debate on important but sensitive health concerns in a compelling, attractive way" (Bamezai and Shukla 1998, 113).

16. Overall there are twenty-four themes featured on *Makgabaneng*. The ones mentioned here are merely samples of the full range.

17. Statistics from the *National Development Plan 9* confirmed that the population was at an estimated 1.6 million and rising at the date of publication (Ministry of Finance and Development Planning 2003, 13).

18. While it is acknowledged that the *National AIDS Policy* was drawn up in 1993, its printing date reads 1998, causing a discrepancy between the actual time of printing. The *Medium Term Plan II*, uses 1993 as the original date, but the *Botswana United Nations General Assembly Special Session on HIV/AIDS (UNGASS) 2005 Progress Report* refers to 1998 as the true date (NACA 2005, 14). Another incongruous date emerges in the ACHAP *Setting the Stage for Scaling Up HIV Prevention—Discussion Paper*, which notes that the Draft Botswana

National Policy on HIV/AIDS was formulated in 2005 (ACHAP, 7). It can be assumed that the policy was set for revision at this final date.

19. It is understood that this response involves the private sector, civil society, and a slew of "multilateral" and "bilateral" organizations working together (NACA 2005, 3). The individuals who prepared policies have also completed the *Comprehensive Health Sector Policy on Care and Treatment* (Government of Botswana 2001) and the *National Policy on HIV Rapid Testing* (Ministry of Health 2005; ACHAP 2006, 7). Pertinent HIV/AIDS policies preceding the formation of NAC include the *National Population Policy* (Government of Botswana 1997) and *National Policy on Women in Development* (Government of Botswana 1997).

20. Botswana's national monitoring and evaluation is conducted by the Botswana HIV/AIDS Response Information Management System (BHRIMS).

21. The *National Strategy for Behavior Change Interventions and Communications for HIV and AIDS* (2006) is also relevant to *Makgabaneng*, however it was not formulated until years after the serial drama was broadcast. Nevertheless, with its focus on "stimulating community response; building capacity for communities to provide environments conducive to HIV prevention, treatment, and care; motivating individual desire to adopt behaviors that protect self and others from HIV infection and related illnesses; enabling individuals with the skills for performing HIV-protective behaviors both in sexual relations and in the provision of care for PLWHA; and creating an institutional culture that relies on evidence-based planning" (NACA 2006, 4–5).

22. For more information on self-efficacy see *Self-Efficacy: The Exercise of Control* by Albert Bandura (1997).

23. The *Makgabaneng* staff summarizes the writing process as "research on programs to be promoted; workshop for material Development and Pathways; individual work (per cycle); group work (for verifying and refining); [script] sent to stakeholders; meet with program officers; Technical Advisory Committee (TAC) meeting; and scripting" (*Makgabaneng*, The Writing Process).

24. This quote originally appeared in Berger's publication *Scripts: Writing for Radio and Television* (1990).

25. Maungo Mooki subscribes to the belief that the drama is best suited for radio because it "makes the listener visualize" what is taking place. Despite the data on the reach of radio in the country, she is convinced that "radio isn't about accessibility"; rather it is about "people internalizing the message" (Interview, Jul. 29, 2004).

26. These serials were all broadcast on television, but Abu-Lughod's analysis is equally relevant for *Makgabaneng*.

27. The questions used during LDGs were elaborated on during a 2003 presentation "Getting Personal: Engaging a Mass Media Audience Through Reinforcement Activities" created by Siphiwe Rametsi et al.

28. There was a dual interpretation of this information regarding female listening patterns. One reading of the information was that there are more female listeners overall. The other one was that women are more inclined to participate in *Makgabaneng* contests (Tembo et al. 2003).

CHAPTER 14

1. I would like to thank Professor William Beinart, Professor Colin Bundy, Rebecca Davis, Dr. Jacqueline Maingard and Dr. Nicoli Nattrass for their numerous helpful comments on earlier drafts of this article.

2. The political controversy over the use of nutrition for treating HIV mounted when lemons and garlic cloves instead of ARVs were displayed in the South African Pavilion at the 2005 International AIDS Conference (IAC). From 2005 onwards, Minister of Health Manto Tshabalala-Msimang was lambasted by the medical and activist communities in South Africa and abroad for claiming that a diet rich in Vitamin C, beetroot, olive oil, and garlic could prevent the onset of AIDS. The role of healthy eating in "positive living" was therefore relegated in later series of *Beat It!* which placed greater emphasis on public education about the benefits of ARVs.

3. The Health Minister praised Uganda's PMTCT successes as an example of the efficacy and necessity of African solutions to HIV/AIDS. The stress on "home-grown" solutions became increasingly notable in the struggle to obtain a national HAART program in South Africa, as political leaders attempted to contrast the western scientific enterprise of 'biomedicalization' with indigenous, "African" solutions. (See Ek 2005, 8, for further analysis of the minister and president's response.)

4. MSF had begun the pilot program to prove that patients in resource-constrained settings could adhere well to antiretroviral treatment in spite of its clinical complexities. The adherence rates documented in the study were the highest on record when the results were published, debunking the notion that patients adhered better to ARVs in rich world contexts (Médecins Sans Frontières 2003, 2).

5. The Medicines Control Council is South Africa's medicines approval body, under the aegis of the Department of Health.

6. The reference to the FDA was misleading as it had not refused to register nevirapine. In March 2002, Boehringer-Ingelheim had withdrawn its registration application for the drug for the purposes of PMTCT of HIV. The reason for this did not concern the drug's efficacy or safety, but rather stemmed from the clinical trials which had taken place in Uganda, and which did not comply with standards of the FDA. For further details, see Heywood (2003, 307). For a discussion of the details around the Health Minister and MCC's opposition to nevirapine, see D'Adesky 2004, 181–84.

CHAPTER 15

1. The author is responsible for all translations from French into English in this article.

2. HIV/AIDS edutainment campaigns in Francophone Africa not covered in this article but that will be addressed in a more developed version of this study include *Yamba-Songo*: Les Clés de la Vie (Keys to Life, http://www.comminit.com/en/node/1699/38); Reaching Men (http://www.jhuccp.org/topics/enter_ed/eeprojects/05-26.shtml), 100% Jeune (100% Young, http://www.reglo.org/), Nous Sommes les Tams-tams (We Are the Drums, http://www.tg.undp.org/tamtam/tamtam.htm), Rien Que la Vérité (Nothing But the Truth, http://www.comminit.com/en/node/301344/38), and Ma Vie, Ma Decision (My Life, My Decision, http://www.comminit.com/en/node/264107/38).

3. In the late 1990s, ORSTOM's name changed to l'Institut de recherche pour le dévelopement (IRD).

4. Jula is one of the core Mande languages—a language family including Maninkakan (Malinké), Mandinka, and Bamanankan (Bambara), among others. These languages are similar enough so as to be (to greater or lesser degrees) mutually intelligible. Thus, some residents of other francophone countries in the West African region (such as Mali, Burkina Faso, Guinea, and Senegal) would likely be able to understand the text of a song in French and Jula. Still, the pairing of French and this particular Mande language suggests a primary target audience of Ivorians.

5. SFPS focuses on health development assistance in Francophone Africa. A central office is located in Abidjan, and regional offices and initiatives have been established in Burkina Faso, Cote d'Ivoire, Togo, Cameroon, Niger, Benin, Mauritania and Congo-Kinshasa (http://www.jhuccp.org/africa/regional/FHA.shtml, accessed October 2, 2009).

6. I wish to offer an expression of thanks to Jane Brown for loaning me archival copies of Wake Up! Africa materials and for agreeing to talk with me about the project. Information from Brown was obtained during an interview conducted on November 2, 2009.

CHAPTER 16

1. A pseudonym.

2. This version was recorded by Canadian journalists at ANC headquarters in Lusaka, Zambia, in 1985 and later appeared as track 7 on the commemorative Radio Freedom CD (Rounder Records USA 11661–4019–2).

3. HIV prevalence in Uganda decreased from 9.5 percent of the population in 1997 to 5 percent in 2001 (UNAIDS 2003 in Barz 2006, 11). Other data from antenatal clinics in Uganda suggest that the figures have fallen from 29.4 percent in 1992 to 11.25 percent in 2000 (O'Manique 2004). It is sobering to compare this to comparable statistics for South Africa; from 12.9 percent in 1997 to 20.1 percent in 2001 (ibid.), although in the two national settings, very divergent nationalisms, economic contexts and market-driven change interact to produce rather different overall settings.

4. See for example Heald 1995, 2006; Ingstad 1990; De Bruyn 1992; McDonald and Shatz 2005. Farmer (1990, 1994, 2006) has documented the ways in which AIDS became incorporated into the preexisting folk model of illness in Haiti. His work is particularly interesting as he conducted research on the subject there before AIDS was known in the area, and documented the ways in which it was incorporated and the role of narrative and rumor in the reaching of consensus. He looks mainly at AIDS as a "sent illness" in terms of sorcery accusations. Although he does provide an analysis of blood related illness and female morality (1988), he does not connect this directly with etiology of AIDS as much of the material on southern Africa has.

5. This extract is taken from McNeill (2007), in which the entire 17 minutes and over 200 lines of "Zwidzumbe" is translated in Appendix B. The line numbers refer to that appendix.

6. *Gokhonya* is usually found in women after a difficult or problematic birth such as that induced by caesarean section. Symptoms include the child refusing the mother's milk and red marks on the child's head and neck. White pimples will be found inside the mother's vagina, and the conventional cure involves the *inyanga* scraping the vaginal sores with a razor and mixing the resultant fluid with the mother's urine and a mixture of three herbs. This is then given to the child in a milky drink and it will be healed. The mother, however, must undergo several more rites of purification. *Gokhonya* often starts with *zwilonda*: open sores on and in the vagina that resemble the third phase of syphilis.

7. This refers to a specific group of traditional healers called *maine*. They are comparable to family doctors and specialize in treating specific ailments.

CHAPTER 17

1. Recorded by Gregory Barz in 2001 with the Namirembe Post-Test Club, a support organization for those who have received the results of HIV blood tests that reveal a positive result.

2. Recorded by the TASO Mbarara Drama Group c. 2004 and distributed on the group's album *Fight Against AIDS/Turwanise Silimu: Songs For Our Community/Ebyeshongoro Byeitu*. Transcribed by Judah M. Cohen. Words in square brackets indicate a choral echo sung overlapping the end of the previous phrase.

CHAPTER 18

1. An earlier version of this article was published in 2007 in *Art South Africa* 5 (2).
2. Quoted from *Cape Times*, May 29, 2002.

CHAPTER 19

1. Transcribed from Barz's original recording and translation (2006).
2. When comparing the stanzas about the ideal woman and man, the only difference is in the placement of statements about loving family members, and that the ideal of cleanliness only appears in the description of an ideal woman in this version of the song.
3. In this analysis I focus largely on the community experience and how this contributes to Vilimina's critical perspective. Attention could also be paid to Vilimina's individual experience. As an HIV-positive woman who has seen explosive social changes in her lifetime, her personal experiences are no doubt deeply relevant to how her critique has developed.
4. "Things are different nowadays" could also be read as related to Westernization. Locally, Westernization is often seen as deeply intertwined with discourses about AIDS and gender; commentary on Westernization at this musical juncture would be extremely relevant.
5. HIV cannot be spread by sharing food or by contact with spittle, but may other viruses can. AIDS does often travel with multiple other infections and viruses. Perhaps that other diseases can be transmitted through food and quotidian contact is one origin of these cultural taboos.
6. Westernization is an intriguing trope in Vilimina's song. In her own life, Vilimina has seen dramatic Westernizing trends, and her song is replete with images that may be seen as commenting on Westernization: drinking from gourds that were already drunk from versus eating with Western-style forks and cups, women crossing their legs, and sitting on Western-style chairs rather than on ground mats. Indeed, even wearing half a *gomesi* could potentially be tied to rural women often not wearing coverings on their torso. Moreover, Vilimina also comments on the age of marriage, which in many areas has been deeply influenced by Westernization. Perhaps most notably, in certain areas of Uganda Western-influenced schooling has begun teaching girls to play men's musical instruments. Westernizing influences have been one cause of dramatic shifts in gender roles in Uganda. In the context of this analysis, it is important to ask whether Vilimina sees women actively choosing these changes for themselves, or whether she sees women's roles being redefined through externally imposed Westernization. Analyzing the dynamics around Westernization may deeply impact how we understand Vilimina's portrayal of women's agency with respect to sexuality and AIDS.
7. The role of Westernization is extremely complex in this interaction. Certainly hierarchical social rank is one dynamic associated with Western traditions, which people who have talked with Vilimina about the song see as important. However, many valences are plausible.
8. Interestingly, the international and medical communities are also beginning to recognize how these dynamics are related, with AIDS infecting those who are poor and marginalized at significantly higher rates.

9. Why does Vilimina focus on abstinence rather than condoms or other approaches to preventing AIDS? One might ask if she feels that women do not have enough power to negotiate using condoms and abstinence is seen as more culturally acceptable or more passive than actively negotiating a male partner's condom compliance. If women do not feel that they can negotiate condom use and therefore Vilimina is resorting to promoting abstinence as more realistic, this paints a more delimited picture of the extent of women's power.

10. Radically, Vilimina uses mostly post-traditional arguments. If a "traditional argument" grounds validity in the presumptive force of history and tradition (e.g. "because my pastor says it is right," or "this is what we have done for years"), a "post-traditional argument" by contrast grounds itself on a rationally accessible argument which all may engage in, and whose claims only have weight in so far as they touch the goals of the participants in the argument. Vilimina's central argument takes the latter form. She sets out her main moral imperatives (saving lives from AIDS and improving the agency of marginalized women) and her whole argument flows from there. Anyone can access and engage with her argument, inside or outside of local custom. In an amusing turn, Vilimina's one authority-based argument does draw on authority—her authority as an HIV-positive woman. Far from reinforcing the traditional loci of communal authority it puts forth herself, one village woman, as a person with the authority to be making claims about how the community should function. This occurs in large part because she sadly has personal knowledge of the ultimate devastation of AIDS—and again her argument comes back to the moral claim of saving lives.

11. Large-scale change can be as important when grappling with marginalization as it is when grappling with AIDS. Since marginalization is a societal phenomenon, to effectively address it a sense not only of individual agency but of collective potency must be gained, and recognized by wider society. For the disenfranchised more than anyone, the ability to see ones' self as part of a greater, powerful collective is indispensable in combating and reversing marginalization. Vilimina's use of symbols to lay the groundwork for a social movement could be extremely potent here.

12. Indeed the power imbued in this musical language may be another reason why Vilimina chose to communicate her message through song. Perhaps as a musician she can "get away" with saying things that otherwise would be too shocking, donning the cultural role of a musician social commentator.

CHAPTER 20

1. Literally, "by he who paid your bride wealth."
2. The word *muteuro* may be interpreted either as a traditional ritual offering or as a Christian prayer, depending on context.
3. Mtukudzi's description of marital rape is given additional cultural depth by the wording he uses in the second iteration of this line, which literally reads, "how does it feel to be raped by he who paid your brideprice?"
4. *Jiti* is a rural drum and dance entertainment genre. It is performed outside at ritual events including funerals and the *kurova guva* post-funerary rite. Thomas Turino has documented the development of *jiti*, and the associated urban popular music of *jit*, in his work on nationalism and popular music in Zimbabwe (Turino 2000, 229). For more on music at *kurova guva*, see Kyker 2010.
5. Mwendamberi is the name of a particular *chidao*, or sub-clan, of the *Shava*, or eland, totem.

6. "Tozeza Baba," a strong condemnation of domestic violence, describes the fear experienced by children who witness their mother's abuse at the hands of their father. "Nhaka Sandibonde" discusses customary practices of wife inheritance, where a brother of the deceased is chosen to inherit his widowed sister-in-law. The song emphasizes that this practice is meant to provide for the family of the deceased, and should not serve as an opportunity for the deceased's brother to claim sexual rights over the widow for whom he is chosen to provide. In the song's title, the image of a reed mat, commonly used as bedding throughout much of Zimbabwe, stands in as a metaphor for sexual relations.

7. Personal communication, August 12, 2006.

8. This stiff maize porridge is Zimbabwe's staple food.

9. For an interpretation of this *tsumo* which predates the AIDS epidemic, see Hamutyinei and Plangger (1974, 63).

10. *Aiwaiwaiwa* is formed by reduplicating the word *aiwa*, or "no." The use of similar interjectives to express grief or misfortune has been noted by Hannan (2000, 948) under the alternate form "haiwaiwa," formed by two repetitions of *aiwa* rather than the three successive iterations in the text of "Mabasa."

11. This figurative use of the word *mabasa* was first brought to my attention by Esau Mavindidze. It is likewise noted in respect to "Mabasa" by Sibanda (Sibanda 2004, 52).

12. The ambiguity of the word *vakuru*, which could refer either to living elders or to ancestral spirits, likewise characterizes the word *muteuro*, used in this song and in "Todii," and which can refer either to a Christian prayer or to a traditional ritual offering.

13. Nicholas Kunaka.

14. Indeed, Silindiwe Sibanda has suggested that in using the term *utachiwana*, Mtukudzi directly references HIV/AIDS (Sibanda 2004, 52–53).

CHAPTER 21

1. Following my research on AIDS and literature in Bukoba Kagera (sponsored by the Kagera AIDS Research Project since 1992), I wrote this play in collaboration with Mgunga Mnyenyerwa of Parapanda Arts in 1993–94. Initially it was intended only for the stage, but the script got into the hands of Medical Aid Foundation personnel, who sent it to a publisher.

2. Ebrahim Hussein (1983) writes that at one time, Aristotle's *Poetics* influenced the art of drama in the whole of Europe. And when Europeans colonialists came to Africa, they brought along this Aristotelian theory of drama.

3. Cf. note no. 1.

4. *Desis*, translated as tying, is "the action in a tragedy leading to climax. Plot threads are craftily woven together to form a more and more complex mess. At the turning point [*peripeteia*] these plot threads begin to unravel in what is called *lusis* or denouement. *Lusis*, translated as untying, is all the action in a tragedy from the climax onward. All the plot threads that have been woven together in the desis are slowly unravelled until we reach the conclusion of the play (online source at http://www.sparknotes.com/philosophy/poetics/).

CHAPTER 23

1. Estimated by UNICEF as 0.1 percent among adults (ages 15–49) in 2009, at http://www.unicef.org/infobycountry/morocco_statistics.html#55.

CHAPTER 24

1. This paper is a product of an ongoing research in South Africa made possible by the Fulbright-Hays Fellowship from the U.S. Department of Education. I am also indebted to the University of KwaZulu-Natal's Theology Department, Alan Paton Center and Struggles Archives, the Killie Campbell Archives and the McCord Hospital, The Diakonia Council of Churches, the Pietermaritzburg Agency for Christian Social Awareness, KwaMashu and Clermont Community Resource Centers, and St. Clement Home Base Care Project for providing me the research space. I am also indebted to all my friends and informants in Durban for their continued help and support.

2. The Church World Service, a sister organization to the National Council of Churches USA, brings churches from a variety of Christian faiths together in the service of humanitarian projects around the world.

3. *Umsebenzi* means "work" in Zulu, but is also used to refer to major ritual events in the family during which cows are slaughtered, especially *ukubuyisa*—the ritual of bringing home the dead commonly referred today as the unveiling of tombs (see Berglund 1989, 41).

4. Ndaba is the great-grandfather of Shaka the founder of the Zulu nation. Thus Nkonyane Kandaba means the "son of Ndaba." It is also used as a praise name for the Zulu as one of the chiefdoms in the Mthethwa confederacy. In the pre-Shaka Zulu nation, military regiments were organized according to chiefdoms, but Shaka changed the formations into Age Grade regiments (from interview with Xolani in Durban, 2007). In this battle song the sons of the chiefdom are urged to proceed into battle with the ferocity of wounded dogs.

5. An example was the speech that Rev. Mdabe gave at the St. Clement Home Based Care Project AIDS Awareness Function in May 2007.

6. An example is the experience I had in Clermont while making a round of home visits with the St. Clement Home-based Care in May 2007. A young man whose sick girlfriend admitted to us that she had AIDS rejected our advice that he and his two children receive HIV counseling and testing. He blamed his girlfriend's sickness on the acts of witchcraft that was being visited upon them by their neighbors who were jealous of them.

CHAPTER 25

1. For Ghanaians, the term "culture group" often indicates a performance ensemble that represents traditional drumming and dance from ethnic groups across the country, imitative of the style and repertoire of well-known national companies such as the Ghana Dance Ensemble.

CHAPTER 26

1. The names of all drama group members have been changed.

2. My experiences in TASO Mbarara's older van confirmed the difficulty involved in transporting both people and props (including a full theatrical curtain in many cases) in a limited space on unpaved roads sometimes riddled with potholes. On another occasion, when I was able to use an associate's hired driver to go to a performance, two TASO drama group members were more than happy to join me, along with extra props.

3. UNICEF, for example, discussed the continuation of programs to "shap[e] artistic [drama, dance, and song] productions to address AIDS related topics" in Uganda—complementing similar programs from the World Health Organization and the Uganda AIDS

Commission—in its 1991 Draft of Plan Operations (UNICEF Response to AIDS 1991, 43). Later, the United States Agency for International Development (USAID) included the training of "more than 200 drama group members from 31 groups in the development and execution of voluntary counseling and testing and condom efficacy scripts" as part of its 2002–2003 HIV/AIDS prevention activities; such performances, USAID claimed, "[r]eached out to more than 200,000 persons." (USAID 2003, 27).

4. For a more detailed account of this period, see Bond and Vincent 1997a and 1997b.

5. http://www.must.ac.ug/medicine/index.htm. Accessed April 12, 2008.

6. A March 16, 2008 PubMed search for the terms "Mbarara" and "HIV" turned up thirty-one articles, several of which were written by local researcher Fred Nuwaha and funded through MUST. In contrast, a search for "Kampala" and "HIV" turned up 325 articles, many funded by international initiatives, including a partnership with Johns Hopkins University.

7. I owe my presence in Mbarara to the Montefiore Medical Center's Primary Care/Social Medicine residency program, where my wife completed her internal medicine residency. At the time, we travelled to Mbarara as part of my wife's international health elective.

8. See http://www.aicug.org/index.php?option=displaypage&Itemid=74&op=page&SubMenu. Accessed April 12, 2008, and http://www.tasouganda.org/mba.php. Accessed April 12, 2008.

9. As opposed to other incarnations of hospice, Hospice Africa Uganda (a division of Hospice UK) identifies its primary mission as serving "cancer and AIDS patients with severe pain" (Hospice Africa Uganda 2003, 3; see also http://www.hospiceafrica.or.ug). The logo gracing the organization's 2002–2003 annual report—a silhouette of a kneeling caregiver reaching out to a kneeling recipient inside a straw-covered hut—emphasizes the organization's mission as a largely rural-based one.

10. Other organizations include the Agency for Cooperation in Research and Development (ACORD). For more, see District Response Initiative 2003, 24.

11. See http://www.thetaug.org. Accessed April 13, 2008. See also Barz 2006, 156.

12. Noticeably absent from this Mbarara AIDS landscape in 2004 was international corporate sponsorship. While Coca-Cola advertisements featured prominently in the town (taking up a good percentage of the MUST welcome sign, for example), health-related materials saw little overt corporate association until 2005, when Pfizer funded half of TASO Mbarara's new $700,000 "AIDS counseling and training center" (New HIV/AIDS Care Center 2005).

13. A 2003 survey of Faith-Based Organizations (FBOs) addressing HIV/AIDS around Mbarara listed two Catholic groups (including the Daughters of Mary and Joseph) and the Anglican Diocese of East Ankole. Surely others existed as well on a less formal basis (New HIV/AIDS Care Center 2005).

14. The Internet café I describe, known as "The Source," prohibited pornography, named its terminals after biblical figures, and requested Christian denomination information on its membership application (Personal observation, July 2004).

15. For more on the expansion of Christian evangelical activity throughout sub-Saharan Africa at the start of the twenty-first century, see Epstein 2007, 185–201. I experienced the extent of the Christian Evangelical presence in Mbarara one Friday night, when my wife and I were invited to a singing group "rehearsal" of MUTH students, only to have that rehearsal turn into a small-scale tent meeting, complete with a sermon given by a visiting minister from Alabama (Fieldnotes, July 10, 2004).

16. In addition to personal observation by Rebecca Cohen (July 2004), see Sprenkle 2007 and "Biblical Holistic HIV Care in Uganda" 2004. I wish to emphasize that the missionary

work of AIDS clinic physicians typically supplemented appropriate clinical care and did not appear to compromise the quality of treatment. The physician present during my time in Mbarara, Dr. Rick Goodgame, earned deep respect among both patients and medical personnel for his decades of experience treating HIV/AIDS patients in Africa.

17. Personal observation, Rebecca Cohen; Mobile Hospice Mbarara Newsletter, December 2003. See also Mobile Hospice Newsletter, v. 11, #1 (April 2004): this issue of the newsletter, which coincided with Easter, included the words "He is risen! Alleluia" on the front page just under the banner.

18. From the 2001 report: "Day Care Centers are places for clients to share experience of living with HIV in order to cope and live positively with the disease. Other activities include skills training, Music, Dance, and Drama rehearsals and Health Education Tasks. In 2001 rehearsals of songs, plays and poems by the drama groups were the main activities. Drama groups are composed of people living with HIV/AIDS and thus have proved very instrumental in AIDS education in the community" (TASO Uganda Limited 2002, 22).

19. In the village performances I viewed (which were attended by people of all ages), questions about sexual activity sometimes received frank responses, though several were referred directly to the village's appointed health educator. In secondary schools, the responses were far more general; with the director avoiding intimate discussions of sex and largely refusing to answer questions about condoms, mostly due to religious concerns. Perhaps in her most forward response in this setting, the director answered a student's questions about condom effectiveness by warning that student should not have sex until marriage; but if they wanted to "sin against God," they should use a condom (Fieldnotes).

20. The TASO Mbarara drama group's cassette tape, which the Centre sold to me for 2000 USh (c. $1.20) had many of the group's songs set to an electronic keyboard's chordal Afropop "fill." This practice also occurred at the end of one rehearsal, when the music master used an electric keyboard to accompanying one of the group's songs.

21. ABC references (A)bstinence, (B)e faithful, and the use of (C)ondoms. This system tended to work far better as a political trope than as a reality, and did ot appear in the drama group's musical repertoire. (And there was no little irony in listening to the chairman introduce the concept in English to a group that appeared to speak almost exclusively in Ranyankole.) Instead, the drama group took it upon itself to present a more nuanced understanding of human relationships in a time of AIDS. Moreover, when the drama group gave its presentation to secondary schools, the group's director played down the use of condoms (largely only deflecting rumors about their ineffectivenes) in favor of an abstinence message (see note 19).

22. Curwen, a Congregationalist minister, developed his Tonic Sol-Fa system in London; but its reach throughout the British Empire could explain its appearance in Uganda.

23. This well-considered proposal came from the member's own past—her husband, who had passed away from AIDS, had been a soldier—and from Uganda's history with the disease, which was first discovered in epidemic proportions through testing of soldiers being trained in Cuba (Bosch 2003).

24. This drama group member has since become a key publicized figure in the same organization's more recent microfinancing initiative.

CHAPTER 27

1. Ethiopia's national language is Amharic, which is written in the same script used for Ge'ez, the liturgical language of the Ethiopian Orthodox Church. No international standard yet

exists for transliterating the script, commonly called *fidel*, into the Roman alphabet. In this chapter, I transliterate Amharic into the Roman alphabet without using diacritical marks and into a form that renders words easily readable and that approximates as closely as possible the way in which they would be pronounced in Amharic.

2. Circus Addis Ababa was founded as Circus Ethiopia, the original name reflecting both the troupe's status as the first to be established and its location in the Ethiopian capital city. Sometime in 2004, the name was changed to Circus Addis Ababa to correspond with most of the other major troupes in the country, which are eponymously named for the cities in which they are based. I shall use Circus Addis Ababa throughout this chapter, although it is important to note that many people still refer to the troupe as Circus Ethiopia. Circus Tigrai has not changed its name to Circus Mekelle, after the city in which it is based, nor do I expect it to do so given the troupe's name recognition and economic security, which free it from having to cooperate fully with Circus in Ethiopia on certain issues, for example, the effort to rename troupes.

3. This chapter is closely based on an introductory article to Ethiopia's circuses that I wrote several years ago (Niederstadt 2009).

4. In this aspect, Ethiopian circuses share many similarities with the forms of performance considered by Kelly M. Askew in her study of cultural performance in Tanzania (2002) as well as the various case studies presented in *The Politics of Cultural Performance* (Parkin et al eds. 1996).

5. My ongoing research into Ethiopian circus performance began in 2000 as part of a project that examined contemporary expressive culture in Ethiopia's urban centers while a doctoral candidate at the Institute of Social and Cultural Anthropology at the University of Oxford. This chapter is based on fieldwork conducted in the country's two largest cities Addis Ababa and Dire Dawa as well as visits to other cities and towns that are home to circuses. I am grateful to the innumerable circus performers, administrators, and fans, both Ethiopian and foreign, whose ideas and opinions about the Ethiopian circus movement have contributed to this research. I am also thankful for the support of my mentors and colleagues at Oxford, the University of Michigan, and Wheaton College, and to the Institute of Ethiopian Studies at Addis Ababa University where I was a Visiting Scholar from 2001–2007. Finally, many thanks to Christopher Hyde, Visual Resource Curator, Wheaton College for his continued patience and help with image production and to Mell Scalzi and Emma Westbrook for research assistance and digital imagery wizardry.

6. I use the term "theatre for development" broadly to refer to forms of performance—however diverse—that address issues of social, economic, or political importance for the community either creating or witnessing the performance. (In doing so, I am subscribing to a definition of the term broader than that normally abbreviated as "TFD.") For more on the topic, see Banham et al. eds. 1999, Boon and Plastow eds. 1998, Boon and Plastow eds. 2004, Etherton ed. 2006, and Kerr ed. 2008.

7. In Ethiopia, *wetatoch*, or youths, comprise a social and legal category that differs from those of children and adults. The Federal Democratic Republic of Ethiopia defines "youth" as an age-based category that extends from fifteen to twenty-seven years of age. Few Ethiopian circus performers in their early twenties live as adults because most of them are still engaged in secondary schooling, live at home with the parents and siblings, and do not function socially as *gorumsewotch*, or adults. It is important to note that in the rural countryside, girls and young women take on the social responsibilities of adulthood when they are married, often around eleven or twelve years of age, usually to older men. The compensation received

by circus performers varied from troupe to troupe and was usually only provided to those members who performed publicly. In the past, this compensation has consisted of a stipend, transport money, food, milk, health care, and/or educational support including tutoring and school materials.

8. Ethiopian circus members regularly perform on a slack rope, which is considered to be more difficult from a tight rope, as it moves from side to side as well as up and down when the performer walks on it.

9. In 2007, an Israeli clowning troupe called Dream Doctor led a clowning workshop in Addis Ababa for members of five circus troupes. I have only witnessed one circus performance and a few rehearsals since that time so I do not yet know what, if any, impact the workshop had on public circus shows ("Dream Doctor" in Addis 2007).

10. Reviews by foreign audience members demonstrate that they perceive an Ethiopian, or even more generic "African," circus. The markers of ethnic identity that are so familiar to Ethiopians are usually not recognized by foreign spectators.

11. For much of the first fifteen years of the Ethiopian circus movement, shows held as part of international tours were usually less overtly didactic, although they occasionally incorporated generic messages about the need for peace and unity or more specific messages about HIV/AIDS, such as spelling out H-I-V with juggling bricks (figure 27.2).

12. Neither is currently involved significantly in the Ethiopian circus movement. Andy Goldman now lives and works as a consultant and photographer in South Africa. Marc LaChance committed suicide in May 1999 following allegations by circus performers seeking asylum in Australia that he had abused them.

13. I use the terms "street children" and *godana tadaderi* to refer to children who both live and work on the streets, not children who work on the streets, for example, selling gum, to help support their families, with which they live, as many circus members have done, and continue to do. For a thorough analysis of the situation of street children in Addis Ababa, see Heinonen 2000.

14. The process of establishing an NGO in Ethiopia is quite complex but it was the only way in which the circus movement could legally operate within Ethiopia, unless it associated itself with an existing institution, such as a school or another NGO. Sometime in 2007 or 2008, the organization changed its name to Circus in Ethiopia for Youth and Social Development (CIEYSD). The reasons for the renaming remain unclear. As nearly everyone still calls the organization Circus in Ethiopia, or CIE, I have continued to do so in this chapter.

15. Circus Jimma was established in western Ethiopia in 1992 by Bereket Tizazu, followed by Circus Nazaret, which was founded in 1995 by Ephrem Haile. (Nazaret was the Amharic name for the town of Adama, which is part of the Oromia Regional State. While the town is now known as Adama, its name in Afaan Oromo, the circus still goes by the name of Circus Nazaret.) Tesfaye Gebreyohannes founded Circus Tigrai in the northern city of Mekelle in 1993, while Circus Dire Dawa was established in eastern Ethiopia in 1996 by Meseret Manni and Deresse Lakew. Although technically an associate member circus until 2003/2004, Circus Dire Dawa functioned as a main branch circus long before then. In 2005, plans were made to elevate two associate circuses to main branch status, but the transition appears not to have been realized, due to funding constraints.

16. After Marc LaChance left Ethiopia, Metmku Yohannes, a longtime Circus in Ethiopia board member, served as executive director, although primarily in an advisory role; other Ethiopian staff handled day-to-day affairs as Metmku then held a full-time position as senior lawyer with the Ethiopian Electric Power Corporation. In the last ten years, at least six Ethiopians

have served sa executive director, some for as little as six months. A Dutch consultant Cees DeGraaf also held the position for several years from 2002–2004.

17. The other exceptions are Circus Dire Dawa and Circus Hargeisa, which were directly funded for many years by Novib, although the Circus in Ethiopia organization administered the funds.

18. For more on Adugna Community Dance Theatre Company, see Plastow 2004.

19. Such engagement of the audience is common in many forms of African performance. See Askew 2002 for several examples.

20. When I asked circus staff about the meaning of the show, I was told that while it appeared to be about two families, in reality, it was about Ethiopia and Eritrea and the need for the two countries to be reunited. Following the downfall of the Derg, Eritrea, which had been an Ethiopian province for nearly forty years, gained independence from Ethiopia in a 1993 referendum. Eritrea's independence left Ethiopia landlocked without a port on the Red Sea and relations between the two countries grew strained. As of 2001, the situation remained difficult, especially after the Ethiopian-Eritrea war that began in 1998 and ended in the summer of 2000. To address their concerns, circus performers and staff developed *Selam*.

21. In Ethiopia, although the husband is socially recognized (and often legally upheld) as the head of household, the federal constitution addresses women's rights and provides for legal equality in all areas, including education, employment, and property ownership. In reality, however, few women (or girls) have the means to pursue their rights if they face discrimination or threat. Even if they do, regional and federal laws often differ significantly from long-standing social practices, thus making enforcement difficult.

22. Due to safety concerns, circus staff, local police and *de facto* security guards quickly disperse crowds following performances, making it difficult to conduct research on what information audience members do take away from a performance or how effectively didactic messages have been conveyed.

CHAPTER 29

1. Not his real name.

2. For general information on kwaito, see Steingo 2005.

3. In the course of a 2006 rape trial against former deputy president Jacob Zuma, Zuma said that after having sexual intercourse with an HIV-positive woman he took a cold shower. Zuma's statement caused much confusion among the public, many of whom were led to believe that a cold shower after unprotected sex decreases the risk of contracting HIV.

4. For more on the issue of the political in kwaito, see Steingo 2005.

5. Bhekezizwe Peterson has also taken issue with Nuttall and Michael's editorial comments to Stephen's chapter. His critique, however, is very different from my own. Writes Peterson: "Commentators can draw our attention to what is perceived to be the aura of wanton criminality that engulfs kwaito, but my unease concerns the analytical and socio-political consequences of the flattening of what is an immensely complex, textured, variegated and historically specific constellation between the zones of kwaito's musical and performance forms, its practitioners and consumers" (2003, 201).

6. In full, Allen's quote reads as follows: "In its early years, *kwaito* was a South Africanized blend of hip hop with European and American dance music, especially house and techno, and pop. The music of the top *kwaito* groups of this period…was generally dominated by an unyielding, pounding bass beat that was marginally mediated by other cyclically repeated

rhythmic modules. The instrumental backing tended to be entirely computer generated. Snatches of catchy melodies were layered and looped around the vocal parts that tended to be the only 'live,' human aspects of *kwaito* performance...Although the rhythmically spoken lyrics were inspired by rap, vocal delivery tended to be much slower in *kwaito*, and the lyrics consisted of a few of the latest catch phrases repeated and played against each other" (see Allen 2004, 82–111).

7. Although Thandiswa continues to say that "Even the kind of House music we like in South Africa is the more kind of soulful stuff," I would suggest that she is referring more to the House music of 2001 (the year she made her statement). Today, House music in South Africa is extremely fast and exhausting to dance to.

8. The notion of "kwaito-speak" has been developed by linguist Sizwe Satyo (2001).

9. Most of the terms offered by Satyo are in a kind of creolized version of Xhosa that he calls "kwaito-speak," or (more conventionally) *tsotsitaal*.

10. Note that the letter "i" is used as a noun prefix in some cases in both Zulu and Xhosa. Note also that both Zulu and Xhosa (along with Swazi) are in the Nguni language group and are fairly similar.

11. Note that even though Dowling calls the group TKZ, the real name is actually TKZee. The two "ee's" are added after the "Z" presumably to clarify pronunciation, since in South African English the letter Z is pronounced "zed." It is likely that TKZee appropriated American English (that is, the letter Z pronounced as "zee") for reasons of identification.

12. Wearing All-Star canvas *takkies* (sneakers), for example, is a warning sign for many parents that their children are being initiated into kwaito culture.

13. Of course this reminds us of the preceding discussion of music as a narcotic.

14. Quoted on Zola's Web page: http://www.zola7.co.za, accessed 2 November, 2009.

15. Note that in South Africa, "platinum" means that an album sold 40,000 copies.

16. See Crowe 2006. Note that Crowe erroneously refers to Zola as a "hip-hop" star.

17. Note that at the concert Zola was introduced as the "unofficial mayor of Soweto."

18. Zola wears a large number seven around his neck, and his TV show is called *Zola 7*. In fact, in casual conversation among black South Africans, Zola himself is often referred to as "Zola 7."

19. Zola said this in an interview in the documentary *Sharp Sharp: The Kwaito Story* (dir. Aryan Kaganof. South Africa-Netherlands. Featuring Zola, TKZee, Oskido, Mzambiya, Don Laka, and Mandoza. Aryan Kaganof, 2003). A transcription of the interview can be found at: http://www.kaganof.com/kagablog/category/films/sharp-sharp-the-kwaito/story.

20. Khabzela's life has been documented in meticulous detail in McGregor 2005.

21. Khabzela also released several albums. After choosing tracks that he liked, those tracks would be licensed and then be released on a compilation under Fana's name. (See McGregor 2005, 124.)

22. In 2005, Yfm's Web site (yfm.co.za) stated: "Gigs and bashes have been powerful players in the history of Yfm and establishing Kwaito music as a viable commercial genre has positioned the station as 'owning' and its artists who dominate the music charts today. Think Kwaito, think Yfm." Since 2005, however, the Web site has changed slightly. Because kwaito has lost some popularity, the Web site now presents Yfm as more diverse and mentions the station's ties to genres such as hip hop, House, R&B, and raga.

23. As McGregor writes: "The theme of [Khabzela's] intervention was an almost biblical redemption. Prisoners were encouraged to confess and apologise on 'Positive Youth of Gauteng'; the community to forgive and embrace them" (2005, 148).

24. Note, however, that Maloka also had this to say about his friend: "He didn't believe in his limitations. He didn't allow the system to fence him in and that mindset might work for you at a certain stage but if it makes you stubborn, it might work against you later on."

CHAPTER 30

1. For a description of "thug rhymes," see the aforementioned in the radio executives' description of rap rife with sexual and violent imagery. Club mixes entail rap music that is not socially conscious, that may or may not contain sexual and/or violent imagery, and is intended for social gatherings.

2. "Lugaflow" is a descriptor that Ugandan MCs coined to describe rap in the Luganda language. Ugandan hip hop group Bataka Squad, credited by many to have been the first professional rap group in Uganda, and now relatively inactive as members have moved away from Kampala, began their careers rapping in Lugaflow.

3. Ironically, Lumix has faired far better by touring in Gulu and in villages outside of Uganda by sticking to the use of his home dialect.

4. These notebooks do in fact exist and not simply as notebooks either—see for example *The Uganda All-Star Aids Struggle* CD featuring Lyrical G; Tshila's "Sipping from the Nile"; the single "One" featuring Eazy Tecs and Lyrical G; and GNL's more recent "Koi Koi" and "Story ya Lukka."

5. All artists retained copies and ownership of their recordings. An agreement was entered that allowed us to have first release rights, after which the complete rights would revert back to the artists.

6. More recently, in his chapter, "The Ethics of Representation," Kofi Agawu, in conversation with Barbara Krader and Mark Slobin, explores what he calls the "impossibility" of establishing normative content for ethics within ethnomusicology. Agawu's assessment can also only provide a point of departure. His categories do not easily map onto thinking about the ethical implications of producing a Ugandan rap album with limited appeal that is arguably derivative of music from the United States. Though Agawu addresses the ironic resistance to popular music studies within ethnomusicological circles, nowhere does he speak of hip hop. Agawu does, however, mention the "potency" of popular music and laments the academy's resistance to take seriously its study within ethnomusicology (2003, 170–71).

7. See for example Lomax 1993 and Work et al. 2005 in this regard.

8. For *Kampala Flow*, beats were made by studios in which the tracks were recorded—those owned by GK (with some beats made by GK's studio technician Daddyskills), Dawoo, and Lumix. Other beats were purchased from beatmakers such as Sam. For work on "beat" production see Walser 1995, which refers to the "beat" as a "groove" and discusses its construction.

9. The initial tracks were recorded and laid down in Kampala, Uganda in several different recording studios based on beats also created in Uganda. The album was mixed down by Quanie Cash, a rap artist and producer in Nashville, TN. The album was published with a label in Los Angeles.

10. Admittedly, the use and definition of the term "religion" has been extensively problematized (see J. Z. Smith 1982, xi). "Religion is solely the creation of the scholar's study." Despite its long history in university education and the continued and pervasive effects of faith and religion in the public sphere, theology's place in the academy has long been questioned. While this longstanding suspicion of theology and these definitional debates and

cautions regarding usage of religion are critical for scholarship that is careful and self-conscious of what Fitzgerald calls its own "semantic and ideological bias[es]" (2000, 53) such discussions exceed the scope of this essay. It should also be noted that definitional debates have likewise problematized the use of the term "ethnomusicology" since the nineteenth century. Without dismissing the complexity of suggesting that Ugandan rap music and rappers have religious dimensions, commitments, and expressions worth analysis, Liu suggests that the theologically based portions of this essay may become more tenable if the line of argumentation in these sections is viewed as another method, as subject to emendation and critique as any other, and if the assertions be seen as catechrestically constructed. This essay at first uses religion, theology, and their cognates interchangeably and uncritically (with the exception of this footnote). As the confessional language of the artist interview becomes more prominent and relevant to the recommendations for more religiously and theologically oriented ethnomusicology, Liu will use theology and its cognates with more frequency for two reasons: (1) to acknowledge an analysis of the artists' statements on their own terms (no pun intended) and (2) to acknowledge interdisciplinary link to his home discipline of Homiletics and Liturgics.

11. Calvinist minister Jean de Léry's 1578 writings about the music of indigenous Brazilians may also be an earlier account of religiously linked ethnomusicology. "De Léry's Calvinist beliefs allowed him to be skeptical of the emerging scientific paradigm. He sought religious truth, not scientific objectivity, and though in his mind the native Brazilains were mistaken, de Léry seemed sensitve to their efforts to express belief systems in ritual forms" (Barz and Cooley 2008, 6).

12. See Wong 2001 and Shelemay 1992. See also Shelemay's writings on Ethiopian Jewish music (1991), and the three volumes of *Ethiopian Christian Liturgical Chant* edited by Shelemay and Peter Jeffrey (1993, 1994, 1997). For the North American context, see also Barz 2003, Bohlman, Blumhofer, and Chow 2006, and Marini 2003.

13. In *Mek Some Noise*, Timothy Rommen develops what he calls an "ethics of style" to assert the importance of belief as a necessary and fruitful starting point for ethnomusicological analysis. He writes, "I am increasingly convinced that belief, values, faith—that is, conviction—have been held for too long, to borrow from Sartre, in bad faith. Belief—whether placed in institutions, theories, cosomologies, or markets—permeates our lives, and yet we often wear our beliefs quite uncomfortably. After all, when it gets right down to it, they configure themselves in terms of right and wrong, good and evil—in terms of ethics" (Rommen 2007, 27). For Rommen, his ethics of style takes the "foundation" of conviction "seriously" to both interpret Trinidadian full gospel lyrics and the culture they effect with more than a political, social, or aesthetic reading, but also "nuance the political, social, and aestethic implications of gospel dancehall" (30). With Rommen, we want to acknowledge the vital link between belief and ethics in its social, political, and aesthetic dimensions. In contrast to him, however, we do not want to reduce ethnomusicological consideration of belief to ethical discourse. Also, though Rommen, by way of Levinas, admits that his analytical framework is an "act of identification" whereby he too becomes "implicated" and a part of the othered "discourses surrounding style in full gospel Trinidad," such admission does not make a claim regarding the believability of the beliefs or ethics of style in musics like "gospelypso" or its participants and performers (168–170). Nor is Rommen's admission expressly theological. It is not expressly theological because ethical discourses surrounding style as he describes seem confined to analysis of dialogue in which only humans participate. The theological trajectory of this chapter, however, aims to suggest that the self-

descriptive language, lyrics, and lives of Tafash and Twig offer ways to reconceive convictions about HIV/AIDS relief, music, and ethics, and the presence or absence of God in their lives and perhaps ours as well.

14. Sarah Coakley writes, "If this is a real possibility [that "dying Christians" enter into 'Christ's pain'] of which contemporary medicine should be taking account, then we need to be asking how its effects could be measured scientifically" (2007, 92). Though Coakley does speak of "secular impoverishment" related to medical meanings, deciphering whether theology functions as an extra or integral ingredient to treating such epistemological lack depends upon how one interprets words such as "plea," "enrich," and "consideration." "To say this in any way is not to condone the continuation of curable pain or to invite medical neglect; rather it is a plea to *enrich* medical reflection on pain and pain management with a deep consideration of the ethical and spiritual questions that narratives such as the Carmelites' lay before us" (ibid.). Though there exists in this chapter a shared concern for addressing what Coakley calls the "secular impoverishment" of medical ways of knowing, our theological analysis differs from one like Coakley's in three ways. First, it begins with the ethnographic, and particularly engages the medical ethnomusicological, rather than the historical, medical, and theological. Second, we also provocatively suggest that theological analysis is requisite for the ethnomusicological study of Tafash and Twig described in this chapter. Thirdly, theological analysis of Tafash and Twig may also suggest ways of knowing God for this chapters' readers as well.

15. Again, Rommen's study is no exception. *Mek Some Noise* focuses upon Trinidadian full gospel worship musics and congregational locations like Mt. Beulah Evangelical Baptist Church in Point Fortin, Trinidad. Other authors outside the field of ethnomusicology, including Jeremy Begbie, Teresa Berger, Ed Foley, and Mary McGann, attempt to make Christian theological claims about God based upon music. McGann's work in particular incorporates congregational ethnography (2004). For writing that makes general claims of spirituality as deriving from music, but does not use ethnography, see Cobussen 2008.

16. Not until the month of June did the artists know that Liu would be conducting exit interviews regarding their theological and spiritual outlooks and whether their perspectives effected their music-making. Neither did the artists know that Liu was a doctoral student in Homiletics and Liturgics or associated with theology at all.

17. Note that GK was uncertain of the spelling of okuhingira or okuhinjere, GK's studio (Interview with Liu, June 17, 2008).

18. Students in Form 6 are typically 17–18 years old.

19. Tshila, mentioned earlier, features as a singer on the compilation. She also does not consider herself a rapper.

20. English translation of " Ukimwi," Barz.

21. Peter Tosh (Winston Hubert McIntosh, Oct. 19th, 1944–Sept. 11th 1987) had a prominent career as a solo reggae performer. He was also a popular advocate of Rastafarianism. He was a former member of reggae group, The Wailers.

22. Liu, exit interview, June, 2008.

23. E-mail correspondence with Gerald Liu Jan. 10, 2009.

24. Though she directs her rap at "you," I am suggesting that it is a plural audience that she has in mind, something like what southern vernacular might phrase as "y'all."

25. Perhaps her point about "jingle" AIDS relief advertising is warranted when considering examples such as the recent theme for World AIDS Day and its accompanying slogan. The

2007 and 2008 theme was "leadership." This theme has been promoted with the slogan, "Stop AIDS. Keep the Promise." See http://www.worldaidscampaign.org/en/Key-events/World-AIDS-Day/World-AIDS-Day-2008, last accessed Nov. 23, 2009.

26. "Coinherence" suggests a type of coalescence between religious belief, personal identity, and musical endeavor for Tafash and Twig. The connection between these three attributes of belief, identity, and musical endeavor do not, however, constitute a seamless unity. Rather, the three are *inherent* to the artists' identities and are made to *cooperate* with one another through the artists' subjective negotiation. Coinherence also contrasts with the theological use of "dialectic." Belief, identity, and musical endeavor are neither suspended in relationship where all three contribute equally to a fulsome sense of self. Nor do they cancel one another resulting in a distillation of some notion of personhood. Rather, for Tafash and Twig, we suggest that they arrive at a sense of self by continually negotiating the related and opposing spheres of religious belief, personal identity, and musical endeavor.

27. Twig then seems to provide her own particular answer to Marion's question, and perhaps another version of his answer. Marion asks, "Does God give himself [sic] to be known according to a more radical horizon than being?" (Marion 1991, xxiv). Marion answers by suggesting the God offers Godself as gift. Though some, in recognizing Marion as a Catholic theologian and the hellenistic roots of terms such as "homiletics" and "liturgics," may now be questioning the academic integrity of mixing Christian-oriented scholarship with African female rappers, I first suggest that far from determining the interpretation of interview responses from Twig and Tafash, the selection of Christian texts in this article intends to emphasize their religious particularity and in no way presumes any type of religious etiology or seeks to prevent religious multivocality. Secondly, though every effort should and will be made to take the artists' words in their own right, but as Bruno Nettl admits, ideology is necessarily a part of ethnomusicology's intellectual history (2005, 4).

28. See Heidegger 1962, 30: "*Theology* is seeking a more primordial interpretation of man's being towards God, prescribed by the meaning of faith itself and remaining within it." [Italics from printed version, masculine language from original.]

29. Barz 2006a, 170. Italicization of *future* from this chapter.

30. What is still needed in academic studies of disease and health care are field-based research studies, such as on the culture of AIDS-specific transinstitutional efforts to study religion, medicine, and music with a focus on the interaction between faith, expressive culture, and healing within local conceptualizations of disease and healing in sub-Saharan Africa (Barz 2006a, 153).

31. There are, however, numerous contributions that explore homologous aspects of religion in prayer/meditation, spirituality, shamanism, Native American healing, and possession in Islamic culture (see especially Roseman 2008, Koen 2008, Bakan 2008, Olsen 2008, During 2008, Locke and Koen 2008).

32. For more on the practice of radical hope in the face of cultural devastation, see Lear 2006.

33. For more regarding "alterity" and the ethical advantages of proceeding from a position of alterity, see Bhabha 1994, 175: "The postcolonial perspective forces us to rethink the profound limitations of a consensual and collusive 'liberal' sense of cultural community. It insists that cultural and political identity are constructed through a process of alterity."

34. See Kampala road interview above.

35. For more on the importance of divergence as a practice of faith, see de Certeau 1998.

CHAPTER 31

1. The dates used in the music citations refer to the date of the recording and may not be the original date of recording in cases of licensed or compilation works.

2. After the arrival of a multiparty dispensation in Malawi, Saleta complained that he had never been paid for composing "public health" songs for *cholea* (cholera) or HIV/AIDS (Saleta Phiri 1995).

3. Constraints of space dictate that I cannot discuss the critical role of radio and DJs in promoting HIV/AIDS awareness in this chapter. The power of DJs and radio stations can make or break a musician.

CHAPTER 32

1. Originally published in the *International Studies Quarterly* (2007) 51, 139–63. Thanks are due to John Ballard, Thomas Bernauer, Gerard Holden, Emma Hutchison, Subhash Jaireth, and Hanspeter Kriesi as well as the ISQ editorial team and their anonymous referees for insightful comments on earlier drafts of this essay. We would also like to acknowledge the generous help of Eric Gottesman, who repeatedly took the time and care to respond to our inquiries. Much of the background information about our case study on pluralist photography is based on these interviews, which took place either by phone or e-mail between June 2004 and July 2006. Rather than citing the interviews individually throughout the text, we acknowledge them here collectively.

INDEX